ESSENTIALS OF
LOW VISION PRACTICE

ESSENTIALS OF
LOW VISION PRACTICE

Richard L. Brilliant, O.D., F.A.A.O.

Associate Professor of Optometry
Pennsylvania College of Optometry
Elkins Park
Senior Low Vision Practitioner
William Feinbloom Vision Rehabilitation Center
The Eye Institute, Philadelphia
Director of Low Vision Services
Moore Eye Foundation, Springfield Hospital Healthplex Pavilion II
Springfield, Pennsylvania
Adjunct Professor
College of Optometry
Waterloo, Ontario, Canada

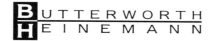

Boston   Oxford   Johannesburg   Melbourne   New Delhi   Singapore

Every effort has been made to ensure that the drug dosage schedules within this text are accurate and conform to standards accepted at time of publication. However, as treatment recommendations vary in the light of continuing research and clinical experience, the reader is advised to verify drug dosage schedules herein with information found on product information sheets. This is especially true in cases of new or infrequently used drugs.

Recognizing the importance of preserving what has been written, Butterworth–Heinemann prints its books on acid-free paper whenever possible.

 Butterworth–Heinemann supports the efforts of American Forests and the Global ReLeaf program in its campaign for the betterment of trees, forests, and our environment.

Library of Congress Cataloging-in-Publication Data
Essentials of low vision practice / [edited by] Richard L. Brilliant.
        p.   cm.
    Includes bibliographical references and index.
    ISBN 0-7506-9307-X
    1. Low vision--Patients--Rehabilitation. I. Brilliant, Richard L.
        [DNLM: 1. Vision, Subnormal--rehabilitation. 2. Vision Tests.
    3. Optometry--methods. 4. Ophthalmology--methods. WW 140 E78
    1999]
    RE91.E86 1999
    617.7--dc21
    DNLM/DLC
    for Library of Congress   98-4114
                                                                        CIP

British Library Cataloguing-in-Publication Data
A catalogue record for this book is available from the British Library.

The publisher offers special discounts on bulk orders of this book.
For information, please contact:
Manager of Special Sales
Butterworth–Heinemann
225 Wildwood Avenue
Woburn, MA 01801-2041
Tel: 781-904-2500
Fax: 781-904-2620

For information on all Butterworth–Heinemann publications available, contact our World Wide Web home page at: http://www.bh.com

10 9 8 7 6 5 4 3 2 1

Printed in the United States of America

This book is dedicated to my family:

In memory of my father, Buddy; my father-in-law, Warren; and my grandmother, Flo. Although no longer with us, they will never be forgotten.

To my mother, Yvette, and her husband, Mike, and to my mother-in-law, Muriel

To my sisters, brother, and their families: Barbara, Gail, Mark, Mitchell, Chandra, Brad, Bodi, Melissa, Blake, Alex, and Ryan

To my wife, Karen, and sons, Scott and Joshua. Without their love and support this project would have been impossible.

Contents

Contributing Authors

Sarah Deborah Appel, O.D.
Associate Professor of Clinical Sciences and Chief of Services, William Feinbloom Vision Rehabilitation Center, Pennsylvania College of Optometry, Elkins Park

Jean Astorino, O.D.
Optometrist, Ophthalmic Surgical Associates, Upland, Pennsylvania

Maryellen Bednarski, M.S., M.Ed.
Coordinator of Low Vision Services, Moore Eye Foundation, Springfield, Pennsylvania

Richard L. Brilliant, O.D., F.A.A.O.
Associate Professor of Optometry, Pennsylvania College of Optometry, Elkins Park; Senior Low Vision Practitioner, William Feinbloom Vision Rehabilitation Center, The Eye Institute, Philadelphia; Director of Low Vision Services, Moore Eye Foundation, Springfield Hospital Healthplex Pavilion II, Springfield, Pennsylvania; Adjunct Professor, College of Optometry, Waterloo, Ontario, Canada

Alvin Byer, M.S., O.D.
Associate Professor of Optics, Pennsylvania College of Optometry, Elkins Park

Bill G. Chapman, B.A., B.D., Ed.D.
Guest Lecturer, University of Houston School of Optometry and Northeastern State University School of Optometry, Talequah, Oklahoma

Elise B. Ciner, O.D.
Associate Clinical Professor, Director of Infant Vision Service, and Co-Director, Special Populations Assessment and Rehabilitation Clinic, Pennsylvania College of Optometry, Elkins Park

Michael Colucciello, M.D.
Retina and Vitreous Specialist, South Jersey Eye Physicians, Moorestown, New Jersey; Clinical Associate in Ophthalmology, University of Pennsylvania School of Medicine, Philadelphia; Active Staff, Department of Ophthalmology, Presbyterian Medical Center of Philadelphia and Children's Hospital of Philadelphia, Philadelphia and Memorial Hospital of Burlington County, Mount Holly, New Jersey

Glenn S. Corbin, O.D.
Private Group Practice, Wyomissing, Pennsylvania; Adjunct Faculty, Pennsylvania College of Optometry, Elkins Park; Consulting Medical Staff, Reading Rehabilitation Hospital, Reading, Pennsylvania

Roger W. Cummings, O.D.
Associate Professor of Clinical Sciences, Pennsylvania College of Optometry, Elkins Park; Staff Optometrist, Department of Surgical Services, Philadelphia Veterans Administration Medical Center, Philadelphia

Edward A. Deglin, M.D.
Associate Professor of Optometry, Pennsylvania College of Optometry, Elkins Park; Attending Ophthalmologist, Scheie Eye Institute, Philadelphia

Maureen A. Duffy, M.S., C.R.T.
Assistant Professor and Director, M.S. Program in Rehabilitation Teaching, Department of Graduate Studies in Vision Impairment, Pennsylvania College of Optometry, Elkins Park

Laura A. Edwards, Ph.D.
Program Coordinator, Master of Science Program in Low Vision Rehabilitation, Pennsylvania College of Optometry, Elkins Park

Kathleen Fraser Freeman, O.D., F.A.A.O.
Optometrist, Santa Rosa Low Vision Clinic, San Antonio

Leonard H. Ginsburg, M.D., C.D.E.
Chairman, Moore Eye Institute, Brandywine and Springfield Hospitals, Springfield and Exton, Pennsylvania

Marcy Graboyes, M.S.W., A.C.S.W.
Associate Professor, Department of Graduate Studies and Coordinator of Social Services, William Feinbloom Vision Rehabilitation Center, Pennsylvania College of Optometry, Elkins Park

Lee A. Hersh, O.D.
Private Practitioner, Hammonton, New Jersey

Charles Hollander, O.D., F.A.A.O.
Clinical Instructor, Department of Ophthalmology, Cornell University Medical College, New York; Professional Associate, Department of Ophthalmology, New York Hospital-Cornell Medical Center

Michele A. Maahs, M.S., O.T.R./L.
Occupational Therapist, Visiting Nurse Association of Delaware, New Castle

Tracy Matchinski, O.D.
Optometric Consultant, Low Vision Department, The Chicago Lighthouse for the Blind and the Visually Impaired

Bruce G. Muchnick, O.D.
Associate Professor of Optometry, Pennsylvania College of Optometry, Elkins Park; Attending Staff, Department of Surgery, John F. Kennedy Memorial Hospital, Philadelphia

John S. Ray, O.D., M.S.
Associate Professor of Optometry and Rehabilitation Optometrist, Pennsylvania College of Optometry, Elkins Park

Michael R. Spinell, B.A., B.S., O.D.
Associate Professor of Optometry, Department of Clinical Sciences and Staff, Cornea and Specialty Contact Lens Service, The Eye Institute, Pennsylvania College of Optometry, Philadelphia

Glenda V. Such, M.Ed.
Manager of Development, AbiliTech, Philadelphia

Jennifer Tasca, O.D.
Staff Optometrist, Bascom Palmer Eye Institute, Miami; Instructor, Departments of Geriatrics and Low Vision Rehabilitation, Nova Southeastern University, Health Professions Division, Division of Optometry, Ft. Lauderdale, Florida

Laurel A. Tucker, M.S.
Blind Rehabilitation Specialist, Department of Veterans Affairs Blind Rehabilitation Program

Stephen G. Whittaker, Ph.D.
Associate Professor, Department of Basic Sciences, Pennsylvania College of Optometry, Elkins Park; Director of Technical Assessment Services, William Feinbloom Low Vision Rehabilitation Service, The Eye Institute, Pennsylvania College of Optometry, Philadelphia

Douglas R. Williams, O.D., F.A.A.O.
Private Practice, Huntington Beach, California; Associate Clinical Professor, Low Vision Rehabilitation Services, Southern California College of Optometry, Fullerton

Preface

Low vision knows no barriers. It affects rich and poor, old and young, all races and ethnic backgrounds. Although visual impairment affects all ages, sight-related problems are most commonly found in the older population.

From 1900 to 1970, the total population of the United States tripled, while the older segment grew by a factor of almost seven times and is still growing faster than the younger than 65 population. It has been estimated that by 2020, 15.5% of the population will be older than 65 years and will therefore include an increasing number of potential low vision patients. There is no doubt that there is a need for eye practitioners, both now and for the future, to become more involved in the field of low vision rehabilitation, by either actively participating or becoming more involved in the referral process. It is with this in mind that this book has been written. For those practitioners who would like to become involved in the field of low vision rehabilitation or for those who are presently optometry or ophthalmology students, this book provides the basic or essential information to begin work in this rewarding field (for both the practitioner as well as the patient) of eye care. It is my hope that the seasoned low vision practitioner will also find the information in this book helpful, perhaps by providing a new slant to his or her routine in working with the low vision patient.

The chapters of this book are based on the lecture notes I use to teach third-year optometry students at the Pennsylvania College of Optometry. They have been arranged in sequential order, so that the reader is able to move from one chapter to the next, gaining the essential knowledge in evaluating the low vision patient and then providing the appropriate remediation. These chapters were written by a team of professionals with many years of experience in patient care. The chapters provide the student or practitioner with both the theoretical aspects of low vision and unique clinical pearls of wisdom. Additionally, much of the optics used in low vision are clearly explained so that the reader is able to see the relationship between theory and clinical practice. The final chapter, Case Studies, presents cases that summarize the previous chapters and demonstrate how closely theory is related to the clinical remediation of the low vision patient.

To be comprehensive, a text such as this must include the many low vision systems or devices available to the practitioner. Therefore, many of the chapters that discuss low vision systems describe most of the major devices currently available. It is expected that many of the devices discussed in this text may change, be improved, or be discontinued over time; however, these systems or devices are part of the history of low vision and should, therefore, be presented. It is impossible to mention every system that has existed or is presently available. This book is not intended to be a low vision catalogue; nonetheless, I apologize if any particular device presently in use was inadvertently excluded.

In conclusion, I hope that the information in this text will be invaluable to you, the student or practitioner, but most of all to the patient with low vision who will benefit from your expertise. It is only through hard work and dedication that the goal of helping others attain improved functional vision will be achieved.

RLB

Acknowledgments

Life is a continual learning process. Over the course of writing and editing this book, I have learned many lessons about the quality of life and about people.

This book could not have been written without the hard work and dedication of all of the authors. There were also many other individuals who helped me through this "adventure" that I would like to thank. I gratefully acknowledge the expertise and assistance of the following individuals:

Gwenn Amos, O.D.
Dawn Bearden, O.D.
Jay Cohen, O.D.
Cathy Czeto
Vivian Descant, O.D.
Krista Davis, O.D.
Bette Homer, M.S.
Patrick Johnson, O.D.
David Jupiter, O.D.
Bruce Kastner, O.D.
James Lewis, M.D.
Paul Pascarella, O.D.
Gail Pontuto, M.S.
Deborah Schreiver
Carl Urbanski, O.D.
James Verkuilen, O.D.

I would be remiss if I did not thank my two mentors, Dr. Randy Jose and Dr. William Feinbloom, who taught me, encouraged me, and believed in me.

And finally, I would like to especially thank Dr. Andrew Gurwood, for his superb graphics, and Ms. Marcy Graboyes, Dr. Lee Hersh, and my wife Karen for all of their hours spent reading, rereading, and making changes to the many chapters with which I bombarded them. Also, I thank my youngest son, Joshua (age 11), who helped to design the cover of this book. I could never have accomplished all this without their unselfish and tireless commitment.

ESSENTIALS OF
LOW VISION PRACTICE

CHAPTER ONE

Historical Overview of Low Vision: Classifications and Perceptions

Richard L. Brilliant and
Marcy Graboyes

HISTORICAL REVIEW

To look to the future, one must review the past. The history of low vision devices extends back to the origin of ophthalmic lenses. Since that time, numerous inventions and developments have paved the way for the evolution of modern low vision devices.

Over the past centuries, optical and nonoptical devices have been developed or adapted for individuals with different visual needs. Although in 1268 Roger Bacon described the convex lens through detailed drawings,[1] it was not until the early 1300s that a small spectacle lens industry began to flourish in the cities of Nuremberg, Germany; Haarlem, the Netherlands; and Venice, Italy. The lenses manufactured during this time were convex lenses used primarily as reading lenses (perhaps the beginning of the low vision microscope). It appears that the concave lens was developed later, with the earliest record of its use occurring in the 1450s. Through the writings of Franciscus Maurolycus (1494–1577) and Johannes Porta (1538–1615), it appears that myopia and hyperopia, as well as the optical lenses needed to correct these conditions, were fairly well understood.[2] A document issued by the Opticians Guild of Regensburg (Bavaria, Germany) in 1600 contained colored drawings of various styles of eyeglasses and reading lenses. In the same journal in 1623, there was a reference to aphakic spectacles.

In 1784, Benjamin Franklin invented the bifocal lens by cutting two different lenses in half and piecing together the upper half for distance and the lower half for near use. In 1796, J. McAllister, Jr. opened the first optical shop in America (Philadelphia). In this shop, he not only provided frames and lenses but also "measured the eyes" to determine the appropriate lenses. He is also credited as being the first to grind lenses for the correction of astigmatism.[1]

During the 1800s, many changes occurred in the examination and correction of the eye. Retinoscopy (Cuignet, 1871), keratometry (Javal, 1882), ophthalmoscopy (Helmholtz, 1851), visual acuity tests (Snellen, 1862), and trial lenses were invented and developed. C. F. Prentice, in 1888, presented the prism diopter to explain the bending of a light ray through a given strength prism. He was also responsible for explaining the need to redesign a lens to account for various vertex distances. To meet the needs of this expanding industry, William Beecher started a company in 1833 to produce frames, lenses, and testing equipment. This company later became known as the American Optical Company of Southbridge, Massachusetts. In 1853, the Bausch & Lomb Company began in Rochester, New York. In the early 1900s, both of these companies manufactured many of the magnifiers and reading lenses used by individuals at that time and also, perhaps, by many of the "low vision patients." Magnifying lenses, however, had been around for hundreds and maybe even thousands of years before this time. Magnifying lenses, probably used initially as "burning lenses" (condensing the sun's light), appear to date back as far as 1600 B.C. There also exists references to Alhazen, an Egyptian-born scientist, who may have designed and used a magnifying lens in A.D. 1038 to aid his "aging eyes" when reading small print from his scrolls.[1]

By the time the telescope was invented, the problems of hyperopia, myopia, and presbyopia were fairly well understood. It appears that Galileo Galilei (1564–1642) was one of the first to design and construct a telescope that bears his name. Johannes Kepler (1571–1630) developed a two-convex-lens telescopic system that created an inverted image. This telescope, named after Kepler, is also known as an *astronomical telescope.*

The first major contribution to the development of telescopic devices for patient care was made by a Jesuit priest, F. Eschinardi, in 1667. He recognized the possibility of changing the distance between the ocular and objective lenses of the Galilean telescope to correct for an individual with myopia. He further recommended that telescopes can be used to view various distances and if the tube length (distance between the ocular and objective lenses) could not be adjusted conveniently, that two telescopes be made, one for distance and one for near. It appears that a few years after Eschinardi's discovery, mechanical adjusting devices to vary the distance between lenses of a telescope were regularly used. As a matter of fact, in 1695, a mathematic relationship had been developed by Christian Huygens that specified the relationship between the tube length, the power of the ocular and objective lenses of the telescope, and the correction of refractive error.

The next major development of the telescopic device was made by H. Dixon in 1785. He suggested the use of two spherical mirrors mounted in a spectacle frame so that the distance between the mirrors could be changed not only to produce magnification but also to correct for refractive errors. The advantage of this mirror system was improved image quality over a telescope composed purely of lenses.[3]

The nineteenth century saw significant strides in improving the quality of the Galilean telescope. This improvement was aided tremendously by the different types of glass lenses that were made available and the ability to correct for chromatic aberration. The redesign of the telescopic mountings was also important in reducing the overall weight of the system.

Steinheil and Seidel designed a small Galilean telescope in 1846 that was composed of an objective lens of crown glass and an ocular of flint glass. This system was designed for individuals with myopia and produced a magnified (1.2–1.3×) and achromatic image. Giron and Mitaine, in 1840, and Dillenseger, in 1849, designed the lenses of a Galilean telescope to be adjusted in and out without any tubular support (Figure 1-1). This construction was lightweight and somewhat comfortable to wear, much like theater spectacles.

The first telescopic use of a doublet objective and ocular lens was in the panorthic monacle, designed and manufactured by Steinheil's sons in Germany in the 1870s. It was a small telescope made with an aluminum mount that produced a magnification of 1.6× and a visual field of 20 degrees. It was intended for use with individuals who were not capable of obtaining good acuity and for those who needed corrective lenses and wanted magnification for distance viewing. Since the discovery of astigmatism and its correction in the early part of the nineteenth century, telescopes were not used as frequently to improve acuity loss due to refractive errors. This undoubtedly contributed to the reduced interest in the further development of telescopic spectacles. It was not until 1910 when Dr. M. von Rohr, working for Carl Zeiss Company of Jena, Germany, developed mathematic formulas (which are still used today) for telescopic systems having different vertex powers. His formulas accounted for the types of lenses and their powers and thickness as well as the number of lenses used in a telescope so as to neutralize the distortion and maximize the field of view. He designed slip-over plus lenses to be used in front of the objective lens to accommodate for different distances closer than infinity. He also designed slip-over lenses for use behind the eyepiece to correct for refractive errors.

To evaluate individuals with amblyopia or myopia, the Zeiss Company produced trial kits of telescopic spectacles with slip-over lenses to correct for refractive error and to create appropriate reading distances. If binocular vision was desired for both distance and near, then two sets of telescopic spectacles had to be prescribed (one for distance and one for near). If binocular vision was to be used at distance but not at near, a frosted glass cap was used over the objective of the unused telescope to occlude its use. After World War I, Zeiss telescopes were used for a large number of wounded soldiers who had reduced vision in both eyes.

In 1928, Dr. William Feinbloom ordered a pair of telescopic lenses from the Zeiss Company after studying von Rohr's work on the development of telescopic spectacles. Feinbloom had been seeing a patient with reduced visual acuity and photophobia secondary to retinal degeneration and incipient cataracts. Although the 1.8× telescopes from Zeiss improved the patient's vision, the improvement was insufficient to meet the patient's needs. Feinbloom designed a 2.5× Galilean telescope with a pin-hole diaphragm that could change the telescopic opening from 2 mm to 5 mm. This telescope not only provided a more significant visual acuity improvement but also helped eliminate some of the patient's photophobic complaints.[4] This spectacle telescope was tilted up pantoscopically by adjusting the temples so that the patient could look below the telescope to see the ground below him when walking (the first bioptic telescope).

In 1930, Feinbloom attempted to provide normal localization of distant objects when looking through a Galilean telescope by producing a meridional magnifying telescope.[5, 6] This system produced 1.7× magnification in the horizontal meridian and 1.3× magnification in the vertical and could be used on a full-time basis (for distant objects). When looking through this system, the patient would see objects that appeared shorter and wider at approximately the same position as the actual object. In other words, a square object would appear rectangular at the same distance.

In 1934, Feinbloom designed microscopic spectacles ranging in power from 2× to 20× for those patients who wanted to read but who could not use a telescopic system with reading caps. He also studied and presented the many problems associated with the lenses' reduced focal distance, such as the need for direct illumination and the

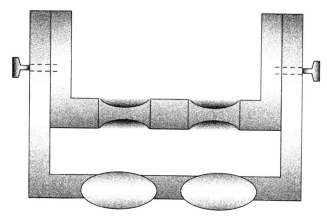

FIGURE 1-1. **Variable focus Galilean telescope initially designed by Giron and Mitaine, and Dillenseger, 1840s.**

difficulty of maintaining fixation when making saccadic eye movements. Feinbloom also demonstrated the importance of a typoscope, a black reading slit designed by Prentice in 1897, when reading with high-powered lenses.

In 1936, Tait and Neil designed telescopic spectacles that provided a combination of magnification at distance and near in the same spectacle system.[5] This system used ordinary spectacle lenses to correct for refractive error, and on the front surface of this lens, two concave lenses were ground. One set of lenses were in the straight-ahead position and the other set in the lower position (similar to a bifocal). These concave lenses served as the oculars of the telescope, whereas another large plano lens with two convex lenses ground into it sat at a given distance away from the spectacle-mounted ocular and provided the objective lenses. The combination of lenses in the upper portion of the system (straight-ahead position) provided for afocal magnifications of approximately 1.7–2.5× and the lower portion combined for a reading distance dependent on the plus power of the objective lens (Figure 1-2).

In the hope of providing greater magnification, Feinbloom produced a 3× Galilean telescope composed of a doublet objective lens and a single ocular lens in 1941. This lens system was mounted in a transparent plastic shell that was then placed in a spectacle "carrier" lens. In 1956, Feinbloom designed a Galilean telescope with concave mirror as an objective lens and a convex mirror as the ocular. This system had the equivalent power of 3.5×.

In an attempt to provide greater magnification for reading, the closed-circuit television (CCTV), an electronic instrument using a camera and a monitor to provide magnification of printed material, was first described by Potts, Volk, and West in 1959.[7] They described a hand-held camera that provided good image quality and magnification. In 1968, Dr. Genensky reported on a CCTV that he had developed at Rand Corporation (Santa Monica, CA), which was available for patient care.[8]

In 1977, Dr. Feinbloom presented the Camera Lens Telescope (Designs for Vision, Inc., Ronkonkoma, NY), a Keplerian system mounted in a spectacle. This telescope, after years of redesigning to a smaller size, consisted of a black

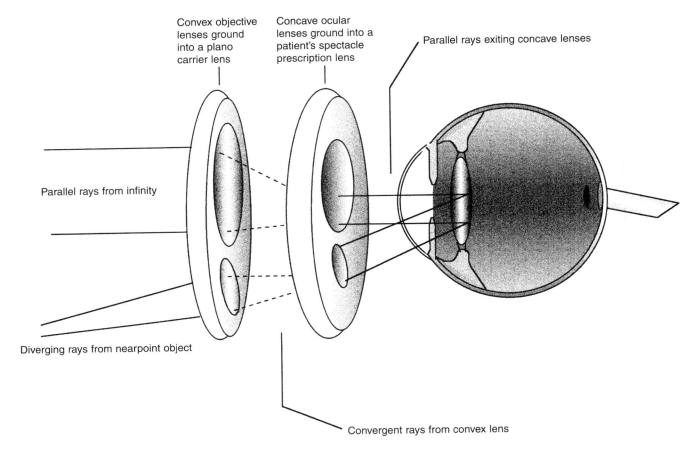

Convex objective lenses ground into a plano carrier lens

Concave ocular lenses ground into a patient's spectacle prescription lens

Parallel rays exiting concave lenses

Parallel rays from infinity

Diverging rays from nearpoint object

Convergent rays from convex lens

FIGURE 1-2.   **Telescopic spectacle lenses designed by Tait and Neil in 1936.**

tube extending approximately 2 in. perpendicular to the spectacle frame. The telescope was initially available in 6× magnification and was the most powerful system mounted in a spectacle. This telescope was later made focusable to allow for near, intermediate, and distance focusing and available in powers of 2× through 10×.

In the hope of providing a spectacle-mounted telescope with as large a field as possible, Feinbloom and Brilliant designed and clinically evaluated the Honey Bee

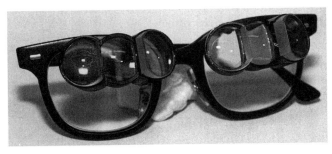

FIGURE 1-3.   **Honey Bee (Designs for Vision, Inc., Ronkonkoma, NY) telescopic bioptic designed by Feinbloom and Brilliant in 1980.**

Lens (Designs for Vision, Inc.) in 1980. This telescope consisted of three Galilean telescopes arranged together in a horizontal array (Figure 1-3). The two outer telescopes had base-in prisms mounted on the objective lenses to help maintain a continuous field of view at distance. Attempts were made to make this system in Keplerian form as well; however, weight and size prevented this from being accomplished.

In 1983, Feinbloom designed the Amorphic Lens (Designs for Vision, Inc.) for patients with reduced peripheral fields. This lens system was a cylindrical, reverse Galilean telescope that created minification in the horizontal meridian and no change in the vertical. Feinbloom hoped that patients with extremely reduced peripheral fields would be able to use this lens for mobility purposes, allowing for increased horizontal fields with no acuity reduction secondary to the minifying system. This full-field Amorphic Lens produced distortion, loss of depth perception, and nausea for patients using it on a full-time basis. To improve patient acceptance, the Amorphic Lens was redesigned into a rectangular shape and mounted in the superior position of the carrier lens (Figure 1-4). This bioptic position enabled the patient to alternate between the cylindrical minifier and the carrier lens while in motion.

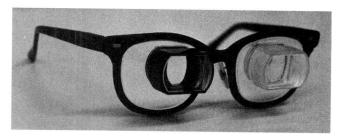

FIGURE 1-4. **The Amorphic Lens (Designs for Vision, Inc., Ronkonkoma, NY) was originally designed by Feinbloom in 1983 as a full-diameter telescope. It was later redesigned into a bioptic telescope.**

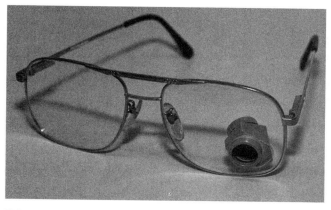

FIGURE 1-5. **Spitzberg developed the Behind-the-Lens telescope (Optical Designs, Inc., Houston, TX) in 1989.**

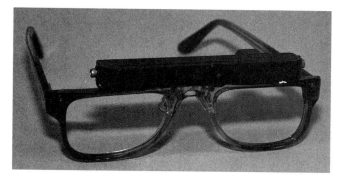

FIGURE 1-6. **Pekar and Greene developed the Horizontal Light Path-Vision Enhancing system (Ocutech, Inc., Chapel Hill, NC) in 1989.**

Since the 1990s, when designing new low vision telescopes, designers have concentrated on making the systems smaller, lightweight, and more cosmetically pleasing. The Bi-Level Telemicroscopic Apparatus, by Edwards Optical Corporation (Virginia Beach, VA), and the Clear View Lens, by Designs for Vision, address the preceding concerns. Both telescopes are lightweight, small, and less noticeable (see Figures 9-B11 and 9-B7, respectively).

In 1989, Dr. Spitzberg developed the Behind-the-Lens telescope (Optical Designs, Inc., Houston, TX) with cosmesis in mind. This telescope is of Keplerian form with the objective lens being an achromatic doublet and the ocular being a biaspheric lens. This miniature telescope is located behind the spectacle carrier lens in an inferior temporal position, and the objective lens (of the telescope) is flush with the front surface of the carrier lens (Figure 1-5).

Pekar and Greene, of Ocutech, Inc. (Chapel Hill, NC), developed the Horizontal Light Path-Vision Enhancing System (HLP-VES) in 1989. This system is a monocular Keplerian telescope that lies parallel to the spectacle plane and is positioned on top of the frame (Figure 1-6). In 1996, the HLP-VES was made available as an autofocus telescope.

In 1995, image-processing technology became available to low vision patients. A head-mounted video display with electronic manipulation known as the *Low Vision Enhancement System* (LVES) (Visionics Corporation, Vadnais Heights, MN) came on the market. This system used tiny electronic cameras to produce a magnified black and white image on a video screen in front of the patient's eyes. In addition to variable magnification, brightness and contrast were also adjustable to the patient's needs. LVES was developed under the direction of Dr. Massof of Johns Hopkins Wilmer Eye Institute (Baltimore, MD) in collaboration with the U.S. National Aeronautics and Space Administration and the Veterans Administration (see Figure 11-7).

The preceding brief historical summary describes, in part, the efforts that were made to design, develop, and produce systems and devices to assist low vision patients. Many others have contributed to this field through lens development, teaching, research, case reports, and clinical practice. Most important, there appear to be many new and promising devices on the horizon that will provide practitioners with even more treatment alternatives. The future holds the promise of major breakthroughs, and

hopefully, more progress will be made in the next 10 years than in the last 100 years.

DEFINITIONS AND EPIDEMIOLOGY

Webster's New World Dictionary defines *blindness* as "without the power of sight; sightless; eyeless," whereas *Dorland's Medical Dictionary* defines the term as a "lack or loss of ability to see; lack of perception of visual stimuli, due to disorder of the organs of sight, or to lesions in certain areas of the brain." These definitions apply to an extremely small portion of the general population. The vast majority of individuals who have a visual impairment have some remaining amount of vision. There have been many names and terms used to describe this population, from *subnormal vision*, to *partially sighted*, to *low vision*. Needless to say, there are many professionals who have different opinions and philosophies regarding the appropriate name and definition for this group of individuals who are visually impaired.

The federal government has provided a legal definition for official purposes and has, therefore, defined *legal blind-*

ness as visual acuity of 20/200 or worse in the better seeing eye with best conventional correction (spectacles, contact lenses, or intraocular lenses), or a visual field of 20 degrees or less in its widest diameter. Most states have adopted this definition to provide benefits to those individuals who fall within this category. Individual variations, however, may exist at the local level.

The benefits that may be available to those individuals who are classified *legally blind* are as follows:

- An Internal Revenue Service (IRS) income tax exemption. The #907 Tax Information for Handicapped and Disabled Individuals publication is available from the IRS.
- Free telephone directory assistance. The telephone company understands that a person who is visually impaired may have difficulty looking up telephone numbers in the telephone book. A person's visual impairment must be confirmed by a healthcare provider.
- Transportation benefits. Transportation services to individuals with impairments are available in some areas. They provide door-to-door transportation to many locations, for example, doctors' offices, grocery stores, and recreational facilities. Transportation is generally at a reduced fare and advanced scheduling is required.
- Free mailing. All materials related to blindness or visual impairment (e.g., educational materials, information regarding support groups) can be mailed without charge. Permission should be obtained through the local post office. A stamp with the words "Free Matter for the Blind" should be purchased so that the envelope can be stamped in the upper right-hand corner. The envelope should also be left unsealed for those occasions when the post office elects to inspect the material.
- Free library services. This service is funded through the Library of Congress and is administered by local regional libraries. This service provides books, magazines, and newspapers in large print or on cassette tapes or long-playing records. These materials are sent free through the mail to the individual's home.
- Vocational rehabilitation services. State services are available to provide funding for low vision evaluations and devices to rehabilitate individuals. Services are also available for job training, orientation and mobility, and instruction in activities of daily living such as cooking, grooming, shopping, and cleaning.

There are, however, some major problems with defining *legal blindness* purely on a visual acuity or visual field loss. It does not account for the following:

1. Chart used.
   a. Number versus letter charts. Number charts may be easier to read because there are fewer numbers to guess from.
   b. Most Snellen charts have optotypes that jump from 100 to 200 with nothing in between. This does not take into consideration a patient with a visual acuity better than 20/100 but worse than 20/200. What about the patient with 20/120 or 20/160 acuity?
   c. Chart illumination and chart contrast are not standardized.
2. Room illumination or glare.
3. Patient motivation.
   a. A patient may not be willing to attempt to guess at a letter or number if it appears "too blurry."
   b. A patient may be malingering.
4. A patient with pendular nystagmus may have an increase in his or her nystagmoid motion when an eye is occluded and therefore demonstrate a decreased acuity.
5. Patient eccentric fixation or eccentric viewing.
6. Doctor motivation. Some doctors may not "push" the patient to obtain threshold or maximum acuity.
7. Field testing equipment not fully specified.
8. Hemianopic field losses.
9. A patient's functional adaptation to vision impairment. A patient with 20/70 acuity may appear as if he or she is totally incapacitated while another patient with the same visual diagnosis and acuities of 20/400 may appear to have minimal visual problems.

The term *low vision* or *visually impaired* encompasses those individuals with less severe vision loss as well as those who are legally blind. Unlike the definition of legal blindness, *low vision* should not always be defined by visual acuity or visual field boundaries. Some practitioners define *low vision patients* as those individuals who exhibit acuities of 20/70 or poorer through standard correction. This definition ignores vast numbers of individuals who possess better acuities but have seriously impaired visual functioning. A realistic definition must consider the level of visual functioning as well as existing acuities or fields. A good example might be seen with a surgeon who had 20/15 acuity and full fields but could not perform microsurgery without the use of a surgical telescope (magnification). In this case, he may be considered a low vision patient because his visual functioning was not adequate for the task at hand. Another example may be seen in a patient who found it impossible to read her textbooks even though she had 20/40 vision in the better seeing eye. On careful visual field testing, it was determined that although there were no limitations in peripheral fields, the patient had small scotomas to the right and left of fixation. These scotomas obscured the beginning and end of words. The patient certainly was not considered *legally blind* nor did she fall into the 20/70 classification of *low vision*, and yet the patient was unable to function in an academic setting and benefited greatly by angling her reading material to read from an inferior to a superior position rather than from left to right. Even though no low vision lenses or devices were involved, the patient was completely satisfied by this simple procedure and thought that the "low vision evaluation" did indeed provide a successful solution.

Other terms commonly used in low vision rehabilitation describe the functional aspects of the individual or the visual system. A *visual impairment* is a reduction in the ability of the eye or visual system to perform. An example is a patient with macular degeneration who has reduced visual acuities. This loss of visual acuity is considered a visual impairment. It does not define how the patient is functioning but rather how the eye or visual system is functioning (i.e., loss of visual acuity). When a patient is not able to perform a particular task because of his or her impairment, the patient is said to have a *visual disability*. A visual impairment may not always cause a visual disability. For example, a patient with macular degeneration and reduced visual acuity will not have a visual disability when it comes to driving a car if he or she had never had a driver's license. A patient would be considered visually disabled, however, if he or she at one time was able to drive but can no longer do so because of impaired vision. The former patient, who never had a license to drive and always depended on public transportation (and still uses this service) may, however, be considered visually handicapped. Even though this patient is not disabled or prevented from getting around, the general public may think that he or she is at a disadvantage and, therefore, label the patient as *handicapped*.

It should be apparent that the term *blindness* is relative. From the legal point of view, this classification is quite broad and includes many people with useful vision. Of the 11.5 million people who are visually impaired (i.e., cannot read standard-size newsprint with conventional lenses), approximately half a million (4%) are considered legally blind.[9] The largest segment of the legally blind population are individuals who are 65 years of age and older. The incidence or number of new cases of legal blindness per year for this population is primarily caused by one of four ocular disorders: macular degeneration, glaucoma, diabetic retinopathy, or cataracts.[9]

The elderly are the fastest growing segment of the U.S. population. In 1985, there were approximately 28.3 million individuals aged 65 years and older. By the year 2035, it is expected that this population will double. It is also predicted by the U.S. Census Bureau that by the year 2050, the number of individuals older than 55 years will increase by 113% whereas the general population will increase by only 33%. As the life expectancy of the general population increases, it is also expected that there will be an increase in the incidence of age-related ocular diseases. This increase in potential patients with low vision is expected to have a significant impact on eye care services, requiring more eye doctors specializing in low vision rehabilitation or offering some form of low vision service in their practice.

It should also be understood that it is difficult to obtain a true number of new cases of legally blind individuals each year because all cases are not reported. Some patients who are visually impaired and who have been told that "nothing else can be done" do not seek further care, thus making it difficult to determine when they might have crossed the line to legal blindness. Young children, perhaps with retinopathy of prematurity, may not be reported until they have been enrolled in school. Nevertheless, Table 1-1 provides the most commonly diagnosed ocular disorders (in descending order) for each age group that are responsible for causing legal blindness as seen at the Feinbloom Vision Rehabilitation Center, Philadelphia, Pennsylvania (1980–1990).

TABLE 1-1
Leading Causes of Legal Blindness

Birth to 19 yrs
    Congenital cataract
    Optic atrophy
    Albinism
    Retinopathy of prematurity
    Cone-rod dystrophy
20–44 yrs
    Albinism
    Cone-rod dystrophy
    Optic atrophy
    Myopia
    Retinitis pigmentosa
    Diabetic retinopathy
    Macular degeneration
45–64 yrs
    Diabetic retinopathy
    Glaucoma
    Retinitis pigmentosa
    Macular degeneration
    Cataracts
65–74 yrs
    Macular degeneration
    Diabetic retinopathy
    Glaucoma
    Cataracts
    Retinitis pigmentosa
75 yrs and older
    Age-related macular degeneration
    Glaucoma
    Cataract
    Diabetic retinopathy

SOURCE: Data from The William Feinbloom Vision Rehabilitation Center of The Eye Institute at the Pennsylvania College of Optometry, Philadelphia, Pennsylvania (1980–1990).

PERCEPTIONS OF BLINDNESS AND VISUAL IMPAIRMENT

The White House Conference on Handicapped Individuals defines an *attitude* as "a positive or negative emotional response to an object; a reaction that is accompanied by specific beliefs and tends to impel the individual to behave in specific ways toward the object of the attitude."[10] In providing services to individuals with visual impairment, it is helpful to have an understanding of attitudes toward blindness and visual impairment. Society has preconceived notions about what it must be like to have a vision problem. These notions shape the reaction to and treatment of those with a vision impairment. Most of the prevailing attitudes toward blindness are negative or unrealistic. A survey conducted by Gallop in 1988 found that blindness was the most feared disability among 42% of the 1,072 individuals surveyed, and the fourth most feared disease after acquired immunodeficiency syndrome, cancer, and Alzheimer's disease.[11] The average person has had little direct contact with individuals who are visually impaired and therefore may base perceptions of blindness and visual impairment on external influences such as the media, literature, and religion.

To understand more fully why these attitudes exist, it is useful to examine the origins of prevailing attitudes toward blindness and visual impairment. One only has to look as far as the Bible, in which blindness was often used as a threat of punishment or as a cross to bear. In 1973, a historical review of blindness was conducted by Michael Monbeck to examine the portrayal of blind characters in literature.[12, 13] He identified 15 traits most frequently connected to characters in literature who were blind. The findings revealed a predominantly negative image often reflecting low social status. Other descriptors of blindness included *miserable, helpless, useless, evil,* and *maladjusted.* Characters played the role of a fool or beggar and were usually feared or avoided. Monbeck also found instances of the blind portrayed as having superhuman powers or insights—again, unrealistic. These themes can be traced through Greek mythology and Shakespeare with a slow evolution of more fully developed and less stereotypic characters not occurring until well into the 1900s. The media through the years have also portrayed blind characters in a negative manner in movies and theater, further perpetuating negative stereotypes.

It is important that professionals in the field of low vision have insight into their own attitudes toward visual impairment. These attitudes may consciously or subconsciously impact on interactions with patients. For example, if a practitioner believes that a person with a visual impairment is helpless, he or she might inadvertently modify a patient's goals or perhaps influence expectations. This, in turn, may lead to a reinforcement of stereotypes and prevent the person with a visual impairment from realizing his or her true potential.

The individual with the visual impairment also enters the low vision process with his or her own attitudes toward vision loss. These may have also been shaped by the family, the media, or religion as well as a host of other influences. These attitudes may also influence the emotional adjustment to vision loss. For example, if the patient believes that a person who is visually impaired is in some way inferior, he or she may develop lower self-esteem, which may impact on the types of goals set during low vision care. It may become a self-fulfilling prophecy for the individual who believes those who are "blind" are helpless. On the other hand, if an individual who loses vision believes that a person with a visual impairment can accomplish any goal, he or she may be more likely to realize his or her potential. Most individuals with a visual impairment may have few, if any, reference groups with which to compare themselves as they search to redefine their self-concept. Individuals with low vision have reported a number of negative encounters with the sighted world during which their behaviors have been misinterpreted. These include being viewed as drunk if they bump into another person, a snob if they fail to say hello, or illiterate if they are unable to read small print and need to ask for assistance.

Patients may also have misconceptions about the use of vision. It is not uncommon to hear a patient express fears of damaging his or her eyes by using vision. In many cases, eye strain or fatigue may be perceived as causing further vision loss. Patients may also assume that low vision devices will work for them in the same way that regular glasses once did. It is also a common misconception that the larger the magnifier the stronger the power. Many individuals state that if they could only find a magnifier large enough, they are certain they could function better. It is therefore essential that patients have realistic expectations regarding low vision services and the benefits and drawbacks of optical devices.

Professionals working in the field of low vision are in a pivotal position to change negative attitudes toward visual impairment. Disseminating realistic information about low vision and its functional implications may help to dispel misconceptions. Introducing a positive role model to an individual who may be struggling with the loss of sight may also provide a means to realistically portray the potential for visual functioning. Most important, by modeling positive and realistic attitudes toward visual impairment to patients and family members, the practitioner can be a powerful conduit of change.

SELF-ASSESSMENT QUESTIONS

1. Certain benefits, such as an IRS exemption on income tax, are available to those individuals who are classified as
   (a) having subnormal vision
   (b) partially sighted
   (c) legally blind
   (d) functionally blind
   (e) visually impaired

2. Legal blindness is defined as
   (a) 20/200 or better in the better seeing eye
   (b) 20/200 or worse in the better seeing eye
   (c) 20/200 or worse in the worse seeing eye
   (d) a 20-degree field loss in the periphery of each eye
   (e) c and d

3. Which ocular condition in the United States is not considered one of the four major causes of legal blindness in the population of 65 years and older?
   (a) retinitis pigmentosa
   (b) diabetic retinopathy
   (c) age-related macular degeneration
   (d) glaucoma
   (e) cataracts

4. Which statement is incorrect?
   (a) It is not possible to obtain an exact number of new cases of legally blind individuals each year in the United States.
   (b) It is important for professionals in the field of low vision to have an understanding of attitudes toward blindness and visual impairment.
   (c) The attitudes of society have very little to no influence on an individual's adjustment to vision loss.
   (d) A visual impairment may lead to a visual disability.
   (e) A visual impairment is a loss in functioning of the visual system.

5. When taking a visual acuity test to determine legal blindness, the following conditions must be considered:
   (a) room illumination
   (b) patient's cooperation
   (c) letter contrast on the acuity chart
   (d) all of the above
   (e) only a and c

REFERENCES

1. Bronson LD. Early American Specs. Glendale, CA: The Occidental Publishing Company, 1974;18–28.
2. Southall JPC. Mirrors, Prisms and Lenses: A Textbook of Geometrical Optics. New York: Dover Publications, 1964;570.
3. Brunner AB. Telescopic lenses as an aid to poor vision. Am J Ophthalmol 1930:13;667–674.
4. Feinbloom WA. A Review of My Past Fifty Years in Low Vision Development and My Thoughts for Future Work. Paper presented to the annual Academy of Optometry at Houston, TX, Dec. 1985.
5. Tait EF, Neill JC. A new sub-normal vision appliance. Am J Optom 1936;13:55–60.
6. Feinbloom W. A new wide angle telescopic spectacle. Optom Wkly 1933:24;685.
7. Potts AM, Volk D, West SS. A television reader as a subnormal vision aid. Am J Ophthalmol 1959;47:580–581.
8. Genensky SM, Baran P, Moshin PL, Steingold H. A Closed Circuit TV System for the Visually Handicapped (RM-672-RC). Santa Monica, CA: The Rand Corporation, Aug. 1968.
9. Vision Problems in the U.S.: Facts and Figures. New York: National Society to Prevent Blindness, 1990.
10. The White House Conference on Handicapped Individuals. Awareness Papers (Vol 1). Washington, DC, May 23–27, 1997.
11. Augusto CR, McGraw JM. Humanizing blindness through public education. J Vis Impair Blindness 1990;84:397–400.
12. Monbeck M. The Meaning of Blind: Attitudes Toward Blindness and Blind People. Bloomington, IN: Indiana University Press, 1973.
13. Kent, D. Shackled Imagination: Literary Illusions About Blindness. J Vis Impair Blindness 1989;83:145–150.

CHAPTER TWO

Psychosocial Implications of Visual Impairment

Marcy Graboyes

Mrs. Jones is a 75-year-old woman with macular degeneration. She has come in for a low vision evaluation with entering acuities of 20/200 in each eye. She reports that her main area of difficulty is reading, and she is hoping that low vision glasses will help her return to this activity. Through the course of the evaluation, every device that is presented to her is rejected, despite the improvement in her clinical acuity. She appears angry and expresses feelings of frustration.

The previous scenario is not that uncommon. It is a classic example of functional versus clinical success: a patient who appears to have enough vision to benefit from low vision services and devices but does not have a successful experience. This chapter examines one of the most critical determining factors in the effectiveness of low vision services: psychosocial implications of visual impairment.

Loss of vision is one of the most emotionally devastating physical problems. According to a survey conducted by Gallup in 1988, blindness was the most feared disability for 42% of the 1,072 adults polled.[1] The impact of visual impairment extends beyond functional vision problems to a myriad of psychosocial issues ranging from grieving the loss of sight to the impact of the loss on the family and significant others. It is virtually impossible to provide low vision care without being cognizant of the psychosocial impact of the loss of sight. When an individual with a visual impairment presents for an evaluation, it is essential to view that individual from a holistic perspective, looking beyond the pathology in considering low vision needs. The low vision practitioner must also attend to the emotional impact of the vision loss on the patient when providing low vision services.

FACTORS AFFECTING ADJUSTMENT TO VISION LOSS

In an attempt to understand more fully the impact of vision loss, the practitioner may use a thorough history to glean important information. A number of factors that affect the adjustment to vision loss may reveal pertinent information about the psychosocial well-being of the patient. These factors would typically be explored while taking the history as well as by observing the patient as he or she interacts with family and friends, the practitioner, and the environment in general. It is important to note that all of these factors are interconnected. When looked at as a whole, they will paint a picture of who the individual is as well as the impact of the visual impairment on that individual.

Type of Loss

The first factor to consider that may reveal significant information is the type of vision loss the individual has experienced. The diagnosis itself and its functional implications can affect the adjustment process. An initial area to explore is how much the patient knows about his or her vision problem. There may be the need to clarify the

meaning of the diagnosis and prognosis. For example, many individuals with macular degeneration are fearful that they will lose all of their sight. Others who have been told that they are legally blind often do not fully understand the meaning and implications of this label. For many, hearing the word *blind* often confirms their fear of losing all of their sight in spite of a stable prognosis. The practitioner can serve a valuable role by dispelling fears about the visual impairment, which in some cases can create feelings as disabling as the eye condition itself.

Another diagnosis-related factor that might influence low vision services is whether the visual impairment is congenital or adventitious. The person with a congenital visual impairment may have learned to adapt many tasks and activities to the necessary level of visual functioning. Having no prior visual experience with which to compare, the person born with a vision problem might not have as clear an idea of how low vision services might be of assistance. A host of influencing factors will help shape this individual's attitude toward visual impairment, which in turn can influence the low vision evaluation. The attitudes toward visual impairment of family members, peers, teachers, and society as a whole all impact on how the individual with a congenital visual impairment's personality develops and his or her level of self-confidence and self-esteem.[2] Cultural and socioeconomic factors as well as attitudes toward blindness that are encountered by the individual will all influence how he or she is affected by the visual impairment.

The individual who has experienced an adventitious (acquired) visual impairment may present with a different set of issues and expectations. The recency of onset as well as the extent of the vision loss may influence the rehabilitation process. For example, an individual who has recently been diagnosed with macular degeneration and comes in for a low vision evaluation may still be hopeful that conventional lenses may correct the problem. This individual may not be ready to part with the hope that he or she may be able to perform visual tasks in the same way as before the loss of vision. The practitioner should take into account the recency of onset if a patient is not successful in using low vision devices despite the clinical potential for visual improvement. It is not uncommon for this individual to return for help at a later date after having time to deal with the emotional impact of the loss.

The meaning of vision loss for an individual with an adventitious visual impairment is shaped by factors similar to those for individuals with a congenital loss of vision. For example, a person with Stargardt's macular degeneration whose only exposure to visual impairment has been a blind person selling pencils on a street corner might assume that individuals with visual impairment are not capable of achieving the same goals as those who are fully sighted. In other words, a person's life experiences will influence his or her own aspirations and goals in vision rehabilitation.

A sudden loss of vision, such as that experienced as a result of head trauma or stroke, may have different implications for adjustment than a slow loss of sight. The person experiencing a sudden onset has had no time to prepare for the myriad changes that often accompany vision loss. The task of coping with physical adaptations as well as the psychological adjustment can be overwhelming for some individuals. A more gradual loss, such as that experienced with age-related macular degeneration or retinitis pigmentosa, may often allow more time for the individual to slowly adapt. If the visual impairment is genetically linked, it is important to consider that the family might be experiencing a range of emotions, including anger, rejection, and guilt. It is essential that accurate information be provided to patients and their family or significant others to ease some of these feelings.

Family Reaction

Family reaction to visual impairment is another important consideration in the adjustment process. "If there is a single universal, it can be assumed that it is the entire family unit that is experiencing a vision loss and not just the individual sustaining blindness."[3] The messages that family members give in terms of expectations and the types of role changes, both voluntary and imposed, that may occur after one family member becomes visually impaired can have a profound impact on the individual's adjustment. Significant role changes occurring as a result of the vision loss, such as a shift in household responsibilities or job roles, may cause anger and resentment among family members. These issues may very well carry over into the low vision examination and may become apparent in the goal-setting phase of service delivery as well as in the use of optical devices. For example, a wife forced into the job market or a husband accustomed to the traditional role of breadwinner having more household responsibilities may be in the process of adjusting to these changes. Pre-existing family problems may become exacerbated by the stresses brought on by visual impairment. If a patient comes to the low vision evaluation alone, it can be useful to ask questions about family composition, frequency of contact with family and significant others, and the perceived quality of these interactions.

Children of all ages are also affected when a parent becomes visually impaired. For example, the adult child of an older parent with a visual impairment may need to assume a number of responsibilities that the parent is no longer able to do. It is important to explore how each family member feels about these changes. Family members may also be confused by fluctuations in vision or by inconsistencies in visual capabilities. For example, it is not uncommon for the family of a person with macular degeneration to wonder why the person is unable to read small print yet can see a thread on the floor or can walk with relatively little difficulty. The use of visual impairment simulators may assist family members to better understand the functional impact of the vision loss. Simulators, while helpful in imitating the functional aspect of loss, do not simulate the psychological aspect of the visual impairment. In other words, the family member knows that the simulator can be removed and therefore does not experience the emotional impact of the loss of sight. Families need time as does the individual with

the visual impairment to adjust to the changes accompanying the vision loss. It is important to note that families can be an important source of emotional support in the adjustment process and should be encouraged to participate during the low vision examination.

Life Stage

The life stage of the patient at the onset of visual impairment as well as life stage at the time of low vision intervention also have potential implications for psychosocial adjustment. A child with a visual impairment may be struggling to keep up with schoolwork or to participate in the same activities as his or her peers. The messages the child receives regarding his or her competence from family, teachers, and peers will be critical in the development of self-esteem and the potential for achievement of life goals.

A teenager faces a different set of life events that also impact adjustment. Adolescence is a tumultuous life stage even without the presence of visual impairment. It is generally important for adolescents to feel similar to their peers. Problems in school that might necessitate the use of low vision devices or other adaptive equipment, such as large print books or a closed-circuit television, might have a negative impact on this quest to "fit in." Rites of passage during this life stage, including dating and driving, may also be impacted by visual impairment. The significance of all of these issues for low vision services is that although a teenager might appear to be an excellent candidate for optical and nonoptical devices, he or she might categorically reject the use of any device that may draw attention to the visual impairment. It is not uncommon for a teenager to initially refuse to use low vision devices while in high school but become more open to various options as he or she begins college or enters the job force. It therefore might be useful to have the teenager view the low vision process as a fact-finding mission, reinforcing that the ultimate decision of whether any devices are prescribed will be left to him or her.

The working-age adult with vision loss might experience role change within the family and community at large. For example, a husband and wife might be forced to switch roles if a husband becomes disabled and the wife enters the job force. This change is especially significant for a family with traditional values and may lead to feelings of anger and resentment. Conversely, a woman who becomes visually impaired might be forced to alter her job or household responsibilities, thus leading to a diminished sense of self-esteem. Children of a parent who is visually impaired may also be affected by the vision loss if activities once done jointly have been affected or if they see that the parent is having a difficult time adjusting to the vision loss.

The older adult faces a unique set of challenges related to the aging process, which can be compounded by vision loss. In addition to the typical problems associated with growing older, such as the loss of a spouse or friends and decline in general health, the impact of visual impairment may have a significant effect both functionally and psychologically. During the "golden years," retirement affords the older person opportunity to do the activities that time did not permit during the working years. A visual impairment may disrupt the individual's ability to participate in leisure activities such as hand crafts, reading, card playing, and golf. The impact of visual impairment may be especially significant for the older person living alone. Often, the most basic activities, such as cooking, cleaning, or even dialing the telephone, seem insurmountable, forcing many older adults to question their ability to live independently. Relationships with adult children may become strained as the need for assistance becomes greater.

Significant Life Events

Another factor affecting adjustment to vision loss that the practitioner should consider is the occurrence of recent significant life events. These may include a recent change in living situation, other health problems, loss of or change in employment, and change in marital status through death, divorce, or separation. If an individual has faced a number of critical stressful events, he or she might not have the mental or physical energy to participate in low vision services. It is therefore important to have an awareness of other events that might have recently occurred in the life of the patient. For example, if a person has recently experienced a catastrophic loss (e.g., death of a spouse or close relative) the stress of this event might impact the available energy that the person has to learn new visual skills. Significant life events should be noted and considered, especially if an individual is exhibiting difficulty concentrating or learning new tasks. This information can easily be collected as part of an initial history.

Patient Expectations

Patient expectations of low vision services are very important to consider. A patient who is still searching for a cure for visual impairment or is seeking conventional glasses to resolve all visual difficulties may not have a complete understanding of low vision services or have fully come to terms with the permanency of the vision loss. Realistic expectations are critical for goal setting and effective low vision service delivery. One of the most important aspects of the history-taking process is listening carefully to the goals expressed by the patient so that low vision services move in a direction that is meaningful and motivating. It is important not to assume that an activity the patient reports having problems performing is necessarily a low vision goal. Some individuals may be relieved to relinquish the responsibility of certain activities, such as shopping or writing checks, to other family members. If at all possible, it is very useful to have direct contact with the patient before the first low vision appointment to discuss the patient's goals and expectations. During this conversation, information regarding the potential of low vision services can be shared so that the patient can begin to formulate

goals that are obtainable. If time does not permit a phone call, a brief questionnaire could be completed by the patient before the first clinic visit so that the practitioner has information regarding patient expectations.

Self-Concept

Another factor that the practitioner should be aware of is the impact of visual impairment on an individual's self-concept. A person's self-concept is composed of both internal and external influences that determine how one views him- or herself. This view of self is in some way impacted by a vision impairment. Self-perception may be altered temporarily or permanently by a disability. Levels of self-esteem may also be affected as the individual's sense of competence in his or her ability to perform tasks and the confidence of others in him or her to accomplish tasks are in some way impacted by vision problems. The individual with low vision has been described as the "marginal man," not belonging to the world of the sighted or the blind, but in a gray area, a no-man's land.[4] This sense of not belonging can feel frightening and confusing to the individual who is struggling to regain a sense of independence. If the feedback received from significant others is that one is unable to perform certain activities, the implied message is that the individual is incapable of being independent.

"Passing" is a strategy that some individuals may use to attempt to fit in. Passing is a behavior in which an individual chooses to conceal critical information about him- or herself.[5] There may be significant rewards for being perceived in a different way. In certain situations, the visually impaired person might think that there is something at risk in allowing others to know of the visual impairment. Some examples might be an employment situation in which job jeopardy may be an issue or a social situation in which rejection is feared if the visual impairment is discovered. By concealing the visual impairment, the individual assumes that others will not pass judgment on him or her based on vision.

Personality

An individual's personality is another consideration. How an individual has coped in the past with stressful life events before the onset of vision loss will help determine the coping pattern for the vision loss. Each person will react to the loss of sight in an individual way. This is why it is so important to treat each person as a unique individual. Factors, such as how a person handles anxiety and stress, attitudes toward independence, and levels of aspiration, will all affect the reaction to the visual impairment and impact on low vision services. For example, an individual who has a history of anxiety and depression may react more intensely to the loss of sight and may perhaps require psychosocial intervention to assist in the adjustment process. An individual who has always valued independence may be more motivated to do whatever it may take to help get back to the desired level of self-sufficiency than someone who has been more dependent on others in having his or her needs met.

EMOTIONAL REACTION TO LOSS

Individuals experience a wide range of emotions in response to loss. A number of theories attempt to describe the process a person might go through in coming to terms with loss. One well-known theory was put forth by Elisabeth Kübler-Ross, who developed her work with individuals who were facing terminal illness.[6] The framework that she used to describe this process is fairly similar to that which an individual with a vision loss might also experience. It is important to note that not all individuals go through all of the stages of loss, nor do they experience them in the same order. It is also important to recognize that the grieving process is not finite: it is possible that as a person faces further loss of sight, there may be a return of feelings that were previously experienced in response to the initial loss.

Shock or Denial

The first of these stages is *shock* or *denial*. This stage usually begins when the individual either realizes that there is a problem with vision that is not correctable or is given the diagnosis. Shock is a normal response to an emotionally painful situation. It allows the individual time to mobilize the necessary resources to deal with the pain of the loss. If this period of shock or denial goes on for a lengthy period and begins to interfere with the individual's moving ahead, other intervention, such as therapy, might be indicated.

Anger

The second stage of grieving is *anger*. At this stage, the individual is beginning to feel the emotional impact of the loss. The person often asks, "Why is this happening to me?" and may feel resentful of others who have not experienced this loss. It is not unusual for some of this anger to be directed to others with whom the individual may be interacting. It may be the doctor, the clerk in the grocery store, a family member, or a bus driver. The angry feelings may come spilling out especially in situations in which the individual is made acutely aware of his or her visual impairment. It can be very helpful to acknowledge the anger when working with the patient by simply stating, "You seem to be very angry. Can you tell me what's going on?" The person may feel the need to vent some of these feelings and know that they are normal. An individual should know that it is legitimate to feel angry about the vision loss and that talking about it might be cathartic. If the anger is out of control or interfering with relationships or the ability to accept help, it may be necessary to refer the individual to a counselor or therapist to address the anger and any underlying causes for the problem.

Depression

The next stage of grieving is *depression*. At this point, the person may be feeling a deep sense of sadness about the loss and a sense of hopelessness about the situation. A number of indicators of depression can be noted by the practitioner to determine whether the person is experiencing depression. For example, if the patient seems noncommunicative, lacks affect, exhibits body posture such as slouched body position, or averts eye contact, further questioning may be indicated to explore more deeply the emotional state of the person. Questions regarding changes in sleeping patterns, eating habits, and activity level may glean critical information about how the person is feeling. It should be noted that depression is a normal response to vision loss. If, however, the depression becomes severe enough to affect the person's ability to perform day-to-day activities, more intensive intervention by a mental health professional may be warranted. For example, a 69-year-old woman reported that she had experienced a rather sudden loss of vision secondary to macular degeneration and that her vision had worsened further after laser treatment. It was evident to both the patient and the social worker during the initial interview that the patient was experiencing acute depression in relation to this sudden loss. On further exploration, the patient revealed a history of depression in response to other significant life changes, such as the death of her parents and her children moving away from home. Although she felt somewhat encouraged by the potential help of low vision devices, she soon realized that she lacked both the physical and emotional energy to continue with services. The patient was referred to a psychiatrist and eventually spent almost 3 weeks in an inpatient psychiatric facility to address the issues related to this most recent loss of vision. With the support of both a psychologist and psychiatrist, the patient soon returned home and eventually resumed low vision services. As she began to find low vision devices helpful in meeting her goals, she developed a sense of hope that she would regain some of the skills necessary to remain independent.

Bargaining

Bargaining is the next grieving stage and is usually the briefest in duration. At this point, the person is seeking to gain control by making deals or pacts to negotiate a change in the situation. This attempt to control and ultimately change the situation usually does not last long because it soon becomes apparent that regardless of what is tried, the situation remains the same. Control is an important issue to a person with a visual impairment because so much of his or her functional abilities may feel beyond control.

Acknowledgment

The last of the grieving stages described by Kübler-Ross is that of *acceptance*. Many visually impaired individuals have taken exception to referring to this last stage by the term *acceptance* because it has a connotation of willingly embracing the vision loss. A more accurate and acceptable term for this stage for many is *acknowledgment*, or making peace with the permanence of the visual impairment to move on with one's life.

It is essential that the low vision practitioner have some level of awareness and an appreciation for the range of emotions experienced by a person with a visual impairment. The ability and willingness to recognize and respond to the emotional needs of the patient during the evaluation will make low vision care much more effective and ultimately contribute to a higher level of patient satisfaction with vision rehabilitation services.

METHODS OF PROVIDING PSYCHOSOCIAL SUPPORT

The discussion so far has dealt with the multitude of issues that shape an individual's response to visual impairment. It is fair to say that it is virtually impossible to provide low vision services without some of these issues affecting this process. It is therefore essential for the practitioner to know how to respond to these issues and to know where and to whom to turn for problems that fall outside the expertise of the eye care practitioner.

Effective Communication

One of the most important factors in providing effective low vision care is good communication. A practitioner who conveys a sense of warmth and genuine caring will establish a trusting doctor-patient relationship. There are several ways to build this rapport.

One method is to listen for and acknowledge feelings. It is common for strong feelings experienced due to vision loss to be expressed during the low vision evaluation. In many cases, the low vision practitioner may be the first professional to really focus in on the problem areas experienced by the patient. It is therefore important to be prepared for the sharing of feelings such as fear, anger, sadness, or depression. At times, the practitioner may be the target of displaced anger and should be aware that the anger is not directed at him or her but at the current life situation.

Active listening is a technique that can be used to communicate to the patient that what he or she is saying or feeling is being understood. By listening to the patient and rephrasing the patient's words, the practitioner demonstrates that he or she has identified the underlying feeling or has grasped the meaning of the patient's statement. For example, if a patient states that some days it is very hard to muster the energy to get out of bed, the practitioner in an effort to actively listen may respond, "It sounds as if you are feeling really down about your life right now." Through this empathetic response, the doctor is communicating an understanding of what the patient is sharing, allowing for the exchange of further pertinent information about this situation. Active listening is an important element of empathy, or feeling with a person, not for a person. This is an important aspect of relationship building and a key element in the helping process.

At times, the most important help that a practitioner can offer is to allow the patient to share feelings. Through this process, a trusting relationship is established through which more effective services can be provided. If a patient continually needs to spend time at each visit discussing the impact of the vision loss and related issues, the practitioner might need to consider a referral for psychosocial intervention before this patient is ready to move through the low vision evaluation.

Family as a Resource

As discussed in Family Reaction, the family and significant others can be important influencing factors in the adjustment to vision loss. The family can also impact the outcome of low vision services and serve as a resource and support system. If sharing difficult news, such as a diagnosis or prognosis, is part of a visit, it is important to try to have a family member or friend present. The patient may be unable to absorb the information being shared due to shock or denial. A family member or friend may be able to take in more of the information and serve as a resource to the patient at a later time. A follow-up visit may be necessary to give the patient time to digest information and provide an opportunity to ask questions. It is important to observe family interactions and encourage family members or friends to be part of the rehabilitation process. If family relationships are not positive, it might be more beneficial to the patient to experience low vision services without family members present.

Resources

Practitioners should be knowledgeable about community resources available to address the potential range of psychosocial needs. One type of resource is support groups. Support groups can be effective in assisting the individual with low vision to adapt to vision loss. As low vision is a relatively low-incidence disability, many individuals who have become visually impaired often mention that they feel alone with their thoughts, feelings, and functional problems and wish they knew others with whom they could compare notes. When the practitioner hears these and similar comments, such as "Nobody understands what I'm going through," or, "My family doesn't understand why I can see some things but not others," it can be valuable to make a referral to a group of individuals with similar issues and concerns, bonded by common experiences. There are many support groups, both on the local and national levels. It is helpful to have information on file, for example, a brochure or the name and phone number of a contact person, so that when a problem is encountered, an appropriate referral can be made. Various national organizations, such as the National Organization for Albinism and Hypopigmentation and the Foundation Fighting Blindness, are excellent sources of information and in many areas have local chapters. The Council of Citizens with Low Vision has chapters throughout the country and meets the needs of many partially sighted individuals. There are groups for parents, such as the National Association for Parents of the Visually Impaired, as well as local parent support groups sponsored by schools, hospitals, and area rehabilitation agencies for the visually impaired. Support groups also exist for older persons. An excellent resource to locate these groups nationally is the Lighthouse publication, *Self Help and Mutual Support Groups for Visually Impaired Older Adults.* Another publication entitled *Agencies Serving the Blind and Visually Impaired* is published by the American Foundation for the Blind in New York. It includes many services and resources related to visual impairment. This book should be part of every low vision practitioner's library.

For patients who might be in need of counseling, it is important that the practitioner be familiar with community mental health resources. A working knowledge of the various professionals trained to provide therapy can be critical in making an effective referral for a patient who is depressed, suicidal, or experiencing any number of other emotional difficulties that might be addressed through therapy.

In conclusion, providing vision care to a person with visual impairment requires that the low vision practitioner have an appreciation for the psychological and social impact of such a loss on the patient as well as on the low vision rehabilitation process. A successful low vision experience for both the practitioner and the patient requires attention to the whole person and not just the physical aspect of vision loss.

SELF-ASSESSMENT QUESTIONS

1. All persons with visual impairment experience the grieving process in the same way.
   True or False

2. List the five stages of grieving that a person with a visual impairment might experience.

3. List four factors affecting adjustment to vision loss.

4. A person experiencing depression may exhibit which of the following behaviors?
   (a) changes in sleeping patterns
   (b) slouched body posture
   (c) flat affect
   (d) loss of appetite
   (e) all of the above

5. An individual's reaction to vision loss may be similar to the reaction to previous losses.
   True or False

REFERENCES

1. Augusto CR, McGraw JM. Humanizing blindness through public education. J Vis Impair Blindness 1990;October:397–400.
2. Vanderkolk C. Assessment and Planning with the Visually Impaired. Baltimore: University Park Press, 1981.
3. Freedman S. Family Reactions to Blindness and Visual Impairment. Presented at the International Conference of American Association of Workers for the Blind, Toronto, July 1981.
4. Ault C. The Low Vision Person: "A Marginal Man" (unpublished manuscript). Palo Alto, CA: Western Blind Rehabilitation Center, 1976;98–122.
5. Goffman E. Stigma. New York: Simon & Shuster, 1963.
6. Kübler-Ross E. On Death and Dying. New York: Macmillan, 1969.

CHAPTER THREE

The Low Vision Examination

Sarah Deborah Appel
and Richard L. Brilliant

There are many approaches to evaluating the low vision patient. Practitioners use varying techniques, charts, and procedures to evaluate the visual status of their patients. The key is that the testing procedures must be appropriate for the patient's ocular condition and visual status, that they yield accurate and useful findings, and that the patient's goals be a key factor in determining a management and rehabilitation plan. The purpose of the following discussion is to explore the components of the low vision examination.

OBSERVATION

The low vision examination process should commence before the visually impaired patient enters the examination room. Observation of visual behaviors in an unfamiliar environment can yield significant preliminary information about visual status that can be used to shape examination and rehabilitation strategies. Observations should begin when the patient enters the office and should continue throughout the evaluation sequence.

Whenever possible, the doctor should greet the patient in the reception area and accompany him or her to the examination room. This provides the practitioner with an excellent opportunity to note how the patient negotiates his or her visual environment. It also allows the practitioner to meet family members and observe family interactions. As the practitioner accompanies the visually impaired patient, observations in postural abnormalities, mobility, and appearance should be noted.

Postural Abnormalities

It is not unusual to encounter an individual who has adapted posturally to slowly progressive field loss and yet is unaware of the extent or even presence of the field defect. Head turns or tilts are frequently found with peripheral field defects that are more pronounced in one hemisphere or quadrant. The turn or tilt is typically in the direction of the field loss. Pronounced head and eye movement while traveling may also indicate the presence of significant field constriction.

Head turns or tilts can also alert the practitioner to other visual implications. A null point or dampening of nystagmus may be easier to achieve and maintain by embedding a head turn. Diplopia resulting from strabismus that is more significant in one direction of gaze can be reduced or eliminated by a head turn or tilt. A downward head tilt may be an adaptation to significant glare or photophobia as the individual attempts to create a visor effect. Head turns may also indicate the presence of a central scotoma and may be the result of an attempt to achieve a consistent point of eccentric fixation. Such central scotoma–induced head turns become more apparent during tasks that require increased visual acuity such as reading, writing, and general identification of visual targets. Head turns related to central scotomas typically are not prevalent during mobility-related activities, as they reduce critical peripheral field information originating on the side from which the head is turned.

Mobility

A tentative gait, postural stiffness, and maintenance of close proximity to walls or handrails while traveling may be indicators of peripheral visual field loss. Excessive reliance on tactile information while traveling by holding onto an individual or trailing a wall may also indicate the presence of significant field loss. During the history, the possibility of physical conditions that adversely affect independent mobility, such as arthritis, stroke, or cerebral palsy, should be explored when mobility-related difficulties are observed.

Appearance

The practitioner should note the individual's overall appearance. The presence of nystagmus, obvious external eye disease, or strabismus should be noted early so that it may be explored further during the history and examination process. Squinting may indicate the presence of photophobia or uncorrected refractive error. Sunglasses worn indoors may also indicate the presence of significant photophobia. Erratic eye movements or lack of central fixation may result from a central scotoma. Eye poking may indicate an attempt to elicit visually stimulating pressure phosphenes by individuals with significant vision loss from conditions such as Leber's congenital amaurosis. Such behavior may also represent an attempt to reduce discomfort in an irritated eye.

Soiled clothing or missing buttons alert the practitioner to the possibility of difficulties in the area of activities of daily living that should be addressed. An overall disheveled, fatigued appearance may be a sign of a serious systemic disorder, depression resulting from recent vision loss, or the impact of other psychosocial factors.

SIGHTED GUIDE

If the patient is unable to walk independently into the examination room as a result of significant visual impairment, the sighted guide technique of mobility assistance should be used by the practitioner. The following is a step-by-step procedure for the sighted guide technique:

1. When the patient stands, the doctor offers his or her arm. If the patient is not aware of the position of the doctor's arm, the doctor should move his or her arm so that his or her elbow contacts the patient's hand. Talking to the patient also provides valuable verbal cues that assist the patient in determining where the doctor is standing.
2. The patient grasps the doctor's arm above his or her elbow with four fingers on the inside of the doctor's

The Low Vision Examination 21

arm and the patient's thumb on the outside of the doctor's arm. This grip should be firm yet comfortable. The doctor's arm should be relaxed by his or her side (Figure 3-1).

3. The doctor and the patient should be standing side by side so both are facing the same direction. As the doctor begins to walk, he or she is one step in front of the patient so that the patient has some time to react when the doctor stops for obstacles (Figure 3-2).

4. The patient should respond to the doctor's body movements while walking and be able to walk around corners without verbal instructions. If the patient seems to have difficulty following the doctor's body movements, the doctor may want to provide additional verbal information while he or she is walking to increase the patient's comfort and confidence. The doctor may also want to warn the patient if a change in the texture of the walking surface is present.

5. When approaching a narrow area, such as a door, that does not allow two individuals to pass through side by side, the doctor should move his or her arm toward the center of his or her back. The doctor then tells the patient to follow single file while moving through the narrow area (Figure 3-3).

6. When traveling on stairs, the doctor should stop at the base of the first step and inform the patient that he or she will be walking up or down. There is no need to count the number of steps. If a handrail is available, the doctor should position the patient so that he or she is in contact with the handrail while holding the doctor's

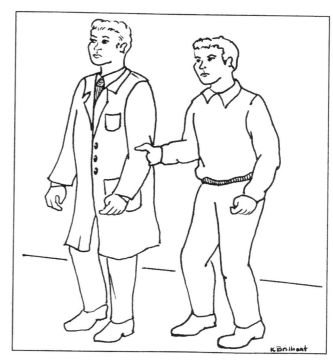

FIGURE 3-2. **When the doctor walks, the patient will be one step behind so that he will be able to react if the doctor stops or avoids an obstacle.**

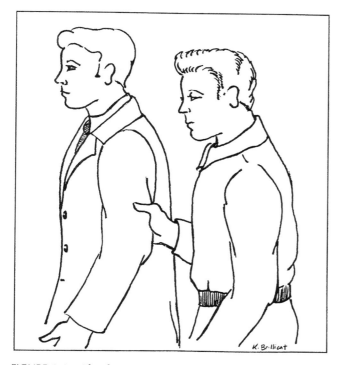

FIGURE 3-1. **The doctor's arm is relaxed by his side. The patient grasps the doctor's arm above his elbow with four fingers on the inside and the patient's thumb on the outside.**

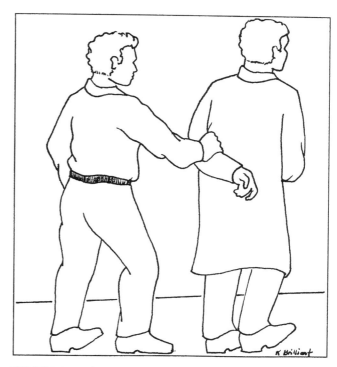

FIGURE 3-3. **When approaching a narrow area, such as a doorway, the doctor moves his arm toward the center of his back. The patient is told to follow him, in single file, while still remaining one step behind.**

arm. As the doctor takes the first step, the patient follows while remaining one step behind. The doctor's body movement should provide information that he or she has reached the top or bottom of the stairs. Providing verbal information about the location of the last step also increases the patient's safety and comfort.

7. When approaching a chair or seat of any kind, the doctor should provide a verbal description of the orientation of the chair. Is the patient facing the chair or standing to the side of the chair? Does the chair have arms or a foot rest that might be an obstacle? If so, the doctor should provide the patient with a verbal description of the chair. As the doctor reaches the chair, the patient's hand should be placed on the chair so that he or she has physical contact with the chair. If needed, the doctor should provide additional verbal instructions that enable the patient to be seated safely.

8. The doctor should inform the patient when he or she leaves the room at any time. This prevents the embarrassing situation of the patient speaking to the doctor when he or she is not in the room. Other members of the staff who are present should always be introduced so that the patient knows who is in the room at any time.

HISTORY

The history provides essential information on the patient's visual and medical status. A comprehensive low vision history, however, should also provide insight into the patient's lifestyle, interests, and concerns. The exploration of all these areas is critical to the development of appropriate and realistic evaluation and management strategies.

General Information

In addition to obtaining all the demographic information common to any history, the low vision history should contain specific information about an individual's current living situation. This provides the doctor with an initial indication of the support system available to the low vision patient. A family member can be invaluable in monitoring progress during home-based instructional sessions as well as in providing assistance and encouragement when needed. The doctor should, however, also be alert to any negative interactions that occur between the patient and accompanying family members. An unsupportive family member can be a significant obstacle to the rehabilitative program. Involving family members in the evaluation and rehabilitation sequence increases their understanding of the patient's visual difficulties and also frequently generates interest and enthusiasm about the patient's success with the devices. Low vision simulators are an excellent means of enabling family members to appreciate how the patient's visual impairment impacts on activities of daily living.

Exploration of marital status may reveal a recent loss of a spouse or a divorce that could negatively affect the patient's emotional readiness for services. A recent change

in living situation necessitated by the visual impairment may also have implications for the patient's psychosocial well-being.

Systemic History

Systemic disorders, such as diabetes, multiple sclerosis, and human immunodeficiency virus, can present with both serious visual impairment as well as significant physical debilitation. Knowledge of a patient's systemic disorder enables the doctor to prepare for associated visual abnormalities as well as to explore if the individual is receiving adequate care, complying with the prescribed treatment regimen, and has adequate support mechanisms. Exploration of systemic health status should include diagnosis, onset, stability, previous surgeries, medication regimen, allergies, and family history. The doctor should also attempt to elicit the patient's understanding of the disease process and prognosis. An individual who is knowledgeable about his or her disorder and its management tends to be more involved in the therapeutic process.

Identification of systemic pathology alerts the doctor to the need for appropriate timing of the examination. For example, diabetic patients should be scheduled so that the examination does not overlap with their lunch time. In addition, patients with physically debilitating conditions, such as multiple sclerosis, tend to require shorter examination sessions, with breaks when needed, to minimize fatigue. Exploration of systemic pathology also identifies therapy-related visual needs that should be addressed during the low vision evaluation. Activities critical to the management of systemic disease, such as distinguishing pills and other medications, self-injection of insulin, monitoring blood glucose levels, and monitoring of blood pressure, are visually demanding and often pose significant difficulty for the patient who is visually impaired.

Visual History

Similar to the systemic history, the visual history should include determination of diagnosis, onset, stability, previous surgeries, medication regimen, allergies, and family history. When there is a family history of visual impairment, hereditary factors and genetic counseling may be considered. The doctor should determine how frequently the patient is being monitored for a visual disorder and look for indications that the patient may not be complying with the medical management plan. In such situations, it may be helpful to work with the primary care physician to improve compliance. Reports of fluctuations in vision and recent changes in vision should be recorded. Such changes may be indicative of pathology-related changes and may necessitate referral to the appropriate health care provider. They may also indicate, however, normal age-related accommodative changes or difficulty in maintaining a consistent eccentric viewing (EV) position. It is not unusual for a 30-year-old individual with a stable disorder, such as albinism, to present with complaints of a progressive vision loss that is causing great concern. On questioning, the patient reveals that the vision reduction is noticed only while reading and may be due to normally reduced accommodative amplitudes. That individual is no longer able to comfortably focus at the 6-cm focal distance necessary to achieve the correct amount of relative distance magnification. In such cases, it is important to differentiate between overall vision reduction and reductions limited solely to near-point activities.

The doctor should also explore the patient's understanding of his or her disorder and obtain the patient's perspective on how the disorder has impacted his or her life. An individual with 20/100 vision who views him- or herself as blind may be at a point in the grieving process at which he or she is not yet ready for low vision rehabilitation. An individual with end-stage glaucoma and visual fields constricted to 5 degrees who is convinced that his or her vision will get better and whose main objective is to resume driving may be in the stage of denial and thus unable to set realistic goals. An individual who reports that no one is aware of his or her visual disorder may be embarrassed or scared to reveal the situation. This patient may benefit from positive reinforcement from others with similar ocular disorders (support groups), thus reducing feelings of isolation and insecurity.

Education

Background information regarding current educational status is helpful in alerting the doctor to the special needs of the patient who is a student. Ascertaining grade level, major, and degree helps the practitioner to determine the student's print size requirements, complexity of reading materials, and distances at which materials will be presented. For example, computer-linked learning activities necessitate magnification at arm's length, whereas those activities involving blackboard or audiovisual presentations require magnification at distances of 20 ft or greater. For individuals who are no longer in school, identifying their educational level may alert the practitioner to the possibility that observed reading difficulties may be due to poor reading skills and not solely to visual factors. Care should be taken, however, not to assume a direct relationship between educational level and reading abilities. Many individuals with limited formal education attain excellent reading skills through self-study.

During questioning about reading methods, the patient may indicate that braille or auditory reading is the preferred mode. The doctor should be sensitive to a concern experienced by some low vision individuals who are not visual readers. These individuals may interpret the introduction of techniques and devices that would enable them to read visually as an implication that this should become their primary mode of reading. In such cases, the doctor should stress that visual reading may be complementary to other modalities and should be regarded solely as an auxiliary mode of reading that can increase

access to a wider range of reading materials. The patient is thus given an opportunity to choose the reading modality that is most efficient for a particular task or activity.

Determination of primary language for reading is important in accurately determining visual demands. A hemianopic or attitudinal visual field defect has different effects on reading languages such as Hebrew (read right to left) or Chinese (vertical reading) than it will on reading English. A central scotoma may have a more significant effect on reading Russian or Japanese due to the complexity of each character and may require greater magnification than standard English characters require. Additionally, if English is a second language, reading difficulties may not be solely due to vision when the patient is presented with English reading materials.

For the student, information on present educational placement provides the doctor with information on visual demands. Some educational programs may present many of their materials in less visually demanding, large-print formats. Tactile and auditory learning may be stressed. Questioning on the range and type of educational services being received alerts the practitioner to situations in which supportive services may be inadequate or nonexistent and may indicate the need for appropriate referral.

It is important to determine if the low vision individual is presently reading print of any size. An individual who reports that he or she can only read large print and reads a large-print Bible and newspaper every day demonstrates excellent motivation and potential. This individual has not given up on visual reading and has successfully adapted to one form of magnification to continue a valued activity. He or she therefore may be a good candidate for other modes of magnification that increase access to all publications.

Vocation

Determination of occupational status provides additional insight into an individual's visual needs. Exploration of current employment status as well as past employment history may uncover a need for low vision devices, vocational rehabilitation, or public advocacy services to ensure maintenance, advancement, or resumption of work. A thorough exploration of the occupational environment may uncover the need for environmental modifications that would improve the individual's efficiency at the work site and increase safety.

Mobility

Information about mobility provides the doctor with the patient's perspective on how his or her visual functioning impacts on mobility-related activities. It alerts the doctor to the possibility of visual field loss or reduction in contrast sensitivity and provides insight into the patient's vision-related concerns. An individual's level of confidence during mobility-related tasks may drastically change under different levels of environmental illumination as well as with different degrees of familiarity with surroundings. Questions exploring the patient's independent use of public transportation, confidence in crossing streets, and negotiation of unfamiliar environments provide insight into mobility-related concerns and to the possible need for orientation and mobility services. The presence of photophobia or light-dark adaptation difficulties highlights the need for exploration of absorptive lenses.

Activities of Daily Living

Information about activities of daily living provides the doctor with the patient's perspective on how his or her visual functioning impacts activities that are performed as part of a daily routine. Grooming, cleaning, cooking, keeping up with personal finances, and correspondence are important daily activities that are essential for independent living. They are also visually challenging. There are numerous optical and nonoptical devices and techniques that can minimize these difficulties. It is important to establish the difficulties a patient is experiencing in performing these tasks. Specificity in describing the problem areas is essential if solutions are to be found. It is also important to obtain as much information about the home environment as possible to determine if an environmental assessment may be indicated.

Leisure Activities

Discussion of leisure activities, such as television viewing and avocational interests, provides both visual information as well as information on activities that are motivating and enjoyable for the patient. Description of television screen size, color, and viewing distance helps in developing appropriate prescribing strategies. This information also may provide clues on visual status. An individual who sits at a 16-ft distance from the television to "see better" may be compensating for significant visual field constriction.

The patient should be encouraged to discuss present leisure activities in addition to those that were abandoned due to vision loss. Unless prompted, the low vision individual may omit discussion of previously enjoyed activities due to the erroneous assumption that vision loss has made continuation of these activities impossible.

Previous Low Vision Evaluations

Questioning about previous low vision evaluations and use of prescribed devices can provide insight into current visual skills and the individual's level of motivation and expectations. The individual who has been consistently using optics and has adapted well to the devices is frequently a good candidate for further exploration of devices directed toward solving new goals. An individual who presents with a shopping bag full of unused devices and reports having been to every low vision facility in the area, however, may have unrealistic expectations. This individual is frequently one whose chief concern is to "get a pair of glasses that will help me to see better." It is important to identify unrealistic expectations early in the process and educate the individual about what is realistically achievable with available optics and rehabilitative instruction.

Visual Goals

A key component of the low vision history is the exploration of the patient's goals and concerns. The practitioner who neglects to ascertain and address a patient's concerns and goals cannot provide a successful rehabilitative plan. The patient's active participation in the rehabilitative process is critical for success, and nowhere is that participation more important than in the setting of realistic goals and objectives. The patient should be asked to prioritize visual goals. Specificity should be stressed due to the specificity of optical and nonoptical devices. A realistic and motivating set of goals greatly enhances the prognosis for success. The practitioner should ensure that the patient has not inappropriately ruled out a goal due to the mistaken belief that the activity is no longer possible due to vision loss.

Throughout the history, the patient should be encouraged to analyze his or her daily routine and favored activities and identify difficulties that should be addressed. Through this process, the patient becomes aware of the need for his or her input and critical assessment of needs and objectives. It also demonstrates the doctor's interest in a holistic approach that seeks to address each patient's unique needs and concerns. In this approach, exploration of the status and effects of ocular pathology, while important, is viewed within the context of overall functioning and not as the primary focus of the evaluation.

PROGNOSTIC INDICATORS

Information obtained from the initial history should provide the practitioner with an initial sense of prognosis for successful rehabilitation. Accurate prognostic indicators include realistic goals, adaptation to vision loss, understanding of visual status, strong motivation, good support mechanisms, and stable visual status. All these areas should be explored in the comprehensive low vision history. This appraisal of prognosis may change as the examination and rehabilitation process progresses. An initial perception of prognosis, however, enables the practitioner to begin to formulate individualized evaluation strategies as well as begin to plan for any necessary rehabilitative and psychosocial intervention that appear to be needed to improve prognosis.

Other factors, such as age, educational level, visual acuity level, and type of pathology, are not as consistent in predicting successful rehabilitation. Psychosocial issues, such as motivation, support mechanisms, self-image, and acceptance of the visual impairment, often play a much more decisive role in determining the potential for success. An individual with 20/60 visual acuity and poor motivation typically is less likely to benefit from low vision rehabilitation than is someone with 20/400 acuity who is highly motivated. Some may argue that severely reduced visual acuity and active pathology indicate a negative prognosis for low vision rehabilitation. That may be true for practitioners whose goals are to improve every patient's visual acuity to 20/20. Keep in mind, however, that the low vision evaluation should be directed toward meeting the patient's goals, which may be quite different than the doctor's goals. Nonoptical devices, large-print materials, adaptive technology, and rehabilitative services can meet the needs of individuals with severe vision loss. Successful low vision rehabilitation occurs in these cases if both the patient's and doctor's goals and expectations are realistic.

INITIAL EVALUATION STRATEGIES

After the low vision history, the doctor should have sufficient information to begin to formulate an evaluation plan. Inconsistencies between the presenting ocular diagnosis and the patient's reported visual status may indicate the need for further diagnostic testing to rule out the possibility of a misdiagnosis. Information obtained from the history may also alert the doctor to concentrate on certain areas during the evaluation. For example, an individual who reports having no problems reading small print but is experiencing significant mobility-related difficulties would benefit from careful examination of peripheral fields and contrast sensitivity. On the other hand, an individual who reports fluctuations of vision during reading may be experiencing eccentric fixation difficulties and require careful mapping of the central visual field to determine if a central scotoma is present. Other causes of visual fluctuations, such as undiagnosed systemic disease or accommodative difficulties, should also be explored. In all cases, a thorough examination of visual and ocular health status is critical to the success of any low vision rehabilitation plan.

Visual Acuities

Measurement of visual acuities during the low vision evaluation accomplishes a number of objectives:

1. It provides the doctor with baseline information from which the course of a pathology may be monitored.
2. It is essential for calculating a patient's magnification needs. Inaccurate information can result in incorrect selection of optical devices for evaluation and often prolongs the duration of the low vision evaluation.
3. Determination of visual acuity levels provides the patient with an appreciation for residual vision.
4. It documents a level of visual acuity that may establish eligibility for services, benefits, and even driving privileges.

The practitioner should recognize, however, that visual acuity information can also be the key factor that deprives a patient of existing benefits, services, and driving privileges. It is therefore critical that the information be accurate and reproducible and that the appropriate techniques and measurement instruments be used during testing. The following factors have a significant impact on visual acuity testing:

1. Visual acuity charts
2. Illumination
3. Visual field status
4. Measurement techniques and procedures

Visual Acuity Charts

A multitude of visual acuity charts are available to the low vision practitioner. Visual acuity findings may actually vary from chart to chart. Such variations are the result of a number of factors. These include the number of optotypes presented per line of acuity, spacing between optotypes and between rows of optotypes, configuration of optotypes and contrast of charts. It is therefore important to use the same chart for each visit to monitor visual acuity status.

DISTANCE VISUAL ACUITY CHARTS
See Table 3-1.

I. Projector charts: The Snellen's projector chart is the most commonly used chart in assessment of distance visual acuity. It is not, however, a recommended chart for low vision patients because of the following factors:
   A. The luminance level of this chart is generally fixed and not easily varied during the patient evaluation.
   B. The contrast level is generally poor, especially in older models. The contrast level also varies with the age of the bulb and quality of the screen or mirror (if a mirrored system is used).
   C. There are large gradations in size of optotypes, especially at poorer acuity levels. For example, if the patient is unable to see the 20/100 line, the next acuity level that the doctor can test is 20/200.

TABLE 3-1
Distance Visual Acuity Equivalents

Feet	Metric	Logarithmic Maximum Angle of Resolution (logMAR)	Decimal
20/400	6/120	1.3	0.05
20/320	6/95	1.2	0.06
20/250	6/75	1.1	0.08
20/200	6/60	1.0	0.10
20/160	6/48	0.9	0.125
20/125	6/38	0.8	0.16
20/100	6/30	0.7	0.20
20/80	6/24	0.6	0.25
20/63	6/19	0.5	0.32
20/50	6/15	0.4	0.40
20/40	6/12	0.3	0.50
20/32	6/9.5	0.2	0.625
20/25	6/7.5	0.1	0.80
20/20	6/6	0.0	1.00
20/16	6/4.8	−0.1	1.25
20/10	6/3	−0.3	2.00

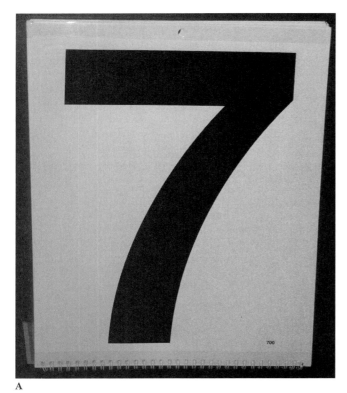

A

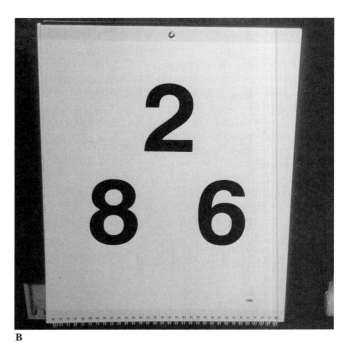

B

C

FIGURE 3-4.   **The Feinbloom Distance Test Chart (Designs for Vision, Inc., Ronkonkoma, NY) uses numerals and has a large number of optotypes beginning with a 700-ft optotype (A). As the size of the optotypes decreases, more numbers are added to each row (B, C).**

This gradation leaves significant gaps in visual acuity levels that cannot be easily refined.

    D. It is difficult to measure acuity at various distances because, in most cases, the patient blocks the projected image as he or she is walked up to the screen.

II. Printed visual acuity charts

    A. Feinbloom Distance Test Chart (Designs for Vision Inc., Ronkonkoma, NY)

        1. The original Feinbloom chart (Figure 3-4), designed by Dr. William Feinbloom, consists of numeric optotypes with the following progres-

sion: 700, 600, 400, 350, 300, 225, 200, 180, 160, 140, 120, 100, 80, 60, 40, 30, 25, 20, 10 ft.

        2. The chart is calibrated for 20 ft but may be used at any distance.

        3. Due to the increased number of optotypes that are available at lower acuity levels, patients are often encouraged by the increased number of lines that they are able to read successfully. For example, an individual with 20/120 vision may only be able to read the 20/200 line on many Snellen's projector charts. On the Feinbloom

chart, however, he or she is able to read 11 lines at a 20-ft distance and 14 lines at a 10-ft distance.

4. It should be kept in mind that because of the reduced number of optotypes, numerals are easier to guess than letters.

B. The redesigned Ferris-Bailey ETDRS (Early Treatment of Diabetic Retinopathy Study) Distance Visual Acuity Chart[1] (The Lighthouse, Inc., Long Island City, NY)

1. The ETDRS chart (Figure 3-5) maintains a consistent number of letters (5) in each row with the optotype metric progression as follows: 40, 32, 25, 20, 16, 12, 10, 8, 6, 5, 4, 3, 2.5, 2 ft. The separation between optotypes and between rows of optotypes has also been standardized to be proportional to the size of the optotype. This results in smaller spacing in the higher visual acuity levels, giving the chart its characteristic triangular configuration.

2. There is a geometric (logarithmic Minimum Angle of Resolution [logMAR]) progression of size differences between lines. Optotypes on each line are 0.1 log unit, or 25% larger, than the preceding line. This progression results in every three rows representing a halving or doubling of visual acuity levels at any viewing distance. For example, if original acuity was 2/16, a decrease in acuity by three lines would result in 2/32 while an increase by six lines would result in 2/4.

3. The logarithmic progression and proportional spacing of optotypes allows for consistent and accurate evaluation of visual acuity levels. It also allows for better interpretation of the significance of noted visual acuity changes, because a three-line difference in the higher acuity ranges would represent the same degree of change as a three-line difference in the lower acuity ranges. As the patient progresses to higher acuity levels, however, he or she experiences increased contour interaction (crowding phenomenon) which, in the case of central scotomas, may result in the measurement of poorer acuity levels than those measured using charts with increased spacing between optotypes.

4. The ETDRS chart may be used at any distance, but testing distances are typically 4 m or 2 m. At the 2-m distance the acuity obtained is easily translatable into Snellen 20-ft equivalent acuity by multiplying the fraction by 10/10. For example, an acuity of 32 M (meter system) at 2 m, or 2/32, corresponds to a 20-ft equivalent acuity of 20/320. Testing at the 2-m distance does require accommodation of 0.50 D.

5. The ETDRS chart is available in Landolt C configuration (Figure 3-6) as well as in numeric optotypes. There is also a LEA Symbol Test System (Figure 3-7) and HOTV chart for pediatric low vision patients.

C. Chronister Pocket Acuity Chart (CPAC) (Gulden Ophthalmics, Elkins Park, PA)

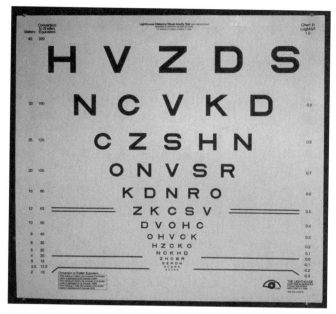

FIGURE 3-5. A logarithmic Maximum Angle of Resolution (logMAR) chart maintains a consistent number of letters in each row, and the separation between optotypes and rows is also standardized. As the size of the optotypes decreases, so does the separation between letters (in a row) and between rows.

1. The CPAC (Figure 3-8) is uniquely designed for use with patients during "out-of-office" examinations in hospitals and nursing homes, and during home visits and screenings.

2. The CPAC consists of letter optotypes with the following progression: 220, 200, 180, 160, 140, 120, 100, 80, 60, 50, 40, 30, 25, 20, 15, 10 ft.

3. The CPAC chart is calibrated for 20 ft but may be used at any distance.

4. The chart also contains a near acuity test in logMAR format. It can be recorded in reduced Snellen at 40 cm or in the meter system.

NEAR ACUITY CHARTS
See Table 3-2.

Similar to the distance visual acuity charts, there are a number of near acuity charts, including

I. Single-letter charts

A. Reduced Snellen's chart

1. This chart was first introduced by Snellen in 1866 as a means of recording near visual acuity.

2. The chart was designed so that a 20/20 letter would subtend a 5-minute angle at a given distance (typically 40 cm). The recording of the acuity would be 20/20 with a 40-cm working distance understood. This can be confusing, especially when testing at different distances is performed to extend the range of the test.

3. As in the standard Snellen distance charts, the levels of acuities are limited.

B. The Meter (M) System—Lighthouse Near Visual Acuity Test, 1st Edition (LHNV-1)

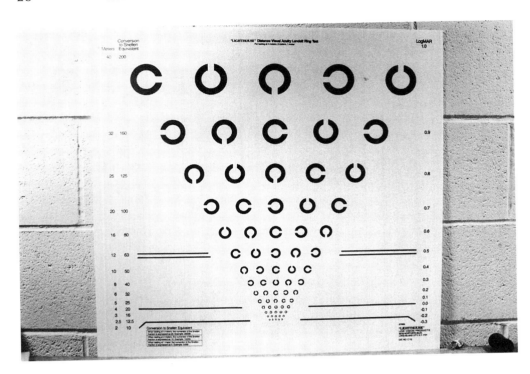

FIGURE 3-6. **A logarithmic Maximum Angle of Resolution (log-MAR) chart using the Landolt C as its optotype.**

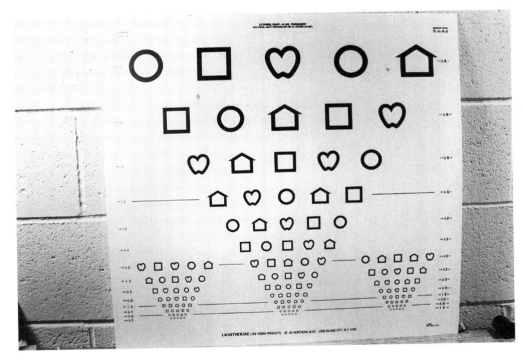

FIGURE 3-7. **A logarithmic Maximum Angle of Resolution (log-MAR) chart using a LEA Symbol Test System (apple, circle, square, and house).**

1. The "meter system" or "meter equivalent" was first advocated by Sloan.[2] A 1-M optotype will subtend 5 minutes of arc at 1 m. A 1-M letter viewed at 1 m may be equated to Snellen acuity in the following manner:

   1.00/1 M = 20/20 Snellen equivalent

   Because near acuity is frequently measured at 40 cm (0.40 m), a 1-M letter viewed at this dis-

   tance appears 2.5 times larger; therefore, 1 M is equivalent to 20/50 at 40 cm (0.40/1 M = 20/50 Snellen equivalent).

2. The optotype progression of the LHNV-1 (Figure 3-9) is as follows: 16 M, 12 M, 10 M, 8 M, 6 M, 5 M, 4 M, 3 M, 2.5 M, 2 M, 1.6 M, 1.2 M, 1 M, 0.8 M, 0.5 M.

3. Testing may occur at any distance. Acuities should be recorded as follows:

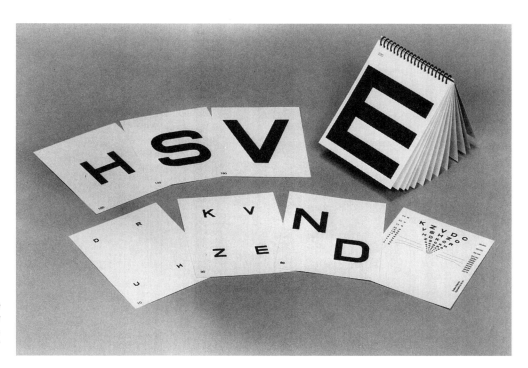

FIGURE 3-8. **The Chronister Pocket Acuity Chart is uniquely designed for "out-of-office" use. (Photo courtesy of Gulden Ophthalmics, Elkins Park, PA.)**

TABLE 3-2
Near Visual Acuity Equivalents*

Snellen Equivalent	Meter Units (M System)	Metric	American Optical Jaeger (approximate)	American Medical Association Notation	Point	Logarithmic Maximum Angle of Resolution (logMAR)	Approximate Height (mm)	Decimal	Usual Type Text Size
20/500	10.00	6/150	J19	14/350	80	1.40	15.00	0.04	½-in. letter
20/250	5.00	6/75	J18	14/175	40	1.10	7.50	0.08	Newspaper headlines
20/200	4.00	6/60	J17	14/140	32	1.00	6.00	0.10	Newspaper subheadlines
20/100	2.00	6/30	J11	14/70	16	0.70	3.00	0.20	Large-print material
20/80	1.60	6/24	J9	14/56	12	0.60	2.30	0.25	Children's books
20/60	1.20	6/18	J7	14/42	10	0.48	1.75	0.33	Magazine print
20/50	1.00	6/15	J6	14/35	8	0.40	1.50	0.40	Newspaper print
20/40	0.80	6/12	J4	14/28	6	0.30	1.15	0.50	Paperback print
20/25	0.50	6/7.5	J1	14/17.5	4	0.10	0.75	0.80	Footnotes
20/20	0.40	6/6	—	14/14	3	0.00	0.58	1.00	—

*If chart read at 40 cm.

$$\frac{\text{Test distance (meters)}}{\text{M notation}}$$

For example, 3 M at 25 cm would be recorded as 0.25/3 M.

4. Conversion of metric print size acuity to Snellen equivalent is as follows:

$$\frac{\text{Test distance (meters)}}{\text{M notation}} \times \frac{100}{100}$$

For example, 0.25/5M acuity would translate into 25/500. The 20-ft Snellen equivalent of this ratio would be 20/400.

5. The LHNV-1 provides 20-ft Snellen equivalent acuities for 40 cm (written on the side of the card).

C. Designs for Vision Number Chart (Point [N] System)
1. An 8-point optotype (N8) subtends 5 minutes of arc at a 1-m viewing distance.

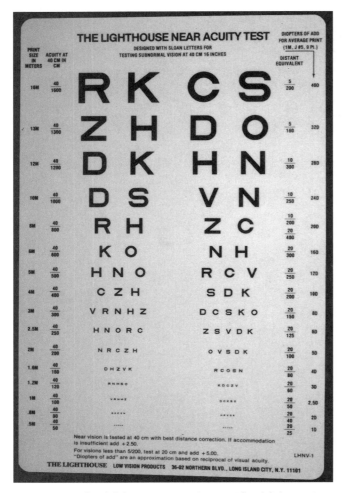

FIGURE 3-9.   **The Lighthouse Near Acuity Test (The Lighthouse, Inc., Long Island City, NY) is recorded in the meter system as well as in the reduced Snellen system.**

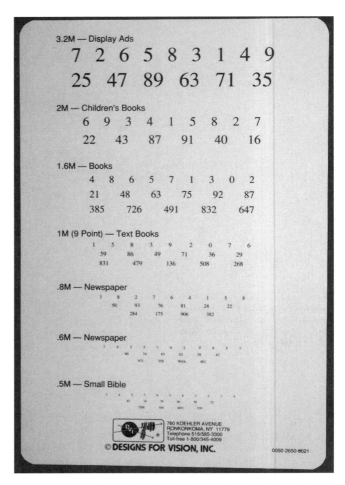

FIGURE 3-10.   **The Designs for Vision Number Chart (Designs for Vision, Inc., Ronkonkoma, NY) uses the point (N) system.**

2. N notations may be converted to M notations by dividing by 8. For example, 4 point (N4) is the equivalent of 0.5 M print (4/8).
3. The optotype progression of the Designs for Vision Number Chart is as follows: 24 N, 18 N, 14 N, 10 N, 7 N, 5 N, 4 N.
4. This chart (Figure 3-10) presents two or three lines for each acuity level. The first is a series of single numbers and is followed by a series of two-, three-, or four-digit numbers. This chart does not use proportional spacing.
5. As with any number chart, numbers vary in legibility and guessing is easier than with letter optotypes due to the reduced number of choices.
D. Reduced Ferris-Bailey ETDRS Chart (logMAR) (The Lighthouse, Inc.)
1. The ETDRS chart (Figure 3-11) maintains a constant number of letters (five) in each row with the optotype (metric) progression in the Lighthouse Near Visual Acuity Test, 2nd Edition, as follows: 8.0 M, 6.4 M, 5.0 M, 4.0 M, 3.2 M, 2.5 M, 2.0 M, 1.6 M, 1.25 M, 1.0 M, 0.8 M, 0.6 M, 0.5 M,

0.4 M, 0.3 M. The separation between optotypes and between rows of optotypes has also been standardized to be proportional to the size of the optotype. This results in smaller spacing in the higher visual acuity levels giving the chart its characteristic triangular configuration.
2. As in the distance ETDRS chart, there is a geometric (logMAR) progression of size differences between lines. Optotypes on each line are 0.1 log unit or 25% larger than the preceding line. This results in every three rows representing a halving or doubling of visual acuity levels at any viewing distance. For example, if original acuity was 0.40/3.2 M, a decrease in acuity by three lines would result in 0.40/6.4 M, whereas an increase in acuity by three lines would result in 0.40/1.6 M.
3. The logarithmic progression and proportional spacing of optotypes allows for consistent and accurate evaluation of visual acuity levels.
4. The ETDRS chart may be used at any distance. The chart provides Snellen equivalent acuities for 40 cm and 20 cm. Recording of acuity at any

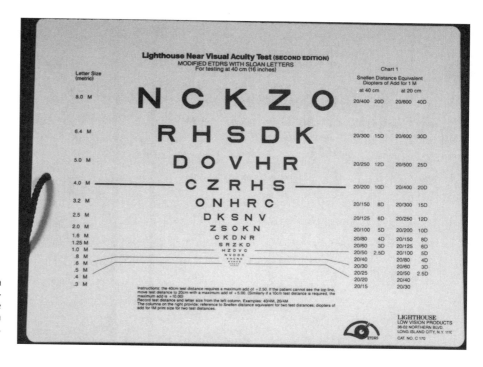

FIGURE 3-11. **A logarithmic Maximum Angle of Resolution (logMAR) chart calibrated for near use. This card uses both the meter system as well as the reduced Snellen system. (Coutesy of The Lighthouse, Inc., Long Island City, NY.)**

distance is the same as that outlined for the LHNV-1 chart.

II. Word and continuous text charts

A. Jaeger chart

1. The Jaeger (J) chart was first introduced in 1857.
2. Paragraphs are numbered from J1 to J20, with J1 representing the smallest print size.
3. There are a number of disadvantages to this chart. The character and form of the type varies from edition to edition. Rows of letters were of unequal height and diameter when compared from edition to edition. Jose and Atcherson[3] found that American Optical's (Southbridge, MA) J1 was approximately 60% larger than Bausch and Lomb's J1 (Rochester, NY).
4. There is no predictable relationship between the rows of Jaeger letters. For example, J4 is not necessarily twice as large as J2.

B. Lighthouse Game Card (The Lighthouse, Inc.)

1. The progression of metric print size of the words on this chart (Figure 3-12A) follows the same logMAR increments as the Lighthouse Near Visual Acuity Test, 2nd Edition. It does not, however, include 3-M print. The Lighthouse Game Card also does not use proportional spacing between words and between lines of acuity.
2. The Lighthouse Game Card uses the same geometric progression as the single-letter chart, with each three-row progression representing a halving or doubling of visual acuity levels at any viewing distance.
3. Visual acuity obtained with this chart may be poorer than that obtained from a single-letter ETDRS chart due to the presence of increased

contour interaction between the letters of each word. As the words decrease in size, individuals with central scotomas with unstable eccentric fixation skills may experience a dimming or distortion of part of the word and may lose their place while reading.

4. The Lighthouse Game Card may be used at any distance, but the Snellen equivalents provided are calculated for 40 cm. As with other metric-print acuity cards, acuity is recorded as a fraction with the numerator recording the metric testing distance and the denominator recording the metric print size. Snellen equivalent is calculated in the same way as previously described for the LHNV-1 chart.
5. A similar format is available in a number card (Lighthouse Number Card) (Figure 3-12B).

C. Lighthouse Continuous Text Card for Adults (The Lighthouse, Inc.)

1. The Lighthouse Continuous Text Card (Figure 3-13A) follows the same geometric progression as the Lighthouse Game Card.
2. As with the Lighthouse Game Card, recorded visual acuity may be poorer than single-letter visual acuity, especially in cases in which central scotomas are present.
3. Snellen equivalents noted on the testing card are calculated for 40 cm, but as with the Lighthouse Game Card, testing may occur at any distance. Recording of acuities and calculation of equivalent Snellen acuities is as described for the LHNV-1.
4. Other logMAR continuous text charts include the Lighthouse Continuous Text Card for Children (Figure 3-13B) (The Lighthouse, Inc.) and

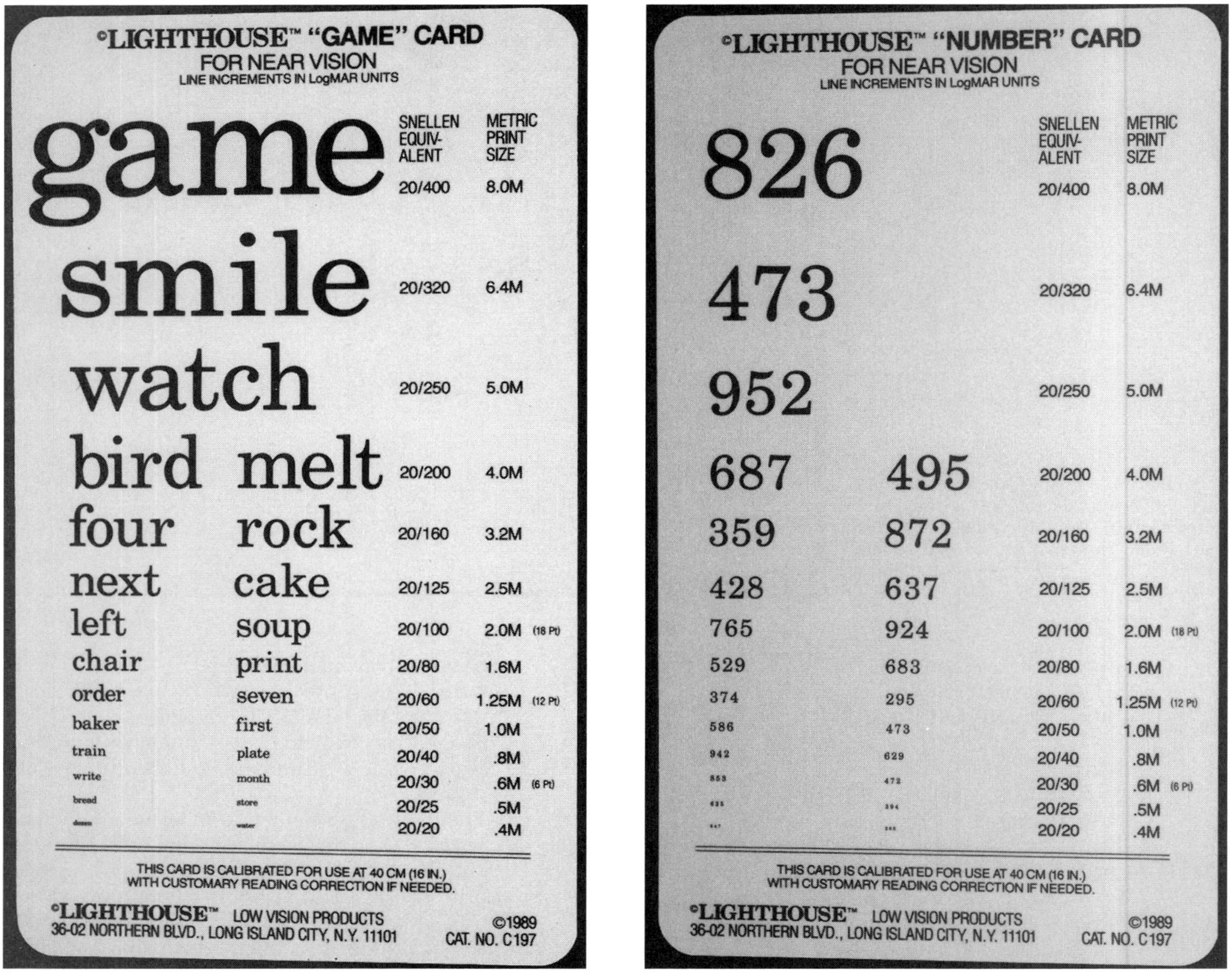

FIGURE 3-12.   **A. The Lighthouse Game Card (The Lighthouse, Inc., Long Island City, NY) follows the same logarithmic Maximum Angle of Resolution increments between rows of words; however, it does not use proportional spacing between words and between lines of acuity. B. A similar format to the Lighthouse Game Card using numbers.**

the University of North Carolina Near Vision Test Chart with words (Figure 3-13C) and with the illiterate E (Figure 3-13D).

D. MNREAD Card (The Lighthouse, Inc.) (Figure 3-14). This test combines a quick reading performance assessment with a reading acuity assessment. Reading passages are printed in decreasing M sizes in logarithmic progression from 8.0 M to below 0.2 M. This test is unique in that each three-line sentence has an identical number of characters (letters and spaces). Thus, with the MNREAD card it is easy to estimate reading speed: One simply measures the time required to read each passage. In this manner, an estimate of reading time for each print size may be recorded until the patient reaches acuity threshold. The MNREAD Card enables the doctor to

determine optimal print size for fluent reading tasks.

Illumination

The field of illumination should be uniform and glare free. The introduction of glare onto an acuity chart can result in a significant underestimation of the level of measured visual acuity due to the degradation of image quality. Back-illuminated charts are useful in the elimination of glare. The illumination system should be capable of producing variable levels of illumination so that the doctor can duplicate the patient's preferred levels of illumination.

Illumination levels can have a significant impact on results. For example, disorders, such as macular degeneration and retinitis pigmentosa, typically exhibit optimal visual acuity responses under bright illumination that is

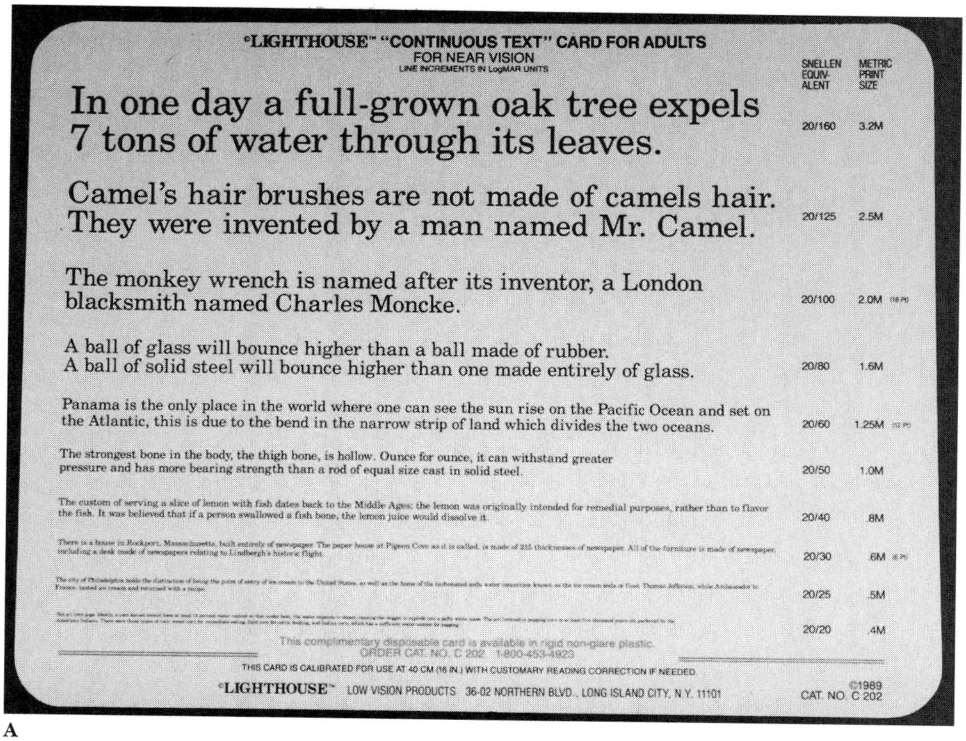

A.

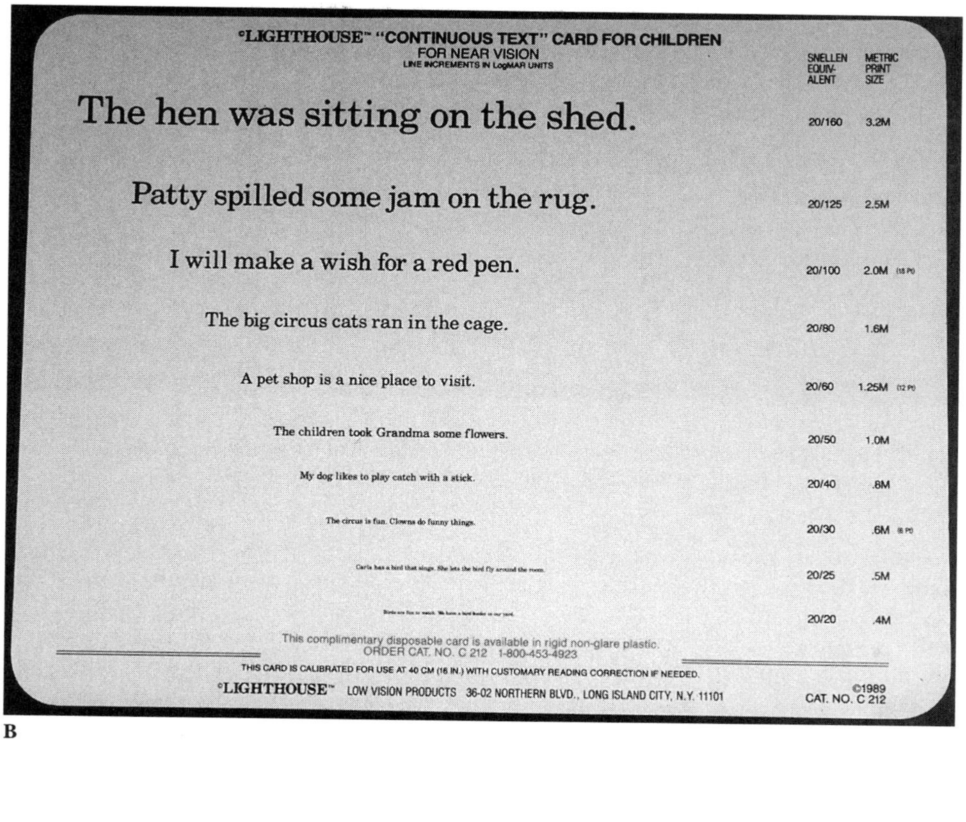

FIGURE 3-13. **A. The Lighthouse Continuous Text Card (The Lighthouse, Inc., Long Island City, NY) for adults is recorded in the meter (M) system as well as the reduced Snellen system. B. The Lighthouse Continuous Text card for children is recorded in the M system as well as the reduced Snellen system.**

B.

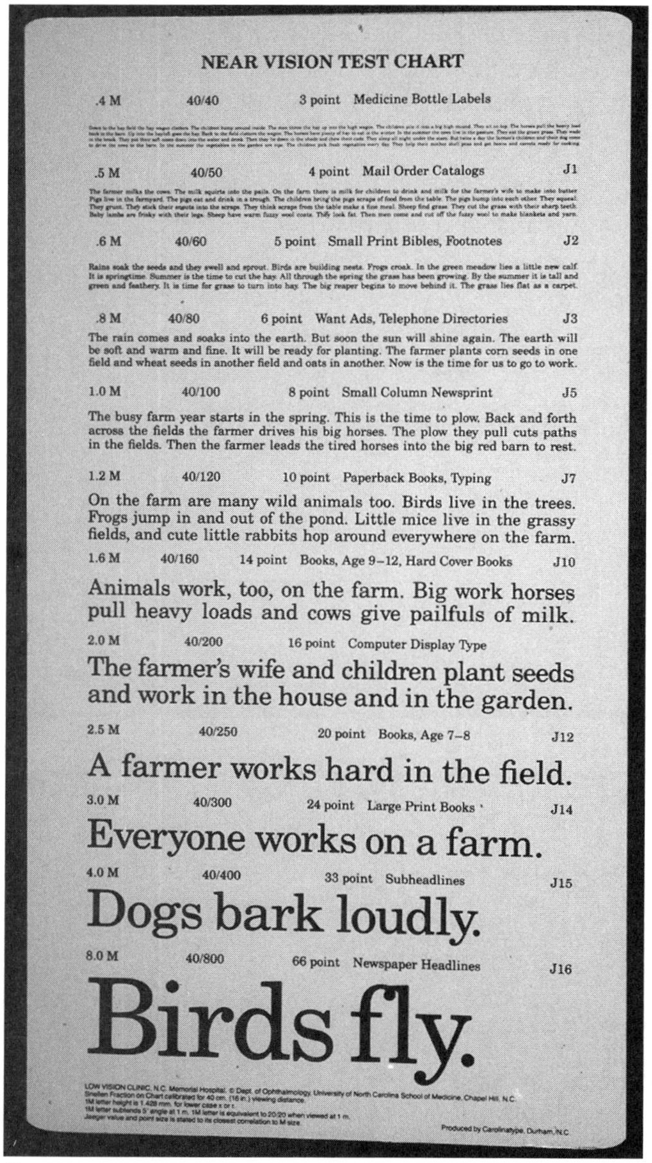

NEAR VISION TEST CHART

.4 M	40/40	3 point Medicine Bottle Labels	
.5 M	40/50	4 point Mail Order Catalogs	J1
.6 M	40/60	5 point Small Print Bibles, Footnotes	J2
.8 M	40/80	6 point Want Ads, Telephone Directories	J3
1.0 M	40/100	8 point Small Column Newsprint	J5
1.2 M	40/120	10 point Paperback Books, Typing	J7
1.6 M	40/160	14 point Books, Age 9–12, Hard Cover Books	J10
2.0 M	40/200	16 point Computer Display Type	
2.5 M	40/250	20 point Books, Age 7–8	J12
3.0 M	40/300	24 point Large Print Books	J14
4.0 M	40/400	33 point Subheadlines	J15
8.0 M	40/800	66 point Newspaper Headlines	J16

(Chart C continuous-text samples:)

Animals work, too, on the farm. Big work horses pull heavy loads and cows give pailfuls of milk.

The farmer's wife and children plant seeds and work in the house and in the garden.

A farmer works hard in the field.

Everyone works on a farm.

Dogs bark loudly.

Birds fly.

LOW VISION CLINIC, N.C. Memorial Hospital. © Dept. of Ophthalmology, University of North Carolina School of Medicine, Chapel Hill, N.C.
Snellen Fraction on Chart calibrated for 40 cm. (16 in.) viewing distance.
Produced by Carolinatype, Durham, N.C.

C

NEAR VISION TEST CHART (illiterate E version)

.4 M	40/40	3 point Medicine Bottle Labels	
.5 M	40/50	4 point Mail Order Catalogs	J1
.6 M	40/60	5 point Small Print Bibles, Footnotes	J2
.8 M	40/80	6 point Want Ads, Telephone Directories	J3
1.0 M	40/100	8 point Small Column Newsprint	J5
1.2 M	40/120	10 point Paperback Books, Typing	J7
1.6 M	40/160	14 point Books, Age 9–12, Hard Cover Books	J10
2.0 M	40/200	16 point Computer Display Type	
2.5 M	40/250	20 point Books, Age 7–8	J12
3.0 M	40/300	24 point Large Print Books	J14
4.0 M	40/400	33 point Subheadlines	J15
8.0 M	40/800	66 point Newspaper Headlines	J16

LOW VISION CLINIC, N.C. Memorial Hospital. © Dept. of Ophthalmology, University of North Carolina School of Medicine, Chapel Hill, N.C.
Snellen Fraction on Chart calibrated for 40 cm. (16 in.) viewing distance.
Produced by Carolinatype, Durham, N.C.

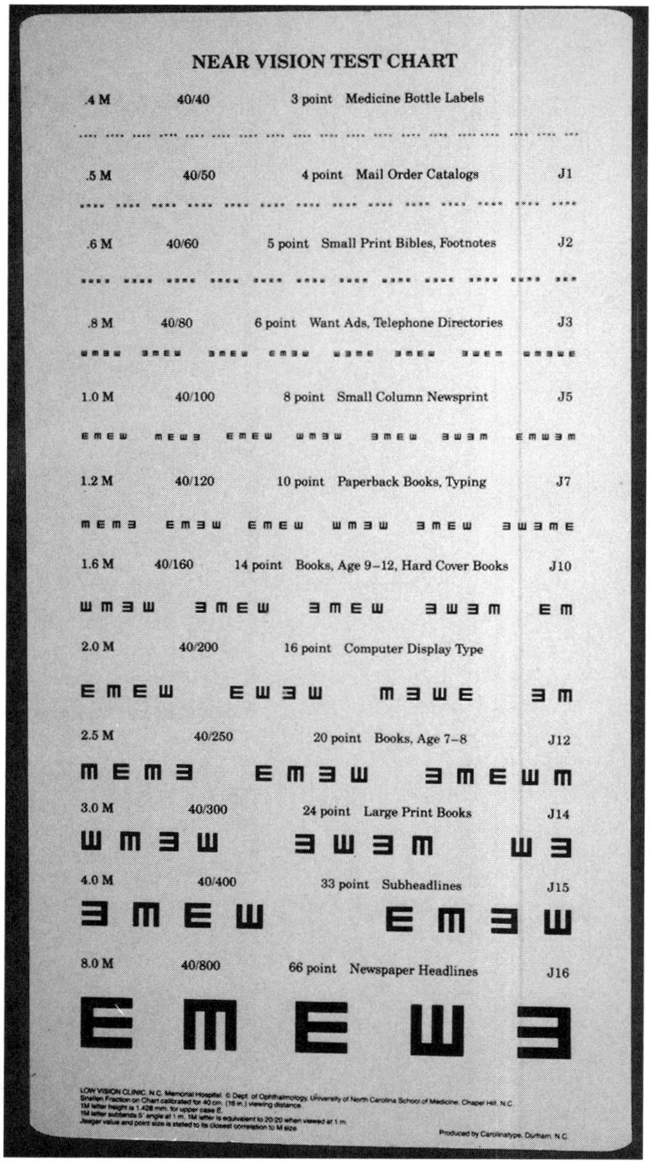

D

FIGURE 3-13.   *Continued* C. The University of North Carolina continuous text is recorded in the M, reduced Snellen, point, and Jaeger systems. D. The University of North Carolina Near Vision Test Chart using the illiterate E.

free of glare. On the other end of the illumination spectrum, some ocular disorders that involve cone abnormalities, such as rod monochromatism, typically show a heightened visual acuity response under more dimly illuminated conditions. To further complicate matters, practitioners frequently encounter situations in which a disorder does not exhibit the typical characteristics or manifestations described in textbooks. It is therefore helpful to establish the optimal levels of illumination for a patient at the beginning of the testing procedure. As the patient begins to read from the chart, the practitioner should vary the illumination levels until the patient reports optimal comfort and image quality. When the threshold of visual acuity is reached, it is also good practice to see if further manipulation of the illumination results in enhanced resolution. Once the optimal illumination level has been attained, the levels of illumination should be measured and recorded. This record aids in ensuring duplication of testing conditions at subsequent evaluations. The information is also beneficial in determining appropriate illumination devices and systems for each patient.

Visual Field Status

Visual field status can have a significant effect on responses during visual acuity testing. Disorders that involve central scotomas can result in varying visual acuity responses during testing, depending on the patient's viewing angle. When fixation occurs without an attempt to foveate because of macular damage but rather occurs

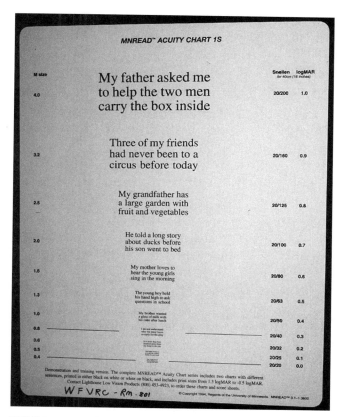

FIGURE 3-14. **The MNREAD Card (The Lighthouse, Inc., Long Island City, NY) enables the doctor to determine optimal print size for fluent reading tasks.**

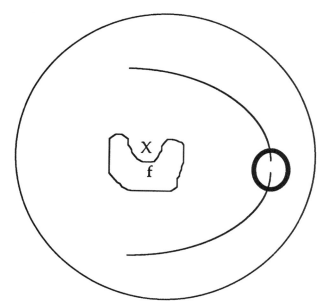

FIGURE 3-15. **A patient with reduced vision (irregular-shaped central scotoma) may attempt to identify an object at distance by using a fixation point (x) as close to the anatomic fovea (f) as possible.**

directly to an extrafoveal point, this is characterized as *eccentric fixation*. When the individual's first response to visual stimuli is an attempt to foveate within a damaged macula, which is then followed by a search for an extrafoveal point that provides visual enhancement, this is characterized as *eccentric viewing*. An individual with long-standing age-related macular degeneration (ARMD) who has an embedded eccentric fixation point should demonstrate more consistent visual acuity responses than someone with recent-onset ARMD with variable EV strategies. In both situations, it is helpful to explore EV and fixation skills. During visual acuity testing, it is important to record any apparent EV angles. EV angles are typically recorded using a clock-dial designation, as viewed from the patient's perspective. For example, a patient who experiences enhanced visual performance when using a superior temporal EV position with his or her left eye is using an 11 o'clock angle of EV.

The doctor should not assume that the patient uses the same eccentric fixation and viewing strategies for distance as well as near visual tasks. In the absence of telescopic optical devices, when an individual with a central scotoma attempts to identify an object at distance, he or she may use a fixation point as close as possible to the anatomic fovea to enhance visual discrimination (Figure 3-15). The configuration of the scotoma is not as significant in this situation

because distance identification tasks are often visual spotting tasks in nature. During near-point activities that require reading, however, it becomes more important to use a parafoveal or paramacular region that is free of scotomatous defects and allows for as uncombed a visual field area as possible. This adaption enables the patient to maintain his or her place while reading much of the line of print unobscured by the scotoma. In this situation, the reader may use a point that is farther away from the anatomic fovea to reduce the areas in which the scotoma overlaps the reading material (Figure 3-16). The reduction in acuity resulting from the use of a point that is more eccentric to the fovea can be offset in young individuals with good accommodative amplitudes or in highly myopic individuals by reducing the reading distance, thereby increasing the amount of relative distance magnification. Clinically, it is not unusual to find low vision individuals who are highly myopic or who have early-onset vision loss manifest multiple eccentric fixation points. Due to the possibility of multiple eccentric fixation points, distance acuity should not be used to determine magnification needs for nearpoint acuities.

Individuals with central scotomas or metamorphopsia typically demonstrate better single-letter visual acuity than continuous text acuity. They may consistently omit letters at the beginning or end of lines. During testing, they may lose their place frequently and repeat lines already read. They also tend to demonstrate higher visual acuity when optotypes are isolated than when presented within a row of optotypes. This finding is consistent with studies that demonstrate more significant contour interaction effects in individuals with macular disorders.[4]

In cases of visual field constriction, resolution may actually appear to improve as optotypes decrease in size. In

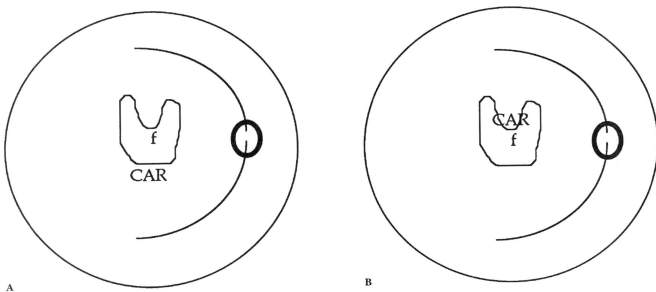

A   B

FIGURE 3-16.   **When reading a word (i.e., car) a patient may prefer to use an area of the retina that affords a wider field of view (no scotomatous area) with reduced resolution (A) than to have better visual acuity (closer to the fovea [*f*]) with some letters or words located in the irregularly shaped scotomatous area (B).**

such situations, optotypes in the 10/600 or 10/400 range may be too large for the remaining visual field area at a 10-ft testing distance, and the visually impaired individual may be unable to identify the optotype without scanning. As the optotypes decrease in size, they become visible in their entirety within the remaining visual field area, and visual acuity responses improve.

Individuals with hemianopic visual field defects typically omit the beginning or end of a line of optotypes. When the defect is a left homonymous hemianopsia, individuals also have a difficult time efficiently progressing to the next line. When the defect is a right homonymous hemianopsia, they may have difficulty determining when they have reached the end of the line. Similar difficulties are exhibited by individuals who, as a result of stroke or brain trauma, manifest a visual field neglect or inattention to a visual field hemisphere (see Chapter 17 for more information).

Measurement of Visual Acuities

When measuring the visual acuity of a patient with low vision, some doctors elect to follow conventional visual acuity measurement protocol and routinely test the right eye first. This strategy is attractive because it facilitates the flow of the examination and reduces confusion when recording visual acuity information. Others may prefer a strategy that considers the patient's reported visual status in determining which eye is tested first. Before visual acuity testing begins, the doctor asks the patient which is the better seeing eye. He or she then initially measures visual acuity in the poorer seeing eye to reduce any memorization of the chart. This sequence also provides the patient with a positive experience, as it emphasizes the increased amount of residual vision in the better seeing eye.

As with all visual acuity measurement procedures, both unaided and aided acuities should be recorded as well as monocular and binocular acuities. The following is a description of procedures for measurement of distance and near visual acuities.

Distance Visual Acuity Testing Procedure

1. Acuities should be tested until threshold is reached. Initial testing distance is typically 10 ft. If the patient cannot resolve the poorest acuity level, the chart is brought to 5 ft, 2 ft, and 1 ft. Progression of testing distances for the ETDRS chart is typically 4 m, 2 m, and 1 m. When testing at closer viewing distances the patient should be appropriately corrected for the accommodative demand induced by the viewing distance.

2. Notations for recording of visual acuity are as follows: NLP (no light perception), LP (light perception), L Proj (light projection), HM (hand motion), Snellen fraction (feet, meters, decimal, logMAR).

3. It is not acceptable to record acuities as finger counting (FC). It is frequently demoralizing to a patient to be asked to count fingers as opposed to identify optotypes on a chart. Many individuals interpret this as an indication that they are so severely visually impaired that they are unable to read a chart. The average adult male hand subtends roughly the same visual angle as the 20/200 optotype. It is frequently of much poorer contrast and is certainly not standardized. It is far more effective to bring an appropriate chart to the equivalent viewing distance and obtain a standardized and reproducible visual acuity.

4. The clock-dial technique is used to determine the optimal EV angle. The patient should be tested monocularly as well as binocularly. The patient is asked to view a threshold line of acuity. The patient is instructed to view

an optotype at the center of the line and to consider that optotype to be at the center of a clock dial. The patient is then asked to view the different positions on the clock dial surrounding that optotype to determine if an enhancement in resolution of the optotype is experienced.

5. If the patient has difficulty in shifting fixation, an alternative technique proposed by Paul Freeman may prove to be effective.[5] The chart is moved while the patient maintains fixation on a target that is straight ahead. The doctor records the deviation of the visual axis from the target in a similar manner to the recording of EV positions. For example, if the preferred chart position is above the line of sight, a 6 o'clock EV position is recorded because optimal viewing angle is below the visual target.

6. The doctor should isolate the optotypes to determine if resolution is enhanced. This may provide higher levels of acuity, as contour interaction is eliminated.

7. Measurement of acuities with a pinhole may reveal the presence of uncorrected refractive errors or significant media abnormalities. Significant field defects can interfere with the effectiveness of this procedure. In such situations, multiple pinholes may be effective.

8. Visual acuities should be recorded with the appropriate distance along with a description of charts and illumination levels used. EV positions should be recorded as well as any acuity changes elicited by isolation of optotypes. For example, 10/40 OS EV 6 o'clock; 10/30 0S EV 6 o'clock (letters isolated).

9. Acuities should be recorded at the test distance that was used for measurement. It is inaccurate to record a 10/30 visual acuity as 20/60. If it is necessary to equate visual acuity to a 20-ft distance for reporting purposes, acuities should be recorded as 20-ft-equivalent acuities. For example, 10/100 can be recorded as 20/200 equivalent (making sure to add the word "equivalent" after the visual acuity).

10. The doctor should record whether a patient consistently loses his or her place or omits sections of the chart. Such information is helpful in establishing strategies for instruction in the use of optical devices and for overall enhancement of visual skills.

11. Visual acuity should be measured with any telescopic device that the patient brings to the office. The type of telescope and its magnification should also be recorded. The telescope should also be examined to determine if any defects are present that would reduce visual acuity responses.

Near Visual Acuity Testing Procedure

1. Single-letter acuities should be evaluated until threshold is reached.

2. Continuous-text acuities should be evaluated until threshold is reached.

3. Eccentric fixation positions should be explored and recorded if present. The patient may have a different position of eccentric fixation for multiple-character reading tasks than for single-character visual identification tasks. This difference becomes most apparent in reading tasks that involve words and continuous-text print.

4. The clock-dial technique should be used to explore any optimal EV angle.

5. Isolation of letters and words through the use of a typoscope (Figure 3-17) should be demonstrated to determine if resolution is enhanced. The typoscope serves a dual purpose. In addition to isolating letters and words, thereby decreasing contour interaction, it also reduces background glare and enhances image quality.

6. Visual acuities should be recorded with any near magnification devices that the patient brings to the office. If several devices are used, acuities should be recorded for each device. A description of the magnifying devices, which includes equivalent power, design, and manufacturer, should also be recorded.

7. Visual acuities should be recorded during each of the preceding steps along with description of charts, illumination levels, and EV positions and how they were elicited. The doctor should also record whether the patient consistently lost his or her place or omitted sections of the chart. As in the case of distance acuities, such information is helpful in determining prescription and rehabilitative instruction strategies. Visual acuities are recorded at the test distance from the spectacle plane. For example, 1.5 M acuity measured at 10 in. (25 cm) should be recorded as 0.25/1.5 M.

Strategies vary for testing distances during near acuity testing. Some practitioners prefer to use a set testing distance, typically 25 or 40 cm, for all patients. Such conventional testing distances increase the likelihood that the accommodative demand can be met by the patient's habitual add or by accommodation. Testing at a set distance may be facilitated by attaching a cord of the determined length to the card. The cord may be used as a measuring device to establish that the card is being held at the appropriate distance. A 40-cm testing distance is also the distance at which the LHNV-1 near acuity chart lists the adds that are necessary to achieve a single-letter acuity of 1.0 M. For example, if a 0.40/2.0 M visual acuity is measured, the chart indicates that a +5.00 add improves single letter acuity to 1.0 M. This simplified approach to prescribing is attractive but also limiting, especially if target acuities differ from a 1.0-M single

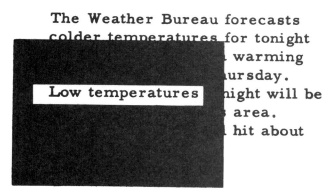

FIGURE 3-17. **A typoscope not only isolates letters and words but also reduces background glare.**

letter, which is frequently the case. As shown in Chapters 7 and 10, the calculations needed to determine magnification needs are easy to understand and execute.

Another strategy is to counsel the patient to bring the near-point visual acuity chart to a distance that provides maximum resolution. The practitioner should measure the distance and ensure that the image is in focus by adding more plus if the present add or accommodative reserves are insufficient. This approach accomplishes several objectives: It evaluates early in the examination process a patient's response to relative distance magnification and his or her tolerance to reduced focal distances. It can also prove to be a motivating factor for the patient as he or she responds to the relative distance magnification and reads smaller print material than he or she had previously thought possible.

Whatever strategy is used for near visual acuity testing, it is critical that the patient be properly corrected for the testing distance. A common error is recording visual acuities at distances that are impossible for a patient's accommodative system to clear. For example, recording an acuity of 0.08/2.5 M for a 75-year-old absolute presbyope with a habitual spectacle prescription of plano/+2.50 ignores the fact that this individual is incapable of producing +10.00 D of the required +12.50 D (8-cm focal distance) of accommodation. The doctor should always rule out uncorrected myopia in such situations. Once that has been ruled out, other factors should be considered. It is not unusual to encounter a low vision patient who habitually views visual targets at a closer distance than his or her accommodative reserves would allow. In such situations, the patient is sacrificing clarity to obtain relative distance magnification. Although miotic pupils may partially compensate for the reduced focal distance by increasing depth of field, the patient still experiences some residual blur. The induced blur reduces the potential improvement in visual acuity resulting from relative distance magnifica-

tion. Had the 75 year old been corrected for the 8-cm viewing distance with a +12.50 D add, the resultant acuities should have improved for the same testing distance. Accurate acuities are critical as they are the foundations on which all calculations for magnification devices are based.

During visual acuity testing, it is good practice to make family members or friends that are in the examination room aware of the visual acuity findings. They can provide valuable reinforcement to the patient that there is significant residual vision present. The patient can also receive confirmation from a trusted companion that there has been an actual improvement in visual acuity when low vision devices are evaluated. Throughout testing, the patient should be given immediate feedback on the results of testing. The amount of residual vision should be emphasized. This feedback helps to relieve anxiety and increase the patient's motivation in the rehabilitation process.

Refractive Procedures

A careful refraction is an essential component of a thorough low vision evaluation. In many cases, however, refractive status is only minimally explored because of the mistaken assumption that the reduced visual acuity is solely the result of ocular pathology. There is a further misconception that correcting refractive error in the presence of ocular pathology does not result in an improvement of visual acuity. Additionally, improvement in visual acuity to a level poorer than 20/200 (i.e., 10/200 to 10/160) may not be considered significant by the doctor. This belief stems from the perception that any acuity below 20/200 (legal blindness) falls within the category of severe visual impairment and therefore provides minimal useful visual information. Such improvement in visual acuity, however, is frequently appreciated by the low vision patient and can impact positively on overall visual functioning as well as on performance with optical devices. Correction of refractive error may be especially helpful for patients who have central scotomas with normal peripheral fields. Because peripheral vision is instrumental in EV as well as during mobility-related visual activities, it is extremely important for the retina to receive properly focused images.

For patients who have congenital disorders, such as albinism or retinopathy of prematurity, associated high refractive errors (Table 3-3) may never have been adequately evaluated. This is not unusual, especially in cases of nystagmus or media opacities, when typical refraction strategies are less effective. In most cases, if the possibility of a high refractive error is not thoroughly explored, it will not be discovered. Therefore, it is in the best interest of the patient that the doctor approach every examination as if the patient has at least 20.00 D of hyperopia or myopia with 8.00 D of astigmatism and then proceed to rule it out by refractive techniques.

Keratometry

Keratometry is of significant benefit in providing information about corneal toricity and integrity. Significant

TABLE 3-3
Refractive Errors Commonly Associated with Low Vision Disorders

Disorder	Refractive Error
Albinism	Moderate[a] to high hyperopia or myopia with moderate to high astigmatism with-the-rule
Cataracts	Myopic shift
Cerebral palsy	Moderate to high hyperopia
Corneal scarring	Moderate to high astigmatism
Degenerative myopia	High[b] myopia
Diabetes	Myopic shift with increase in sugar level
Down syndrome	Moderate to high myopia
Keratoconus	High irregular astigmatism
Microphthalmos	Moderate to high hyperopia
Monochromatism	High myopia; may have moderate with-the-rule astigmatism
Pendular (congenital) nystagmus	Moderate with-the-rule astigmatism
Retinopathy of prematurity	High myopia

[a]Moderate: 3–6 D of myopia; 3–5 D of hyperopia; 2.5–4.0 D of astigmatism.
[b]High: >6 D of myopia; >5 D of hyperopia; >4 D of astigmatism.

amounts of corneal toricity are frequently present in low vision conditions such as albinism, keratoconus, aniridia, and congenital pendular nystagmus. Individuals who have undergone cataract extraction may also have a higher incidence of corneal toricity as a result of surgery.

Procedures for performing keratometry on low vision patients are identical to those for normally sighted individuals. Nystagmus does, however, require the doctor to vary the procedure slightly. Individuals with nystagmus often manifest a position in which the nystagmus may be dampened or, if a null point is present, totally eliminated. Convergence frequently dampens pendular nystagmus. The doctor should attempt to elicit a viewing posture that reduces or eliminates the nystagmoid eye movements. The doctor should also determine if a latent nystagmus component is present, in which the nystagmus increases in frequency or amplitude with occlusion of the other eye. In such cases, keratometry should be performed without occlusion. If some movement of the eyes is present during testing, the doctor can still obtain an approximation of the cylinder amount by aligning the mires as closely as possible. If the nystagmus has a rotary component, the cylinder axis varies with the rotation of the eye, necessitating estimation of the cylinder axis. The key objective is to uncover significant amounts of cylinder and to determine the approximate amount and axis. Refinement of the final prescription occurs during the subjective refraction.

Retinoscopy
A phoropter is generally not used when evaluating the low vision patient. Instead, a trial frame or spectacle trial lens clips (Halberg, Janelli) and lenses are used for the following reasons:

1. These instruments provide more of a habitual situation for the patient than do the phoropter. The larger lens aperture enables the patient to assume a habitual eccentric fixation position in cases of central scotomas.
2. Use of these instruments enables the doctor to more easily observe the patient's head and eye turns. In cases in which pendular nystagmus is present, the larger lens aperture enables the doctor to visualize the reflex throughout the entire extent of the nystagmoid eye movements.
3. These instruments allow for comparison of lenses more easily and quickly. For example, the doctor is able to compare +10.00 D to −10.00 D with ease and speed.
4. These instruments allow for a more stable and normal vertex distance. The doctor is able to achieve a closer vertex distance than with the phoropter, an important consideration when evaluating high refractive errors.
5. With these instruments, the doctor can incorporate other lenses into the prescription that would not be available if a phoropter is used. Examples might include tinted trial lenses, high-powered doublet microscopes, and telescopes.

When the testing distance during objective refraction is closer than 20 ft, the accommodative stimulus should be considered in determining the objective refractive error. The acuity target used should be larger than the measured

visual acuity threshold. A large aperture lens rack used in conjunction with a trial frame may be very helpful in reducing retinoscopy time.

When an overrefraction is performed with a Halberg clip and trial lenses and a change in cylinder axis is found, the total dioptric power of the habitual spectacle–trial lens combination can be easily determined. The resultant back vertex power is measured by placing the spectacles lenses, combined with the trial lenses, in a lensometer, and a new sphere, cylinder, and axis result.

In situations in which a reflex cannot be visualized at the habitual retinoscopy distance due to medial opacities, radical retinoscopy can be performed.[6] With this procedure, the doctor may need to use a different retinoscopy angle as well as significantly reduce the working distance. As with all standard retinoscopic procedures, the working distance must be factored into the final prescription. When performing radical retinoscopy, the doctor should keep in mind that the speed and brightness of the reflex are a function of the closeness to neutralization. As neutrality is approached, the brightness of the reflex should increase as should the speed of the retinoscopic reflex. One must keep in mind, however, that the closer one is to the eye, the shorter the range of neutrality and the greater the chance of miscalculation of neutrality.

When performing off-axis radical retinoscopy, it is also important to keep in mind that cylinder power and axis may change. It is therefore important to follow up the objective refraction with a careful subjective refraction. When patients demonstrate a significant eccentric fixation point due to the presence of macular defects, off-axis refractive findings may actually be prescribed. Frequently, however, the doctor finds that the prescription found during radical retinoscopy is modified during the subjective refraction.

Retinoscopy may be repeated after dilation if significant nuclear lens changes prevent the visualization of the retinoscopic reflex. Either a spot or streak retinoscope may be used, depending on the doctor's preference. The streak retinoscope facilitates the determination of the major meridian of astigmatism, whereas the spot retinoscope may be more useful in determining the refractive error in cases of medial opacities.[7]

Subjective Refraction
As mentioned in the preceding section, the subjective refraction should be performed with a trial frame. The chart is typically located 10 ft away from the patient. Providing relative distance magnification by placing the acuity chart at 10 ft may enhance the patient's sensitivity to dioptric lens changes during the refraction. If the chart is placed at a distance closer than 20 ft, it is necessary to factor the accommodative stimulus into the final refractive findings. Illumination of the chart is very important and may impact significantly on results of testing. Therefore, the entire chart should have equal illumination. The chart should also be placed perpendicular to the patient and not propped up against a wall. This positioning reduces glare and minimizes differences in testing distances as the patient reads each line on the chart. When possible, a rheostat on the light source should be used to obtain the

illumination that the patient subjectively prefers. The starting point for the subjective refraction is the keratometry and objective refraction findings. When objective retinoscopy or keratometry is not possible, a habitual spectacle prescription that improves the patient's visual acuity may be used as the starting point.

If objective refractive information does not appear to be reliable, then assume each patient has severe myopia or hyperopia with a significant cylindrical component. Determination of the refractive error may be accomplished by the bracketing technique, in which plus and minus lenses of equal powers are compared until a favorable response is elicited. This technique can also be used with cylinder lenses, comparing one cylinder lens at the four major meridians to another cylinder lens and so on. A handheld cross cylinder may also be used to refine the final cylinder and axis. In cases of significant acuity loss (worse than 20/200), a ±1.00 D cross cylinder should be used because these patients are typically not sensitive to a lower-power cross cylinder. With visual acuities higher than 20/200, ±0.75 D, and ±0.50 D cross cylinders may enable further refinement of cylinder axis and power.

To determine the strength of the power changes in the preceding bracketing technique, a simple concept of just noticeable difference (JND) is used.[8] JND helps the doctor determine the interval between the two lenses that are being compared and is based on the patient's best visual acuity at 10 ft. To calculate the dioptric interval of JND, the denominator of the acuity at 10 ft is divided by 100. For example, if the patient's best acuity is 10/200, then lens changes of 2.00 D would be presented (200/100 = ±2.00 D). The patient would have difficulty responding to smaller dioptric changes at that acuity level. If during the subjective evaluation visual acuity improves, JND must be modified to reflect the improvement in acuity. For example, if the preceding individual's acuity improved from 10/200 to 10/120, the JND lenses are modified to ±1.25 D.

The subjective refraction is a slow process, and it is important for the doctor to proceed at a level at which the patient can respond with accuracy. It is also important to provide reassurance and encouragement when needed. If the patient appears to tire or lose interest in responding, a short rest is recommended. The doctor should continue to impress on the patient how important these results are and how an accurate prescription enhances the effectiveness of low vision optical devices.

Telescopic Subjective Refraction

A telescopic subjective refraction is a means of subjectively refining the sphere, cylinder, and axis by having a patient view a distance chart through a low-powered telescope. This technique is most useful when determining whether to incorporate a refractive error correction into a telescope of a spectacle-mounted telescopic system. It may also be used by some practitioners to refine a spectacle correction, because the introduction of magnification may increase the patient's sensitivity to changes in dioptric power.

Many low vision practitioners elect not to perform a telescopic subjective refraction because of the reduced field, vergence amplification,[9] and reduced illumination of a telescopic system. They prefer to reduce the viewing distance of the chart by a factor of two (i.e., 20 ft to 10 ft, or 10 ft to 5 ft), thereby achieving the same magnification objective. When it is not possible to change the viewing distance, the following telescopic subjective technique may be used:

1. The patient is asked to view a chart at a distance of 20 ft and to read the optotypes at his or her acuity threshold.
2. A 2.2× full-diameter afocal telescope is placed in the front cell of the trial frame.
3. A subjective refraction is performed behind the ocular of the telescope with both spheres and cylinders being evaluated. It is essential that lenses be introduced behind the telescopic ocular lens to eliminate lens-induced vergence amplification that would occur if the lens was placed in front of the telescopic objective lens.
4. When testing at 20 ft with a 2.2× afocal telescope, the practitioner must introduce approximately –0.75 D into the findings. This factors out the +0.75 D needed to compensate for telescopic vergence amplification of the divergence created by the 20-ft viewing distance. If testing occurs at 10 ft with the same telescope, approximately –1.50 D should be incorporated into the findings. Vergence amplification is further discussed in Chapter 9.

Stenopaic Slit

The stenopaic slit is used to help determine the cylindrical component of the refractive error. It can also be useful in determining the total refractive error of the patient. This technique can be very useful for patients who may have large amounts of astigmatism or irregular astigmatism. It can also be useful in patients who have a poor or nonexistent retinal reflex when performing retinoscopy (i.e., cloudy media, corneal distortion, miotic pupils). It should be noted that the patient's choice of the slit position may not always identify the axis of astigmatic correction. In some patients, it may represent an area of unobstructed vision. It should be clearly understood that the stenopaic slit is helpful only as a guide to the subjective refraction. Retinoscopy, if it can be performed, is the preferred procedure due to the reduced time needed to perform the procedure and the greater accuracy of the objective data.

The following are the steps for performing a stenopaic refraction:

1. The stenopaic slit is placed in a trial frame and the untested eye is occluded. The patient fixates on a distance chart (a letter or number that is at the threshold of acuity) with best spherical correction in place.
2. The slit is rotated until the patient reports that the target is clearest. This is recorded as "position 1." If the patient claims that there is no optimal position, there are several possibilities:
   a. No astigmatism is present.
   b. The astigmatic interval is equally mixed (equally spaced around the circle of least confusion).
   c. The patient is incapable of recognizing changes in image quality.

To test the possible existence of any of the preceding, a ±2.00 D sphere is placed behind the slit and the slit is again rotated. If the patient still cannot determine a difference, the optimal spherical correction determined previously by bracketing is prescribed.

3. When the patient identifies a position of optimal image quality (position 1), plus and minus lenses are added (bracketing technique) until optimal acuity is achieved. The total spherical power in position 1 is the corrective sphere of the prescription.
4. Rotate the slit again 90 degrees from position 1 to position 2.
5. Add plus or minus spheres to obtain the best visual acuity. This additional sphere is the cylindrical power that must be added to the corrective sphere of step 3. The resultant cylinder is plus if the added sphere is plus and minus if the added sphere is minus. The corrective lens cylinder axis is parallel to the slit in position 1. An optical cross may be set up with the two sphere powers from position 1 and position 2 to determine the tentative prescription.

Binocularity

Binocularity at distance and near should not be overlooked when evaluating the low vision patient. Most low vision patients lack the highest form of binocularity: depth perception by parallax or stereopsis. Some, however, may demonstrate gross stereopsis. Other patients may exhibit "biocular vision"—that is, alternating vision while suppressing the fellow eye.

When two dissimilar images are presented by the two eyes and neither one is suppressed, then *retinal rivalry* exists. This retinal rivalry tends to exist with those patients who have experienced recent macular changes in one eye and attempt to use both eyes together, especially when reading. The patient generally complains about words running together or that the print appears blurry even when the print is at the exact focal point of the patient's low vision system. When this occurs, it is best to occlude one eye for that particular task.

Many low vision patients who lack binocularity, and therefore stereopsis, may still appreciate depth perception. They may use monocular cues present in the visual environment. Some examples of these cues are the following:

1. Objects that appear larger are assumed to be closer.
2. If one object appears to be hiding parts of another, then the object that is partially hidden would appear to be farther away.
3. Objects that appear to be clear or more distinct are assumed to be closer.
4. Objects that appear to be brighter are often reported to be closer.
5. Near objects appear to move opposite to head movement whereas distant objects appear to move in the same direction (monocular parallax).

For those patients who have acuities that differ no more than a factor of 1.5 (i.e., 20/40 OD and 20/60 OS),

investigation of binocularity is important. There are certain advantages to allowing the patient to be binocular when possible. Some advantages are as follows:

1. It is frequently important psychologically for patients to use both eyes.
2. Visual acuity may be better in a binocular state.
3. Visual fields are larger when binocular. Binocularity may allow the visual system to compensate for scotomatous areas by the overlap of nonscotomatous regions from the companion eye.
4. Contrast sensitivity may be enhanced in a binocular state.
5. Depth perception is generally enhanced when in a binocular state. Stereopsis is only possible in a binocular state.
6. Prescribing binocular optical devices in cases in which there is a potential for some level of binocular vision provides better assurance that the eyes maintain alignment.

A number of techniques may be used to determine if binocularity exists in the low vision patient. The practitioner should evaluate both motor binocularity as well as sensory binocularity. Ocular alignment may be evaluated through motor binocularity testing (cover test, Hirschberg's test, vergence testing). Central scotomas and nystagmus, however, may interfere with the interpretation of these tests. Once it has been determined that motor alignment is present, sensory binocularity testing should follow.

Sensory Binocularity Testing

A number of tests are available for sensory binocularity testing of the patient with low vision, including

1. *Worth's four-dot test:* This test can be performed at any distance from the patient. The patient should be tested with the best correction for the testing distance. The test is performed under ordinary room illumination. The patient is asked to view through a red-green filter and is asked to look at a light source with four circles (two green circles, one red circle, and one white circle). If the patient reports four light circles, he or she is demonstrating some form of gross fusion. A jumbo Worth's four-dot test is available for testing low vision patients at an increased distance.

2. *Red-filter and Maddox's rod test:* These tests can be performed at any distance from the patient. A red filter is placed before the nondominant or poorer-acuity eye and the patient is asked to view a muscle light with both eyes. The best correction is in place for the given testing distance. If the patient reports a pink streak, there is suggestion of binocularity.

3. *Prism test:* This test may be performed at any distance under standard room illumination. The patient views through corrective lenses for the testing distance. A prism (approximately 4 prism diopters) is placed before one eye and rotated while viewing a visual target. If the patient reports diplopia, the patient demonstrates some form of

binocularity. The significant exception to this is individuals with central scotomas. In such situations, the prism may shift the image out of the scotomatous area and induce diplopia even though in a normal state it would fall within the scotoma, thereby preventing binocularity.

4. *Stereopsis testing:* This testing is performed at near under high levels of glare-free illumination. The appropriate near-point lenses are worn along with Polaroid three-dimensional vectographic lenses. Line or contour stereo tests, such as the Stereo Fly test or Reindeer test, can test ranges to approximately 2,000 seconds of arc. If the patient reports that the fly or reindeer is protruding from the page, then gross stereopsis is present. If that response is present, then testing can continue for finer levels of stereopsis using the animals or Wirt's circles. Random dot stereopsis testing tends to be more difficult for low vision patients with central acuity loss resulting from macular pathology, hypoplasia, or nystagmus. Typically, patients with low vision are not capable of achieving fine stereopsis because macular integrity is essential for the existence of fine stereopsis.

Visual Fields

Visual field testing is frequently not performed by practitioners who see the low vision evaluation as being driven primarily by a patient's visual acuity status. It is not unusual, however, for central and peripheral visual field status to be the critical factor in determination of magnification, minification, and prismatic needs as well as the development of an appropriate rehabilitative program.

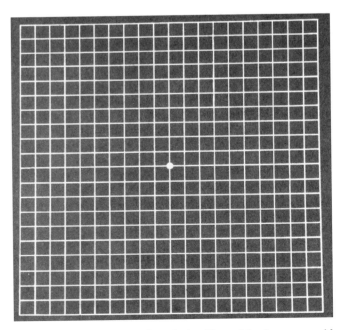

FIGURE 3-18. **The standard Amsler's grid consists of a square grid of white horizontal and vertical lines.**

There are three visual field regions that are typically tested during a low vision evaluation: (1) the central 10-degree radius as tested by the Amsler's grid, (2) the central 25-degree radius typically tested by tangent screen campimetry, and (3) the peripheral field typically tested by arc or bowl perimetry. Automated field testing, which includes mapping out threshold levels, is typically less reliable in cases of significant central scotomas and nystagmus unless a fixation stabilization mechanism is included. Use of a scanning laser ophthalmoscope (microperimetry) provides the most accurate method for monitoring fixation during testing (see Chapter 5 for microperimetry testing).

Amsler's Grid Testing

Amsler's grid testing can provide useful information in cases of metamorphopsia and small (<5-degree radius) central scotomas. It is not useful in cases of hemianopic defects as it cannot establish that the defect extends beyond a 10-degree radius. It is also not useful in cases in which central scotoma size (>5-degree radius) occupies a significant portion of the grid. In such cases, an individual tends to eccentrically fixate to view more of the grid because a majority of the grid's area is obliterated by the scotoma. This individual frequently reports either that there are no defects in the grid (the scotoma has been displaced outside of the grid area) or that the area of the defect is at the border of the grid whereas the central area is free of defects. Although this may provide information on the habitual eccentric fixation patterns of the patient, it does not enable the practitioner to determine the size and configuration of the scotoma. In some cases, such results may lead the practitioner to erroneously conclude that there is no central involvement or to misjudge the size and location of the scotoma or area of metamorphopsia.

The testing distance is 13 in. from the spectacle plane and is typically performed monocularly. Binocular testing, however, may provide useful information when deciding whether to prescribe a device for near to a patient with central scotomas or metamorphopsia. The standard chart consists of a square grid of white horizontal and vertical lines, each 0.5 mm apart (Figure 3-18). Presbyopic patients should be looking through an appropriate add. The patient is asked to fixate on a central dot and to report if all the corners are visible and if any areas of the grid are distorted, faint, discolored, or missing. For individuals who cannot view the central dot due to a central scotoma, a grid is available with intersecting lines crossing at the center (Figure 3-19). The patient is asked to view where he or she thinks the lines intersect, even if the center is not visible. The patient is then asked to describe the area of involvement. A 1-mm visual target may be used to outline the area of involvement if a patient has a difficult time in describing the configuration of the macular defect.[10]

Tangent Screen Testing

Tangent screen testing is useful during the low vision evaluation for determining the size and location of larger scotomas. It can also be useful in determining the habitual EV point of an individual with a central scotoma. The techniques vary depending on the practitioner's objectives for the test.

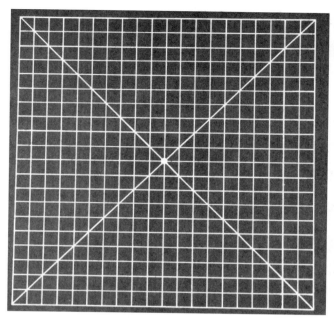

FIGURE 3-19. **When patients have difficulty viewing the central fixation target of an Amsler's grid, intersecting lines forming a cross at the central fixation target should be used to help maintain the patient's fixation.**

FIGURE 3-20. **When patients have difficulty viewing the central fixation target of a tangent screen, intersecting lines forming a cross at the central fixation target should be used to help maintain the patient's fixation.**

Unlike Amsler's grid testing, tangent screen testing enables the doctor to vary target sizes during testing as well as to more precisely explore the configuration of the scotoma.

Testing distance is typically 1 m but may be varied to magnify a defect. As in Amsler's grid testing, tangent screen testing is initially performed monocularly with the patient instructed to view a central fixation dot. The doctor then explores the visual field region with a number of targets typically beginning with a 3-mm white target unless visual acuity reductions necessitate the use of a larger target. In the latter situation, the practitioner uses the smallest target that the patient can see. If the patient cannot see the center fixation dot due to the presence of a central scotoma, two lines of opaque white tape that cross at the fixation dot may be used (Figure 3-20).[11] If the diagnosis indicates the possible presence of a central scotoma, it is important that the doctor instruct the patient on appropriate fixation strategies. The patient should not be instructed to look directly at the intersection point, as that may be interpreted by the patient as a need to eccentrically view so that the intersection is not obscured or distorted by the central scotoma. Instead, the patient should be instructed to fixate "straight ahead" at a point where he or she thinks the two lines cross, even if that region is obscured or distorted. The doctor can then explore the visual field area using standard campimetry procedures.

If the practitioner wishes to explore the patient's EV posture, however, a different technique is needed. In such cases, a visual target, such as a letter that is at the threshold of the patient's visual acuity at 1 m, is placed at the center of the screen (Figure 3-21). The patient is then asked to identify the letter and then maintain fixation on

the letter. These instructions encourage the patient with a central scotoma to eccentrically view to optimally discriminate the visual target. The practitioner then begins to explore the location and configuration of any scotoma or scotomas with the testing targets. The practitioner can use this technique to elicit the patient's initial EV point and chart a patient's progress in maintaining an optimal EV position throughout the rehabilitative process. This technique can also be used to educate the patient on the benefits of EV by providing visible evidence of increased resolution when the appropriate EV angle is achieved.

Arc Perimetry Testing

Arc perimetry testing can provide a quick estimation of the extent of peripheral field constriction. With this test, the practitioner can evaluate all meridians but typically only the 45-, 90-, 135-, and 180-degree meridians are evaluated. As in other field tests previously described, an X pattern may be placed on the fixation dot to facilitate central fixation by an individual with a central scotoma (Figure 3-22). The extent of the visual field is mapped by the doctor moving a wand along the curve of the arc toward the fixation dot until the patient reports seeing the target. This technique enables the doctor to present a target size appropriate for each patient's visual capabilities. As in previous field tests, the initial target presented should be the smallest target that is visible to the patient.

Bowl Perimetry Testing

Bowl perimetry is an excellent tool for obtaining peripheral field information for the widest range of low vision

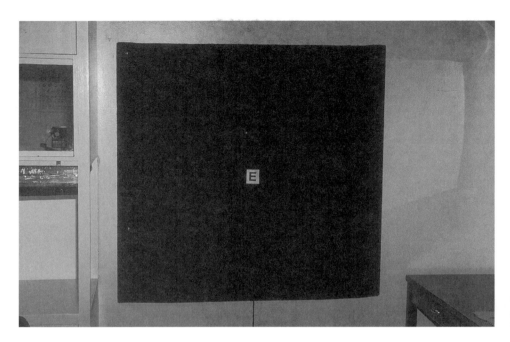

FIGURE 3-21. **A different technique used in maintaining fixation by a patient with poor fixation is placing a visual target that is at the threshold of a patient's visual acuity at the center of the tangent screen.**

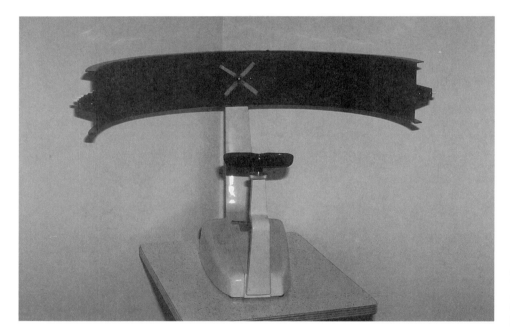

FIGURE 3-22. **When patients have difficulty viewing the central fixation target of an arc perimeter, intersecting lines forming a cross at the central fixation target should be used to help the patient's fixation.**

conditions and visual levels. It enables the practitioner to explore the extent of peripheral field constriction using targets that can be varied in terms of their size, intensity, speed, and degrees of eccentricity. Again, an X target may be used to facilitate central fixation during testing. Steadiness of fixation can be evaluated by viewing through the observation telescope during testing. The doctor should not habitually present only large targets to low vision patients with central scotomas due to the assumption that they would only respond to larger targets. The target size may be determined by the presentation of targets of ascend-

ing sizes at an approximate eccentricity of 15 degrees while the patient views the central fixation target. Therefore, the smallest target that the patient is able to detect, at 15 degrees from the fixation target, is used as the initial testing target.

Functional Field Testing

In cases of significant field constriction or with patients who are not testable with the previously mentioned fields, functional field testing may provide valuable information. Chapter 17 provides a discussion of various functional field testing procedures that may be helpful for the previously mentioned cases.

OCULAR HEALTH EVALUATION

An ocular health evaluation is an integral component of a comprehensive low vision evaluation. It is critical to assess the ocular health status to determine the nature, extent, and stability of the ocular pathology or disorder. This information guides the practitioner in designing appropriate management strategies.

Evaluation of external ocular health indicates the presence of any structural or functional abnormality that would interfere with the use of optical devices. Conditions, such as ptosis, restrictions in eye movements, corneal opacification, or pupillary distortion, may indicate a need for specialized modifications, such as ptosis crutches, reduced aperture contact lenses, or prism systems, to compensate for these defects.

The doctor should note the presence of nystagmus as well as any null points or areas where the nystagmus is dampened. This information may be very helpful in instructing the patient on proper positioning of visual targets. For example, an individual who has a null point on down-gaze may benefit from positioning reading material in his lower field. Latent nystagmus (nystagmus that is present or worsens when an individual is patched) alerts the doctor not to use monocular occlusion when designing a spectacle-mounted telescope or microscope. End-point nystagmus may reduce the effectiveness of Fresnel prism systems used to enhance peripheral field awareness in patients with peripheral field defects.

Tonometry should be performed at each visit in patients who present with a diagnosis of glaucoma. Significant variations in intraocular pressure may indicate that the individual is not compliant with the prescribed medication regimen or that the regimen is not adequately controlling the intraocular pressure. In either case, the information should be given to the managing primary care practitioner or glaucoma specialist so that the problem may be addressed.

Fundus evaluation should be performed to obtain a baseline on retinal status. The low vision practitioner frequently encounters patients with active retinal pathology. Conditions, such as ARMD and proliferative diabetic retinopathy, may change at any time and necessitate close monitoring. A fundus evaluation may also alert the doctor to the possibility of an alternative diagnosis. Although most individuals present with the correct diagnosis, it is not unusual for an individual with ocular albinism to present only with a diagnosis of congenital nystagmus. Other commonly undiagnosed or misdiagnosed retinal conditions include rod monochromatism, cone dystrophy, cone rod dystrophy, and Leber's amaurosis. Color vision testing, exploration of family history, and electrodiagnostic testing can help to determine the nature of the ocular disorder. If any changes are noted during the ocular health evaluation, the patient should be referred back to the primary care practitioner or ocular disease specialist for evaluation and management before further low vision services are provided.

Acknowledgments
We would like to thank Susan Parthosarathy for her help in writing the section on the sighted guide technique. The authors would also like to acknowledge Dr. Stephen Whittaker's input on adopting tangent screen testing procedures to evaluate eccentric fixation in individuals with central scotomas.

SELF-ASSESSMENT QUESTIONS

1. The sighted guide technique involves the use of an opaque slotted card used as a guide while reading.
   True or False

2. Four-point print is equal to 0.5-M print.
   True or False

3. For reporting purposes, 10/100 acuity should be reported as 20/200.
   True or False

4. Visual field abnormalities can have a significant effect on response to visual acuity testing procedures.
   True or False

5. Just noticeable difference for a visual acuity of 20/400 is ±2.00 D.
   True or False

6. The Snellen equivalent of a 2.0-M letter read at 40 cm is 20/100.
   True or False

7. When performing a telescopic subjective, the trial lenses are compared in front of the telescopic objective lens.
   True or False

8. A patient with ARMD and best-corrected visual acuity of 10/100 reports no metamorphopsia or scotomas on Amsler's grid testing. These findings rule out the possibility of a central scotoma.
   True or False

9. Individuals with rod monochromatism typically demonstrate higher levels of visual acuity under dimmer testing conditions.
   True or False

10. Visual acuity level is not the most accurate prognostic indicator of successful rehabilitation.
    True or False

REFERENCES

1. Ferris L, Kassoff A, Bresnick GH, Bailey IL. New visual acuity charts for research purposes. Am J Ophthalmol 1982;94:91–96.
2. Sloan LL. New test charts for the measurement of visual acuity at far and near distances. Am J Ophthalmol 1959;48:807–813.

3. Jose R, Atcherson R. Standardization of near point acuity tests. Am J Optom Physiol Optics 1977;54:634–638.
4. Lovie-Kitchen JE, Bowman KJ. Senile Macular Degeneration. Boston: Butterworth, 1985.
5. Freeman P, Jose RT. The Art and Practice of Low Vision (2nd ed). Boston: Butterworth–Heinemann, 1997.
6. Mehr E, Fried A. Low Vision Care. Chicago: Professional Press, 1975.
7. Bailey IL. The Optometric Examination of the Elderly Patient. In AA Rosenbloom, MW Morgan (eds), Vision and Aging. Boston: Butterworth–Heinemann, 1993
8. Rosenthal BP. The Structured Low Vision Evaluation. In BP Rosenthal, RG Cole (eds), Problems in Optometry. A Structured Approach to Low Vision Care (Vol 3). Hagerstown, MD: Lippincott, 1991.
9. Bailey IL. Refracting Low Vision Patients. Optom Monthly 1978; 69:131–135.
10. Faye EE. Evaluating Near Vision: The Amsler Grid and Field Defects. In EE Faye (ed), Clinical Low Vision. Boston: Little, Brown, 1984.
11. Bailey IL. Visual Field Measurement in Low Vision. Optom Monthly 1978;60:84–88.

CHAPTER FOUR

Specialized Testing in Low Vision

Roger W. Cummings,
Bruce G. Muchnick,
and Stephen G. Whittaker

Low vision patients have serious visual problems that have caused their vision loss. In many instances, the underlying cause of the vision loss is not easily determined. In these circumstances, electrodiagnostic and psychophysical tests may provide invaluable information concerning the diagnosis. In other cases, the doctor may want to provide prognostic information for problems, such as the potential for cataract surgery in patients with both age-related maculopathy and cataracts or in patients who are multiply impaired. Color vision testing may be very important in low vision patients to determine the presence of monochromatism or to aid in the diagnosis of specific cone degenerations.

In many visually impaired patients, the standard ways of predicting magnification through the use of low vision charts using single letters or continuous text result in successfully choosing a device that is acceptable to the patient. In a number of cases, however, even with the predicted magnification, a patient is unable to achieve his or her goals. When this happens, the doctor should routinely test the patient's contrast sensitivity (CS) and visual fields. These tests, along with the patient's visual acuity, produce a variety of information that effectively describe a patient's visual function.

This chapter describes tests that are performed when there are unanswered questions at the conclusion of the initial low vision evaluation. These tests may measure the psychophysical, sensory, electrical, or structural aspects of the patient's visual system. There is a progression of complexity of these tests. Some are performed when a patient cannot achieve an expected level of function, whereas others are used only when a specific diagnosis is being considered.

CONTRAST SENSITIVITY TESTING

Assessment of CS should be performed routinely when the patient's performance does not match the expected results. For example, when a patient reports that he or she is having greater difficulty seeing in the rain and fog and measurement of visual acuity remains consistent from visit to visit, loss of CS should be suspected. A similar problem may be found when a low vision patient reports that he or she is no longer able to read the newspaper with his or her present microscope. Assuming that a number of factors (e.g., correct focal point maintained, lighting remains the same, microscopic lens not scratched or dirty) and the visual acuity have remained unchanged, a reduction in the patient's CS should be evaluated.

A reduction in CS provides information to the practitioner that a patient may benefit from one or more of the following:

- A lighting evaluation (along with elimination of any glare)
- Environmental modifications to help a patient with activities of daily living
- Orientation and mobility services
- The use of a closed-circuit television (CCTV) or computer display to enhance contrast of letters when reading
- A typoscope to reduce glare and contour interaction (crowding phenomenon)

- Filters to reduce glare and enhance contrast
- Greater magnification than initially predicted for low vision devices

Significant loss of CS is common among low vision patients. Advanced diabetic retinopathy and glaucoma are strongly associated with significantly reduced CS, and maculopathies often, but not always, result in significant loss in CS. Assessment of CS is no longer a "specialized test" requiring a separate visit and lengthy testing with sophisticated technology. Using letter charts, a doctor can measure CS as quickly and reliably as he or she measures visual acuity. An important question is how to interpret the results of CS testing. Although clinical research has not been completed, various experimental studies and clinical experience have provided the guidelines that are presented.

Terms and Concepts

A common measure of contrast is known as *Weber contrast*, calculated as the difference between the luminance of an object and its background divided by the brighter of the two. For example, if the object is dark on a light background, contrast is the difference between the luminance of the object and the luminance of the background divided by the background luminance. Contrast varies from 0% (no contrast) to 100% (the highest contrast). The highest quality print has 85–95% contrast. U.S. paper currency is printed with 55–60% contrast. A gray car approaching an intersection on a shaded street has approximately 30% contrast, whereas a dark car on a sunny street has approximately 80% contrast. See Tables 4-1 and 4-2 for the contrast of text and common objects.

Contrast threshold (CT) is defined as an object with the lowest contrast that a patient can recognize. *CS* is the complement (reciprocal) of CT and is usually expressed as a logarithm of $1/CT$, where CT is expressed as a percentage. As vision improves, CS increases and CT decreases. Both terms, *CT* and *CS*, are used clinically.

CT depends on the size of objects. As stimulus size approaches acuity threshold, CT increases until the maximum CT approaches 100% (CS = 2.0). When stimulus

TABLE 4-1
Contrast of Common Reading Materials

Weber Contrast (%)	Object
55–60	U.S. currency
71–75	Daily newspapers
76–80	Paperback books
81–85	Large-print newspapers
86–90	Large-print paperback books, large-print *Reader's Digest*, xerography telephone books (yellow and white pages)
88–93	Glossy periodicals, xerography high-contrast quality hardcover print

TABLE 4-2
Contrast of Common Objects

Object	Contrast (%)
Maroon chair on maroon carpet	5
Maroon chair, light gray carpet	74
Wood door, light wall	64
Red exit sign (back illuminated)	80
Black automobile on sunny street	82
Gray automobile on shady street	32

size is at acuity threshold, one needs the highest contrast (100%) to identify letters. When letters are enlarged to approximately 10× acuity threshold (a 20/200 or 4/40 letter), a normally sighted patient is able to recognize a letter of only 2–3% contrast. For this reason, the size of the stimulus letters on the contrast chart and a person's best visual acuity must be specified along with the measured CT.

Functional Effects of Reduced Contrast Sensitivity

Normal CTs for regular-size (12-point) print or objects, such as chairs at approximately 10 ft (3 m) and cars at approximately 30 ft (10 m), would be approximately 1–3% (CS = 0–0.5), well below the contrast of nearly all of the objects described in Tables 4-1 and 4-2. Because print and most objects in the environment are well above normal CT, a low vision patient's CS, although abnormally low, may still not be low enough to create functional problems. The practitioner, in many cases, may need to decide when CS is low enough to cause functional difficulties for the patient. To make such a decision, the doctor must conduct a careful interview to identify what objects the patient is trying to read or recognize.

The effects of poor CS are obvious in cases in which objects are below the patient's CT: Patients cannot recognize them. Even if objects are above CT, reduced CS will slow the speed with which patients detect obstacles or recognize faces and words. A patient with CT of approximately 4–5% print contrast will be able to read a newspaper (print contrast of approximately 75%) because the print is 15 times CT. Further reductions in print contrast or poor lighting, however, will significantly reduce reading rate (and probably comfort). Even the poorest quality newsprint is well above (20–40 times) normal CTs. Thus, variations in lighting and print contrast have little effect on reading rate in normally sighted individuals. These factors, however, will have significant effects on the reading rates of visually impaired patients with reduced CS.

The ratio of contrast of an object to the CT is referred to as *contrast reserve*. Normal contrast reserves for regular print have print contrast–to-CT ratios ranging from 20 to 1 to greater than 40 to 1. A patient with a 5% CT would read 75% contrast newsprint with approximately 15 to 1 contrast reserves. Contrast reserves below 20 to 1 slow recognition reaction time somewhat, but below 10 to 1 the effects

become very obvious. Contrast reserves less than 3 to 1 result in significant reductions in recognition accuracy.

Contrast Sensitivity Assessment

CT is most easily measured using a letter contrast chart with letters of the same size but decreasing contrast. As the patient reads down the chart, the CT is determined by the last line in which characters can be recognized. Two contrast charts that use letters are presently available: a distance chart developed by Pelli and Robson (Pelli-Robson Contrast Sensitivity Chart, Clement Clark, Dayton, OH) and the LEA Vision Screening Card (Precision Vision, Villa Park, IL) developed by Lea Hyvarinen. The Pelli-Robson chart has more lines and is better suited for research application, whereas the LEA Vision Screening Card is easier to use when office space is limited.

Before CT is measured, the distance of the chart must be set so that the letters on the chart are the same angular size as the optotype that the patient is capable of recognizing. To ensure adequate acuity reserve, the chart distance should be set so that the letters are twice the acuity threshold. The chart distance, D (in m), is set by the following formula:

$$D = Scc(Dat/Sat)/2$$

where Scc is the size of the contrast chart letters in meter system (M) units (34 M for the Pelli-Robson chart; 9.5 M and 3 M for the LEA Vision Screening Card), and Dat/Sat is the acuity ratio. Table 4-3 lists the appropriate test distance for each chart based on the patient's visual acuity and the preceding formula. Table 4-4 lists the CTs for each line of the Pelli-Robson chart. CT is supplied with the LEA Vision Screening Card. Illumination of the chart must be uniform and consistent at all distances. The illumination

TABLE 4-3
Test Distance (m) of Contrast Charts to Achieve 2× Acuity Threshold[a]

Visual Acuity (ft)	Visual Acuity (m)	Pelli-Robson 34-M Chart[b]	LEA Vision Screening Card 9.5-M Chart[c]	LEA Vision Screening Card 3-M Chart[c]
20/600	6/190	0.56	0.16	—
20/500	6/150	0.68	0.19	—
20/400	6/120	0.85	0.23	—
20/320	6/95	1	0.30	—
20/250	6/75	1.4	0.38	—
20/200	6/60	1.7	0.48	0.15
20/160	6/48	2.1	0.59	0.18
20/120	6/38	2.8	0.79	0.25
20/100	6/30	3.4	0.95	0.30
20/80	6/24	4.2	1.2	0.38
20/60	6/19	5.6	1.6	0.50
20/50	6/15	6.8	1.9	0.60
20/40	6/12	—	2.3	0.75
20/20	6/6	—	4.7	1.5

[a]One-half this distance for 4× acuity threshold.
[b]Clement Clark, Dayton, OH.
[c]Precision Vision, Villa Park, IL.

TABLE 4-4
Pelli-Robson Chart Contrast Threshold (CT) Values:
Contrast of Letters on the Pelli-Robson Chart*

		Chart Letters	
Level of Function	CT (%)	Form 1	Form 2
Severe loss	90.0	V R S	H S Z
	63.0	K D R	D S N
	44.0	N H C	C K R
	31.0	S O K	Z V R
Significant loss	22.0	S C N	N D C
	15.0	O Z V	O S K
Noticeable loss	11.0	C N H	O Z K
	7.8	Z O K	V H Z
	5.6	N O D	N H O
	3.9	V H R	N R D
Normal	2.8	C D N	V R C
	1.9	Z S V	O V H
	1.4	K C H	C D S
	1.0	O D K	N D C
	0.7	R S Z	K V D
	0.5	H V R	O H R

*Clement Clark, Dayton, OH.

should be checked with a light meter according to the instructions supplied by the chart. The doctor may also test the effects of varying the room illumination or compare different color filters when evaluating a patient with the CS chart. A patient's subjective preference should be recorded in his or her record for future recommendations.

CS or threshold should be specified with the test distance—for example, OD: 8.9% at 2 m, 4.5% at 1 m. The doctor determines the print contrast that the patient intends to read as well as the patient's CT. The contrast reserve is then calculated by dividing print contrast by CT. For example, a patient with 9% CT would be reading the highest quality print (90% contrast) with 10 to 1 contrast reserves. This same patient could read, with approximately 11 to 1 reserves, any print that was enhanced by a CCTV to approximately 100% contrast.

In certain instances in which CS testing materials are not available or when there is potential for the patient to become fatigued, a determination of the patient's response to increased contrast and illumination can be made using a CCTV. Also, when the doctor encounters patients who do not respond to near point magnification as expected, it may be appropriate to empirically evaluate the patient with a CCTV as well. The patient should be allowed to set the polarity, contrast, illumination, and magnification level to achieve the maximum reading level. Again, this information should be recorded in the patient's record for future consideration in determining the final recommended low vision device(s) (see Chapter 11 for more information on the CCTV).

Interventions that Increase Contrast Reserves

Contrast reserves can be increased and performance enhanced by either decreasing CT (i.e., increasing sensitivity) or increasing the contrast of the objects to be recognized.

Closed-Circuit Television or Computer Displays

CCTV systems and special print enhancement systems for computers not only enlarge print but also enhance print contrast to better than 95%. For example, a CCTV increases newsprint contrast from 75% to nearly 100%. These systems are also able to enlarge text substantially, in some cases up to 60 times larger than the original text. A patient may often choose to magnify text 6–10 times above his or her acuity threshold. Magnification usually increases contrast reserve because CS tends to improve as objects increase in size. In addition, the monitor of a CCTV enables the patient to obtain optimum contrast and illumination on the screen. It is especially important to provide glare-free screens when patients with poor CS use a CCTV or computer display.

Environmental Modifications

A patient's home and work environment may be modified to compensate for poor CS. Utensils, furniture, doorways, light switches, and steps should be modified so that they stand out with high contrast. For example, steps can be marked with reflective tape or lights. One can use furniture covers, slipcovers, doilies, and table cloths to lighten or darken a background to enhance contrast. Dangerous objects should have sufficient contrast to attract the patient's attention. In most cases, it is best to recommend that the patient's home or work environment be evaluated by a low vision rehabilitation specialist and that both verbal and written recommendations be provided to the patient.

Lighting Evaluation and Instruction

Lighting can be a critical factor for a patient with reduced CS. The best light levels are a matter of individual preference; there are no known rules or general guidelines for selecting the best light levels, bulb types, or tints. Moreover, preferred lighting may change with the task or the objects being read or viewed. Properly performed, a lighting evaluation is time-consuming because it involves trial and error with different light sources and tints for each task that the patient wishes to perform. A minimal lighting evaluation should include testing with directional and diffuse incandescent and fluorescent lights. Directional lighting should be shaded and positioned to the side or above the material so that the bulb is never in the patient's field of view. Each of these four lighting situations should be used to evaluate performance with samples of the actual task that the patient intends to perform (including a sample of the same reading materials).

Mobility Instruction

Patients with severe CS loss (greater than 30% CT [CS = 1.5]) should be routinely referred for mobility training because their personal safety is at risk. A more adventurous patient may have good mobility skills but be unaware of specific hazardous situations that involve low-contrast obstacles. The ability to detect low-contrast obstacles is essential for safe and independent travel, because it is not uncommon to encounter obstacles such as curbs, steps, and irregularities in street and sidewalk surfaces.

Levels of Contrast Sensitivity Loss and Recommended Interventions

For objects or letters that are magnified 2–4 times the patient's acuity threshold, a CT worse than approximately 35% should be considered a severe loss for most activities. In Table 4-2, one can appreciate that poorly contrasting furniture or a gray car speeding toward an intersection on a shady street would be below a 30% threshold and, therefore, would not be seen by a patient with severe loss. Even with the highest quality print, these patients still read slowly. They would make errors reading paper money because contrast reserves would be less than 3 to 1. Patients with severe CS loss would be good candidates for a CCTV for all reading needs and perhaps use books on tape for casual reading. They would be poor candidates for optical magnification, requiring much greater magnification than initially predicted. They would certainly have special lighting needs and would require mobility instruction and an assessment of the home and work environment to ensure that utensils, tools, furniture, and light switches, among other objects, have high contrast.

A patient with CTs worse than 8.9% present a significant loss, mostly for reading activities and in some mobility situations in which quick reaction times are important, such as avoiding a speeding car. One can see from Tables 4-1 and 4-2 that print and most objects are above the CT of these patients and, although objects will be recognized, reserves will be low and response times slowed. A lighting evaluation, instructions regarding glare avoidance, and special directional lighting would be helpful. Patients with intensive reading needs would probably benefit most from the higher contrast of a CCTV and computer systems. CTs worse than 4.5% may present a small but noticeable loss under some lighting situations. Performance speed may be compromised. A lighting evaluation or consideration of a CCTV or computer system would be a reasonable response if the patient complains about lighting, glare, or dissatisfaction with reading speed or comfort with optical devices.

Contrast Sensitivity Testing with Sinusoidal Gratings

Contrast can also be measured with sinusoidal gratings produced electronically or printed as a chart, such as the Vistech Contrast Test System (Dayton, OH). Measurement of the contrast sensitivity function with these gratings will give rise to a curve representing the visual system's sensitivity to the different spatial frequencies of the grating (Figure 4-1). The left side of the curve will provide the doctor with information concerning the patient's ability to detect large objects, which would be important for orientation and mobility tasks. Patients with advanced retinitis pigmentosa or glaucoma would have a loss in these low spatial frequencies. The high spatial frequencies, on the right side of the curve, would correspond to higher levels of visual acuity. Patients with maculopathies would have a loss in these high spatial frequencies and, in many cases, have normal middle and low spatial frequencies.

Summary

The practitioner can use a number of tests to measure different aspects of CS. As there is no consensus as to which test is best for evaluating patients with low vision, the practitioner should use the test with which he or she feels most comfortable. There is valuable information that can be obtained through CS testing. The following points may be of some help when evaluating the contrast sensitivity of patients with low vision:

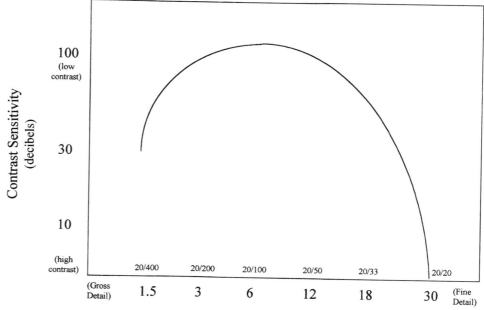

FIGURE 4-1. **Contrast sensitivity testing curve representing the visual system's sensitivity to different spatial frequencies.**

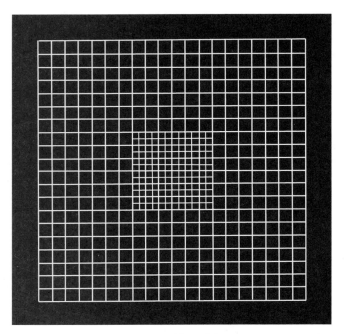

FIGURE 4-2. **Amsler's grid test with each large square representing 1 degree (total of 10 degrees from central fixation target) when the grid is held 13 in. from the patient.**

1. Loss of high spatial frequency contrast usually indicates problems with near-point and reading tasks. A patient may require increased magnification, increased contrast of materials, and increased illumination.
2. Loss of low spatial frequency contrast usually indicates problems with mobility and nighttime travel. A patient may require orientation and mobility services and perhaps a flashlight for nighttime travel.
3. In normally sighted binocular patients, binocular CS is higher than monocular sensitivity across all spatial frequencies. This is called *binocular summation.*
   a. If a low vision patient demonstrates binocular summation, then binocular devices should be encouraged at distance and near when possible.
   b. Low vision patients who do not demonstrate binocular summation should be encouraged to be monocular and use the eye with the better CS (assuming that other factors, such as visual acuity and visual field, do not contraindicate the use of this eye).

VISUAL FIELD TESTING IN LOW VISION

Visual field testing for low vision patients is used for the following reasons:

- Determining legal blindness
- Determining eligibility for privileges such as driving
- Calculating compensation for functional loss

One important aspect of field testing, however, is to determine if a field defect is the principal cause of a patient's inability to achieve a particular goal. In most low vision cases, calculating magnification will result in an appropriately powered device, allowing patients to achieve their vision goals. In some instances, however, field testing should be performed to adequately characterize the patient's vision loss and design devices and strategies to allow the patient to achieve maximum potential.

In patients with intact central fixation, field testing can be done with methods similar to those for patients with normal vision. The majority of low vision patients, however, have some loss in macular function, often resulting in eccentric fixation. This loss in macular function can also result in a decrease in the steadiness of fixation. As a result of research done by Timberlake et al.,[1] Schuchard with the scanning laser ophthalmoscope,[2] and Whittaker et al.,[3] it is now known that most patients with a maculopathy use a point adjacent to the scotoma to observe objects of interest (preferred retinal locus [PRL]). Depending on the position of the scotoma relative to the retinal area used for fixation, the PRL may be placed in any direction and will result in a compensatory eccentric viewing position.

Standard Amsler's Grid Testing

The standard Amsler's grid test includes seven different charts to test the quality of central vision within a field of 20 degrees (Figure 4-2). The chart is held 13 in. from the patient while the patient is wearing the appropriate add. The standard chart consists of a central white horizontal and vertical grid, with each line 0.5 mm apart. The large square grid is 10 cm on each side of the fixation target. The patient occludes one eye, stares at the center of the grid, and is asked if he or she can see all four corners of the square. The patient is then asked if any of the vertical or horizontal lines are missing or distorted. Distortions of the Amsler's grid reflect the presence of metamorphopsia, caused by macular elevations or depressions. The patient should also be asked if the actual white grid seems to have any color or tint. If so, this effect may be due to fresh hemorrhaging or exudative mechanisms (see Chapter 3 for more information on Amsler's grid testing).

Threshold Amsler's Grid Testing

A variation on standard Amsler's grid testing is *threshold Amsler's grid testing* (Stereo Optical Co., Chicago, IL) (Figure 4-3). In this test, crossed polarized filters are used in a trial frame to reduce the contrast of a standard Amsler's grid. Relative metamorphopsias or scotomas that would not be obvious to a patient under normal high-contrast situations may be elicited under low-contrast conditions. The threshold Amsler's grid kit comes with threshold Amsler's grid polarizers, a black plastic Amsler's grid, and a white Amsler's grid pad.

The patient is instructed to hold the white Amsler's grid (on black background) 16 in. from the unoccluded eye. The polarized glasses are put over the patient's near prescription. The patient is instructed to stare at the center dot and to

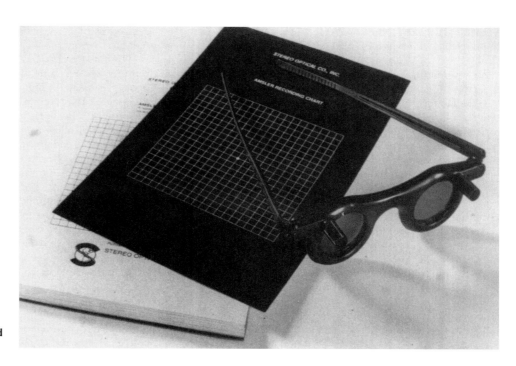

FIGURE 4-3.   **Threshold Amsler's grid test using crossed polarized filters.**

take note of any distortions or scotomas within the grid. If the patient does not notice any metamorphopsias within the grid, the practitioner begins to increase the polarization, thus dimming the light entering the patient's eye. Some macular irregularities may be elicited under dim illumination that would not be visualized in bright light conditions.

Interpretation of Amsler's Grid Results

The Amsler's grid is used to examine the central 10 degrees on all sides of fixation. It may be useful for detecting central and paracentral scotomas as well as metamorphopsias. The Amsler's grid is not intended to accurately evaluate a low vision patient; however, in some cases, the test may provide valuable information regarding the patient's potential for using magnification for near-point tasks such as reading and writing. A patient who has learned to eccentrically view and is able to fixate on the central fixation target may report a scotoma to any side of fixation. If the scotoma is to the right of fixation, it may hamper the patient's reading or writing because the patient is reading or writing into a blind spot. If the scotoma is large and absolute, the prognosis is poorer for using optical magnification (relative distance and angular magnification) than when compared to a scotoma that may be small and relative. In this situation, the patient may function better for reading and writing with a CCTV. If the scotoma is to the left of fixation, the patient may experience problems in locating the beginning of the next line. A typoscope, ruler, or the patient's finger (positioned at the beginning of the line just read) may be helpful in pointing out the beginning of the line. In this situation, the patient would be instructed to follow the same line that

he had just read back to his finger, or the end of the ruler, and then drop down one line to begin the next sentence.

There have been some questions as to the validity and reliability of Amsler's grid testing on some patients with low vision. From the work of Schuchard,[2] it is now known that patients with well-established eccentric viewing techniques use their PRL to fixate the center dot of the Amsler's grid, regardless of the instructions they are given. When the doctor tests a patient with a well-adapted PRL, it is often difficult for that patient to use any point other than that which has been well established. There are also some patients who report that the grid appears complete due to the phenomenon of "perceptual completion"[2] or "filling in." Therefore, in these instances, the patient may not see any defect in the grid, or he or she may interpret the grid as being blurred or distorted rather than having sections missing, even though the doctor suspects the presence of a dense scotoma.

Goldmann's Visual Field Perimeter Testing

The Goldmann's perimeter is one of the best instruments to test the entire field of a low vision patient. It allows targets of a variety of sizes and intensities to be presented in any order or speed to positions 90 degrees eccentric to a patient's fixation. A separate projector can be used to position a letter appropriate to the patient's acuity at the center of the bowl as a fixation target. Because individuals with maculopathies will commonly adopt an eccentric fixation position, the practitioner can use this characteristic by asking the patient to view the central fixation target as clearly as possible. The practitioner's observation telescope can then be used to determine if the patient is holding his or her fixation steady.

SUBJECTIVE TESTING OF PATIENTS WITH MEDIA AND RETINAL LOSS

When evaluating low vision patients, doctors must consider the effects of medical abnormalities on overall vision loss. When cataracts, corneal scars, or vitreal opacities make it difficult or impossible to perform a fundus examination, testing for retinal functioning and pathology can proceed through other means. The instrumentation and tests described in this section enable the practitioner to perform subjective testing to determine retinal functioning.

Potential Acuity Meter

The potential acuity meter, or PAM unit, measures the retinal visual acuity behind mild to moderate media opacities such as cataracts. The PAM unit, manufactured by Mentor (Norwell, MA), is called the *Guyton-Minkowski Potential Acuity Meter*. It attaches to a slit-lamp and projects a Snellen's visual acuity chart through a "window" in the cataract. Retinal pathology should be considered if the PAM test reveals

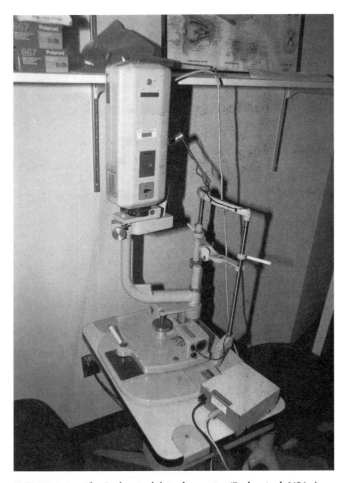

FIGURE 4-4.   **The Rodenstock interferometer (Rodenstock USA, Inc., Danbury, CT) uses dual coherent laser beams to generate the interference pattern viewed by the patient.**

a true loss of visual acuity despite the presence of a media opacity.

The PAM works best on immature cataracts because it requires a clear zone through which the narrow beam of light is projected. The effect is similar to pinhole testing except that the Snellen's chart projected onto the retina is very bright. Obviously, denser cataracts without these windows will not allow for transmission of the Snellen's chart, and the scattered light will reduce or eliminate the predictive value of the test. Because of this effect, patient selection is of critical importance to the efficacy of this test.

The visual acuity chart that is projected by the PAM unit is designed to be brighter than the standard Snellen's chart and has black letters or numbers set against a white background. The chart can test visual acuity from 20/20 to 20/400. The instrument can be focused to compensate for a patient's refractive error between +13.00 and −10.00 D.

To perform potential acuity assessment with the Mentor Guyton-Minkowski Potential Acuity Meter, the patient should be placed comfortably at the slit-lamp (which has a mounted PAM unit attached) in a dimly lit room. The patient's approximate refractive error should be set on the spherical power control. The doctor should move the slit-lamp around to find the clearest window and focus the chart until the patient reports that the clearest image has been obtained. The patient then reads the smallest line of letters possible. There is a strong likelihood that surgical intervention is appropriate when the PAM visual acuity is three lines better than standard visual acuity.

White Light and Laser Interferometry

Another way to perform an acuity test is by using interferometry. Three examples are the Randwal interferometer (no longer manufactured), the Rodenstock laser retinometer (Rodenstock USA, Inc., Danbury, CT), and the Visometer (Haag-Streit, Bern, Switzerland) (Figures 4-4 and 4-5). Typically, the interferometer projects stripes of coherent light through media opacities. The Haag-Streit Visometer and the Randwal interferometer use white incandescent light while the Rodenstock laser retinometer uses a neon-helium laser. The better the true retinal vision, the finer the stripes (spatial frequency) the patient can detect. Again, if visual acuity remains reduced when testing by interferometry, there is a greater possibility of the reduction being caused by a retinal pathology. The interferometer works on the principle of optical interference fringes between two beams of light and is less affected by a patient's refractive error. Furthermore, because the interference fringe patterns depend more on the amplitude of the electromagnetic wave and less on the intensity of the light transmission, the interferometer may be more helpful in evaluating retinal function through more dense media opacities.

Randwal Interferometer

The advantages of the Randwal interferometer are that it can be both slit-lamp mounted and handheld, it uses white light, and it can easily be used on children or multiply impaired patients. The patient is placed in a room with just enough lighting to be able to visualize the pupil. The patient is seated comfortably and pupil dilation, particularly in cataractous eyes, is recommended (Figure 4-6). Refractive error does not need to be corrected in most cases.

Testing begins with the widest line pattern (lowest spatial frequency), and the patient is asked to describe the direction of the lines, which can be oriented horizontally, vertically, or obliquely. Every time the patient reports the correct line orientation, the practitioner decreases the width of the lines. This procedure continues until the patient can no longer identify the line orientation. The Snellen visual acuity that is equivalent to the finest lines that the patient can perceive is recorded as the interference acuity. The entire test is repeated with a different field size and then performed again in the other eye.

Rodenstock Laser Retinometer

The Rodenstock laser retinometer is a slit-lamp–mounted instrument that uses two neon-helium (red) laser beams to produce an interference pattern. The patient will either

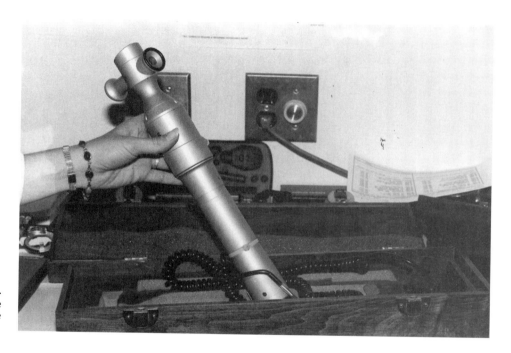

FIGURE 4-5. **The Randwal interferometer uses white light to produce the interference (bar) pattern seen by the patient.**

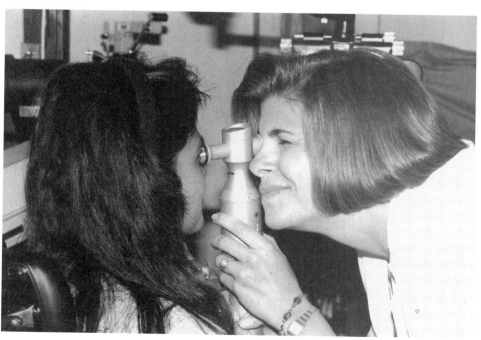

FIGURE 4-6. **The Randwal interferometer being used on a patient with cataracts.**

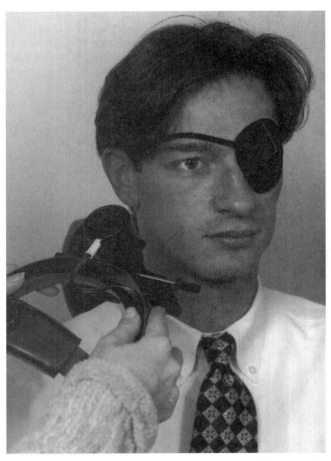

FIGURE 4-7. **The photostress recovery test using the bright light of a binocular indirect ophthalmoscope to initially bleach the patient's retina.**

report seeing just a red light or will report black and red lines oriented in one of four directions: horizontal, vertical, 45 degrees, or 135 degrees.

Haag-Streit Visometer
The Haag-Streit visometer is slit-lamp mounted, and the evaluation procedure is the same as in the Randwal unit. Again, the finest stripe that can be visualized by the patient is recorded as a Snellen visual acuity equivalent. The clearest zone through the cataract should be used.

Interpretation of Interferometry Results

In patients with reduced visual acuity, there are retinal conditions that produce better interference acuity than Snellen acuity. These conditions include cystoid macular edema, macular cyst and hole, amblyopia, and some cases of age-related macular degeneration. In the presence of a cataract, if the interference acuity is superior to the standard acuity, then there is a strong likelihood that surgical intervention will help to improve acuity. In patients without a clear section of the cataractous lens, as in patients with very dense, mature cataracts, it may be impossible to obtain a better acuity esti-

mate with a white light or laser interferometer, even though the acuity after surgery may be significantly improved.

Photostress Recovery Test

To further evaluate macular disease, the photostress recovery test can help diagnose disruption of normal macular physiology from early optic nerve disease. Early optic nerve disease will show normal recovery whereas slow recovery from a bright light may mean macular pathology. During testing, the patient is dark-adapted for 1 minute, then is instructed to stare at a bright light for 10 seconds with only one eye (Figure 4-7). The light is then turned off and the practitioner measures the time it takes until the patient can read one line less than his or her best visual acuity. This procedure is subsequently repeated with the other eye. The average or normal recovery time is 50–60 seconds. If the recovery time is substantially longer, or there is a large difference in recovery time between the two eyes, macular disease is the most probable cause. Recovery time, however, may also be decreased by the age of the patient (older patients may show "normal" slower rate), poor visual acuity (generally less than 20/100), and dense media opacities.

Glare Testing

The brightness acuity test (BAT) is useful in measuring the reduction of visual acuity in the presence of glare when a cataract or corneal opacity is present. Glare can be caused by intraocular light scattering, and therefore, glare testing is likely to be more specific in evaluating anterior segment media opacities. To perform this test, the patient is instructed to wear his or her best spectacle correction. The BAT encloses the unoccluded eye in a small sphere with an exit hole along the visual axis. The visual acuity is measured in nonilluminated conditions. A small light inside the sphere is then turned on to create glare conditions and the visual acuity is reassessed. If there is a decrease of two or more lines of visual acuity, then media opacities or other ocular pathology may be significantly interfering with the patient's ability to see under bright light conditions. The effect of absorptive filters on improving the glare problem may be tested by placing tinted lenses between the BAT and the patient's eye.

Color Vision Testing

Color vision testing can be extremely valuable in making the correct diagnosis concerning the cause of a patient's decreased vision. In addition, color vision testing can help monitor the progression of a disease as well as gauge the level of difficulty a patient may have in performing tasks that require processing of color information such as in activities of daily living (i.e., coordinating clothing colors).

Several color vision tests are available to the practitioner. The most commonly used tests are the color plate tests, such as the Ishihara, pseudoisochromatic, or Dvorine color plates, and the color arrangement tests, such as the Farnsworth dichotomous test (D-15). Color plate tests are quite valuable in identifying the presence of a color vision defect and confirming the diagnosis of a congenital defect. The Farnsworth D-15 test, Farnsworth-Munsell 100-hue test, and the Nagel anomaloscope are more sophisticated tests and are used to help diagnose both congenital and acquired disorders.

Farnsworth Dichotomous Test

The D-15 test (Figure 4-8) is a color arrangement test. The patient is asked to arrange 14 test chips according to hue, using a stationary blue test chip as a reference point. This test should be performed monocularly when any color vision defect is suspected that is not due to classic inherited defects (protan or deutan). In addition, the test must be administered under the proper illumination. This can be accomplished in three ways. The preferred illumination uses a MacBeth lamp giving illuminant "C." An alternative is to use a suitable blue Wrattan filter, and another option is to use northern skylight.

The D-15 test is helpful in determining whether the color vision defect is typical of a protanope or deuteranope, or whether it shows the classic errors of an X-linked blue cone monochromat or rod monochromat. The important clinical decision is to determine if there are multiple error lines that parallel the axes that are indicated. If a patient has inherited protanomaly or deuteranomaly, these major error axes will not be present. In these instances, there may be minor alterations, or the error pattern may be the normal inverted C (see Figure 4-8). The Farnsworth Panel D-15 test can be extremely valuable in differentiating macular pathologies as well. Maculopathies due to diabetes, hypertension, and age-related macular degeneration usually cause blue-yellow defects, whereas dystrophies, such as central areolar, vitelliform, and Stargardt's, usually cause red-green defects.

For the practitioner who may want to determine the color vision of young patients (cognitive age of 3 years and older), two simple tests are available. The Portnoy plates and the Berson plates use Munsell colors similar to the Farnsworth Panel D-15 test. The Portnoy plates are arranged with four colored circles and the child is asked to choose the one color that is different. The Portnoy plates identify protan, deutan, and tritan anomalies. The Berson plates help to differentiate between rod monochromatism and blue cone monochromatism.[4, 5]

Nagel Anomaloscope

A more advanced color test is the Nagel anomaloscope (Figure 4-9). This instrument uses prisms that separate white light into the spectral colors. It provides a circular split field creating two equal semicircle fields: One field is a mixture of red and green and the other is yellow (589 nm). The red and green half can be adjusted by the patient to form different color combinations. The yellow half is not variable except for brightness. The patient is asked to subjectively match the red and green semicircle to the yellow semicircle. This test is performed monocularly. The patient who is protanomalous matches the yellow with too much red, whereas the deuteranomalous patient matches with too much green. Finally, individuals with rod or blue cone monochromatism demonstrate a classic error pattern that distinguishes them from all other X-linked inherited color vision defects.[5] The monochromatic patient would match an intense red color with the yellow standard. This lack of color discrimination matches the typical subjective complaint of this patient—the inability to distinguish in daylight conditions whether a red light is shining. It is only under mesopic or scotopic conditions that he or she can determine if a red light (stop light or brake light) is on.

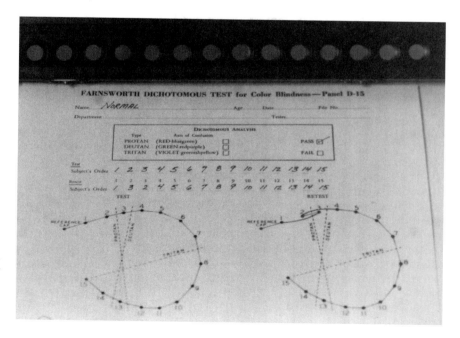

FIGURE 4-8. **The Farnsworth dichotomous (D-15) test is helpful in determining the type of color vision defect that may be present in a low vision patient. Normal-sighted patients will show a reversed C pattern or possibly minor misplacement of a test chip.**

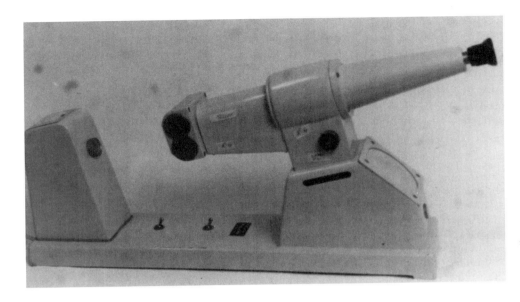

FIGURE 4-9. **The Nagel anomaloscope is an advanced form of color testing that can categorize all forms of red-green inherited color vision defects.**

Dark Adaptometry

Patients with stationary night blindness or some form of tapetoretinal degeneration will commonly complain of decreased sensitivity when in dimly lit environments. Dark adaptometry allows the doctor to quantify the classic complaints of these patients concerning their adaptation when going from a light to a dark environment. This finding may be particularly valuable in monitoring patients with tapetoretinal degenerations who have an extinguished electroretinogram (ERG) but have remaining vision.

The standard instrument that is used for clinically testing dark adaptation is the Goldmann-Weekers dark adaptometer (Haag-Streit, Bern, Switzerland) (Figure 4-10). This apparatus uses a Ganzfeld or bowl into which the patient views. Within the bowl are lights for bleaching the patient's retina and a dim red fixation light and a flashing white test light.

The patient is first light-adapted for 5 minutes, which essentially bleaches the retina. Immediately after these bright lights are extinguished, the patient views a superiorly located red fixation light and taps on the examination table when he or she detects the flashing stimulus light. For each measurement, the doctor increases the intensity until reaching the patient's threshold. This measurement is repeated as often as possible in the first few minutes and every minute thereafter. The test proceeds for approximately 45 minutes.

The recording sheet plots time versus sensitivity (measured on a logarithmic scale). Patients who are visually normal usually have a 5-log-unit change in sensitivity over the course of the test. Initially, there is a steeper drop in sensitivity corresponding to the patient's cone system. After 5–10 minutes, the patient's rod system will become more sensitive than his or her cone system, and therefore, the latter increase in sensitivity is due to the rod system.

Patients with even moderately advanced retinitis pigmentosa usually display no more than a 2-log-unit change in sensitivity, corresponding to a response in their cone system (Figure 4-11).

OBJECTIVE TESTING OF RETINAL FUNCTIONING

Objective testing of the visual system is theoretically less biased than subjective testing and therefore may be more effective as a diagnostic strategy. Objective testing, however, does not take into account how the patient functions in his or her own environment. Therefore, objective tests, although excellent for diagnosis, are sometimes poor prognosticators of low vision management.

B-Scan Ultrasonography

If a media opacity is present and prevents satisfactory views of the fundus, then diagnostic ultrasound can be a benefit in detecting changes in structure of the retina. B-scan ultrasonography may help detect retinal detachment, retinoschisis, staphylomas, buried drusen, or retinal tumors.[6]

The technique is accomplished by using a handheld probe, which both transmits ultrasonic energy and receives the reflections of this energy from the ocular structures. The probe is held against the patient's closed lids and produces an image of a section through the ocular structures (Figure 4-12). The orientation of the probe is changed to investigate the entire globe and orbit. The image is stored on the computer and displayed on a video monitor (Figure 4-13). A final Polaroid picture or high-resolution print of the B-scan ultrasound is produced for the record. Sample results from two patients, one with a long-standing retinal detachment and another with a posterior staphyloma, are shown in Figures 4-14 and 4-15.

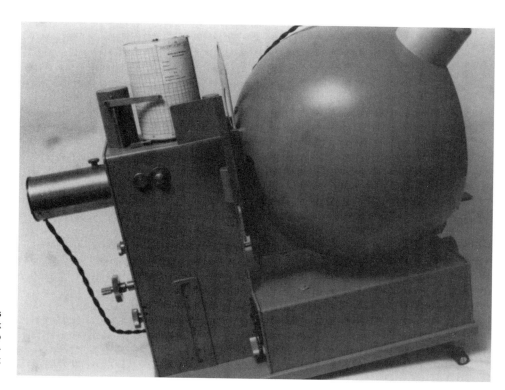

FIGURE 4-10. **The Goldmann-Weekers (Haag-Streit, Bern, Switzerland) dark adaptometer is an instrument used to clinically test patients for decreased sensitivity when changing from light to dark environments.**

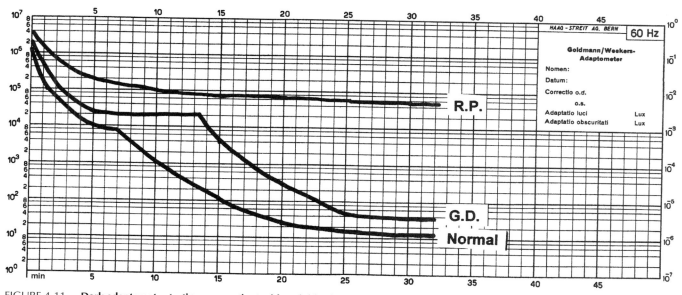

FIGURE 4-11.   **Dark adaptometry testing on a patient with retinitis pigmentosa (RP) usually displays no more than a 2-log-unit change in sensitivity. In comparison, normal-sighted individuals usually demonstrate a 5-log-unit change in sensitivity. The patient, GD, who had suspicious retinal pigmentary changes showed normal dark adaptation.**

Electrodiagnostic Testing

ERG and visual evoked potential testing (VEP) are the most valuable electrodiagnostic tests used in assessing the electrical processing of the ocular structures in low vision patients. These two tests measure the function of different anatomic structures. ERG is most important in cases of family history of tapetoretinal degenerations in which there are observable pigmentary or other suspicious retinal findings, or when the patient has unexplained loss of field or prolonged dark adaptation. VEP testing is most valuable in cases of unexplained visual acuity loss, pallor, or

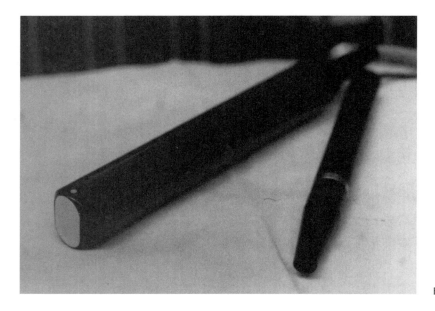

FIGURE 4-12.   **The probe of an ultrasound instrument.**

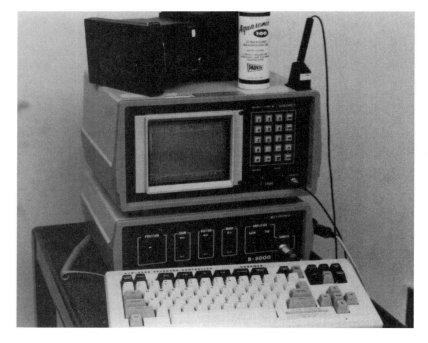

FIGURE 4-13.   **The computer and video monitor used with a B-scan ultrasonography instrument.**

other suspicious changes in the appearance of the optic nerve, or as a rough gauge of visual acuity in patients who are unable to cooperate for standardized tests. Often, patients who require these tests will need further monitoring of their condition. Fundus photographs taken near the time of the electrodiagnostic tests can be quite valuable when evaluating these patients in the future.

Electroretinography
ERG is an electrodiagnostic test that measures the electrical activity in the patient's retina. It is a valuable test in cases of tapetoretinal degenerations, which usually show a

decrease in the patient's ERG before there are clear ophthalmoscopic changes or before the patient has distinct complaints. The ERG reflects the composition of the photoreceptive elements of the retina. Because there are many more rods than cones, the ERG is rod dominant—that is, the majority of the response is produced by the rods. The rod, or scotopic response, is enhanced by dark adaptation. The cone response is measured under light-adapted and fast-flicker conditions. At a 30-Hz stimulation rate, only the cone system can respond.

PATIENT PREPARATION AND TEST PROCEDURE.   A number of steps are required before performing the actual test. The

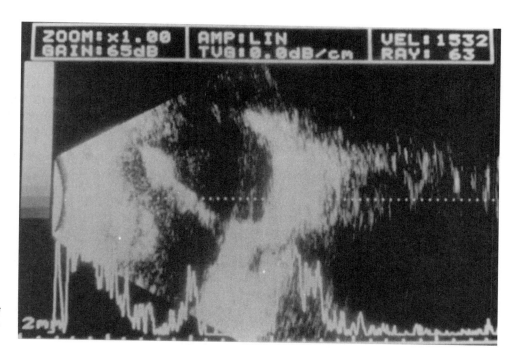

FIGURE 4-14. **B-scan ultrasound of a patient's eye with a retinal detachment.**

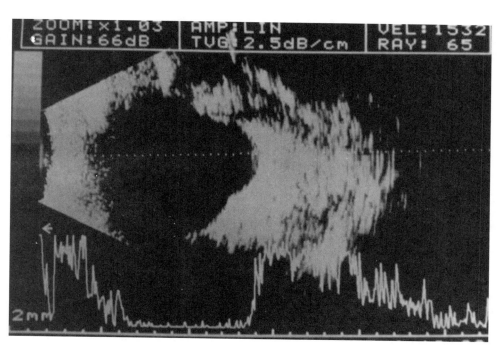

FIGURE 4-15. **B-scan ultrasound of a patient's eye with a posterior staphyloma.**

patient is initially dilated and is then completely dark-adapted in a room under a dim red light. The patient's corneas are anesthetized and a special electrode, similar to a contact lens, is placed on the cornea. The most common electrode is the Burian-Allen electrode (Ophthalmic Development Laboratory, Iowa City, IA) (Figure 4-16). This electrode contains a speculum that holds the patient's eyelids open during the test. Although the speculum will reduce blink artifacts, the patient is less comfortable with this electrode than with others. In addi-

tion, care must be taken to ensure that the corneas remain moist during the test. Other electrodes, such as gold foil, Mylar, or platinum wire embedded in plastic, fit over the lower lid of the patient's eye (Figure 4-17). These electrodes will still allow the patient to blink or close his or her eye, thus providing less risk of corneal injury. During the test, the patient will look into a Ganzfeld (similar to the bowl in Goldmann's or Humphrey's perimeter) with a photostimulator mounted to uniformly stimulate the retina. The patient is tested under dark- and light-adapted conditions at slow flash rates and under 30-Hz conditions.

The ERG generated is a relatively small electrical signal. Thus, it must be amplified, much like a stereo amplifier is needed to amplify signals from a tape recorder, record turntable, or compact disk player. These amplifiers are either battery powered or specially designed to isolate the patient from any risk of electrical shock from equipment powered with 120-V alternating current.

The results of the ERG are usually stored in the digital memory of the computer, displayed on a video monitor, and printed out on either a printer or an X-Y plotter. A calibration pulse is used to compare the timing and amplitude of the response. The normal ERG (Figure 4-18) shows a negative deflection (A-wave) at approximately 18–20 ms and a subsequent positive deflection at approximately 40–50 ms (B-wave). The amplitude of the dark-adapted ERG is approximately 300–500 µV. In cases of retinitis pigmentosa and similar disorders, the A- and B-waves of the ERG become slightly delayed and reduced in amplitude and are finally extinguished (see Figure 4-18).

CLASSIC RETINITIS PIGMENTOSA. Classically, retinitis pigmentosa presents as a field loss in the midperiphery along with a decrease in sensitivity in a scotopic environment. Typically, patients will have initial complaints of seeing under twilight conditions. The important triad of ophthalmoscopic signs are bone spicule pigmentation in the midperipheral retina, attenuation of retinal vessels, and pallor of the optic disc. For example, KC is a 15-year-old girl, with 20/20 acuity and mild complaints of poor vision in the dark. There is no history of blindness in her family. Ophthalmoscopy reveals slight attenuation of the retinal vessels, slight pallor of the nerve head, and distinct retinal pigment epithelium pigmentation in the midperiphery (Figure 4-19). A diagnosis of retinitis pigmen-

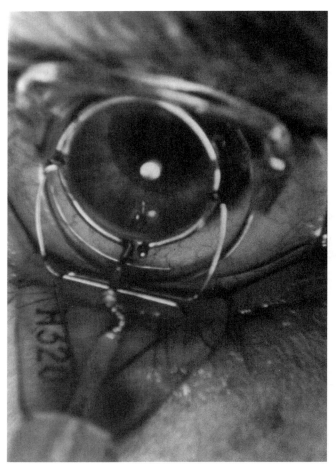

FIGURE 4-16. **The Burian-Allen electrode (Ophthalmic Development Laboratory, Iowa City, IA) commonly used in electroretinography.**

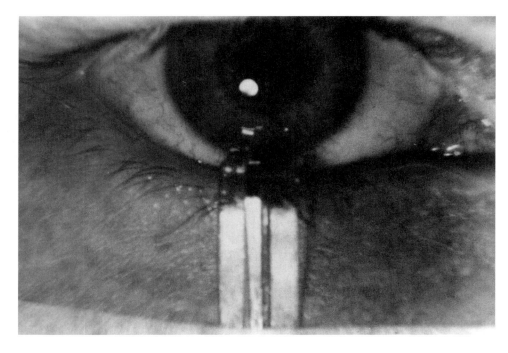

FIGURE 4-17. **Compared to the Burian-Allen electrode (Ophthalmic Development Laboratory, Iowa City IA), platinum wire imbedded in plastic provides less risk of a corneal injury and allows the patient to close his or her eye during dark adaptation before electroretinography.**

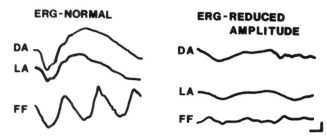

ERG-NORMAL

DA
LA
FF

ERG-REDUCED
AMPLITUDE

DA
LA
FF

FIGURE 4-18. **Comparison of a normal electroretinogram (ERG) wave to an abnormal ERG wave (i.e., retinitis pigmentosa) in which the A- and B-waves are reduced in amplitude. ERGs are recorded under dark adapted (DA), light adapted (LA), and fast-flicker (FF) conditions.**

tosa was confirmed with electroretinography, which revealed an extinguished ERG under dark-adapted, light-adapted, and fast-flicker conditions (Figure 4-20).

INVERSE RETINITIS PIGMENTOSA. There are numerous variations of retinitis pigmentosa. One such case is represented by BH, a 45-year-old woman who first noticed a decrease in acuity at age 15 years. Her initial ocular examinations yielded a diagnosis of Stargardt's macular degeneration. Since that time, she has noticed an increase in the size of her central scotoma as well as a decrease in visual acuity. In later ocular examinations, her original diagnosis was questioned because of the progressive nature of the signs and symptoms. These included bone-spicule pigmentation throughout the macula in each eye along with vessel attenuation and slight optic nerve pallor (Figure 4-21).

Electrodiagnostic testing was performed to determine whether the patient had Stargardt's degeneration or inverse retinitis pigmentosa. The results of the electroretinogram showed an extinguished ERG in each eye, which would be consistent with a diagnosis of inverse retinitis pigmentosa.

JUVENILE X-LINKED RETINOSCHISIS. In certain instances, a unique combination of ophthalmoscopic findings and electrodiagnostic results is helpful in making a diagnosis.

AS was a 17-year-old boy of Middle Eastern descent who was enrolled in his senior year of high school. He reported that his vision had been reduced since age 10 years. His chief complaint was his inability to see the blackboard. His best visual acuity was OD 10/100 and OS 10/120. Ophthalmoscopy (Figure 4-22) showed wrinkling of the internal limiting membrane in each eye. Specialized testing revealed ERGs with reduced amplitudes and delayed B-wave implicit times under both light-adapted and fast-flicker conditions (Figure 4-23). The combination of the structural changes in the inner retina along with the electrophysiologic changes supported the diagnosis of juvenile X-linked retinoschisis.

Monochromatism

The battery of ERGs, D-15, and Nagel anomaloscope testing can be used to make a diagnosis of monochromatism with certainty.

RM, an 8-year-old white boy, was initially diagnosed as having albinism with associated nystagmus and congenital myopia when he was referred for low vision services. His parents reported that his vision had been stable since birth. His best acuity was 10/60 in each eye. He had approximately 3.00 D of myopia in each eye. Amsler's grid and tangent screen testing revealed no field defects. External examination was normal. There was no iris trans-illumination detected with slit-lamp examination. Ophthalmoscopy revealed clear media, normal maculae, and

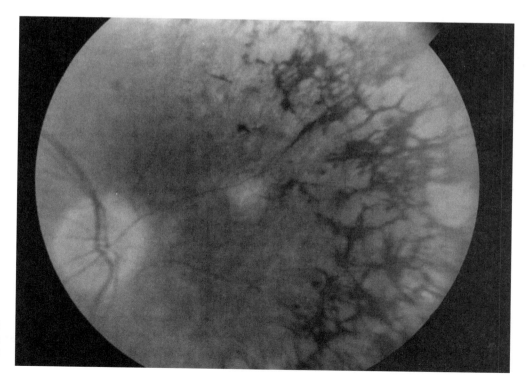

FIGURE 4-19. **Ocular fundus of a patient with retinitis pigmentosa shows bone spicule pigmentation in the midperipheral retina.**

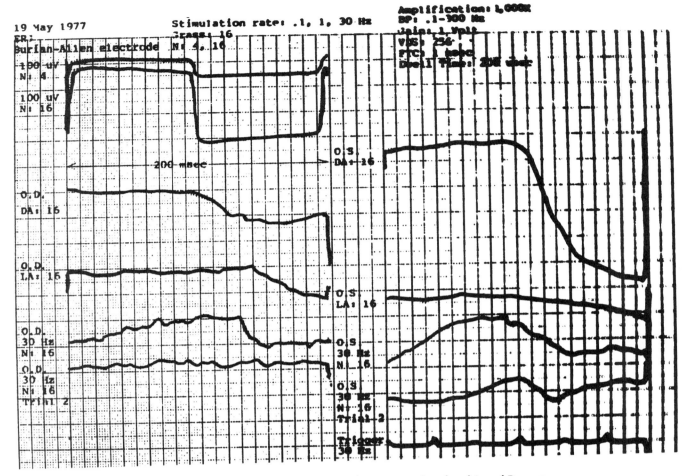

FIGURE 4-20.   Electroretinogram of a patient with retinitis pigmentosa shows extremely reduced A- and B-waves.

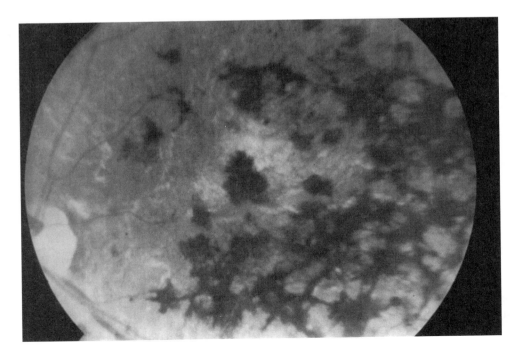

FIGURE 4-21.   Ocular fundus of a patient with inverse retinitis pigmentosa shows bone spicule pigmentation in the macula area.

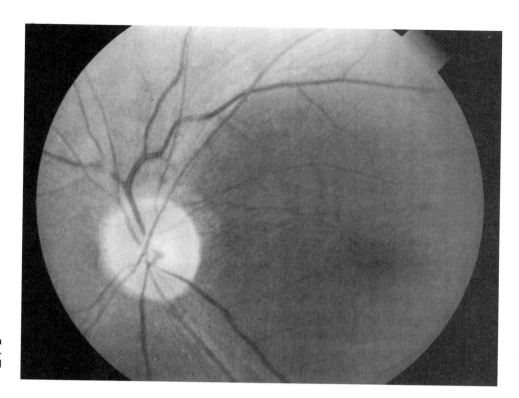

FIGURE 4-22. **Ocular fundus of a patient with juvenile X-linked retinoschisis shows wrinkling of the internal limiting membrane.**

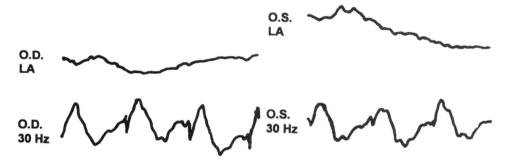

FIGURE 4-23. **Reduced and delayed electroretinogram recorded under light adapted (LA) and fast-flicker conditions support the diagnosis of juvenile X-linked retinoschisis.**

a foveal reflex in both eyes. The cup-to-disk ratio was 0.3 to 0.3 in each eye. The arteriole-to-venule ratio was 2 to 3 in each eye. There was relative loss of retinal pigment epithelial pigmentation around the disc in each eye. In addition to providing RM low vision care, a battery of tests was performed to determine the cause of his vision loss.

ERG revealed normal results under dark-adapted conditions. He did, however, demonstrate abnormal photopic and fast-flicker ERGs, which are indicative of monochromatism (Figure 4-24). D-15 testing revealed major color vision errors with an axis between the protan and deutan error lines (Figure 4-25). The Nagel anomaloscope showed the classic error pattern consistent with some form of monochromatism (Figure 4-26).

When comparing patients with rod monochromatism to patients with blue cone monochromatism, the latter demonstrates some residual cone function that provides the basis for some color perception. A patient with rod monochromatism would have no color perception; all colors would appear as

shades of gray. Therefore, the results from the ERG and color testing confirm a diagnosis of monochromatism, more specifically, a diagnosis of blue cone monochromatism.

Visual Evoked Potential

VEP is a measure of the electrical activity at the visual cortex. Because of the orientation of the cortical cells corresponding to the macula and the relative number of ganglion cells representing the macular area, the VEP tends to emphasize a patient's central vision. For low vision patients, in whom the practitioner has little information about where the defect is, the combination of ERG, emphasizing retinal electrical activity, and VEP, emphasizing the macula, optic nerve, and cortical processing, can be a very powerful probe of the patient's visual status. VEP is especially sensitive to pattern information. VEP is a much smaller electrical signal than ERG and requires additional amplification and computer summation to extract the signal from the ongoing electroencephalogram.

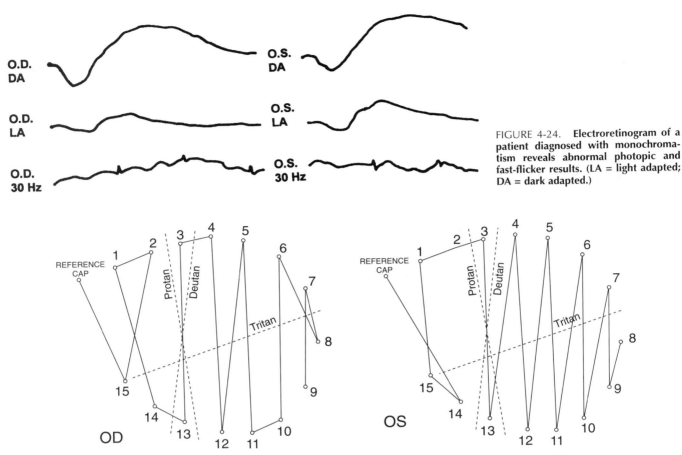

FIGURE 4-24.   **Electroretinogram of a patient diagnosed with monochromatism reveals abnormal photopic and fast-flicker results. (LA = light adapted; DA = dark adapted.)**

FIGURE 4-25.   **Farnsworth dichotomous (D-15) test shows abnormal color vision results in a patient with monochromatism.**

PATIENT PREPARATION AND TEST PROCEDURE.   It is important to inform the patient that this test does not involve any pain but does require cooperation by remaining still and looking at the target. When patients cannot cooperate, as in cases of children or patients with mental retardation, the doctor should monitor the patient to ensure that the VEP is being recorded only when the patient is looking at the stimulus. The active signal is recorded from a skin electrode placed on the patient's scalp, usually several centimeters above the inion (the prominence at the back of the skull). Before electrode placement, the patient's skin is cleaned with alcohol or acetone to remove any dead skin and oil. Reference and ground electrodes are placed over visually inactive areas of the patient's skull.

The patient then looks at a video monitor that displays a repetitive stimulus such as a checkerboard, square wave, or sinusoidal grating. When testing a patient's visual acuity or form perception, the overall luminance of the stimulus remains constant while the individual elements or patterns (i.e., checks) change from black to white and vice versa. In instances in which a pattern VEP cannot be recorded, such as with patients who have severe media opacities, a flash stimulus (similar to that used for an ERG) can be used (flash VEP).

VEP is designated by sequential negative and positive deflections. These are either labeled negative 1 (N1) and

positive 1 (P1) or, because there is a major positive wave at approximately 100 ms, it may be labeled by the corresponding implicit time (P100). Sample normal results are shown in Figure 4-27. The major changes that can occur in VEP are either monocular or binocular delays or reductions in amplitude. These are most common in cases of optic nerve lesions but may also be found in cases of maculopathies. In cases of patients with cataracts, comparing the VEP recorded in the cataractous eye to that of the eye having clear media provides important information concerning the retina (especially macula), optic nerve, pathways, and cortex.[6, 7] In instances of multiply handicapped patients or those with cortical blindness, even positive VEPs to light may provide valuable information concerning the basic transmission of visual information to the cortex.

In most instances, the stimulus pattern is some type of video display with a time-locked trigger signal. This signal is commonly produced by a computer with the ability to change both amplitude and check or bar size. These systems use computer displays to generate the pattern alternation while the overall luminance on the monitor remains the same. Other, more sophisticated systems have the ability to display sine wave gratings or more complex waveforms. When patients have very poor vision (less than 20/400), a pattern VEP may be impossible to record. In

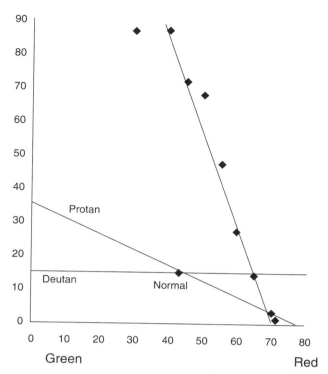

FIGURE 4-26. **Nagel anomaloscope testing shows the steeply sloped line that is the classic error pattern of a patient with mono-chromatism. This can be easily distinguished from error patterns of a protanope or deuteranope.**

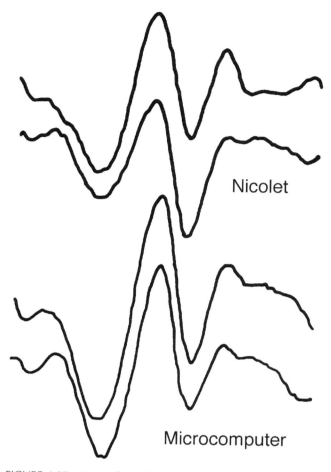

FIGURE 4-27. **Normal results on visual evoked potential testing. These results show the repeatability of subsequent recordings on the same individual using a stimulus produced by either a Nicolet Pattern generator or a microcomputer (Nicolet Instrument Corp., Madison, WI).**

such an instance, a diffuse-flash VEP may be tested, using an apparatus similar to that used for ERG testing.

SAMPLE RESULTS. The following case report illustrates how VEP testing assists in the management of a low vision patient who is unresponsive to routine testing. In patients with multiple impairments, it is often difficult to determine the extent to which a patient can see or use visual information. Patients who have a substantially normal afferent visual system (retina, optic nerve, visual radiations, and cortex) and respond favorably to electrodiagnostic testing may be helped by visual stimulation.

MB is a 4-month-old boy who was born 1 month prematurely. The chief complaint his parents express is that he exhibits no visually guided behavior. He could not cooperate for any visual acuity testing. Pupillary responses were normal, with no afferent defects noted. Ophthalmoscopy revealed grossly normal retina and optic nerves. Both ERG (using external electrodes) and VEPs with large checks (88-ft check size) were performed to determine both retinal and higher visual functioning. In this instance, ERG showed normal waveforms, implicit times, and amplitudes. VEP showed a repeatable response with normal P100 latencies (Figure 4-28). In the case of MB, one would expect that he had the basic structure and function to receive and process visual information. A program of visual stimulation was undertaken to improve the patient's response to visual stimuli. Three months after the initial electrodiagnostic examination, the patient was exhibiting visually guided behavior.

CONCLUSION

Low vision patients often have complicated ocular conditions requiring a variety of tests to determine the diagnosis, prognosis, or functional implications of their vision loss. The testing that has been described will assist the practitioner in providing the most efficient and comprehensive service for his or her low vision patients.

SELF-ASSESSMENT QUESTIONS

1. Contrast sensitivity testing will help the practitioner determine the need for _____ when evaluating his or her low vision patient.
   (a) increased illumination
   (b) decreased contrast
   (c) orientation and mobility services
   (d) all of the above
   (e) a and c

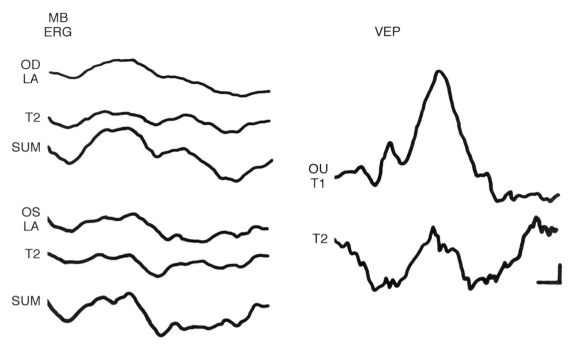

FIGURE 4-28.   **Electroretinogram (ERG) and visual evoked potential (VEP) testing results show that the patient (MB) has basic retinal and visual processing still functioning. ERGs were recorded under light adapted (LA) conditions for two trials (T1 and T2) before being computer summated (SUM). The VEP was recorded binocularly (OU) for two trials (T1 and T2).**

2. Information provided by CS testing may be helpful in determining
    (a) monocularity versus binocularity
    (b) dominant eye
    (c) need for increased magnification
    (d) all of the above
    (e) a and c

3. The ratio of an object to the CT is referred to as *Weber contrast.*
True or False

4. Advanced macular degeneration will most likely show a decrease in high spatial frequency with contrast sensitivity testing.
True or False

5. When a patient consistently has difficulty finding the beginning of the next line when reading, the following test(s) should be performed.
    (a) contrast sensitivity testing
    (b) Goldmann's field test
    (c) Amsler's grid test
    (d) potential acuity meter test
    (e) all of the above

6. When performing a brightness acuity test on a low vision patient, a decrease of two or more lines of visual acuity may indicate glare problems.
True or False

7. The greatest advantage of using white light interferometry is that the light will penetrate totally dense cataract.
True or False

8. ERG testing provides valuable information concerning the structure of the retina.
True or False

9. ERG testing provides valuable information concerning the function of the retina.
True or False

10. In patients with retinitis pigmentosa, the ERG is usually decreased only after ophthalmoscopic signs are visible.
True or False

11. VEP testing is valuable in patients with suspect optic nerve lesions.
True or False

12. A-scan is the preferred ultrasound method for determining the lateral extent of a retinal detachment.
True or False

13. D-15 testing is helpful to differentiate patients with rod monochromatism from those with protanopia or deuteranopia.
True or False

14. Rod and blue cone monochromatism can be differentiated by the results on the Nagel anomaloscope.
True or False

15. Dark adaptometry would be of no value to help determine the sensitivity or disease progression in patients with retinitis pigmentosa.
True or False

16. Laser interferometry, bright-flash electroretinography, visual evoked potentials, and B-scan ultrasonography all have a place in evaluating the potential visual function of low vision patients who are possible referrals for cataract surgery.
True or False

REFERENCES

1. Timberlake GT, Mainster MA, Pelli E, et al. Reading with a macular scotoma: I. Retinal location of scotoma and fixation area. Invest Ophthalmol Vis Sci 1986;27:1137–1147.

2. Schuchard RA. Validity and interpretation of Amsler grid reports. Arch Ophthalmol 1993;111:776–780.

3. Whittaker SC, Budd JM, Cummings RW. Eccentric fixation with macular scotoma. Invest Ophthalmol Vis Sci 1988;29: 268–278.

4. Berson E, Sandberg M, Rosner B, Sullivan PL. Color plates to help identify patients with blue cone monochromatism. Am J Ophthalmol 1983;95:741–747.

5. Haegerstrom-Portnoy G, Schneck ME, Verdon WA, Hewlett SE. Clinical vision characteristics of the congenital achromatopsias. II. Color vision. Optom Vis Sci 1996;73:457–465.

6. Fuller G, Hutton W. Presurgical Evaluation of Eyes with Opaque Media. New York: Grune & Stratton, 1982;29–88.

7. Knighton R, Blankenship G. Electrophysiological evaluation of eyes with opaque media. Int Ophthalmol Clin 1980:20;1–19.

CHAPTER FIVE

Scanning Laser Ophthalmoscope: A New Frontier for Low Vision Rehabilitation

Leonard H. Ginsburg and Michael Colucciello

The scanning laser ophthalmoscope (SLO) has created much interest by its ability to produce high-contrast dynamic images and by its ability to perform psychophysical tests with simultaneous visualization of the fundus. The SLO's macular perimetry function enables characterization of illuminance sensitivities in the macular region. This allows the practitioner to follow the course of macular disease, allows for prediction of scotoma post–laser surgery and post–macular surgery, and facilitates low vision training in patients with macular scotomata. This chapter describes the SLO, how it works, and how it relates to low vision rehabilitation.

OVERVIEW OF THE SCANNING LASER OPHTHALMOSCOPE

The SLO allows for real-time confocal and nonconfocal imaging of the retina. It uses a laser source (infrared or helium-neon) to scan over an area of the retina to be imaged on a video monitor.[1, 2] Consecutive laser scanning of the fundus allows for a small spot on the retina to be illuminated at any point. The light returned from this focused spot inside the eye determines the brightness of a corresponding pixel on the video monitor.[3] Consecutive scanning used in a raster fashion, using a spinning mirror and an oscillating mirror, enables successive points on the fundus to be built up as an array of pixels (voxels) on the video monitor. The angle through which the laser beam is scanned determines the field of view (either a 20-degree or a 40-degree mode may be chosen).

The photodetector in the scanning laser ophthalmoscope assesses returned light from the illuminated spot on the fundus. If the photodetector accepts all of the light returning from the eye, then the image is said to be nonconfocal. Images that are nonconfocal have decreased contrast due to scattering of light. To improve the contrast of the image, the photodetector can receive light that is scattered back directly from the laser focus by placing a confocal aperture pinhole in front of the detector conjugate to the laser focus (Figure 5-1). The confocal SLO uses a double scanning system in which the same scanning system is used in reversed directions for the illumination and detection systems. This setup enables the detection system to scan in synchrony with the laser illumination directing these systems on the same point on the fundus. In the confocal mode, reflected light that is not conjugate (focused in the same plane) to the confocal aperture will not contribute to the image, therefore allowing for a tomographic image (Figure 5-2). This process is contrasted with conventional imaging, in which objects outside the field depth contribute a blurred image. The thickness of the optical section in the SLO depends on the confocality of the image. A smaller confocal aperture provides a narrower optical section. The plane of focus may be moved by using the ametropic corrector to alter the plane that is conjugate to the confocal aperture.

The use of an annular aperture produces a nonconfocal mode by blocking out light directly scattered back from the laser while allowing light that has been rescattered from an area adjacent to the laser focus to pass through (Figure 5-3). Objects that have many scattering centers will appear bright in this mode (e.g., drusen).

As a device allowing for the imaging of retinal tissue, the SLO will provide the following advantages:

- A thin collimated laser beam transmits easily through even a small pupillary aperture or around lenticular opacities, yielding far superior retinal images compared

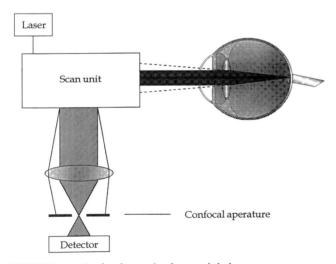

FIGURE 5-1. **Confocal scanning laser ophthalmoscope.**

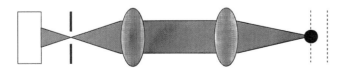

FIGURE 5-2. **Confocal mode of the scanning laser ophthalmoscope yielding tomographic image.**

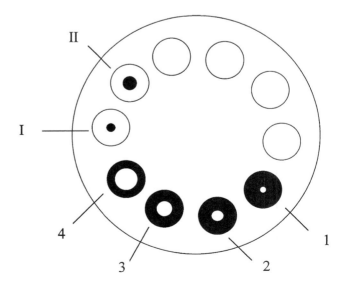

FIGURE 5-3. **Confocal (1–4) and annular (I and II) apertures.**

to standard photography in the setting of small pupils or cataracts.

- Owing to monochromaticity and consecutive scanning with a collimated thin beam, there is far less scattering of light from media opacities and the optic nerve with SLO acquisition as compared to standard photography. This yields an image with much higher contrast.
- Tomographic images may be obtained with an SLO.
- Annular apertures and infrared imaging yield better choroidal detail than standard images.

The SLO does have some disadvantages as well, including the following:

- Cost
- Resolution is limited by the number of pixels that the current television monitor technology allows for

APPLICATIONS

The SLO has been used for a number of functions, including intravenous fluorescein[4] and indocyanine green video angiography,[5] quantitative measurement of erythrocyte flow velocities in perifoveal capillaries,[6] dynamic and morphologic analysis of the perifoveal capillary network,[7] measurement of optic nerve head topography,[8, 9] analysis of visual evoked response,[10] and stereoscopic photography.[11] An additional development has been the use of the confocal SLO tomographic images at different depths of the fundus, yielding three-dimensional information useful in the monitoring of glaucoma patients.[12] Retinal densitometry[13] and fundus tracking[14] measurements using the SLO have also been made.

PSYCHOPHYSICAL TESTING

In addition to the applications of the SLO mentioned in the previous section, evaluations of perimetry by modulation of the intensity of the scanning laser have been described.[15, 16] The low vision practitioner may use the perimetry function of the SLO for macular perimetry, localized retinal acuity testing, and low vision instruction and rehabilitation.

Macular Perimetry

The import of the measurement of the visual field of patients with glaucoma, retinitis pigmentosa, and optic neuritis is well known, but in general, central visual field testing of patients with macular degeneration or other maculopathies has not been as well appreciated. The most challenging aspect of macular perimetry is obtaining steady and accurate fixation. Patients with macular disease often have unsteady, eccentric, and inconsistent fixation patterns.[17, 18] Although many macular perimetry protocols are based on experience with peripheral visual field test-

ing, this disturbed fixation behavior often makes the results inaccurate or incomplete. The fixation monitoring technique of using the physiologic blind spot allows for a 5-degree unsteadiness in fixation without detection, and this method is used in the standard perimetry equipment. Studies have shown that the SLO macular perimetry function is more sensitive in detecting small, localized scotomas than is standard clinical perimetry.[19] Obtaining a very accurate assessment of the central visual field enables the practitioner to predict functional difficulties and possibly plan appropriate adaptation strategies.

During perimetry with the SLO, the retina is stimulated with a modulated, visible, 633-nm red light laser. The patient sees the stimulus, and it is also observed directly on the patient's retina by the doctor, enabling more accurate fixation monitoring, as the practitioner directly observes each retinal point that is stimulated at a given time. The resolution of the SLO is approximately 20 µ for measurement of the retinal areas and the positioning of targets. The targets can be varied from a small dot of light to letters, words, and even sentences. The illumination of the stimuli are adjustable by 256 steps, from 100 trolands to 100,000 trolands. This resolution restricts the SLO to projecting stimuli with a minimum resolution of approximately 20/40. Kinetic, static, or hybrid testing techniques are possible with the SLO macular perimetry method to evaluate light sensitivity in the central 20 degrees of the visual field.

A threshold of light levels may be obtained at the most sensitive macular area, determining the presence and location of any macular scotomata. Macular scotomas are retinal areas of decreased light sensitivity. These areas are located within the central 20 degrees of visual field, and are classified as either central or paracentral. Central scotomas involve the fovea, whereas paracentral scotomas are within the central 20 degrees but spare the fovea. Dense (or absolute) scotomas are retinal areas that are insensitive to the brightest target of the perimeter. Relative scotomas may be mapped for any stimulus intensity between the threshold and the brightest stimulus. Physical and functional borders of lesions can be defined for rehabilitation purposes or therapeutic interventions such as photocoagulation.

Methods of Macular Perimetry Testing

Visual stimulation is produced in the laser beam raster by means of the computer and graphics board coupled to a modulator on the SLO. The modulator can change the intensity of the scanned laser beam in response to electronic signals from the graphics generator in the SLO computer. The pattern produced by the SLO computer and projected onto the patient's retina is displayed simultaneously on the monitor. The SLO obtains retinal images in real time with a near infrared laser (780 nm) and scans graphics on the retina with the modulated visible helium-neon laser (633 nm). The SLO provides the fundus image with a minimum resolution of 4 minutes of arc (20 µ) for measurement in positioning of targets.

Fixation location with the SLO is evaluated by having the patient gaze at a stationary as well as a moving cross. Preferred retinal locus location is determined by instructing the patient to look directly at the cross (99% contrast relative to background illumination of 15×15 pixels—approximately 40×40 minutes of arc). The doctor notes the location and the patient is then instructed to follow a moving cross. The doctor now notes whether the patient can maintain pursuit within a discreet retinal location. The anatomic location of the preferred retinal locus (PRL) is recorded directly on fundus images. In this way, the PRL is located by actually monitoring the retinal location of the cross stimulus. This evaluation is performed before macular perimetry.

Macular perimetry is often performed via a "hybrid perimetry" technique that combines kinetic and static visual field testing. Stationary flash stimuli, as in static perimetry, are presented, but successive flashes are moved progressively across the retina, as in kinetic perimetry, to map isopters. Hybrid perimetry is measured on a background illumination produced by a 633-nm helium-neon laser. Stimuli intensity varies from 5 dB to 40 dB, measuring approximately 24×24 minutes of arc presented for 367 ms. The stimulus is presented at regular intervals and is positioned on the retina by a mouse connected to the SLO computer. Five "rows" of five stimuli are initially presented across the macular region in a grid fashion. Other special areas of interest can then be tested based on the specific anatomy and clinical situation.

Localized Acuity Testing

The SLO can also be used to project an acuity target on a specific retinal locus, which is again directly observed by the doctor, enabling him or her to manually position stimuli, in the form of optotypes, on the patient's fundus and to adjust the intensity and size. This technique enables measurement of visual acuity at individual retinal positions, which can be combined with macular perimetry findings to more effectively help patients in optimizing their visual function.

Low Vision Instruction and Rehabilitation

Activities of daily living may be affected by macular scotomata. Patients with macular scotomata may have impairment of both visual performance and visual function, which can make activities of daily living difficult. Visual performance areas that may be affected include spatial perception,[20] visual search,[21] face recognition,[22, 23] and reading.[24–26] Visual functions that may be impaired are visual acuity, contrast discrimination,[27] contrast sensitivity,[28] stereoscopic depth perception,[29] and stability and precision of fixation.[17, 18, 30]

Patients with a central scotoma often develop a PRL or even multiple PRLs. The PRL is the area of the retina that has been chosen by the patient as the retinal location for fixation. This term usually indicates a visual system that has chosen an extrafoveal retinal area for visual tasks normally performed within the fovea. Multiple preferred retinal loci can affect clinical tests, such as acuity and contrast sensitivity, by reporting over two or more retinal loci. The instability of PRL for fixation makes accurate mapping of scotomatous boundaries difficult. The SLO has shown that persons with low vision can have a PRL as small as that of persons with normal vision (1–2 degrees) and as large as 9 degrees. Therefore, pericentral fixation targets may be very helpful.[17]

It is important to realize that the location of a PRL cannot be determined by visual acuity alone. The SLO macular perimetry function allows for more accurate detection of the PRL, and therefore, provides important information on a patient's eccentric fixation or eccentric viewing position. *Eccentric fixation* refers to use of an extrafoveal retinal locus in which the object of regard is perceived as being straight ahead. In this case, the patient is using the PRL as a pseudofovea. With *eccentric viewing*, however, a retinal locus is used that results in the visual object being perceived as above, below, or to either side of fixation. When the patient eccentrically views, he or she is attempting to compensate for his or her central scotoma.

Once the PRL is determined via the SLO, instruction with regard to eccentric fixation could facilitate stability in fixation behavior and enable use of the eccentric retinal area to optimize vision. This may allow for possible improvement in activities of daily living. The Rodenstock SLO provides specific software localized visual acuity testing of different macular loci called *visumetry*. The patient can be trained to use the retinal locus of best visual function for reading and other activities of daily living. To accomplish this, targets are projected onto the patient's retina with the hope of teaching the patient to use a PRL with consistency that will also provide maximum acuity. Many low vision practitioners think that patients with eccentric preferred retinal loci benefit greatly from eccentric viewing instruction; however, some patients do not improve with instruction.[31] The SLO may prove to be very valuable in providing answers as to why a patient does not respond to eccentric viewing instruction as well.

Adaptation of the Visual System

Most studies regarding a PRL have been done monocularly, and little is known about how preferred retinal loci interact binocularly. Furthermore, monocular characteristics of preferred retinal loci and macular scotomas cannot always be extrapolated to binocular viewing tasks.[32] Preferred retinal loci characteristics are, however, important in their relationship to activities of daily living for low vision patients and need to be assessed. It has been shown that the visual system chooses PRL regions that avoid scotomatous borders below fixation or to the left of fixation.[16, 33] From a functional standpoint, this preference makes sense because visual field defects below the PRL may interfere with visual tasks such as walking, reading, writing, and eating. These tasks require information from the inferior visual field, and reading behavior proceeds from left to right in Western cultures.

Macular perimetry on the SLO has documented that many patients with small macular scotomas do not perceive them during their activities of daily living yet have more difficulty than one would expect.[19] Perceptual completion is a poorly understood phenomenon in which objects appear complete or filled in, without missing visual information, when part of the object falls in a scotoma.

IMPLICATIONS FOR THE LOW VISION PRACTITIONER

Most (four-fifths) of the common low vision conditions are associated with macular scotomata.[34] These macular scotomas may substantially affect activities of daily living. There are obvious implications regarding the information that may be derived from central visual field testing using SLO macular perimetry. This information is very important in obtaining an assessment of central visual function to predict functional difficulties and determine residual capacities. The information obtained from the SLO may be effectively used to plan appropriate rehabilitation strategies.

For example, the presence of a central scotoma predicts the reading speed in the low vision patient more powerfully than does visual acuity.[26, 35] Also, a scotoma to the left of a PRL would predict that the patient may have difficulty with a saccadic eye movement to the left hand margin of the page after completing a line of reading. Patients with a PRL encumbered by surrounding scotomas may have a limited response to magnification because magnifying the letter to a degree that is larger than the available field is of no benefit. Also, knowing the threshold sensitivity of the PRL and the threshold sensitivities of the regions around the PRL may indicate the need for extra illumination. The effective size of a visual island may be increased with optimal lighting (i.e., halogen-illuminated magnifiers).

The SLO macular perimetry function is important in understanding the central visual function of patients with macular disease. Although questions regarding the binocular integration of monocular measurements do exist, the low vision practitioner is aided greatly in the evaluation and treatment of patients by the capabilities of the SLO and the information derived from its use.

SELF-ASSESSMENT QUESTIONS

1. If the photodetector in the scanning laser ophthalmoscope accepts all of the light returning from the eye, the image is said to be *confocal*.
   True or False

2. The eye care practitioner can use the scanning laser ophthalmoscope for which of the following functions:
   (a) fluorescein and indocyanine green angiography
   (b) measurement of optic nerve head topography and electrodiagnostic testing
   (c) microperimetry and visumetry
   (d) all of the above
   (e) a and c

3. During perimetry with the scanning laser ophthalmoscope,
   (a) the retina is stimulated with visible white light
   (b) the light stimulus is visible to the patient as well as the examiner
   (c) the target can have varied illumination levels and is therefore capable of performing static testing only
   (d) all of the above
   (e) a and b

4. The scanning laser ophthalmoscope allows for measurement of visual acuity at individual retinal positions and is capable of obtaining a minimum resolution of 20/20.
   True or False

5. Patients with a central scotoma may often develop one or more preferred retinal locus (loci).
   True or False

6. In most cases, the position of a preferred retinal locus can be determined by the patient's best visual acuity.
   True or False

REFERENCES

1. Webb RH, Hughes GW, Delori FC. Confocal scanning laser ophthalmoscope. Appl Opt 1987;26:1492–1499.
2. Mainster MA, Timberlake GT, Webb RH, Hughes GW. Scanning laser ophthalmoscopy: clinical applications. Ophthalmology 1982; 89:852–857.
3. Woon WH, Fitzke FW, Bird AC, Marshall J. Confocal imaging of the fundus using a scanning laser ophthalmoscope. Br J Ophthalmol 1992;76:470–474.
4. Tanaka T, Muraoka K, Shimizu K. Fluorescein fundus angiography with scanning laser ophthalmoscope; visibility of leukocytes, platelets, and perifoveal capillaries. Ophthalmology 1991;98: 1824–1829.
5. Scheider A, Nasemann JE, Lund OE. Fluorescein and indocyanine green angiographies of central serous choroidopathy by scanning laser ophthalmoscopy. Am J Ophthalmol 1993;115:50–56.
6. Wolf S, Arend O, Toonen H. Retinal capillary blood flow measurement with a scanning laser ophthalmoscope, preliminary results. Ophthalmology 1991;98:996–1000.
7. Arend O, Wolf S, Jung F. Retinal microcirculation in patients with diabetes mellitus: dynamic and morphological analysis of perifoveal capillary network. Br J Ophthalmol 1991;75:514–518.
8. Cioffi GA, Robin AL, Eastman RD. Confocal laser scanning ophthalmoscope; reproduce ability of optic nerve head topographic measurements with the confocal laser scanning ophthalmoscope. Ophthalmology 1993;100:57–62.
9. Chihara E, Takahashi F, Chihara K. Assessment of optic disc topography with scanning laser ophthalmoscope. Graefe's Arch Clin Exp Ophthalmol 1993;231:1–6.
10. Katsumi O, Van de Velde FJ, Mehta MC, Hirose T. Topographical analysis of peripheral versus central retina with pattern reversal visual evoked response and the scanning laser ophthalmoscope. Acta Ophthalmologica 1991;69:596–602.
11. Frambach DA, Dacey MP, Sadden A. Stereoscopic photography with a scanning laser ophthalmoscope. Am J Ophthalmol 1993; 116:484–488.
12. Weinreb RN, Dreher AW. Reproduceability and Accuracy of Topographic Measurements of the Optic Nerve Head with the Laser Tomographic Scanner. In JE Nasemann, ROW Burk (eds), Scanning Laser Ophthalmoscopy and Tomography. Munich: Quintessenz Verlags, 1990;177–182.
13. Van Norren D, Van de Kratts J. Imaging retinal densitometry with a confocal scanning laser ophthalmoscope. Vision Res 1989; 29:1825–1830.

14. Worson DP, Hughes GW, Webb RH. Fundus tracking with the scanning laser ophthalmoscope. Appl Opt 1987;26:1500–1504.
15. Sturmer J, Schrodel C, Rappl W. Scanning Laser Ophthalmoscope for Static Fundus-Controlled Perimetry. In JE Nasemann, ROW Burk (eds), Scanning Laser Ophthalmoscopy and Tomography. Munich: Quintessenz Verlags, 1990;133–146.
16. Fletcher DC, Schuchard RA, Livingstone CO. Scanning laser ophthalmoscope macular perimetry and applications for low vision rehabilitation clinicians. Ophth Clin North Am 1994;7:257–265.
17. Schuchard RA, Raasch TW. Retinal locus for fixation: pericentral fixation targets. Clin Vis Sci 1992;7:511–620.
18. White JM, Bedell HE. The oculomotor reference in humans with bilateral macular disease. Invest Ophthalmol Vis Sci 1990;31: 1149–1161.
19. Schuchard RA. Validity and interpretation of Amsler grid reports. Arch Ophthalmol 1993;111:776–780.
20. Turano K, Schuchard RA. Space perception in observers with visual field loss. Clin Vis Sci 1991;6:289–299.
21. Schuchard RA. Retinal Locus for Identification and Observers with Vision Loss. Non-Invasive Assessment of the Visual System. In Technical Digest on Non-Invasive Assessment of the Visual System (vol 1). Washington, DC: Optical Society of America 1991:46–49.
22. Peli E, Goldstein RB, Young GM. Image enhancement for the visually impaired. Invest Ophthalmol Vis Sci 1991;32:2337–2350.
23. Schuchard RA, Rubin GS. Face identification of band-pass filtered faces by low vision observers. Invest Ophthalmol Vis Sci 1989;S30:396.
24. Cummings RW, Whittaker SG, Watson GR. Scanning characters and reading with a central scotoma. Am J Opt Phys Optics 1985;62: 833–843.
25. Fletcher DC, Schuchard RA, Warren ML, et al. A scanning laser ophthalmoscope preferred retinal locus scoring system compared to reading speed and accuracy. Invest Ophthalmol Vis Sci 1993;S34:787.
26. Legge GE, Rubin GS, Pelli DG. Psychophysics of reading II. Low vision. Vision Res 1985;25:253–266.
27. Schuchard RA. Contrast Discrimination in Observers with Visual Loss. Non-Invasive Assessment of the Visual System. In Technical Digest on Non-Invasive Assessment of the Visual System (vol 1). Washington, DC: Optical Society of America 1991:100–103.
28. Mitra S. Spatial contrast sensitivity in macular disorder. Doc Ophthalmol 1985;59:247–267.
29. Raasch TW. A Method for Assessing Stereopsis and Positional Sensitivity in Normally Sighted and Low Vision Observers. In Technical Digest on Non-Invasive Assessment of the Visual System (vol 1). Washington, DC: Optical Society of America 1991:109–112.
30. Whittaker SG, Budd JM, Cummings RW. Eccentric fixation with macular scotoma. Invest Ophthalmol Vis Sci 1988;29:268–278.
31. Culham L, Silver J, Bird A. Assessment of low vision instruction in age-related macular disease. Proceedings of the International Conference on Low Vision, Sydney, Australia, 1990;162–165.
32. Schuchard RA, Fletcher DC. Preferred retinal locus: a review with applications in low vision rehabilitation. Ophth Clin North Am 1994;7:243–256.
33. Guez JE, Francois JF, Rigaudiere F. Is there a systematic location for the pseudo-fovea in patients with central scotoma? Vision Res 1993;33:1271–1279.
34. Schuchard RA. Adaption to macular scotomas in persons with low vision. Am J Occup Ther 1995;49:870-876.
35. Legge GE, Ross JA, Isenberg LM. Psychophysics of reading-clinical predictors of low-vision reading speed. Invest Ophthalmol Vis Sci 1992;33:677–687.

CHAPTER SIX

Common Disorders Encountered in Low Vision

Jennifer Tasca and
Edward A. Deglin

To holistically treat a patient with an eye condition that causes a visual impairment, a general understanding of the pathology is necessary. The low vision practitioner must be familiar with systemic as well as ocular signs and symptoms, level of visual acuity, visual field defects, and syndromes that are associated with each condition. In addition, information regarding inheritance patterns of the ocular condition should be made clear to the patient so that appropriate decisions can be made and family history can be recorded for the benefit of future generations. Finally, patients should be aware of the visual prognosis of their condition, with and without medical treatment, so that they will be cognizant of the expected outcome.

GENETICS

In attempting to understand the various disorders involved in low vision patients, it is important to have a basic understanding of genetics. An individual is born with 23 pairs of chromosomes with each chromosome containing thousands of genes. The first 22 pairs of chromosomes are called *autosomal*, whereas the twenty-third pair makes up the *sex chromosome*. The genes are responsible for specific physical features of the individual, such as color of the iris. This feature (iris color) will depend on how the chromosomes from each parent were aligned as the embryo developed; it will also depend on how the genes in one chromosome of a pair link up with their opposites in the other chromosome. One or more contrasting genes, situated at the same locus in homologous chromosomes, are called *alleles*. These alleles actually determine the characteristics in inheritance (i.e., blue eyes versus brown eyes). The assumption in genetics is that these allelic genes work independently of other genes on the chromosomes. The only exception would be with the sex chromosome of the male, who receives the X chromosome from the mother and the Y chromosome from the father. The mode of inheritance from genes in the sex chromosome will obviously be different than that seen in the autosomal genes.

To understand how certain disorders are caused by genetic transmission, it is important to define two other terms: *autosomal dominant genes* and *autosomal recessive genes*. A dominant gene is one in which the feature it determines will appear in the next generation regardless of the character of the state of the corresponding gene (on the paired chromosome). A recessive gene will produce an effect on the individual only when it is transmitted by both parents.

Geneticists have also divided the modes of transmission into classifications of which single-gene disorders and multiple-gene disorders are commonly described modes. *Single gene disorders* are a relatively simple example of how inheritance works. In this case, the disease is caused by a single defective gene (the gene can be autosomal recessive, autosomal dominant, or sex-linked) and is easier to predict. Many disorders are not inherited through a defective single gene but through more than one, and here the picture becomes much more complex.

It can be said that a particular disorder "tends to run in families" (e.g., age-related macular degeneration [ARMD]), which means that there is probably a genetic element present in the particular disorder but that it is difficult to isolate and define. Furthermore, the interaction between genes may be influenced or modified by diet or environmental factors.

A summary of the characteristics of a single gene inheritance pattern is as follows:

1. Autosomal recessive
   a. Parents of an affected child are usually clinically normal; however, they both carry the defective gene.
   b. Both males and females are at equal risk.
   c. Two carrier parents of the same defect can expect a 25% chance of producing the disorder in their offspring. One affected parent and one carrier parent will have a 50% chance of affected offspring and two affected parents will have 100% of the offspring at risk.
2. Autosomal dominant
   a. In all cases, the affected individual has an affected parent; however, in some cases, the affected parent may have a very mild form that goes undetected. In cases in which the affected individual has very mild manifestations, other family members should be examined.
   b. Both males and females are at equal risk.
   c. Families typically show affected individuals in each generation. In those cases in which the disorder is mild, the trait may appear to skip a generation.
   d. An individual with the affected gene married to an unaffected individual will have a 50% chance of producing affected offspring.
3. Sex-linked transmission
   a. The male carries an X chromosome and a Y chromosome, whereas the female has two X chromosomes. The Y chromosome carries only genes characteristic of male traits; the X chromosome carries female traits and genes for other characteristics, such as color vision loss and ocular albinism. Therefore, when these sex-linked chromosomes produce disorders, transmission may be referred to as *X-linked*.
   b. X-linked transmission affects males predominantly, with the female carriers of a single chromosome with the X-linked trait being unaffected. An affected male will not transmit the disorder to a male offspring, but all of his female offspring will be carriers.
   c. The affected child's mother, who is a carrier, will have a 50% chance of having a brother who is affected by the disorder.

As science and medicine expand the knowledge of inherited disorders, genetic counseling becomes more important. The purpose of such counseling is to help couples who are concerned about their offspring inheriting a disorder. With some inherited disorders, risks are more difficult to calculate because information on the carriers is not completely reliable. Tests are continuously becoming available to determine whether a parent is a potential carrier. Also, the counselor may have to make an extensive study of all family lines before estimating the risks. In all cases, however, the advice from a genetic counselor is based only on percentages, and the final decision will always be at the discretion of the couples.

ACHROMATOPSIA

Description

Achromatopsia is a hereditary condition in which the cones have not developed properly, therefore leading to an absence of color discrimination. There are two types of achromatopsia: (1) rod monochromatism, which is true color blindness; and (2) blue cone monochromatism, which is caused by a loss of red and green cones.

Etiology

Rod monochromatism is the most common form of achromatopsia and is transmitted as an autosomal recessive trait. Blue cone monochromatism is transmitted as an X-linked recessive inherited pattern and symptoms tend to be milder than with rod monochromatism.[1, 2]

Incidence

This hereditary condition is found in 3 of 100,000 males. Occurrence in females is slightly less.[1]

Visual Acuity

Distance visual acuity ranges from 20/60 to 20/200. Vision is somewhat better at near distances and in dim illumination and worse in bright illumination.[1, 2]

Visual Fields

Visual fields are usually normal but can be slightly constricted, particularly to colors.[3]

Ocular Signs and Symptoms

Achromatopsia, or absence of cones, results in reduced central acuity in bright light, pronounced decrease in color perception, and photophobia. Pendular nystagmus also results from the diminished acuity and may decrease at near. Nystagmus and photophobia may diminish after the age of 15 years.[4]

Pupils react sluggishly to light and paradoxical responses have been reported during dark adaptation.

These patients typically have blond fundi and fine disturbances of retinal pigment epithelium (RPE) in the macula.

Adjunct Testing

Electrodiagnostic testing reveals normal electro-oculogram (EOG) and scotopic electroretinogram (ERG) responses and subnormal photopic ERG responses. Color testing, with a Farnsworth dichomatous test (D-15) or Nagel anomaloscope, is helpful in diagnosing this condition. Blue monochromat plates can be used to distinguish rod monochromatism from blue monochromatism.

Fluorescein angiography (FA) may show mild hyperfluorescence when disturbance of RPE is present.

Low Vision Management

The patient will function better in an environment with reduced illumination. Filters, tints, and sun lenses aid in decreasing levels of illumination both indoors and outdoors. Side shields on a spectacle frame along with hats with large brims may be helpful for outdoors. Red tinted contact lenses and red sun lenses have been used to decrease photophobia with some success.

Magnification devices for distance and near are also beneficial for these patients.

Prognosis

The prognosis for rod monochromats is favorable because it is a nonprogressive condition. Nystagmus and photophobia may decrease by mid-teenage years; however, diminished central acuity remains.

AGE-RELATED MACULAR DEGENERATION

Description

ARMD is an acquired retinal disorder that is caused by degenerative changes in the RPE with subsequent degeneration of the overlying cones and rods. ARMD results in progressive, irreversible loss of central vision from fibrous scarring or geographic atrophy of the macular area.[5-7]

Etiology

At this time, the exact causes of ARMD are not known. Pathogenic studies demonstrate that there are defects in the processing of photoreceptor outer segments by the RPE as well as a deposition of abnormal material within the RPE and underlying Bruch's membrane. It appears that hereditary and genetic factors predispose certain eyes to this degenerative process.[7, 8] Other potential causes may include excessive light exposure,[9–12] nutritional factors,[13, 14] and other as yet undetermined biological,[15, 16] toxic, or vascular elements.[17]

Risk Factors

A number of ocular, systemic, behavioral, and genetic risk factors for the development or severity of ARMD have been identified from the results of epidemiologic studies.[5, 13, 18]

Hyperopia was the most common refractive error found in patients with ARMD.[5, 18, 19] A lower risk of ARMD with increased cup-to-disk ratio has also been observed. In addition, dark ocular pigmentation has been reported as a protective mechanism in some but not all studies.[7, 8, 20]

Systemic conditions, such as elevated serum cholesterol and hypertension, are reported in association with ARMD.[18, 21] However, these findings may be anecdotal with respect to the age group affected by ARMD.[7, 8, 21, 22] Smoking and sunlight exposure have also been associated with ARMD.[8, 9, 23] Conversely, dietary intake of fruits and vegetables high in lutein/zeaxanthin (carotenoids) has been shown to decrease the development of exudative ARMD.[8, 13, 24] No reduction in risk of ARMD was seen with increased intake of selenium, and there was no protective effect with increased levels of zinc.[13, 18]

Associated family history of ARMD is likely due to the role of shared environmental risk factors and genetic factors.[5, 7, 8, 11, 20, 25]

Prevalence and Incidence

ARMD is the second leading cause of legal blindness in the United States and other developed countries[5, 9, 13] and is the leading cause in individuals older than 65 years.[6] The prevalence of ARMD increases with age, and approximately 30% of patients aged 75 years and older are affected.[5–7] There is a greater prevalence in women than men in this age group.[5, 6]

Reports relating prevalence to race have varied in the confirmation of the clinical impression of ARMD, although it seems to be more frequently seen in whites than in blacks, and the more severe stages appear to be less common in blacks.[26, 27]

Visual Acuity

Visual acuity may vary with the extent of the degeneration. With dry-stage ARMD, acuity can range from 20/20 to 20/400. With wet-stage (exudative) ARMD, the acuity can show loss worse than 20/400. Approximately 750,000 Americans have visual acuity worse than 20/200 in one eye or both as a result of ARMD, of which 90% of these individuals experience the exudative form of the disease.[25]

Visual Field

Visual fields demonstrate a central or paracentral scotoma with normal peripheral findings.

Ocular Signs and Symptoms

Patients with ARMD may be completely asymptomatic or may have varying degrees of functional loss. Blurred vision, metamorphopsia, micropsia, or a central scotoma are the first symptoms usually noted with wet-stage disease. Patients with either dry- or wet-stage disease, however, may volunteer no symptoms or offer vague visual complaints, including the need for increased light intensity to read, fading of vision after a few minutes in bright light, and easy fatigability while doing close work.

Visual hallucinations characterized by appearances of people, animals, or objects is a complaint of some patients with bilateral ARMD (due to sensory deprivation). This hallucination or phenomenon is known as *Charles-Bonnet syndrome*.[28] This type of hallucination may occur secondary to some external factor, such as bright illumination, or may occur spontaneously with no known external cause. The majority of patients are aware that this type of hallucination is harmless; however, those patients who are concerned about a possible mental dysfunction should be assured of its benign nature.[29]

Dry Stage

Dry-stage ARMD may include drusen and RPE abnormalities, or both. The exact extent of these abnormalities necessary to be considered as pathologic as opposed to "normal aging" changes remains controversial.

Hard (nodular) drusen are typically small, sharply outlined, yellow-white nodules consisting of globular hyaline bodies.[30] Soft drusen are usually larger, with relatively indistinct borders, which may coalesce into small RPE detachments. Due to an abnormal underlying Bruch's membrane associated with soft drusen, these patients are predisposed to the development of choroidal neovascularization (CNV).[30, 31]

Calcified (glistening) drusen are often due to dystrophic calcification and may be associated with other types of drusen. This type of drusen often heralds the onset of geographic atrophy.

Cuticular (basal laminar) drusen are seen in younger patients. They appear as small yellow nodules representing focal nodular thickening of the basement membrane of the RPE. Some eyes may develop a vitelliform-like yellowish detachment of sensory retina, usually without subretinal neovascularization, which usually spontaneously regresses.[7, 30, 31–33]

RPE alterations occurring as manifestations of dry ARMD consist of geographic atrophy, reticular degeneration, and other pigmentary changes.[34–36]

Wet Stage (Exudative)

Wet-stage ARMD is characterized by the development of neovascularization from the choroid, which passes through Bruch's membrane. Although CNV is not always visible due to its sub-RPE location, clinically visible changes alerting the observer to the likelihood of its presence include gray RPE discoloration, localized sub-RPE elevation, subretinal or retinal exudate or hemorrhage, subretinal fluid, and radial choroidal folds in the macular area. CNV may not be apparent on clinical examination, however, and in many cases FA or indocyanine green (ICG) angiography is required for confirmation of its presence (Figure 6-1).[37]

RPE detachment (PED) may occur in conjunction with or as a result of CNV. Serous PED results from the leakage of choroidal neovascular proliferation that ophthalmoscopically appears as a discrete, dome-shaped, subretinal elevation.[35] An accompanying overlying neurosensory retinal detachment that typically extends beyond the boundaries of the PED may be present as well. Occasionally, other blood products may compose the PED. This hemorrhagic PED typically appears with a red or dark green hue. RPE detachments accompanied by drusen increase the risk for severe visual loss from CNV.[38]

In many eyes, the end-stage finding consists of fibrovascular tissue scar formation within Bruch's membrane or under the retina, known as a *disciform scar*, with the overlying retina undergoing cystic degeneration.

Adjunct Testing

Areas of scotoma or distortion can often, but not always, be mapped on an Amsler's grid. Each patient should be instructed in the methods of home self-testing performed at least once or twice weekly.

FA aids in determining the presence and extent of CNV. Early in the angiogram, classic CNV is characterized by well-demarcated areas of hyperfluorescence, while in the late phases, there is progressive leakage of fluorescein dye, which usually obscures the boundaries of the membrane.[39]

ICG angiography is used to better define CNV in instances in which fluorescein angiography alone provides an indeterminate result. ICG angiography may be indicated in certain cases of occult CNV (poorly defined margins); CNV associated with PED; recurrent CNV; and eyes with poor media quality due to cataract, blood in the vitreous, and exudative or serosanguinous material.[40, 41]

Angiography results help to determine whether the patient would benefit from laser treatment of CNV. FA should be performed within 72 hours of treatment because of the rapid growth of CNV. A repeat angiogram is typically required to determine the treatment efficacy and to rule out persistent or recurrent CNV.

Medical Treatment

Patients with unfavorable prognostic signs should be closely monitored at 6-month intervals with stereoscopic ophthalmoscopic evaluation or urgently if the patient reports decreased vision or changes on the Amsler's grid. The practitioner's reception desk staff must be educated in the need for prompt evaluation of any patient with ARMD who calls in complaining of new symptoms. Indications for referral to a retinal specialist for clinical evaluation and FA include signs of CNV or suspicious change in visual function.[7]

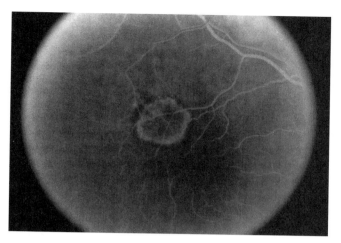

FIGURE 6-1. **Angiogram of new vessel membrane in age-related macular degeneration.**

Photocoagulation Therapy

The Macular Photocoagulation Study (MPS) was a multicenter trial to determine the efficacy of laser photocoagulation treatment for CNV.[42–45] First, the MPS prospectively evaluated the benefit of argon green laser treatment in preventing severe vision loss in patients with well-defined, extrafoveal membranes. Results demonstrated a reduction in the risk of severe vision loss (more than six lines of vision) with treatment (Table 6-1). The mean visual acuity at 5 years was 20/200 in untreated eyes and 20/125 in treated eyes. In this arm of the study, the recurrence rate was high, at 54% by 5 years. Eighty-six percent of recurrences were noted within 1 year of initial treatment, with the highest rate between 6 and 12 months. Recurrent disease was found to be correlated with cigarette smoking, large or confluent drusen in the fellow eye, and the presence of disciform scar in the fellow eye.[42, 44]

The second arm used krypton red laser for treating juxtafoveal CNV. The relatively longer wavelength of the krypton laser was thought to cause less absorption by macular xanthophyll pigment while allowing absorption on the RPE or hemoglobin within the membrane. Results of this arm of the study confirmed the benefit of krypton red treatment (Table 6-2).[46–48] As was the case for treated CNV in the argon arm of the study, recurrence rate was high, at 47% over 5 years. Patients with a fellow eye with CNV, a scar, 20 or more drusen in the macula, or nongeographic atrophy at the initial visit were more likely to have recurrences in

TABLE 6-1
Macular Photocoagulation Study Results: Extrafoveal Choroidal Neovascularization

Post-Treatment Period	Severe Vision Loss in Treated Eyes (%)	Severe Vision Loss in Untreated Eyes (%)
18 mos	33	51
5 yrs	46	64

TABLE 6-2
Macular Photocoagulation Study Results:
Juxtafoveal Choroidal Neovascularization

Post-Treatment Period (yrs)	Severe Vision Loss in Treated Eyes (%)	Severe Vision Loss in Untreated Eyes (%)
3	49	58
5	15	26

TABLE 6-3
Macular Photocoagulation Study Results:
Subfoveal Choroidal Neovascularization

Post-Treatment Period (mos)	Severe Vision Loss in Treated Eyes (%)	Severe Vision Loss in Untreated Eyes (%)	Reading Speed in Treated Eyes (words per min)	Reading Speed in Untreated Eyes (words per min)
3	20	11	33	44
24	20	37	28	12

treated eyes.[47] In view of these findings, patients should now be informed that it is likely that they will need at least two laser treatments.

Laser photocoagulation of subfoveal neovascular lesions was evaluated by the MPS as well.[49–51] When strict eligibility criteria and a well-delineated treatment protocol is adhered to, a definite treatment benefit was demonstrated for a selected group of patients. The benefit was not realized immediately because initially treated eyes are worse than are untreated eyes but function better over time (Table 6-3). Patients must be made aware of the expected immediate decrease in visual function and presence of a central scotoma in the region of laser treatment.[49–52]

Although laser treatment of RPE detachments is usually not recommended at present, treatment is often considered when there is a defined extrafoveal CNV adjacent to an RPE detachment.[53] ICG angiography may increase the number of potentially treatable cases in the future.

Surgery
The value of surgical excision of subfoveal CNV with or without RPE transplantation is unproved at present. In ARMD, the CNV often completely disrupts Bruch's membrane and invades overlying RPE, which may explain the disappointing results regarding surgical excision of membranes in ARMD. The Submacular Surgery Trial is underway, and it is expected that the results will provide guidelines for the use of this potential treatment in the future.[54–59]

Systemic Inhibitors of Neovascularization
Systemic inhibitors of neovascularization have been under evaluation. There are none with proved value at present. Interferon alfa-2a was among the first drugs stud-

ied. Despite the hopeful results of the initial investigators involved in small pilot studies, a large prospective, randomized, placebo-controlled clinical trial demonstrated no benefit.[60, 61]

Other drugs under consideration include interferon beta, retinoic acid, amiloride, AGM-1470 (a synthetic analogue of fumagillin), platelet factor IV, thrombosporin, TGF-beta, thalidomide, and neutralizing vascular endothelial growth factor antibodies.

Radiation Therapy
Low-dose radiation therapy to the macula has been studied. To date, preliminary data suggest that doses of 12 Gy or more result in a course more favorable than would be expected by the natural history. Follow-up for these series is limited at this time, and the role for radiation therapy remains unproved.[62–64]

Photodynamic Therapy
In photodynamic therapy, a photosensitizing dye is administered intravenously followed by light irradiation using nonthermal, low-intensity laser light at the absorption peak of the dye. Excitation of the dye is followed by generation of free radicals and reactive intermediates, resulting in tissue effects, including cellular damage to endothelial cells and vessel thrombosis. A phase III trial is in process at the time of this writing.[65]

Prophylaxis

It is currently unknown whether it is possible to offer preventative treatment against the development of ARMD or against the progression of established ARMD to a more advanced stage. The Age-Related Eye Disease Study has been initiated and is currently in progress to evaluate whether dietary supplementation with high-dose antioxidants slows the onset or progression of macular degeneration or lens opacities, or both.

Ultraviolet- and visible blue-blocking lenses can be prescribed for aphakia, pseudophakia, and young patients with a family history of ARMD, even though the role of light toxicity in the pathogenesis of this condition is unproved.

Other Future Strategies

Other future strategies may include free radical inhibitors or regulators, angiostatic intravitreal steroids, antisense oligonucleotides, integrins inhibitors, RPE and photoreceptor "en bloc" transplantation, and gene therapy.[59]

Low Vision Management

Many patients with long-standing ARMD have not had a recent, thorough refractive evaluation and may benefit from a change in prescription. Increased direct illumination should be recommended for all near tasks. Most patients respond well to magnification at distance and near. Nonoptical systems, filters, tints, and sun lenses for improved contrast, glare, and photophobia should be evaluated. In addition to optical and nonoptical devices, patients or family involvement, or both, in a support group may be beneficial.

Prognosis

The progression of vision loss in dry-stage ARMD is variable. Most patients with ARMD never develop the wet (exudative) form of the disease. Smiddy and Fine found that the incidence of progression to the wet stage over 5 years for patients with bilateral dry-stage disease was 14–20%.[32] Lower estimates have been reported by others, depending on the presence or absence of risk characteristics.

In the wet-stage form of the disease, the incidence of fellow-eye involvement is approximately 28–36% during the first 2 years, and the annual rate of bilateral involvement is 6–12% per year for the next 5 years.[7, 66, 67]

Patients will, in most cases, maintain useful peripheral vision indefinitely.

ALBINISM

Description

Albinism is a congenital condition characterized by lack of pigment or the body's inability to produce pigment. It can occur as oculocutaneous albinism, in which the skin, hair, and eyes are affected, or as ocular albinism, which only involves the eyes.

Etiology

The mode of transmission depends on the type of condition present. Oculocutaneous albinism may be inherited as either an autosomal recessive or autosomal dominant trait. Patients with the recessive form of the disease can have either the tyrosinase-negative or the tyrosinase-positive form, the latter having more ocular pigmentation and fewer visual symptoms.

Ocular albinism is usually inherited as an X-linked recessive trait. Therefore, males are affected by the condition and females are carriers. Carriers have characteristic areas of hypopigmentation scattered among areas of normally pigmented retina. Autosomal recessive inheritance of ocular albinism has also been described.[68, 69]

The pathophysiology of oculocutaneous albinism is reduction in the amount of pigment (melanin) in each of the pigment organelles (melanosomes). In ocular albinism, there is a reduction in the number of melanosomes, although some may be fully pigmented.

It is interesting to note that the offspring of albino parents of different subtypes (tyrosinase positive and tyrosinase negative) have produced only pigmented children.

Incidence

Oculocutaneous albinism occurs in 1 in 20,000 individuals in the general population. Ocular albinism occurs in 1 in 40,000.[69]

Visual Acuity

Tyrosinase-negative oculocutaneous albinism has the most severe effect on visual acuity, ranging from 20/200 to 20/400. Tyrosinase-positive patients generally have better acuity, which may improve over time as they tend to show increasing pigmentation as they grow older. This form is the most common in the United States.[69]

More ocular pigment is present in ocular albinism compared with the oculocutaneous forms. Visual acuity is usually 20/25 to 20/100. Visual acuity does not appear to improve greatly with age.

Visual Field

Visual fields are full, without defects in all forms of albinism.[69]

Systemic Signs and Symptoms

Albinism is the result of decreased pigmentation that can affect the skin, hair, and eyes and therefore predisposes these patients to actinic damage.

Ocular Signs and Symptoms

Oculocutaneous albinotic patients have white eyebrows and eyelashes. Irises are light blue and transilluminate markedly, causing photophobia. Patients with albinism have macular hypoplasia or complete aplasia resulting in decreased visual acuity and pendular sensory nystagmus. These patients have a tendency toward high hyperopic, myopic, or astigmatic (with-the-rule) refractive error. Also, these patients typically demonstrate poor stereopsis, due to abnormal chiasmal nerve fiber decussation, resulting in a high incidence of strabismus.

Fundus appearance includes prominence of choroidal vessels, seen through the depigmented fundus, and absence of a foveal reflex.

Associated Syndromes

Albinism has several associated subtypes and syndromes, which include

1. *Yellow mutant oculocutaneous albinism.* This form is most commonly seen among the Amish. These patients gradually accumulate pigment and may develop yellow-

red hair with cream yellow skin. Black patients may possess this form as well as demonstrate dark cream color skin with hair color ranging from dark yellow to light red. Pigmented nevi are common in these patients.

2. *Albinoidism.* Patients with albinoidism generally have a lighter complexion when compared to their unaffected siblings. They often sunburn easily but have good visual acuity and no nystagmus. Iris transillumination and fundus hypopigmentation with a dull foveal reflex are common.

3. *Hermansky-Pudlak syndrome,* which is most commonly found in the Puerto Rican population and characterized by albinism, easy bruising, epistaxis, and profuse bleeding on injury due to a serum platelet defect. These patients must avoid all medications (i.e., aspirin) that block prostaglandin synthase needed for platelet aggregation.

4. *Chédiak-Higashi syndrome,* which is a rare condition in which the patient has metallic gray hair and skin color and a progressive peripheral neuropathy and an increased susceptibility to infection.

Adjunct Testing

The hair bulb test can be performed to distinguish between tyrosinase-negative and tyrosinase-positive oculocutaneous albinism. Hairs epilated from the scalp are incubated in tyrosine solution. Tyrosinase-negative albinos will show no darkening of the hair bulb. In contrast, the hair bulbs of tyrosinase-positive albinos will become much darker.

Low Vision Management

Initially, therapy of the albinotic patient should be directed toward correcting refractive errors, which may improve visual acuity and reduce nystagmus. Controlling illumination with sun lenses, tints, ultraviolet protection, aperture or colored contact lenses, visors, and hats can often reduce photophobia. Albinotic patients are ideal candidates for magnification due to the absence of central or peripheral visual field defects. Because oscillopsia is absent, nystagmus is not a contraindication for telescopic distance magnification. Genetic counseling is also indicated.

Some albinotic patients have found that it is easier to read if the material is rotated or angled, whereas others may assume a compensatory head tilt as it is believed that the horizontal component of the nystagmus is less bothersome in this fashion.

Prognosis

Albinism is a nonprogressive condition that remains stable throughout the patient's lifetime. Some improvement of vision may be expected in tyrosinase-positive patients with increasing pigmentation as they grow older.

ANIRIDIA

Description

The term *aniridia* implies an absence of iris. However, in the majority of cases a small stump of iris tissue exists at the iris root. This is a bilateral anomaly, which has a tendency to form peripheral anterior synechia.[70]

Etiology

Aniridia is a congenital anomaly that develops at approximately the twelfth week of gestation. Two-thirds of the cases are inherited in the autosomal dominant fashion. The remaining one-third of the cases appear as a result of spontaneous mutation. No sexual or racial predilection for aniridia has been described.[71]

Incidence

Aniridia is found in 1 in 50,000–100,000 of the population.[72]

Visual Acuity

Visual acuity is usually decreased to levels of 20/100 to 20/400 due to an associated macular hypoplasia.[73, 74]

Visual Field

Visual field defects may occur due to secondary glaucoma.[73, 74]

Systemic Signs and Symptoms

There is a significant association with Wilms' tumor of the kidney in children with aniridia. One-fifth of spontaneous aniridic patients develop Wilms' tumor.[71, 75–77] Genitourinary abnormalities and mental retardation are also found with aniridia.

Ocular Symptoms and Signs

Photophobia is the principal subjective symptom experienced by patients with aniridia due to their enlarged pupillary aperture.[73, 74]

Microcornea with peripheral corneal pannus, which extends centrally causing corneal opacification, congenital polar cataracts and lens dislocation are frequent anterior segment findings.[78, 79]

Approximately 28% of patients with aniridia develop progressive glaucoma.[80] The development of glaucoma is dependent on the extent of blockage caused by the attachment of iris stump to the trabecular meshwork.[70, 80]

Macular hypoplasia, which is present at birth, results in decreased vision and sensory nystagmus.[70] Optic nerve hypoplasia may also be seen due to the smaller number of neurons extending from the hypoplasic macula.[70, 81]

Associated Syndrome

Miller's syndrome, or *WAGR*, is the name given to describe the relationship between *W*ilms' tumor, *a*niridia, *g*enitourinary abnormalities, and mental *r*etardation.[70, 77]

Medical Treatment

In cases of aniridia that progress to development of glaucoma, medical therapy should be implemented initially to control intraocular pressure. It has been suggested that early goniotomy be performed to prevent blockage of the trabecular meshwork by iris adhesions.[70] Filtering surgery may be performed but generally gives poor results.[82] Cyclocryotherapy may be of value for advanced glaucoma that is unresponsive to other treatment.

Corneal transplantation may be indicated due to opacification but often yields poor results.[83] Cataract extraction is often performed but not without complications.[84]

Low Vision Management

Pupillary aperture control contact lenses reduce photophobia and may improve visual acuity and decrease nystagmus. In some patients, however, contact lenses may be contraindicated if the cornea is compromised. Photophobic complaints should also be addressed with use of directed illumination, filters, and sun lenses.

Magnification devices for visual enhancement for distance and near are beneficial for these patients.

Genetic counseling is extremely important for patients with aniridia due to its dominant inheritance.

Prognosis

Secondary glaucoma in patients with aniridia is difficult to manage and can lead to blindness despite extensive effort.

CATARACT

Description

Cataract formation is defined as opacification of the crystalline lens, which is classified by anatomic locations of the opacity. The types include anterior and posterior subcapsular, anterior and posterior cortical, equatorial, and nuclear.

Etiology

The etiology of cataracts is variegated: traumatic, metabolic, toxic, pharmacologic, inflammatory, hereditary, and, most commonly, age-related.

In the normal lens, metabolic activity includes transport of amino acids and cations across the lens epithelium and synthesis of protein in the lens fibers. Any disruption of this metabolic process may lead to opacification of the lens and associated decreased vision.

Incidence

Approximately 95% of individuals older than the age of 65 years have some form of lens opacification.[85]

Visual Acuity

The effect of cataracts on visual acuity varies greatly depending on the degree and location of opacification. Acuity ranges from normal to severe vision impairment. Most often, cataracts are bilateral but asymmetric.

Early nuclear sclerotic cataracts are generally not associated with a decrease in visual acuity. Instead, the higher refractive power of the sclerotic lens causes a myopic shift with return of near vision and is referred to as *second sight*.

Posterior subcapsular cataracts often have a profound effect on visual acuity. Because of the central location of the opacity, decreased acuity is noted more in situations in which there are high levels of illumination, which cause pupillary constriction.

Visual Field

Central and peripheral field testing generally show a relative generalized depression without focal defects.

Ocular Signs and Symptoms

Retinoscopy may reveal a dull or abnormal reflex while refraction may yield an increase in myopia due to nuclear changes.

Biomicroscopic evaluation is essential to determining cataract severity and location. In addition, leukocoria is seen in cases of mature cataracts.

Glare and subsequent decreased acuity are the most common complaints for patients with cataracts, especially those in the posterior subcapsular location. Distortion and monocular diplopia can be experienced as well as

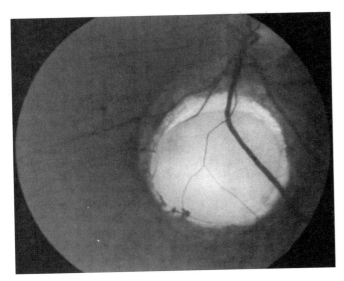

FIGURE 6-2.   **Retinochoroidal coloboma.**

alteration of color perception from nuclear yellowing of the lens.

Adjunct Testing

Interferometry or the use of the potential acuity meter (PAM), or both, can be performed to assess expected postoperative potential visual acuity. Ultrasonography can provide information regarding retinal integrity in the presence of dense media opacification, which obscures visualization of the retina.

Medical Treatment

Some patients with small central cataracts may eliminate glare and blur with use of mydriatics. Surgical removal of the lens is indicated when the decreased vision is interfering with the patient's lifestyle.

Low Vision Management

For patients with cataracts, direct lighting is generally required for near-point activities. Glare can be reduced by use of filters, tints, and sun lenses. Patients respond to magnification at distance and near, which may postpone the need for cataract surgery. Nonoptical systems, such as large-print reading material, bold-line writing paper, and a typoscope may be helpful.

Prognosis

A cataract is a disorder that can lead to severe visual impairment. However, successful lens removal usually results in complete visual recovery.

COLOBOMA

Description

Coloboma is a congenital "notch" that is the result of a defect in the closure of the embryonic cleft. The optic nerve, choroid, and retina can be involved posteriorly (Figure 6-2). Anteriorly, the defect can extend forward and affect the iris.

Etiology

The mode of inheritance of this congenital condition is not completely understood. It is thought to be transmitted as an autosomal dominant trait with variable penetrance.[86] There are also a number of cases in which sporadic, noninherited colobomas can be acquired in association with chromosomal abnormalities.[87]

Incidence

Colobomas are most commonly bilateral.

Visual Acuity

Visual acuity can range from normal to 20/400, depending on the extent and location of the coloboma. If the coloboma involves the optic nerve, vision is usually 20/200 or worse.

Visual Field

Coloboma located in the posterior pole may result in superior visual field loss.

Ocular Signs and Symptoms

Anteriorly, iris coloboma appears as an inferior, keyhole-shaped pupil that may cause the patient to experience glare. Posteriorly, optic nerve coloboma appears as an excavation within the nerve head from which 50% of patients develop nonrhegmatogenous retinal detachments.[87] Retinochoroidal coloboma appears as a white or yellow defect with pigmented borders inferior to the optic nerve head. With retinochoroidal coloboma, the sensory retina is present (visualized with blood vessels transversing through it), whereas the RPE and choroid are absent. Rarely, subretinal neovascularization can occur at the edge of the coloboma.[86, 87] In addition, sensory deprivation commonly causes strabismus and nystagmus.

Associated Syndromes

Coloboma can occur in association with various systemic diseases, including

1. *Trisomy 13* (D trisomy, Patau's syndrome). Coloboma is associated with this chromosomal disorder in almost 100% of cases. Failure to thrive results in death within the first months of life.[88]

2. *Aicardi's syndrome.* Coloboma and gray optic disk coloration are fundus findings that are associated with severe mental retardation and hypsarrhythmic electroencephalogram.[89]

3. *Goldenhar's syndrome* (oculoauriculovertebral dysplasia). Coloboma, dermoids, microphthalmia, and preauricular skin tags are prominent features of this disorder. Vertebral, cardiovascular, renal, and genitourinary anomalies may also be present.[90]

4. *CHARGE.* *C*oloboma, *h*eart disease, *a*tresia choanae, *r*etarded growth, *g*enital hypoplasia, and *e*ar anomalies.[91]

Medical Treatment

Retinal detachment and retinal breaks associated with colobomas require surgical repair.

Low Vision Management

Initially, refractive error should be investigated. Aperture-control or painted-iris contact lenses can help with cosmesis and glare caused by iris coloboma. Corning Photochromatic Filters (CPFs; Corning Medical Optics, Elmira, NY) and sun lenses are also helpful for control of glare and photophobia. Patients may function better in environments with reduced illumination.

Although mobility is generally unaffected by the superior field loss caused by posterior colobomas, patients can be instructed to scan the environment to avoid superior obstructions.

When visual acuity is affected, patients will respond well to magnification at distance and near.

Prognosis

Colobomas are generally stable, but potential complications, such as retinal detachment and neovascularization, should be monitored routinely.

CORNEAL DYSTROPHIES

Description

Corneal dystrophy is a bilateral inherited entity that begins early in life and is usually progressive. There are many types and presentations of corneal dystrophies[92]; therefore, only general information will be provided for the purpose of this text.

Etiology

Most corneal dystrophies are inherited in an autosomal dominant fashion.[93]

Visual Acuity

Visual acuity ranges from normal to light perception depending on the type of dystrophy and the severity of the condition.[92, 94]

Visual Field

Visual fields are usually unaffected by corneal dystrophy but may show generalized depression depending on severity.

Systemic Signs and Symptoms

Lattice dystrophy and *central crystalline dystrophy of Schnyder* may be associated by systemic disease. Lattice dystrophy, characterized by amyloid deposits between the epithelium, Bowman's layer, and throughout the stromal layers, is a sequela to systemic amyloidosis. Central crystalline dystrophy of Schnyder, represented by ring-shaped crystalline opacities in the central cornea, may be associated with systemic hyperlipidemia.

Ocular Signs and Symptoms

Ocular signs vary depending on the particular dystrophy. Common signs include corneal opacification, recurrent corneal erosion, astigmatism, and nystagmus and strabismus caused by visual deprivation.

Symptoms experienced by patients with corneal dystrophy vary in severity and duration. Lacrimation, photophobia, monocular diplopia (ghost images), foreign body sensation, and pain are common symptoms that occur due to corneal dystrophy.

Medical Treatment

Corneal erosions may be treated with antibiotics, cycloplegics, and a bandage contact lens or pressure patch. Lubricating drops or hyperosmotic agents may be necessary to prevent recurrent erosions.

Penetrating keratoplasty may be indicated when the sequelae of corneal dystrophy becomes severe.

Low Vision Management

Refractive error should be investigated carefully. Pinhole spectacle lenses and aperture-control contact lenses can reduce aberrations and ghost images caused by corneal dystrophy as well as reducing glare. In addition, sun lenses, tints, filters, and visors are helpful in reducing glare and photophobia for these patients both indoors and outdoors.

Magnification may be beneficial to some patients but detrimental to others because the ghost image can become magnified as well.

Nonoptical systems, such as large-print reading material, bold-line writing paper, and a typoscope, may be helpful.

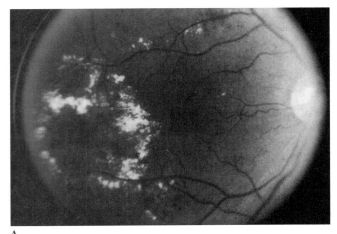

A

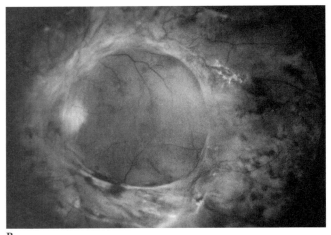

B

FIGURE 6-3.   A. Nonproliferative diabetic retinopathy. B. Proliferative diabetic retinopathy.

Prognosis

Corneal dystrophy is generally a slow progressive condition, which can be visually devastating if severe.

DIABETIC RETINOPATHY

Description

Diabetic retinopathy is a highly specific vascular complication of both type I (juvenile or insulin-dependent) and type II (age-related or non–insulin-dependent) diabetes mellitus. It is the leading cause of new cases of blindness in the United States in patients aged 20–64 years.[95, 96]

Etiology

The exact cause of diabetic microvascular disease is unknown.

In diabetic retinopathy, the supporting cells of the retinal capillaries (pericytes) die off, thereby weakening the capillary wall and allowing formation of microaneurysms. With progression, there is a breakdown of the blood-retina barrier, which allows blood constituents to leak or rupture into the retina. This decreases the retinal integrity both by a physical change (i.e., edema) or nutritional deprivation, or both, which leads to ischemia and subsequent neovascularization.

Morphologic changes include microaneurysms, dot hemorrhages, cotton-wool spots, venous caliber abnormalities, intraretinal microvascular abnormalities (IRMAs), and retinal and iris neovascularization.

Acellular capillaries are nonfunctional and lead to ischemia. The ischemic area produces vasoformative factors and neovascularization results.

Incidence

After a 20-year duration of diabetes, nearly all patients with insulin-dependent diabetes mellitus (type I) and more than 60% of patients with non–insulin-dependent diabetes (type II) have some degree of retinopathy.[96]

Visual Acuity

Depending on the severity of retinopathy, visual acuity ranges from 20/20 to total blindness. Diabetics experience decreased vision for many reasons. Most commonly, decreased vision is a result of lens changes (due to fluctuations in blood sugar level) or macular edema.

Visual Field

In proliferative disease, retinal ischemia, laser scars, and retinal detachment can cause corresponding field loss.

Systemic Signs and Symptoms

Typical signs and symptoms of diabetes mellitus may include the following: excessive thirst, excessive urination, excessive hunger, excessive fatigue, weight loss, recurrent infections, and slow healing.

Ocular Signs and Symptoms

Diabetic retinopathy is broadly classified as nonproliferative diabetic retinopathy (NPDR) and proliferative diabetic retinopathy (PDR) (Figure 6-3) with varying degrees of severity.[97]

Early NPDR is characterized by microaneurysms, hemorrhages or microaneurysms, venous beading, and IRMAs.

Severe NPDR is characterized by any one of the following: hemorrhages and microaneurysms in all four quadrants, venous beading in two or more quadrants, or IRMAs in at least one quadrant.

The hallmark of PDR is neovascularization, presenting either by new vessel growth on or within one disk diameter from the nerve head (NVD) or occurring elsewhere on the retina (NVE).

Vitreous traction on these new vessels may cause rupture leading to vitreous hemorrhage. As NVD and NVE progress, fibrous proliferation develops. Contracture of this fibrovascular complex can cause tractional detachment of the retina.

Three clinically recognizable situations are characteristic of high-risk PDR requiring immediate treatment:

1. Moderate to severe NVD (one-third to one-fourth disk area) with or without vitreous hemorrhage.
2. Less extensive NVD with preretinal or vitreous hemorrhage.
3. Moderate to severe NVE (greater than one-half disk area) with preretinal or vitreous hemorrhage.

Anterior segment neovascularization or rubeosis is also an indication for treatment.

Macular edema may be present at any stage of retinopathy. Clinically significant macular edema as defined by the Early Treatment for Diabetic Retinopathy Study (ETDRS) includes any one of the following lesions: thickening of the retina at or within 500 μ of the foveal center, hard exudates at or within 500 μ of the foveal center associated with thickening of the adjacent retina, or a zone or zones of retinal thickening one disk area or larger within 1 disk diameter of the foveal center.[97–100]

Subjective symptoms experienced by patients with diabetic retinopathy are decreased, fluctuating, or distorted vision; accommodative insufficiency; increased time required for dark adaptation; loss of color vision; and floaters.

Adjunct Testing

FA risk factors for the progression of NPDR to PDR have been identified. Capillary loss and dilation and leakage of fluorescein are risk factors for progression. Although these angiographic abnormalities provide additional prognostic information, clinical fundus examination can allow the doctor to identify the risk of progression.

Medical Treatment

Three major clinical trials have been carried out by the National Eye Institute to investigate the course of diabetic retinopathy and establish guidelines for treatment of the disease.

1. Diabetic Retinopathy Study[101–106]
2. ETDRS[97–100, 107–114]
3. Diabetic Retinopathy Vitrectomy Study[115–119]

According to the American Academy of Ophthalmology guidelines for management, patients with minimal NPDR and patients without macular edema are followed at yearly intervals. Also, patients with macular edema that is not clinically significant are examined at 6-month intervals.[97]

Focal laser photocoagulation is the mainstay of treatment in patients with clinically significant macular edema. The ETDRS demonstrated that this procedure reduces the risk of moderate vision loss by 50% or more.[97–100]

Panretinal photocoagulation significantly reduces the risk of severe vision loss from high-risk PDR. For cases of less severe retinopathy, photocoagulation should be deferred until high-risk characteristics develop.[114, 115] Although laser photocoagulation substantially reduces the risk of moderate to severe vision loss, PDR in a certain number of eyes may progress to tractional retinal detachment and subsequent vision loss.

Standard laser therapy cannot be performed in eyes with vitreous hemorrhage. Vitrectomy may be indicated for cases in which severe hemorrhage persists for several months if vision is impaired and the retina cannot be visualized. Vitrectomy is also used in certain cases of severe proliferative retinopathy when laser treatment cannot be completed or is not effective in eradicating high-risk proliferative changes. Vitrectomy remains the only treatment available for certain cases with traction or rhegmatogenous retinal detachment involving the macula, or both.[115–119]

Low Vision Management

Refractive error should be checked during at least two different visits because fluctuations in refraction may occur along with changes in blood sugar level. Use of contact lenses to correct refractive error in diabetics is controversial because of possible corneal desensitivity and relative high risk of corneal infections.

CPFs and sun lenses that block blue wavelengths may improve contrast and eliminate glare and photophobia. Direct illumination for near tasks is generally helpful. A flashlight is helpful if a patient is experiencing poor night vision. Orientation and mobility training is indicated as the condition progresses and peripheral visual field as well as central vision becomes affected.

Eccentric viewing techniques along with magnification devices for distance and near may be beneficial. Patients should be advised of the possible need for multiple magnification devices as their visual status may change.

Nonoptical devices, such as glucose monitor and insulin-syringe aids, are helpful for these patients. Other nonoptical systems, including talking books and vocalization devices (e.g., vocalization computer systems [see Chapter 14]), and support groups are also available options.

Prognosis

Timely diagnosis and proper treatment offer the prospect of virtual elimination of the 5-year risk of severe vision loss from proliferative diabetic retinopathy for the 7 million Americans who have been diagnosed with diabetes mellitus.[120]

DISLOCATED LENS

Description

Subluxation of the lens is a partial dislocation that is caused by weakened, stretched, or broken zonules. Upward, downward, or lateral displacement can occur.

Etiology

Lens dislocation can be hereditary and may be associated with systemic abnormalities of mesodermal tissue.

Ocular trauma can cause rupture of the zonules resulting in lens dislocation. Intraocular inflammation, buphthalmos, and hypermature cataract can cause a secondary "spontaneous" lens dislocation.

Visual Acuity

Visual acuity ranges from normal to severe impairment depending on lens position. Functional aphakia can be produced if the lens is dislocated beyond the line of sight.

Visual Field

Visual field defects may occur due to lens-induced secondary glaucoma.

Ocular Signs and Symptoms

Blurred vision from acquired spherical and astigmatic refractive error, monocular diplopia, and loss of accommodation can occur due to lens dislocation. Secondary glaucoma may result from phacomorphic pupillary block or inflammatory phacolysis. Iridodonesis is evident due to zonular disruption.

Associated Syndromes

A dislocated lens may be associated with several ocular and systemic disorders, including

1. *Marfan's syndrome*, which is associated with upward lens dislocation in 80% of patients. Other ocular findings include blue sclera, strabismus, myopia, and retinal detachment. Systemic manifestations are arachnodactyly, tall stature, joint hyperextensibility, skin hyperelasticity, and aortic valvular disease.[121, 122]

2. *Homocystinuria*, which is usually associated with downward lens dislocation. Enzyme deficiency causes high levels of homocystine in the blood and urine. Systemically, osteoporosis, mental retardation, and thrombosis of intermediate sized vessels may occur.[123]

3. *Weill-Marchesani syndrome*, which is associated with microspherophakia and anterior dislocation of the lens leading to pupillary block glaucoma. Short stature, stubby digits, joint stiffness, carpal tunnel syndrome, and mental retardation are seen systemically.[124]

Medical Treatment

Treatment of pupillary block glaucoma is to break the attack, followed by iridectomy and lensectomy. Lensectomy is also indicated if anterior lens displacement poses threat of corneal compromise.

Low Vision Management

High plus lenses may be indicated if an aphakic situation is created by lens dislocation. This correction can be provided in the form of spectacle lenses or aphakic contact lenses. Plus addition lenses or magnifiers may be necessary for near tasks due to loss of accommodative ability. Aphakia also allows for increased transmission of ultraviolet light, which can be compensated for by ultraviolet coating of spectacle lenses. In addition, filters and sun lenses may be used to reduce illumination levels.

If diplopia exists, it can be eliminated by pinhole lenses, stenopeic slits, or aperture-control contact lenses.

Prognosis

Lens subluxation is generally a stable condition. However, patients are advised against participating in contact sports or any activity that could cause total lens dislocation.

GLAUCOMA

Description

Glaucoma is an optic neuropathy caused by reduced blood flow to the optic nerve resulting in peripheral visual field loss progressing to central vision loss when severe. This disorder is classified as *open-angle* or *angle closure glaucoma*. In addition, each type may be subclassified as primary or secondary.

Primary open-angle glaucoma, the most common type, can occur with normal or elevated intraocular pressure. The underlying etiology is unknown. In secondary open-angle glaucoma, physical blockage or damage of the trabecular meshwork is a result of another condition, such as uveitis, trauma, pigmentary dispersion, or pseudoexfoliation.

With primary angle closure, relative pupillary block causes an increase in aqueous pressure in the posterior chamber, pushing the peripheral iris forward over the trabecular meshwork. In secondary angle closure, the trabecular meshwork is occluded by the iris being pushed or pulled forward by another condition such as neovascularization of the iris or enlargement of the lens.

Developmental glaucoma is caused by maldevelopment of the anterior segment.

Etiology

Several risk factors predispose a patient to developing glaucoma, including: family history, advanced age, African-American descent, and systemic vascular disease. Ocular risk factors include blunt ocular trauma, pigmentary dispersion, pseudoexfoliation, rubeosis iridies, uveitis, use of steroid pharmaceutical agents, and glaucoma in the fellow eye.

Incidence

Glaucoma is the second leading cause of blindness in the United States. It is the leading cause of blindness in the African-American population. Approximately 1 of 50 Americans older than the age of 40 years have glaucoma, with approximately 1 million unaware that they have the condition.[125]

Visual Acuity

Central visual acuity is generally unaffected until the end stage of this disease.

Visual Field

Early glaucomatous visual field defects include paracentral scotomas, arcuate scotomas, nasal steps, and temporal wedges. Progressive visual field loss from these areas occurs as the disease worsens.[126]

Ocular Signs and Symptoms

Glaucomatous damage is determined by both the level of intraocular pressure and the optic nerve axons' resistance. In most cases, progressive glaucomatous damage is related to increased intraocular pressure. In a minority of cases, intraocular pressure in the "normal" range is too high for proper functioning of the optic nerve axons.

Early glaucomatous changes can be subtle. They include generalized optic nerve cup enlargement, localized vertical notching or narrowing of the optic nerve head rim tissue, superficial splinter hemorrhage, loss of nerve fiber layer, and asymmetric cupping. Progressive damage is characterized by atrophy of the temporal disk margin and the disappearance of the nasal rim. Collateral disk vessel formation may occur when prolonged elevation of intraocular pressure causes stasis in the retinal vessels. Eventually, the optic nerve appears pale and excavated, indicating destruction of neural disk tissue.

Generally, patients with open-angle glaucoma remain asymptomatic until later stages of the disease at which time they may notice decreased central acuity and peripheral field loss. Glaucoma patients with restricted fields report difficulty locating objects, which affects basic functions such as orientation and mobility and reading continuity.

Associated Syndromes

Glaucoma can occur in association with a variety of ocular and systemic disorders, including

1. *Pigmentary dispersion syndrome*, characterized by dispersion of pigment from the pigment epithelium of the iris throughout the anterior segment. It is thought that the shed pigment is a result of mechanical rubbing of the posterior iris by the lens zonules. This condition typically occurs in young, white, myopic males. Approximately 10% of patients with pigmentary dispersion syndrome go on to develop pigmentary glaucoma from pigmentary blockage of the trabecular meshwork.

2. *Pseudoexfoliation syndrome*, which is due to secretion of gray-white "dandruff-like" material that deposits throughout the anterior segment. Approximately 60% of affected eyes go on to develop glaucoma from obstruction of the trabecular meshwork.[127]

3. *Iridocorneal endothelial syndromes* (ICE), which are typically unilateral and affect young to middle-aged women. Abnormal endothelium overgrowth in the anterior chamber causes the formation of peripheral anterior synechiae, which leads to secondary nonpupillary-block angle-closure glaucoma. Essential iris atrophy, Chandler's syndrome, and iris nevus syndrome (Cogan-Reese syndrome) probably represent a continuum of the same clinical disease.

4. *Plateau iris syndrome*, which is a cause of acute angle closure secondary to anatomic anterior iris insertion in the angle in conjunction with a patient's peripheral iridectomy.

5. *Reiger's syndrome*, which is a congenital anterior chamber cleavage dysgenesis that includes prominent Schwalbe's line, peripheral iris anomalies, iris atrophy, and glaucoma as well as dental, skeletal, and structural abnormalities.

6. *Peter's anomaly*, which is characterized by a central corneal opacity due to absent corneal endothelium and iridocorneal adhesions.

7. *Axenfeld's syndrome*, which is characterized by a prominent Schwalbe's line that is associated with a large peripheral synechia.

8. *Sturge-Weber syndrome* (encephalotrigeminal angiomatosis), which is characterized by unilateral facial port-wine stain (nevus flammeus), seizures, hemiparesis, hemianopia, mental deficiency, conjunctival and episcleral vascular lesions, iris heterochromia, choroidal hemangioma, and glaucoma.

Adjunct Testing

The criteria for making a diagnosis of glaucoma involves intraocular pressure measurement, gonioscopic examination of the anterior chamber angle, stereoscopic optic nerve evaluation, and threshold visual field assessment.

Measurement of intraocular pressure is an essential part of evaluation when glaucoma is suspected. Pressures above 21 mm Hg should be considered suspicious for glaucoma. Asymmetry in intraocular pressure between eyes greater than 5 mm Hg should be considered suspect. Some advocate the practice of serial tonometry reading and provocative testing.[128]

Gonioscopic assessment of the anterior chamber angle can be performed to identify individuals who are predisposed to angle closure or to detect the presence of debris or structural changes that may adversely affect the trabecular meshwork.

Appearance of the optic nerve head is critical in the diagnosis of glaucoma. Magnified stereoscopic viewing techniques must be used to detect asymmetric disk size and neural retinal rim thinning. Photodocumentation is helpful for monitoring progression of optic nerve damage.

Visual field changes can occur before noticeable optic nerve damage. Thus, threshold visual field testing is crucial to both the diagnosis and management of glaucoma.[129]

Computerized optic nerve analyzers provide sensitive evaluation of glaucomatous damage by also measuring optic nerve head status in terms of topography, and NFL thickness.[130, 131]

Medical Treatment

In open-angle glaucoma, initial treatment is traditionally aimed toward medically lowering intraocular pressure with aqueous suppressants supplemented by agents that enhance outflow. Typically, laser trabeculoplasty, filtering surgery, or cycloablative procedures may be required when medical therapy fails.

The goal in the treatment of pupillary block angle-closure glaucoma is to medically break the attack, perform a peripheral iridectomy, and protect the fellow eye.

Low Vision Management

Low vision management of the glaucoma patient can be challenging. These patients often are not referred until the end stage of the disease at which time they are experiencing both central visual acuity and peripheral field loss.

Magnification devices can be beneficial for these patients but extent of visual field loss must be taken into consideration. Electronic magnification systems, such as a closed-circuit television (CCTV), are useful because they allow for increased contrast and brightness along with magnification (see Chapter 11). Excessive or bright illumination, at both distance and near, is generally bothersome. CPFs are beneficial in reducing glare and improving contrast for patients with glaucoma. Nonoptical systems should be explored.

For those patients with intact central acuity and peripheral visual field loss, minus lenses or reverse telescopes can be used to enhance the patient's visual field. Prism or mirror systems may stimulate peripheral awareness. Visual field loss in end-stage glaucoma patients creates problems with orientation and mobility. Instruction in long cane travel can also be beneficial to patients with end-stage disease. Use of a flashlight can be helpful for night travel. Support groups should be considered.

Prognosis

Most forms of glaucoma can be controlled with medical treatment if diagnosed and treated in a timely manner. In patients who have intraocular pressure that is poorly controlled, slowly progressive vision loss may eventually result in total blindness.[132]

KERATOCONUS

Description

Keratoconus is a bilateral, noninflammatory, progressive ectasia of the cornea characterized by thinning and steepening of the cornea. The conelike protrusion produces progressive decrease in vision due to irregular myopic astigmatism.

Etiology

Keratoconus is thought to be familial in nature, although no definitive pattern of inheritance has been established.[133] An association with atopic disease has been observed, leading to speculation that excessive eye rubbing can induce, aggravate, or accelerate the condition.[134, 135]

Incidence

The incidence of keratoconus in the general population has been estimated between 1 and 600 per 100,000, but diagnostic criteria vary among studies.[136–138]

Visual Acuity

Keratoconus usually presents as a progressive decrease in visual acuity. Acuity ranges from normal to markedly diminished, depending on the extent of the condition.

Visual Field

There is no definitive visual field defect in keratoconus, but general distortion of field is noted.

Systemic Signs and Symptoms

Studies have shown keratoconus to be associated with atopic disease, such as atopic dermatitis, vernal catarrh, asthma, and hay fever.[134, 135]

Ocular Signs and Symptoms

Slowly progressive myopia with irregular astigmatism occurs secondary to thinning of the cornea. Distortion of retinoscopic reflex ("scissor reflex") and keratometric mires are apparent in the early stages.

Vertical striae of the posterior stroma, fine anterior stromal scars, pronounced corneal nerves, and iron deposition around the base of the cone (Fleischer's ring) occur as the condition progresses. Munson's sign, a V-shaped conformation of the lower lid produced by the bulging central cornea in downward gaze, is found in advanced keratoconus.

Corneal hydrops are ruptures in Descemet's membrane that disrupt the integrity of the corneal endothelium. Acute hydrops cause profound edema and pain. The edema usually resolves after several months, but residual scarring may result in decreased visual acuity.

Patients in the earlier stages of the disease experience spectacle blur, image distortion, and starbursts around objects, necessitating the use of rigid gas-permeable contact lenses. Monocular diplopia may occur as the disorder progresses.

Associated Syndromes

Keratoconus can occur in association with various systemic disorders, including

1. *Down syndrome* (trisomy 21), which is the most common chromosomal anomaly associated with keratoconus. Findings include the following: mental deficiency, small stature, epicanthus, telecanthus, esotropia, and high refractive error.
2. *Marfan's syndrome*, which is an inherited connective tissue disorder associated with keratoconus, subluxated lens, blue sclera, myopia, and retinal detachment. Arachnodactyly, tall stature, laxity of joints, sternal deformities, and mitral valvular disease are found systemically.
3. *Ehlers-Danlos syndrome*, which is an inherited connective tissue disorder associated with keratoconus, blue sclera, angioid streaks, and retinal detachment. Hyperelasticity of skin, hyperextensibility of joints, and fragility of tissue are characteristic of this condition.
4. *Osteogenesis imperfecta*, which is an inherited connective tissue disorder associated with keratoconus, blue sclera, and glaucoma. Bones are fragile and easily fracture.

Adjunct Testing

Keratometry, placido disk (keratoscope), and computerized corneal topography are used to document topographic changes. Central or paracentral corneal steepening with irregular astigmatic changes are common topographic findings in keratoconic patients.[139, 140]

Medical Treatment

Penetrating keratoplasty is indicated when the patient is unable to obtain clear, comfortable vision with contact lenses or is unable to tolerate wearing a contact lens. There is a 90% success rate with this procedure; however,

residual astigmatism may cause poor postoperative visual acuity.[141–143]

Lamellar keratoplasty and epikeratophakia are alternative procedures but have been shown to have greater technical difficulty and less satisfactory visual results.[144–146]

Low Vision Management

A careful refraction should be performed. Contact lenses are considered when the condition reaches the stage at which spectacle correction no longer provides good visual acuity. Rigid gas-permeable contact lenses can provide a regular anterior refractive surface to eliminate much of the irregular astigmatism. A combination piggyback lens system consisting of a rigid lens fit on top of a soft lens is used in cases of rigid lens intolerance. Many contact lens alternatives and frequent changes in design may be necessary (see Chapter 8).

Pinhole lenses, stenopeic slit, and aperture control contact lenses may be indicated to limit the refractive area of the cornea to prevent "ghost images."

CPFs, tints, and sun lenses are helpful due to glare and photophobia. Excessive lighting should be avoided.

Patients will respond to some magnification at distance and near, with greater success occurring at near using electronic magnification systems (i.e., CCTV).

Prognosis

Keratoconus manifests in adolescent years and can progress slowly, stabilizing during middle age, or can advance rapidly, requiring keratoplasty.

MACULAR HOLE

Description

A macular hole appears as a round red lesion in the fovea, usually from one-third to two-thirds of a disk diameter in size, with a gray halo of surrounding (marginal) retinal detachment (Figure 6-4).[147]

Etiology

Macular holes may be caused by trauma, myopia, cystoid macular edema, or inflammation, although most are idiopathic, which will be reviewed here. Idiopathic holes may be due to tangential vitreous traction on the macula.[147, 148]

Incidence

Idiopathic macular holes occur more commonly in middle-aged to elderly women, which suggests a possible hormone influence.[149, 150] They tend to occur unilaterally, but bilateral involvement has been reported in 3–31% of patients.[149]

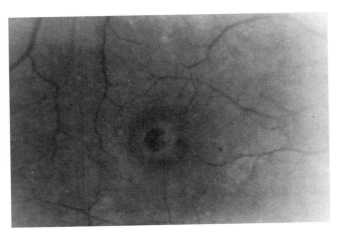

FIGURE 6-4.   **Macular hole.**

Visual Acuity

Patients with stage 1 or 2 lesions will have visual acuity ranging from 20/25 to 20/80. Visual acuity for stage 3 and 4 lesions usually stabilizes at the 20/200 level.[150]

Visual Field

Full-thickness holes result in dense central scotomas.[149]

Ocular Signs and Symptoms

Idiopathic macular holes are classified by stages of development according to Gass.[147]

Stage 1. Foveal detachment or impending hole. There is a loss of the foveal depression.
Stage 1A. A yellow dot lesion appears due to the increased visibility of xanthophyll.
Stage 1B. Appears as a yellow halo lesion.
Stage 2. Early hole formation. The yellow ring enlarges in a can opener fashion, producing a small, full-thickness macular hole.
Stage 3. Fully developed macular hole. A full thickness hole, with or without an overlying operculum, is seen. There is subretinal fluid surrounding the hole, and cystoid edema may be present within the surrounding retina. Yellow deposits can be seen in the base of the hole in some cases.
Stage 4. Macular hole with posterior vitreous separation. An annulus from the optic nerve head, called a *Weiss ring*, is evident if a posterior vitreous detachment has occurred.

Patients with macular holes report distortion or decreased vision, or both.

Medical Treatment

Preliminary studies on the potential role of vitrectomy with fluid-gas exchange to relieve traction have shown favorable results when treated early.[151–153] The management of macular holes, however, is controversial.[154]

Low Vision Management

Refractive error should be thoroughly evaluated. Patients with macular holes respond well to magnification at near and distance with microscopes, magnifiers, and telescopic devices. Eccentric viewing techniques and direct lighting in conjunction with low vision devices may be beneficial.

Prognosis

The majority of stage 1 and 2 holes progress to full-thickness macular holes within several weeks or months. As many as one-third of these patients will develop spontaneous vitreo-foveal separation and foveal reattachment without full thickness hole formation.[147, 148]

With developments regarding the treatment of macular holes, the prognosis for this condition is favorable in cases that are not long-standing.[151–153]

MULTIPLE SCLEROSIS

Description

Multiple sclerosis (MS) is a demyelinating disease of the central nervous system (CNS). Demyelinated nerve fibers have an impaired ability to conduct impulses at physiologic frequencies. The clinical diagnosis of MS can only be made after at least two episodes of neurologic dysfunction and the presence of lesions in at least two sites of the CNS.[155]

Etiology

MS is a chronic demyelination disease of unknown etiology. The pathologic process involves destruction of myelin and oligodendrocytes. Resulting patches of demyelination are found throughout the white matter of the CNS, sometimes extending into the gray matter. Studies hypothesize that MS is of viral etiology from exposure in late childhood. Other studies hypothesize that MS is an autoimmune disease initiated by a virus.[156] There is evidence that a combination of environmental and genetic factors is involved.[156]

In MS, the lesions are infiltrated by T lymphocytes and macrophages that result in the release of lymphokines and monokines to mediate the inflammatory response. This response causes a breakdown of the blood-brain barrier, edema, and macrophagic engulfment of myelin. Remission may occur as edema resolves and partial remyelination allows for recovery of nerve conduction. In chronic cases, proliferation of cells leads to scarring, which gives a sclerotic appearance.

Incidence

MS affects approximately 300,000 young adults in the United States. Age of onset is between 10 and 59 years, with maximum age-specific prevalence at age 30 years.[155] Women are generally affected more than men.[156]

MS is found more frequently in temperate zones compared to the tropics and subtropics. There seems to be an inverse relationship between mean annual temperature and the incidence of MS.[156]

Visual Acuity

Visual acuity in patients with MS ranges from normal to severely impaired depending on the extent of ocular manifestations.[157]

Visual Field

Several patterns of visual field loss occur in patients with optic neuritis secondary to MS. Central and cecocentral scotomas may be present, although altitudinal defects occur most commonly.[158, 159]

Systemic Signs and Symptoms

Systemic manifestations of MS encompass a multitude of signs and symptoms because the entire pathway of the CNS can be affected by this disease.

Paresthesias of extremities, muscle spasticity, and hyperreflexia occur as a result of corticospinal tract lesions. Decreased sense of touch, pain, and temperature is characteristic of posterior column lesions. Bladder dysfunction, constipation, and impotence may result from spinal cord lesions.

Depression, memory loss, and dementia are all associated with cerebral lesions. Seizures may be the presenting sign of MS, indicating involvement of gray matter.

Uhthoff's sign is decreased neurologic function occurring on elevation of body temperature. General weakness, blurred vision, and bladder dysfunction occur due to decreased axonal conduction with raised body temperature.

Lhermitte's sign is a moderate pain sensation that occurs when the neck is flexed.

Ocular Signs and Symptoms

Acute optic neuritis occurs in a significant number of MS patients during the course of their disease and often is the presenting sign. Patients complain of unilateral vision loss with associated pain on eye movement. In retrobulbar optic neuritis, the nerve head will appear normal because the demyelination is present behind the nerve head. Papillitis does occur in approximately 35% of patients affected by optic neuritis. Patients will exhibit an afferent pupillary defect and color vision disturbance due to optic nerve involvement. Visual impairment may be caused by resultant optic atrophy secondary to the optic neuropathy.

Cranial nerve palsies of the third, fourth, and sixth cranial nerves can lead to diplopic complaints. Involvement of the seventh cranial nerve results in a Bell's palsy. Damage to cranial nerve VIII results in nonspecific nystagmus. In addition, bilateral nuclear ophthalmoplegia is commonly seen in patients with MS.

Less common ocular signs include uveitis and retinal periphlebitis.

Adjunct Testing

Magnetic resonance imaging (MRI) with T1- and T2-weighted images reveals the presence and location of plaques.[160]

Visual evoked potentials are a noninvasive method of detecting conduction blockage within the optic nerve.[161]

Evaluation of cerebrospinal fluid may reveal high levels of immunoglobulin G and myelin base protein in patients affected by MS.[162]

Medical Treatment

Treatment for MS includes the following: high-dose corticosteroid therapy for acute exacerbations; potassium channel blockers to restore conduction; interferons for their antiviral, antineoplastic, and immunomodulating properties; cyclophosphamide for immunosuppression; and hyperbaric oxygen, which has been indicated to have an immunosuppressive effect.[163]

According to the results of the Optic Neuritis Treatment Trial, there are two principal treatment recommendations for cases of acute optic neuritis.[158] First, it appears that treatment with oral steroids alone may be associated with increased recurrence of optic neuritis compared to intravenous methylprednisolone for 3 days followed by oral steroids for 11 days. Secondly, patients should undergo MRI scans to rule out MS and be treated with intravenous corticosteroids if their scans show two or more abnormalities.

Low Vision Management

Magnification devices for distance and near are beneficial for patients with central visual acuity loss. Spectacle-mounted devices work best because the stability of handheld devices may be difficult due to the systemic manifestations of this disease.

CPFs, tints, and sun lenses help to eliminate glare. Direct lighting is helpful as are nonoptical systems. Services, such as occupational or physical therapists, may be recommended. Support groups should be considered.

Prognosis

The course of MS is usually prolonged, with remissions and exacerbations over a period of many years. The visual prognosis for patients with acute demyelinating optic neuritis is favorable. The natural history is to worsen over several days to 2 weeks and then improve. Improvement can occur 1 year after onset of visual symptoms. There is a small percentage of patients who experience persistent, severe vision loss after a single episode of optic neuritis.

MYOPIC DEGENERATION

Description

Degenerative myopia occurs when there is excessive stretching and expansion of the posterior segment of the eye associated with increasing axial length. Gradual degenerative changes occur as the sclera, choroid, and retina become thinner.

Etiology

There is strong belief that degenerative myopia may be genetically inherited, but the mechanism of transmission is poorly understood.[164]

Incidence

The prevalence of degenerative myopia is approximately 2% and is the seventh leading cause of blindness in the United States.[165]

Visual Acuity

Initially, visual acuity may be correctable to 20/20. As the condition progresses, gradual decrease in central acuity occurs as a result of structural changes. In more advanced stages, subretinal neovascular membrane formation may occur, causing further decrease in central acuity.

Visual Field

High degrees of myopia can result in a variety of visual field defects. Central ring-shaped scotoma, as well as hemianopic and quadrantic defects, can arise in the presence of posterior staphyloma.

Ocular Signs and Symptoms

Fundus changes associated with degenerative myopia are variable. Diffuse tessellation of the fundus can be seen due to thinning of the pigmented epithelium. Peripapillary scleral crescent results from failure of the choroid and RPE

to extend to the disk margin. Posterior staphylomas may develop, represented as an outpouching of the posterior eye wall. Lacquer cracks, which are yellowish-appearing linear breaks in Bruch's membrane, are a manifestation of axial length changes. A round black lesion, known as *Fuchs' spot*, is a result of hyperplasia of the RPE usually overlying a previous choroidal neovascular membrane. Peripheral retinal changes associated with thinning predispose affected eyes to retinal detachment. These pathologic changes in the fundus typically occur in patients with a refractive error of greater than 6.00–8.00 D of myopia.

Associated Syndromes

Myopic degeneration can occur in association with various systemic and ocular disorders, including

1. *Down syndrome* (trisomy 21), which is a chromosomal anomaly that is associated with mental deficiency, small stature, high myopia, epicanthus, telecanthus, and esotropia.
2. *Marfan's syndrome*, which is a connective tissue disorder that is associated with high myopia, keratoconus, subluxated lens, blue sclera, and retinal detachment. Systemic signs include arachnodactyly, tall stature, laxity of joints, sternal deformities, and mitral valvular disease.
3. *Stickler's syndrome*, which is a hereditary hyaloideoretinopathy with skeletal dysplasia, cleft palate, flattened facies, and mental retardation. High myopia, liquefied vitreous, RPE changes, and retinal detachment are among the ocular manifestations of this condition.

Adjunct Testing

FA may be indicated if CNV is suspected.

Medical Treatment

In cases of CNV, laser photocoagulation may be helpful. Due to the progressive spread of laser scars in patients with degenerative myopia, however, photocoagulation of CNV within 200 μ of the fovea is not recommended.

Prophylactic treatment with cryopexy or photocoagulation to symptomatic, peripheral retinal breaks or tears may be warranted in an effort to prevent retinal detachment.

Low Vision Management

Optical correction of refractive error with conventional spectacles or contact lenses usually improves visual acuity. In myopia, spectacle lenses produce minification compared to contact lenses. The relative magnification produced by a contact lens serves as an advantage over a spectacle lens of the same power. Also, contact lenses eliminate peripheral distortion and prismatic effects experienced with high-powered spectacles. Because spectacles provide minification relative to contact lenses, theoretically a larger field of view is expected. Considering peripheral spectacle lens distortion and frame limitations, however, no difference in field may be noticed.

When using spectacle lenses, a small round frame, high-index lenses, and antireflective coating will help to reduce edge thickness and peripheral distortions. For higher prescriptions (greater than −15.00 D), a myodisc or blended myodisc should be considered.

For magnification at near, the patient can simply remove the spectacle correction and use his or her myopic system as a built-in microscope at the appropriate working distance. This option is an advantage for a patient who wears spectacles compared to contact lenses. A contact lens wearer may choose to wear microscopic spectacles over contact lenses. Other magnification devices for distance and near are effective as well. In addition, sun lenses can eliminate photophobia outdoors. Direct illumination at near is helpful. If night vision is poor, a flashlight may be helpful.

Prognosis

Myopia may progress by as much as 4.00 D yearly. Increases in myopic refractive error usually stabilize at approximately age 20 years but can progress until the mid-30s. Degrees of myopia may be as high as 20.00 D or more.[166]

The visual prognosis in patients with neovascularization depends on the extent and location of the subretinal vessels relative to the fovea.[167]

NYSTAGMUS

Description

Nystagmus is an involuntary, rhythmic, to-and-fro oscillation of the eyes. Nystagmus is described by amplitude, frequency, and wave form. If the eyes move with equal speed in both directions, it is called *pendular nystagmus*. If the eyes move faster in one direction, it is called *jerk nystagmus* and is defined by the fast component. Dual nystagmus consists of the simultaneous mixture of waveforms.

Intensity of nystagmus is defined by amplitude and frequency. Changes in intensity, which occur in various positions of gaze, should be noted as well. The null point is the field of gaze in which the frequency of the nystagmus is minimal. The neutral zone is the field of gaze in which a reversal in direction of jerk nystagmus occurs. In most cases, the null point and neutral zone overlap.

There are more than 45 classifications of nystagmus. Nystagmus can be congenital or secondary to a variety of other conditions. For the purpose of this chapter, only congenital nystagmus is discussed.

Etiology

Congenital nystagmus is present at birth and may be transmitted as an X-linked recessive or autosomal dominant trait.[168] The etiology is poorly understood, but is due to a defect in the efferent visuomotor system.

Visual Acuity

Visual acuity is variable among patients with congenital nystagmus.

Visual Field

Visual field is usually unaffected in patients with nystagmus.

Ocular Signs and Symptoms

Congenital nystagmus is usually binocular with multiple waveforms. The direction of the nystagmus remains horizontal in upgaze. Compensatory head oscillations are generally associated with congenital nystagmus and often demonstrate an increase with visual attention.

Intensity of the nystagmus increases on attempted fixation, resulting in decreased acuity. Nystagmus intensity decreases on convergence and is absent during sleep.

Superimposition of a latent component is often present, meaning that when one eye is covered, the amplitude of the nystagmus increases.

Inversion of the optokinetic reflex occurs with congenital nystagmus. When optokinetic stimuli are presented, the nystagmus is in the opposite direction from what would be expected. This reversal may be simply due to a null point shift.

Patients with congenital nystagmus do not experience oscillopsia.

Low Vision Management

Correcting high refractive error will sometimes reduce nystagmus and improve acuity. Increased acuity is achieved by increased foveation time. In most cases, this increase occurs when the patient is fixated at the null point. In some patients, however, best acuity is achieved in a particular gaze position that yields the best waveform, not particularly the least amplitude. Patients may develop eye or head turns to position fixation in the null area or position of best acuity. These patients may benefit from prism spectacles to permit optimal acuity in primary gaze.

Magnification devices at distance and near are beneficial to patients with congenital nystagmus. Binocular devices work best to alleviate consequences of the latent component that are induced by monocular systems.

Prognosis

Congenital nystagmus initially presents itself at 3–6 months of age and persists in a stable manner throughout life.

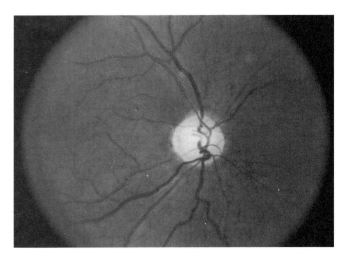

FIGURE 6-5.   Optic atrophy.

OPTIC ATROPHY

Description

Optic atrophy can be classified into three categories. Heredodegenerative optic atrophy should be considered when there is insidious, bilateral loss of central vision in childhood. Primary optic atrophy is the most common form, resulting from a number of conditions that cause damage to retinal ganglion cells. Secondary optic atrophy occurs subsequent to disk edema.

Etiology

The heredodegenerative optic atrophies are transmitted in three ways. Dominant optic atrophy is also known as *Kjer's infantile optic atrophy*.[169] Recessive optic atrophy is further divided into simple, complicated, and juvenile forms.[170, 171] Leber's hereditary optic neuropathy has an unknown etiology, but cytoplasmic DNA mutations are believed to be partially responsible.[172]

Primary optic atrophy occurs after many conditions, including inflammatory, infiltrative, toxic, ischemia, trauma, demyelination, and compressive lesions. These conditions are associated with loss of retinal ganglion cells, resulting in optic nerve atrophy.

Secondary optic atrophy is present after acute or chronic episodes of papillitis and papilledema that disrupt the NFL.

Visual Acuity

Visual acuity ranges from 20/20 to hand motion.

Visual Field

Visual field defects generally affect central vision. Paracentral, cecocentral, or central scotomas may be present.

Ocular Signs and Symptoms

Ophthalmoscopic appearance of the nerve head demonstrates temporal, sectorial, or diffuse pallor (Figure 6-5). Associated nerve fiber layer thinning may be apparent. The optic nerve damage causes secondary signs, including decreased vision, diminished color perception, sluggish pupillary response to light, photophobia, and possible nystagmus.

Low Vision Management

Magnification at both distance and near with the use of low vision devices is indicated for patients with decreased vision due to optic atrophy. Excessive lighting should be avoided. Sun lenses, tints, and filters may help to eliminate glare, both indoors and outdoors. Nonoptical systems should be demonstrated.

Genetic counseling is indicated for the heredodegenerative forms of optic atrophy.

Prognosis

Most forms of optic atrophy are stable. Dominant optic atrophy is mildly progressive, however,[169] and the juvenile recessive form tends to be progressive.[171]

PRESUMED OCULAR HISTOPLASMOSIS SYNDROME

Description

Presumed ocular histoplasmosis syndrome (POHS) is a clinical entity consisting of disciform maculopathy, and peripheral and peripapillary punched-out lesions and is believed to be caused by the fungus *Histoplasma capsulatum*.[173]

Etiology

POHS is a mycotic infection that is thought to be contracted by inhalation of spores from the exogenous organism *H. capsulatum* and disseminated through the bloodstream, including that of the choroid. Presence of the fungus in soil is usually associated with excreta of bats, pigeons, and birds. Individuals with POHS do not have evidence of active, systemic histoplasmosis at the time of diagnosis.[174]

Incidence

Histoplasmosis is commonly found in association with large river valleys. The disease is found around the world in temperate and tropical areas. One adult in 1,000 in an endemic area will develop decreased vision due to POHS.[175]

Visual Acuity

Level of acuity is dependent on the location of the fundus lesions. Macular lesions cause severe central vision impairment.

Visual Field

Field defects correspond to the area of fundus lesions.

Systemic Signs and Symptoms

Pulmonary histoplasmosis is usually benign and asymptomatic. Symptoms may include cough, fever, and malaise. POHS is rarely associated with symptomatic pulmonary histoplasmosis, however.

Ocular Signs and Symptoms

The clinical appearance of POHS includes the presence of histo spots. These small, yellowish, punched-out lesions represent disseminated choroiditis and are found predominantly in the midperiphery. Histo spots located in the macular area may cause damage to Bruch's membrane and may allow for growth of a subretinal (choroidal) neovascular membrane with subsequent sensory retinal detachment. Macular CNV creates the symptoms of metamorphopsia and decreased vision. Streak lesions are seen in 5% of patients with POHS. They appear as depigmented lines with sharp margins and are likely the result of confluent histo spots.[176]

Peripapillary atrophy occurs in most cases of POHS. The ring is thought to be a result of granulomatous atrophy from the active stage of the disease.

Adjunct Testing

FA is indicated if there are new symptoms or clinical findings suggesting the presence of potentially treatable subretinal neovascularization.

The diagnosis of histoplasmosis can be assisted by chest x-ray and the histoplasmin skin test; however, it is usually made on the basis of the clinical findings alone.[177]

Medical Treatment

Patients should self-monitor macular changes with an Amsler's grid. Systemic steroids may be indicated in cases of acute maculopathy with an active choroiditis. Argon or krypton laser photocoagulation is used to eradicate extrafoveal or juxtafoveal subretinal neovascular membrane. A clinical trial is under way to attempt to establish the usefulness of surgical extraction of certain subfoveal neovascular membranes.

Low Vision Management

Magnification at distance and near with low vision devices, in conjunction with eccentric viewing techniques, is helpful for patients with macular involvement.

High levels of direct illumination may be helpful for near tasks.

Prognosis

Visually devastating affects of POHS are caused by subretinal neovascular membrane formation. Five-year results of the Macular Photocoagulation Study concluded that visual acuity of 20/200 or worse was found in 36% of untreated eyes compared to 9% in eyes treated with laser photocoagulation.[178] Recurrence rate of neovascularization was 26% and most often occurred within 1 year of the initial treatment.

Another study showed that 12% of patients with decreased vision in one eye develop symptoms in the second eye within 5 years and 22% will develop symptoms in 10 years.[179]

RETINAL DETACHMENT

Description

Retinal detachment results from accumulation of fluid between the sensory retina and the RPE. This fluid collection occurs in three ways. A rhegmatogenous retinal detachment results from a break in the retina, allowing fluid to escape from the vitreous cavity into the subretinal space. Exudative retinal detachment occurs as a result of damage to the RPE or retinal blood vessels, allowing fluid to pass into the subretinal space. Tractional retinal detachment results from vitreous membranes, caused by penetrating injury or by proliferative retinopathy pulling the neurosensory retina away from the pigment epithelium.

Etiology

Rhegmatogenous retinal detachment is the most common of the three types. It can be precipitated by posterior vitreous detachment, an atrophic hole, an operculated tear, or most commonly, a horseshoe tear. Predisposing factors include blunt trauma, high myopia, aphakia, lattice degeneration, other inherited degenerations of the retina and vitreous, and choroidal coloboma.

Causes of exudative retinal detachment include the following: choroidal tumors, chorioretinal inflammation, scleritis, and retinal vascular disease.

Neovascularization resulting in tractional retinal detachment is caused by retinal vascular diseases, such as diabetic retinopathy, branch vein occlusion, Eales' disease, and retinopathy of prematurity (ROP).

Visual Acuity

Visual acuity in retinal detachment can be severely reduced if there is involvement of the macular area.

Visual Field

Field defects develop corresponding to the site of retinal detachment.

Ocular Symptoms and Signs

An acute posterior detachment, the precursor of a retinal tear in most instances, is heralded by the symptoms of new floating spots or flashing lights. Once a retinal detachment develops and extends far enough posteriorly, the patient may become aware of a "curtain or shadow" extending from the periphery toward the center of his or her field of vision.

In most cases of rhegmatogenous retinal detachment, a definite retinal break can be found. "Tobacco dust" pigment in the vitreous or vitreous hemorrhage, or both, is highly suggestive of a retinal tear. The detached retina has a corrugated appearance and fixed folds.

With exudative detachments, because there is no break, shifting of fluid is seen. The elevated retina appears smooth.

Vitreous membranes from neovascularization can be seen with tractional retinal detachments. The retina appears smooth and immobile, with the detachment extending concave toward the front of the eye.

Associated Syndromes

Retinal detachment can occur in association with a variety of ocular and systemic disorders, including

1. *Ehlers-Danlos syndrome*, which is a hereditary condition with skin hyperelasticity, joint hyperextensibility, and fragility of tissue. Ocular manifestations include keratoconus, microcornea, blue sclera, angioid streaks, and retinal detachment.
2. *Marfan's syndrome*, which is an inherited condition with tall stature, arachnodactyly, sternal deformities, laxity of joints, and aortic valvular disease. Ocular findings include lens subluxation, blue sclera, strabismus, myopia, and retinal detachment.
3. *Stickler's syndrome*, which is a hereditary hyaloideoretinopathy with skeletal dysplasia, cleft palate, flattened facies, and mental retardation. Ocular abnormalities include high myopia, liquefied vitreous, retinal pigmentary changes, and retinal detachment.

Adjunct Testing

Diagnostic ultrasound is important in the evaluation of patients with opaque media and possible retinal detachment.

Medical Treatment

Scleral buckling or pneumatic retinopexy are the most common treatments for rhegmatogenous retinal detachment. During scleral buckling surgery cryotherapy, diathermy or photocoagulation is performed to create a chorioretinal adhesion at the site of the localized break. Subretinal fluid may be surgically drained. Sponge or solid silicone buckling material is sutured to the sclera, pushing the eye wall and retina toward the vitreous to relieve vitreal traction. A pigmented scar forms around the tear so that fluid can no longer get under the retina. Vitrectomy may be needed if a giant retinal tear or proliferative vitreoretinopathy is present.

Treatment of exudative retinal detachment is aimed toward managing the underlying etiology.

Treatment of tractional retinal detachment involving the macula is pars plana vitrectomy with membrane dissection.

Low Vision Management

Photophobia and glare can be eliminated with tints, filters, or CPF lenses. Direct illumination for near-point tasks is recommended.

If central vision is affected, refractive error may change and a new correction may be indicated. A final prescription should not be issued until the eye has fully stabilized, however.

Magnification devices for distance and near may be helpful. Nonoptical systems should be demonstrated.

If bilateral temporal detachments occur, prisms may be considered for improved mobility along with orientation and mobility services.

Prognosis

If detected early, retinal repair is usually successful. Detachment involving the macula has a poorer visual prognosis.

RETINOPATHY OF PREMATURITY

Description

ROP is an abnormal proliferation of the developing retinal blood vessels in eyes of newborn infants in whom retinal vascularization is incomplete. This condition is commonly seen in low birth-weight infants, premature infants, and infants who received oxygen therapy, although it occasionally occurs in full-term infants.

Etiology

During normal development, the retinal vasculature is built from the optic nerve outward. At 8 months' gestational age, it is usually complete out to the nasal periphery but will take approximately 1 month postpartum for the vessels to reach the temporal periphery. Therefore, there will be a broad area of nonvascularized retina in an infant who is born prematurely. Also, exposure of immature peripheral retina to high levels of oxygen results in failure of normal development of the retinal vasculature. With this failure of vascularization, ischemia results, causing neovascularization. If spontaneous regression of neovascularization does not occur, cicatricial changes may develop, causing mild to severe dragging of the retina.

Incidence

Approximately 450–500 babies are blinded by ROP each year in the United States. The incidence of ROP varies according to birth weight and gestational age. Infants at risk for developing ROP are those who weigh less than 1,500 g or those born before 30 weeks' gestational age. The incidence of ROP in infants at risk ranges from 16% to 56%.[180–183]

Ocular Signs and Symptoms

ROP is classified by severity, location, and extent.[184]

Severity
The degree of abnormal vascular response is recognized in the following stages:

Stage 1 appears as a sharp demarcation line between vascularized and nonvascularized retina.
Stage 2 is defined by the formation of an elevated ridge at the site of the demarcation line.
Stage 3 includes extraretinal fibrovascular proliferative tissue extending from the ridge onto the vitreous from the surface of the retina.
Stage 4 is defined by a subtotal retinal detachment without foveal involvement (stage 4A) or with foveal involvement (stage 4B).
Stage 5 is a total funnel-shaped retinal detachment.

If dilation and tortuosity of posterior blood vessels is present in any stage, a plus (+) is added to the number of the stage.

Location
To define location, the retina is divided into the following three zones, with the optic nerve as the center.

Zone I consists of a circle, the radius of which extends twice the disk-fovea distance in all directions from the disk.
Zone II extends from the edge of zone I out to the ora serrata on the nasal side and slightly anterior to the equator temporally.
Zone III is a crescent that involves the remaining temporal, inferior, and superior retina.

Extent
The extent of the condition is simply specified in terms of the clock hours involved.

Associated Ocular Findings

There is an increased incidence of high myopia in patients with ROP. Other complications include microphthalmos, glaucoma, cataract, leukocoria, uveitis, shallow anterior chamber, dragged macula, retinal pigmentary changes, retinal folds, amblyopia, anisometropia, strabismus, nystagmus, and retinal detachment. Subjective symptoms include decreased visual acuity and photophobia.

Visual Acuity

Visual acuity ranges from 20/20 to no light perception, depending on the severity.

Visual Field

Visual field defects are variable, most common nasally, correlating with the area of nonvascularized temporal periphery.

Medical Treatment

Premature infants at risk for developing ROP should be examined at 4–6 weeks of age and then every 2–3 weeks thereafter until vascularization has occurred. If ROP develops, the patient should be followed more closely according to the severity of the disease process.

The Cryotherapy for Retinopathy of Prematurity study indicated that treatment with cryotherapy should be performed on at least one eye in patients with symmetric disease at threshold.[185, 186] *Threshold disease* is defined as five or more contiguous clock hours or eight cumulative clock hours of stage 3 ROP in zone I or II in the presence of "plus" disease. At threshold, 25% will regress spontaneously, but with cryotherapy, 50% will regress.[185] After 1 year, the rate of an unfavorable outcome is reduced from approximately 50% without treatment to approximately 25% with treatment.[186]

Photocoagulation therapy for eyes with threshold disease has been shown to result in outcomes similar to those found after cryotherapy.

Treatment for stage 4B includes scleral buckling with drainage of subretinal fluid. Stage 5 ROP may require vitrectomy, lensectomy, and membrane peeling to reattach the retina.[187]

Patients with any stage of ROP should be monitored indefinitely for development of retinal breaks.

Large dosages of vitamin E have been speculated to reduce the severity of ROP. This has not been proved, and complications from high-dose vitamin E can occur.[188, 189]

Low Vision Management

High amounts of myopic refractive error can be corrected with conventional spectacles or contact lenses. In spectacles with high prescriptions, antireflective coating should be considered. Patients may also benefit from magnification with microscopes, magnifiers, electronic magnification systems, and telescopic devices. Various tints and filters may be useful in decreasing photophobia. Increased, direct, nonglare illumination is helpful at near.

Patients with ROP may also benefit from field awareness systems and mobility services if their peripheral fields have been affected.

Prognosis

The prognosis is guarded due to secondary complications of glaucoma, cataracts, and retinal detachments. The improved anatomic success rates of surgery rarely correlate with improved visual function.[190]

RETINITIS PIGMENTOSA

Description

Retinitis pigmentosa (RP) is the name given to a group of diseases characterized by progressive visual field loss, night blindness, and abnormal ERG recording. It is the most common of the hereditary retinal dystrophies.[191, 192]

Etiology

Heredity is extremely important in RP. Approximately 60–80% of the population affected by RP has inherited it autosomal recessively. Autosomal dominant transfer is the second most prevalent (10–25%) form. The X-linked form is the least prevalent (5–18%). The simplex mode of inheritance only affects one offspring, with no previous family history of RP, and has often been grouped with the autosomal recessive type. An X-linked mode of inheritance, however, is possible for males in this situation as well. As a general rule, dominant inheritance is often associated with milder and later onset disease, whereas X-linked cases are often the most severe and become apparent at an earlier age.[192, 193]

Pathogenesis

Mutations in the rhodopsin gene and in the peripherin/*RDS* gene result in an abnormal amino acid composition of the specific proteins whose production is regulated by those genes. Abnormalities in rhodopsin can affect the first stage of phototransduction by several different mechanisms, depending on the specific mutation in the rhodopsin gene. It is believed that peripherin/*RDS* is important to the structural stability of the outer segments.

With outer segment instability caused by abnormalities in this protein, outer segment renewal may be accelerated, increasing the pigment epithelial metabolic load and causing clinically recognizable changes in the RPE.

Incidence

The occurrence of RP varies with definition but has been reported to be between 1 in 2,000 to 1 in 7,000. It is more common in males.[193, 194]

Visual Acuity

Central vision ranges from 20/20 to no light perception. In early stages of the disease, acuity usually remains normal. In later stages, acuity may become moderately to severely decreased secondary to lens or macular changes.

Visual Field

Visual field loss begins in the midperiphery, extending inward and outward, creating a "donut-shaped" field defect. Many patients are unaware of the field loss because its slow progressive nature allows for long-term adaptation to the constriction.

Ocular Signs and Symptoms

Many fundus changes can occur with RP (Figure 6-6). Pigment and degenerated retinal cells migrate into the neural retina causing bone spicule pigment formation. With loss of pigment, the RPE appears moth-eaten. Also, because pigment is dispersed, the underlying choroidal vasculature becomes prominent, giving the fundus a tessellated appearance. Attenuated retinal arterioles are another diagnostic feature of this disease.

The optic nerve appears to have a waxy pallor, most likely due to gliosis on the disk. Patients with RP tend to have smaller cup-to-disk ratios compared to the normal population.[195, 196] Optic nerve head drusen are commonly present in RP patients.

Although loss of peripheral vision is the most visually devastating symptom for RP patients, loss of central acuity may occur as well. Leakage from disruption in the blood-retinal barrier can manifest as cystoid macular edema, causing decreased acuity. In addition, posterior subcapsular cataracts are a common anterior segment finding that affects central vision.

High amounts of myopia and astigmatism have been found in association with RP. Patients usually present with symptoms before fundus changes are seen. Nyctalopia is experienced during the first or second decade of life. Another common symptom is delay in dark and light adaptation speed. Patients also may notice decreased color sensitivity. Because the RPE can no

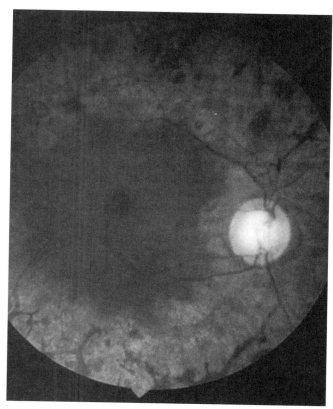

FIGURE 6-6. **Retinitis pigmentosa.**

longer absorb light, photophobia is experienced due to light scatter.[195, 196]

Unusual Findings of Significance

Sector RP describes bilateral retinal changes involving any quadrant or sector of the retina. Most commonly, the inferonasal quadrants are symmetrically involved. The incidence of this condition appears to be low, either because it is uncommon or because it is infrequently diagnosed due to lack of characteristic symptoms.[197, 198]

The existence of unilateral RP is controversial. Most authors believe that the condition is more appropriately termed *unilateral retinal pigmentary degeneration*. The ERG may remain normal over time with this condition. The etiology is usually unknown, but a number of conditions have been documented, including transient ophthalmic artery occlusion, trauma to the eye, and other structural defects of the retina.[199, 200]

Associated Syndromes

The following are the most common systemic conditions associated with RP:

1. *Usher's syndrome*, which is an autosomal recessively inherited condition in which the cochlear and vestibular systems are involved. It is the most common cause of deaf-blindness in the United States.[201]

2. *Laurence-Moon-Biedl syndrome*, which is an autosomal recessive condition characterized by RP, polydactyly, obesity, hypogonadism, and mental retardation.

3. *Alström's syndrome*, which is an autosomal recessive condition associated with childhood blindness due to RP. Obesity, diabetes, deafness, and renal disease are characteristic of this syndrome.

4. *Kearns-Sayre syndrome*, which begins in childhood and is associated with RP, progressive external ophthalmoplegia, and cardiac defects.

5. *Bassen-Kornzweig syndrome* (acanthocytosis), which is an autosomal recessive condition characterized by serum abetalipoproteinemia and spinocerebellar degeneration. The associated pigmentary retinopathy can be reversed in the early stages by vitamin A.

6. *Refsum's disease*, which is an autosomal recessive condition in which there is an increase of phytanic acid in the blood. Pigmentary retinopathy, peripheral neuropathy, deafness, and cerebellar ataxia are associated with this disease.

Adjunct Testing

Electrodiagnostic testing can provide useful information in diagnosing RP. The ERG shows decreased A- and B-waves that eventually flatten in late stages.

Medical Treatment

At this time, there is no treatment for RP. There is evidence that megadoses of vitamin A palmitate may be of some benefit in slowing the progression of the electrophysiologic changes associated with the disease process.[202]

Cystoid macular edema secondary to RP responds to treatment with acetazolamide in approximately 50% of patients.[203] Cataract surgery, when indicated, may be helpful as well.

Low Vision Management

Refractive error should be evaluated carefully. Enhancement of visual field may be accomplished by use of a minus lens held at arm's length or a reverse telescope. Peripheral awareness may also be enhanced with prism or mirror systems.

Magnification can be provided at distance and near with low vision devices for patients who experience central loss. It must be kept in mind, however, that relatively high amounts of magnification may expand the image outside of the visual field for those patients with advanced disease. Electronic magnification systems, such as a CCTV, are useful because they allow for increased contrast and brightness along with magnification (see Chapter 11). Excessive or bright illumination at both distance and near is generally bothersome. CPF lenses are especially helpful for improving contrast and reducing glare in patients with

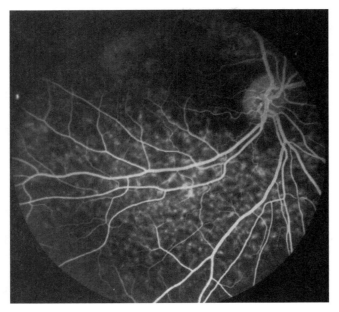

FIGURE 6-7.   **Angiogram of Stargardt's disease demonstrates dark choroid.**

posterior subcapsular cataracts. The photochromatic properties of these lenses allow for greater transition between light and dark environments. Nonoptical systems should be explored.

Visual field loss creates problems with orientation and mobility. Instruction in long cane travel and use of a flashlight for night travel can help patients to travel more efficiently.

Genetic counseling and support groups may be necessary to aid RP patients in coping with the psychological aspects of this condition.

Prognosis

RP is a slowly progressive condition that eventually results in total blindness. Patients with X-linked inheritance are affected earlier in life, with blindness generally occurring by the fifth decade. Autosomal recessive patients may show a loss of vision by the sixth or seventh decade. Patients with autosomal dominant inheritance may lose their vision by the eighth decade.[196, 204]

STARGARDT'S DISEASE

Description

Stargardt's disease and fundus flavimaculatus are now used interchangeably by most authors to describe a condition characterized by a vermilion fundus caused by excessive lipofuscin storage with macular atrophy or "flecks" at the level of the RPE in a typical distribution.[205, 206]

Etiology

Stargardt's disease in most patients is inherited autosomal recessively. There are some reports of a similar spectrum of clinical findings showing dominant inheritance.[205, 206]

Visual Acuity

Patients usually present with bilateral, decreased central vision in childhood or young adulthood. Initially, visual acuity may be at the 20/40 level and can last for several years. By the second decade, visual acuity declines and stabilizes at the 20/200 level or slightly worse.[207]

Visual Field

Visual field testing can reveal a relative central scotoma that may progress to an absolute scotoma.

Ocular Signs and Symptoms

Initially, the fundus may appear normal. Loss of the foveal reflex may be the only initial sign. The fundus appearance of yellow flecks that have been described as having a pisciform (fishlike) shape, may be confined to the macula, or may extend into the equator. The degree and pattern of RPE atrophy may not correlate with the degree of vision loss.

The RPE may be heavily pigmented from abnormal lipofuscin storage, thereby obscuring the choroidal detail. In the central macula, the RPE may atrophy, giving a beaten-metal appearance.

Patients with Stargardt's disease complain of a variety of symptoms, including decreased vision, abnormal color vision, photophobia, and nyctalopia.

Adjunct Testing

FA shows prominent retinal vessels on a dark background of the "silent" choroid. Hyperfluorescence will occur in areas of RPE atrophy. Angiographically the yellow flecks appear either nonfluorescent or show an irregular pattern of fluorescence (Figure 6-7).[208]

Full-field ERGs are typically normal, whereas foveal ERGs are often abnormal, even in patients with near normal visual acuity. The EOG is more likely to be subnormal in patients with widespread flecks, suggesting a defect in the RPE.[206]

Low Vision Management

A careful refraction should be performed to rule out any refractive error causing a decrease in acuity. Eccentric viewing techniques and magnification devices for near and distance are beneficial for these patients. Direct illumination may be very helpful for near tasks. Filters and sun lenses can be prescribed for patients who experience photophobia. Nonoptical systems should be demonstrated.

Prognosis

Visual status usually stabilizes at the 20/200 level during the second decade.

STROKE

See Chapter 17 for a description of stroke and how it relates to vision and vision rehabilitation.

TOXOPLASMOSIS

Description

Toxoplasmosis is the most common cause of chorioretinitis in the Western world. It is a parasitic disease caused by the organism *Toxoplasma gondii*. The term *toxo* is derived from the Greek word *toxon* or *arc* because of the shape of the parasite. The species name, *gondii*, is given because the organism was first found in the rodent *Ctenodactylus gondi*.[209, 210]

Etiology

Ocular toxoplasmosis is acquired most often congenitally from exposure to the organism prenatally but may be acquired through inhalation of oocytes from cat feces or ingestion of contaminated meat.

T. gondii is transmitted within circulating leukocytes and has a predilection for the retina and CNS. The organism multiplies within the infected host cell. If the cell bursts, the organism is liberated and inflammation occurs. If the host cell does not burst, cysts may form. The encysted *T. gondii* is susceptible to compromise in the immune system, with reactivation of infection and renewed inflammation.

Prevalence and Incidence

The prevalence of congenital toxoplasmosis is estimated between 1 in 1,000 and 1 in 10,000.[209–211] The incidence of transplacental transmission varies with the trimester during which the pregnant woman becomes infected. The incidence of infection is 15–20% during the first trimester and increases to 59% during the third trimester.[210, 211]

Visual Acuity

Visual acuity can be severely reduced depending on the extent and involvement of chorioretinitis in the macular area, which is common in congenital toxoplasmosis.[212]

Visual Fields

Visual field defects are variable, depending on number, size, and location of chorioretinal scars.[213]

Systemic Signs and Symptoms

Congenital toxoplasmosis may be associated with CNS disturbances such as convulsions and intracranial calcifications. Infection in the mother is usually asymptomatic.

Acquired toxoplasmosis presents with fever, myalgia, and lymphadenopathy in 10–20% of infected patients.[211]

Ocular Signs and Symptoms

Congenital toxoplasmosis may or may not be active at birth. The first sign of a previous retinitis may be the presence of strabismus or decreased acuity from macular involvement. Symptoms of acquired ocular toxoplasmosis or reactivated congenital infection include blurred vision and floaters.

Both forms can result in an acute necrotizing retinitis. The lesions appear white and elevated, with indistinct borders. Multifocal, gray-white, punctate lesions at the level of the pigmented epithelium may also be seen. Overlying vitreous haze occurs due to vitritis. Iritis, arteritis, periphlebitis, optic neuritis, and papillitis may be evident as well.

Inactive lesions typically appear as white scars with pigmented borders. Encysted organisms remain latent in the retina adjacent to the scars. If reactivated disease occurs next to an old scar, it is termed a *satellite lesion*.

Adjunct Testing

The indirect fluorescent antibody test is helpful in the diagnosis of congenital toxoplasmosis. Enzyme-linked immunosorbent assay detects IgG and IgM toxoplasma antibodies.[214]

Medical Treatment

Active lesions in the macular or peripapillary area, or severe vitritis are indications for treatment. A combination of systemic corticosteroids and antitoxoplasmic agents is the treatment of choice. Commonly used antitoxoplasmic agents include sulfadiazine, pyrimethamine, tetracycline, and clindamycin. The patient's platelet count must be monitored closely if pyrimethamine is used.[209, 215]

Cryotherapy and laser photocoagulation have been used in an effort to prevent recurrences but are not without potential complications.[216]

Low Vision Management

Refractive error should be carefully evaluated. Magnification at both near and distance with optical devices and eccentric viewing techniques are beneficial for patients with central vision loss due to toxoplasmosis. Direct illumination is especially helpful for near tasks. Absorptive lenses are helpful in reducing glare and photophobia. Nonoptical devices should be demonstrated.

Prognosis

Toxoplasmosis is usually a nonprogressive condition, but reactivation is possible. The compromised immune system of patients with acquired immunodeficiency syndrome or those on immunosuppressive therapy increases the risk of reactivation. Patients in these categories should be closely monitored.

SELF-ASSESSMENT QUESTIONS

1. Which of the following is *not* true regarding albinism?
    (a) Males are affected more often than females by ocular albinism.
    (b) Associated nystagmus creates difficulty in using telescopic devices for these patients.
    (c) Albinotic patients have a tendency toward high refractive errors.
    (d) Albinism is a stable condition.

2. Pupillary aperture control contact lenses are appropriate management for
    (a) aniridia, coloboma, and dislocated lens
    (b) coloboma, keratoconus, and glaucoma
    (c) dislocated lens, congenital nystagmus, and albinism
    (d) albinism, corneal dystrophy, and keratoconus

3. Decreased central acuity in patients with RP is caused by
    (a) cystoid macular degeneration
    (b) posterior subcapsular cataracts
    (c) a and b
    (d) none of the above

4. The most challenging pathology in terms of low vision management is
    (a) albinism
    (b) glaucoma
    (c) macular hole
    (d) congenital nystagmus

5. Which ocular disorder would demonstrate congenital nystagmus, photophobia, decreased acuity, and iris transillumination?
    (a) rod monochromatism
    (b) keratoconus
    (c) albinism
    (d) aniridia

6. Which ocular disorder, in its advanced stages, would respond best to minification?
    (a) ARMD
    (b) aniridia
    (c) toxoplasmosis (chorioretinal degeneration)
    (d) RP

7. Which ocular disorder would probably respond best to a multiple pinhole lens?
    (a) corneal dystrophy
    (b) ARMD
    (c) advanced glaucoma
    (d) advanced RP

8. Which ocular sign or symptom is most likely *not* associated with retinopathy of prematurity?
    (a) high myopia
    (b) glaucoma
    (c) corneal dystrophy
    (d) retinal detachment

9. When evaluating a patient who has a diagnosis of diabetes who is complaining of fluctuating vision, all of the following management plans may be considered except
    (a) Question the patient regarding stability of blood sugar level.
    (b) Refer the patient back to his or her internist or endocrinologist.
    (c) Recommend a change in his or her spectacle distance correction.
    (d) Recommend the use of an inexpensive magnifier until his or her vision has stabilized.

10. A patient who has an ocular diagnosis of heredodegenerative optic atrophy may benefit from which of the following?
    (a) magnification at distance and near
    (b) tinted lenses, both indoors and outdoors
    (c) genetic counseling
    (d) all of the above
    (e) b and c

REFERENCES

1. Nathans J, Piantanida TP, Eddy RL, et al. Molecular genetics of inherited variation in human color vision. Science 1986;232:203.
2. Nathans J, Davenport CM, Maumenee IH, et al. Molecular genetics of human blue cone monochromacy. Science 1989;245:831.
3. Nathans J, Thomas D, Hogness DS. Molecular genetics of human color vision: the genes encoding blue, green, and red pigments. Science 1986;232:193.
4. Neuhann T, Krastel K, Jaques W. Differential diagnosis of typical and atypical congenital achromatopsia. Graefes Arch Clin Exp Ophthalmol 1978;209:19.
5. Leibowitz HM, Krueger DE, Maunder LR, et al. The Framingham Eye Study monograph: an ophthalmological and epidemiological study of cataract, glaucoma, diabetic retinopathy, macular degeneration, and visual acuity in a general population of 2631 adults, 1973–1975. VI. Macular degeneration. Surv Ophthalmol 1980;24(suppl):428–457.
6. Klein R, Klein BEK, Linton KLP. Prevalence of age-related maculopathy. The Beaver Dam Eye Study. Ophthalmology 1992;99:933–943.
7. Hyman LG, Lilienfeld AM, Ferris FL III, Fine SL. Senile macular degeneration: a case-control study. Am J Epidemiol 1983;118:213–227.
8. Hyman L, He O, Grimson R, et al. and the Age-Related Macular Degeneration Risk Factors Study Group. Risk factors for age-related maculopathy. Invest Ophthalmol Vis Sci 1992;33(suppl):801.
9. Cruickshanks KJ, Klein R, Klein, BEK. Sunlight and age-related macular degeneration: the Beaver Dam Eye Study. Arch Ophthalmol 1993;111:514–518.

10. Taylor HR, West S, Munoz B, et al. The long-term effects of visible light on the eye. Arch Ophthalmol 1992;110:99–104.
11. West SK, Rosenthal FS, Bressler NM, et al. Exposure to sunlight and other risk factors for age-related macular degeneration. Arch Ophthalmol 1989;107:875–879.
12. Taylor HR, Muñoz B, West S, et al. Visible light and risk of age-related macular degeneration. Trans Am Ophthalmol Soc 1990;88:163–173.
13. Eye Disease Case-Control Study Group. Antioxidant status and neovascular age-related macular degeneration. Arch Ophthalmol 1993;111:104–109.
14. Seddon JM, Umed AA, Sperduto RD, et al. Dietary carotenoids, vitamins A, C, and E, and advanced AMD. JAMA 1994;272:1413–1420.
15. Frank RN, Amin RH, Eliott D, et al. Basic fibroblast growth factor and vascular endothelial growth factor are present in epiretinal and choroidal neovascular membranes. Am J Ophthalmol 1996;122:393–403.
16. Friedlander M, Theesfeld CL, Sugita M, et al. Involvement of integrins alpha v beta 3 and alpha v beta 5 in ocular neovascular diseases. Proc Natl Acad Sci U S A 1996;93:1764–1769.
17. Klein R, Klein BE, Franke T. The relationship of cardiovascular disease and its risk factors to age-related maculopathy. The Beaver Dam Eye Study. Ophthalmology 1993;100:406–414.
18. The Eye Disease Case-Control Study Group. Risk factors for neovascular age-related macular degeneration. Arch Ophthalmol 1992;110:1701–1708.
19. Sandberg MA, Tolentino MJ, Miller S. Hyperopia and neovascularization in age-related macular degeneration. Ophthalmology 1993;100:1009–1113.
20. Weiter JJ, Delori FC, Wing GL, Fitch KA. Relationship of senile macular degeneration to ocular pigmentation. Am J Ophthalmol 1985;99:185–187.
21. Li S, Lam TT, Fu J, Tso MO. Systemic hypertension exaggerates retinal photic injury. Arch Ophthalmol 1995;113:521–526.
22. Klein R, Klein BEK, Franke T. The relationship of cardiovascular disease and its risk factors to age-related maculopathy. The Beaver Dam Eye Study. Ophthalmology 1993;100:406–414.
23. Seddon JM, Hankinson S, Speizer F, Willett WC. A prospective study of cigarette smoking and age-related macular degeneration in women. JAMA 1996;276:1141–1146.
24. Goldberg J, Flowerdew G, Smith E, et al. Factors associated with age-related macular degeneration. An analysis of data from the first National Health and Nutrition Examination Survey. Am J Epidemiol 1988;128:700–710.
25. Marshall J. The aging retina: physiology or pathology. Eye 1987;1:282–295.
26. Jampol LM. Race, macular degeneration, and the Macular Photocoagulation Study [editorial]. Arch Ophthalmol 1992;110:1699–1700.
27. Klein R, Rowland ML, Harris MI. Racial/ethnic differences in age-related maculopathy. Third National Health and Nutrition Examination Survey. Ophthalmology 1995;102:371–381.
28. Siatkowski RM, Zimmer B, Rosenberg PR. The Charles-Bonnet syndrome. J Clin Neuroophthalmol 1990;10:215–218.
29. Rosenbaum F, Harati Y, Rolak L, et al. Visual hallucinations in sane people: Charles-Bonnet syndrome. J Am Geriatr Soc 1987;35:66–68.
30. Sarks SH. Drusen and their relationship to senile macular degeneration. Aust J Ophthalmol 1980;8:117–130.
31. Kenyon KR, Maumenee AE, Ryan SJ, et al. Diffuse drusen and associated complications. Am J Ophthalmol 1985;100:119–128.
32. Smiddy WE, Fine SL. Prognosis of patients with bilateral macular drusen. Ophthalmology 1984;91:271–277.
33. El Baba F, Green WR, Fleischmann J, et al. Clinicopathologic correlation of lipidization and detachment of the retinal pigment epithelium. Am J Ophthalmol 1986;101:576–583.
34. Schatz H, McDonald HR. Atrophic macular degeneration: rate of spread of geographic atrophy and visual loss. Ophthalmology 1989;96:1541–1551.
35. Maguire P, Vine AK. Geographic atrophy of the retinal pigment epithelium. Am J Ophthalmol 1986;102:621–625.
36. Sarks JP, Sarks SH, Killingsworth M. Evolution of geographic atrophy of the retinal pigment epithelium. Eye 1988;2:552–577.
37. Hayashi K, Hasegawa Y, Tazawa Y, deLaey JJ. Clinical application of indocyanine green angiography to choroidal neovascularization. Jpn J Ophthalmol 1989;33:57–65.
38. Elman MJ, Fine SL, Murphy RP, et al. The natural history of serous retinal pigment epithelium detachments in patients with age-related macular degeneration. Ophthalmology 1986;93:224–230.
39. Macular Photocoagulation Study Group. Subfoveal neovascular lesions in age-related macular degeneration. Guidelines for evaluation and treatment in the Macular Photocoagulation Study. Arch Ophthalmol 1991;109:1242–1257.
40. Guyer DR, Yannuzzi LA, Ladas I, et al. Indocyanine green–guided laser photocoagulation of focal spots at the edge of plaques of choroidal neovascularization. Arch Ophthalmol 1996;114:693–697.
41. Lim JI, Sternberg P Jr, Capone A Jr, et al. Selective use of indocyanine green angiography for occult choroidal neovascularization. Am J Ophthalmol 1995;120:75–82.
42. Macular Photocoagulation Study Group. Argon laser photocoagulation for senile macular degeneration: results of a randomized clinical trial. Arch Ophthalmol 1982;100:912–918.
43. Macular Photocoagulation Study Group. Argon laser photocoagulation for neovascular maculopathy after five years. Results from randomized clinical trials. Arch Ophthalmol 1991;109:12109–12114.
44. Macular Photocoagulation Study Group. Recurrent choroidal neovascularization after argon laser photocoagulation for neovascular maculopathy. Arch Ophthalmol 1986;104:503–512.
45. Macular Photocoagulation Study Group. Five-year follow-up of fellow eyes of patients with age-related macular degeneration and unilateral extrafoveal choroidal neovascularization. Arch Ophthalmol 1993;111:1189–1199.
46. Macular Photocoagulation Study Group. Krypton laser photocoagulation for neovascular lesions of age-related macular degeneration. Results of a randomized clinical trial. Arch Ophthalmol 1990;108:816–824.
47. Macular Photocoagulation Study Group. Persistent and recurrent neovascularization after krypton laser photocoagulation for neovascular lesions of age-related macular degeneration. Arch Ophthalmol 1990;108:825–833.
48. Jampol LM. Hypertension and visual outcome in the Macular Photocoagulation Study. Arch Ophthalmol 1991;109:789–790.
49. Macular Photocoagulation Study Group. Laser photocoagulation of subfoveal neovascular lesions in age-related macular degeneration. Results of a randomized clinical trial. Arch Ophthalmol 1991;109:1220–1241.
50. Macular Photocoagulation Study Group. Subfoveal neovascular lesions in age-related macular degeneration. Guidelines for evaluation and treatment in the Macular Photocoagulation Study. Arch Ophthalmol 1991;109:1242–1257.
51. Macular Photocoagulation Study Group. Laser photocoagulation of subfoveal neovascular lesions of age-related macular degeneration. Updated findings from two clinical trials, Arch Ophthalmol 1993;111:1200–1209.
52. Macular Photocoagulation Study Group. Occult choroidal neovascularization. Influence on visual outcome in patients with age-related macular degeneration. Arch Ophthalmol 1996;114:400–412.
53. Maguire JI, Benson WE, Brown GC. Treatment of foveal pigment epithelial detachments with contiguous extrafoveal choroidal neovascular membranes. Am J Ophthalmol 1990;109:523–529.
54. Berger AS, Kaplan HJ. Clinical experience with the surgical removal of subfoveal neovascular membranes. Short-term postoperative results. Ophthalmology 1992;99:969–972.
55. Lambert HM, Capone A Jr, Aaberg TM, et al. Surgical excision of subfoveal neovascular membranes in age-related macular degeneration. Am J Ophthalmol 1992;113:257–262.
56. Maas S, Deutman AF, Bandhoe F, Aandekerk AL. Surgical removal of subretinal neovascular membranes. Eur J Ophthalmol 1995;5:48–55.
57. Thomas MA, Dickinson JD, Melberg NS, et al. Visual results after surgical removal of subfoveal choroidal neovascular membranes. Ophthalmology 1994;101:1384–1396.
58. Valentino TL, Kaplan HJ, Del Priore LV, et al. Retinal pigment

epithelial repopulation in monkeys after submacular surgery. Arch Ophthalmol 1995;113:932–938.

59. Machamer R, Steinhorst UH. Retinal separation, retinotomy, and macular relocation: II. A surgical approach for age-related macular degeneration? Graefes Arch Clin Exp Ophthalmol 1993;231:635–641.

60. Fung WE. Interferon alpha-2a for treatment of age-related macular degeneration. Am J Ophthalmol 1991;112:349–350.

61. Guyer DR, Tiedeman J, Yannuzzi LA. Interferon-associated retinopathy. Arch Ophthalmol 1992;111:350–356.

62. Finger PT, Berson A, Sherr D, et al. Radiation therapy for subretinal neovascularization. Ophthalmology 1996;103:878–889.

63. Hart PM, Archer DB, Chakravarthy U. Asymmetry of disciform scarring in bilateral disease when one eye is treated with radiotherapy. Br J Ophthalmol 1995;79:562–568.

64. Valmaggia C, Bischoff P, Ries G. [Low dosage radiotherapy of subfoveal neovascularizations in age related macular degeneration. Results after 6 weeks and 6 months.] Klin Monatsbl Augenheilkd 1996;208:315–317.

65. Kramer M, Miller JW, Michaud N, et al. Liposomal BPD verteporfin photodynamic therapy: selective treatment of choroidal neovascularization in monkeys. Ophthalmology 1996;103:427–438.

66. Bressler SB, Bressler NM, Maguire MG, et al. for the Macular Photocoagulation Study Group. Drusen Characteristics and Risks of Exudation in the Fellow Eye of Argon SMD Patients in the Macular Photocoagulation Study. Invest Ophthalmol Vis Sci 1989;30(suppl):154.

67. Bressler SB, Maguire MG, Bressler NM, Fine SL. Relationship of drusen and abnormalities of the retinal pigment epithelium to the prognosis of neovascular macular degeneration. Arch Ophthalmol 1990;108:1442–1447.

68. O'Donnell FE, Hambrick GW, Green WR, et al. X-linked ocular albinism: an oculocutaneous macromelanosomal disorder. Arch Ophthalmol 1976;94:1883–1892.

69. Jay B, Carrol W. Albinism: recent advances. Trans Ophthalmol Soc UK 1980;100:467.

70. Nelson LB, Spaeth GL, Nowinski TS, et al. Aniridia. A review. Surv Ophthalmol 1984;28:621.

71. Hittner HM, Riccardi VM, Franks U. Aniridia caused by a heritable chromosome 11 deletion. Ophthalmology 1979;86:1173.

72. Shaw MW, Falls HF, Neel JV. Congenital aniridia. Am J Hum Genet 1960;12:389.

73. Elsas FJ, Maumenee IH, Kenyon KR, et al. Familial aniridia with preserved ocular function. Am J Ophthalmol 1977;83:718.

74. Hittner HM, Riccardi VM, Ferrel RE, et al. Variable expression in autosomal dominant aniridia by clinical electrophysiological and angiographic criteria. Am J Ophthalmol 1980;89:531.

75. Flanagan JC, DiGeorge AM. Sporadic aniridia and Wilms' tumor. Am J Ophthalmol 1969;67:558.

76. Fraumani JF Jr, Glass AG. Wilms' tumor and congenital aniridia. JAMA 1968;206:825.

77. Miller RW, Fraumeni JF Jr, Manning MD. Association of Wilms' tumor with aniridia, hemihypertrophy, and other congenital formations. N Engl J Med 1964;270:922.

78. Mackman G, Brightbell FS, Optiz JM. Corneal changes in aniridia. Am J Ophthalmol 1979;65:497.

79. David R, MacBeth L, Jenkins T. Aniridia associated with microcornea and subluxated lenses. Br J Ophthalmol 1978;62:118.

80. Grove JH, Shaw MW, Bourgue G. A family study of aniridia. Arch Ophthalmol 1961;65:81.

81. Layman PR, Anderson DR, Flynn JT. Frequent occurrence of hypoplastic optic discs in patients with aniridia. Am J Ophthalmol 1974;77:513.

82. Berlin HS, Rich R. The treatment of glaucoma secondary to aniridia. Mt Sinai J Med 1981;48:111.

83. Kremer I, Rajpal RK, Rapuano CJ, et al. Results of penetrating keratoplasty in aniridia. Am J Ophthalmol 1993;115:317.

84. Johns KJ, O'Day DM. Posterior chamber intraocular lenses after extracapsular cataract extraction in patients with aniridia. Ophthalmology 1991;98:1698.

85. National Advisory Eye Council, Cataract Panel. Vision Research—A National Plan: 1983–1987 (Vol 1). Publication no. 83-2470. Washington, DC: National Institute of Health, 1983.

86. Pagon RA. Ocular coloboma. Surv Ophthalmol 1981;25:223.

87. Maumenee IH, Mitchell TN. Colobomatous malformations of the eye. Trans Am Ophthalmol Soc 1990;88:123.

88. Hoepner J, Yanoff ML. Ocular anomalies in trisomy 13–15: an analysis of 13 eyes with two new findings. Am J Ophthalmol 1972;74:729.

89. Denslow GT, Robb RM. Aicardi's syndrome: a report of four cases and review of the literature. J Pediatr Ophthalmol Strabismus 1979;16:10.

90. Poswillo D. Pathogenesis of craniofacial syndromes exhibiting colobomata. Trans Ophthalmol Soc UK 1976;96:69.

91. Pagon RA, Graham JM Jr, Zonana J, et al. CHARGE association: coloboma, congenital heart disease, and choanal atresia with multiple anomalies. J Pediatr 1981;99:223.

92. Brown NA, Bron AJ. Superficial lines and associated disorder of the cornea. Am J Ophthalmol 1976;81:34.

93. Laibson PR, Krachmer JH. Familial occurrence of dot (microcystic), map, fingerprint dystrophy of the cornea. Invest Ophthalmol 1975;14:397.

94. Fogle JA, Green WR, Kenyon KR. Anterior corneal dystrophy. Am J Ophthalmol 1974;77:529.

95. Klein R, Klein BEK, Moss SE, et al. The Wisconsin Epidemiologic Study of Diabetic Retinopathy. II. Prevalence and risk of diabetic retinopathy when age at diagnosis is less than 30 years. Arch Ophthalmol 1984;102:520–526.

96. Klein R, Klein BEK, Moss SE, et al. The Wisconsin Epidemiologic Study of Diabetic Retinopathy. III. Prevalence and risk of diabetic retinopathy when age at diagnosis is less than 30 years. Arch Ophthalmol 1984;102:527–532.

97. Early Treatment Diabetic Retinopathy Study. Fundus photographic risk factors for progression of diabetic retinopathy. Report Number 12. Ophthalmology 1991;98:823–833.

98. Early Treatment Diabetic Retinopathy Study. Early Treatment Diabetic Retinopathy Study design and baseline characteristics. Report Number 7. Ophthalmology 1991;98:741–756.

99. Early Treatment Diabetic Retinopathy Study. Early photocoagulation for diabetic retinopathy. Report Number 9. Ophthalmology 1991;98:766–785.

100. Early Treatment Diabetic Retinopathy Study. Detection of diabetic macular edema. Ophthalmoscopy verses photography. Report Number 5. Ophthalmology 1991;96:746–751.

101. Diabetic Retinopathy Study. A modification of Airlie House Classification of Diabetic Retinopathy. Report Number 7. Invest Ophthalmol Vis Sci 1981;21:210–226.

102. Diabetic Retinopathy Study. Four risk factors for severe visual loss in diabetic retinopathy. Report Number 3. Arch Ophthalmol 1979;97:658.

103. Diabetic Retinopathy Study. Indications for photocoagulation treatment of diabetic retinopathy. Report Number 14. Int Ophthalmol Clin 1987;27:239–253.

104. Diabetic Retinopathy Study. Preliminary report on effects of photocoagulation therapy. Report Number 1. Am J Ophthalmol 1976;81:1–14.

105. Diabetic Retinopathy Study. Photocoagulation of proliferative diabetic retinopathy. Report Number 2. Ophthalmology 1978;85:82.

106. Diabetic Retinopathy Study. A short report of long-range results: proceedings of the 10th Congress of International Diabetes Federation. Report Number 4. New York: Excerpta Medica, 1980.

107. Early Treatment Diabetic Retinopathy Study. Classification of diabetic retinopathy for fluorescein angiograms. Report Number 11. Ophthalmology 1991;98:807–822.

108. Early Treatment Diabetic Retinopathy Study. Fluorescein angiographic risk factors for progression of diabetic retinopathy. Report Number 13. Ophthalmology 1991;98:834–840.

109. Early Treatment Diabetic Retinopathy Study. Photocoagulation for diabetic macular edema. Report Number 1. Arch Ophthalmol 1985;103:1796–1807.

110. Early Treatment Diabetic Retinopathy Study. Treatment techniques and clinical guidelines for photocoagulation for macular edema. Report Number 2. Ophthalmology 1987;94:761–774.

111. Early Treatment Diabetic Retinopathy Study. Techniques for scatter and local photocoagulation of diabetic retinopathy. Report Number 3. Int Ophthalmol Clin 1987;27:254–264.

112. Early Treatment Diabetic Retinopathy Study. Photocoagulation for diabetic macular edema. Report Number 4. Int Ophthalmol Clin 1987;27:265–272.

113. Early Treatment Diabetic Retinopathy Study. Effects of aspirin treatment on diabetic retinopathy. Report Number 8. Ophthalmology 1991;98:757–765.

114. Early Treatment Diabetic Retinopathy Study. Grading diabetic retinopathy from stereoscopic color fundus photographs—an extension of the Airlie House Classification. Report Number 10. Ophthalmology 1991;98:786–806.

115. Diabetic Retinopathy Vitrectomy Study. Two-year course of visual acuity in severe proliferative diabetic retinopathy with conventional management. Report Number 1. Ophthalmology 1985;92:492–502.

116. Diabetic Retinopathy Vitrectomy Study. Early vitrectomy for severe vitreous hemorrhage in diabetic retinopathy. Two-year results of a randomized trial. Report Number 2. Arch Ophthalmol 1985;103:1644–1652.

117. Diabetic Retinopathy Vitrectomy Study. Early vitrectomy for severe proliferative diabetic retinopathy in eyes with useful vision. Report Number 3. Results of a randomized trial. Ophthalmology 1988;95:1307–1320.

118. Diabetic Retinopathy Vitrectomy Study. Early vitrectomy for severe proliferative diabetic retinopathy in eyes with useful vision. Clinical application of results of a randomized trial. Report Number 4. Ophthalmology 1988;95:1331–1334.

119. Diabetic Retinopathy Vitrectomy Study. Early vitrectomy for severe vitreous hemorrhage in diabetic retinopathy. Four-year results of a randomized trial. Report Number 5. Arch Ophthalmol 1990;108:958–964.

120. Paz A, Smith RE. The ETDRS and Diabetes 2000. Ophthalmology 1991;98:739–740.

121. Pyeritz RE, McKusick VA. The Marfan syndrome: diagnosis and management. N Engl J Med 1979;300:772.

122. Maumenee IH. The eye in Marfan syndrome. Trans Am Ophthalmol Soc 1981;79:684.

123. Henkind P, Ashton N. Ocular pathology in homocystinuria. Trans Ophthalmol Soc UK 1965;85:21.

124. Jensen AD, Cross HE, Paton D. Ocular complications in the Weill-Marchesani syndrome. Am J Ophthalmol 1974;77:261.

125. Bengsson B. The prevalence of glaucoma. Br J Ophthalmol 1981;65:46.

126. Sommer A, Duggan C, Auer C, Abbey H. Analytic approaches to the interpretation of automated threshold perimetric data for the diagnosis of early glaucoma. Trans Am Ophthalmol Soc 1985;83:250.

127. Blumenthhal M, Floman N, Treister G. Laser iris retraction for narrow-angle glaucoma. Glaucoma 1982;4:47.

128. Mapstone R. Provocative tests in closed-angle glaucoma. Br J Ophthalmol 1976;60:115.

129. Werner EB, Drance SM. Early visual field disturbances in glaucoma. Arch Ophthalmol 1977;95:1173.

130. Cioffi GA, Sarafarazi F, Perell HF. Computerized optic nerve image analysis with the confocal scanning ophthalmoscope. Ophthalmology 1990;97:144.

131. Sheilds MB. The future of computerized image analysis in the management of glaucoma. Am J Ophthalmol 1989;108:319.

132. Hiller R, Kahn HA. Blindness from glaucoma. Am J Ophthalmol 1975;80:62.

133. Redmond KB. The role of heredity in keratoconus. Trans Ophthalmol Soc N Z 1968;27:52.

134. Spencer WH, Fisher JJ. The association of keratoconus with atopic dermatitis. Am J Ophthalmol 1959;47:332.

135. Gasset AR, Hison WA, Frias JL. Keratoconus and atopic disease. Ann Ophthalmol 1978;10:991.

136. Applebaum A. Keratoconus. Arch Ophthalmol 1936;15:900.

137. Hofstetter H. A keratoconic survey of 13,395 eyes. Am J Optom Am Acad Optom 1959;36:3.

138. Kennedy RH, Bourne WM, Dyer DA. A 48-year clinical and epidemiologic study of keratoconus. Am J Ophthalmol 1986;101:267.

139. Maguire LJ, Bourne WD. Corneal topography and early keratoconus. Am J Ophthalmol 1989;108:107.

140. Rabinowitz YS, McDonald PJ. Computer-assisted corneal topography in keratoconus. J Refract Corneal Surg 1989;5:400.

141. Keates RH, Falkenstein S. Keratoplasty in keratoconus. Am J Ophthalmol 1972;74:442.

142. Payne JW. Primary penetrating keratoplasty for keratoconus: a long-term follow-up. Cornea 1982;1:21.

143. Paglen PG. The prognosis for keratoplasty in keratoconus. Ophthalmology 1982;89:651.

144. McDonald MB, Kaufman HE, Durrie DS. Epikeratophakia for keratoconus. The nationwide study. Arch Ophthalmol 1986;104:1294.

145. Richard J, Paton D, Gasset A. A comparison of penetrating keratoplasty and lamellar keratoplasty in the surgical management of keratoconus. Am J Ophthalmol 1978;86:807.

146. Gasset AR. Lamellar keratoplasty in the treatment of keratoconus: conectomy. Ophthalmic Surg 1979;10:26.

147. Gass JDM. Idiopathic senile macular hole: its early stages and pathogenesis. Arch Ophthalmol 1988;106:629–639.

148. Johnson RN, Gass JDM. Idiopathic macular holes. Observations, stages of formation, and implications for surgical intervention. Ophthalmology 1988;95:917–924.

149. McDonnell PJ, Fine SL, Hillis AI. Clinical features of idiopathic macular cysts and holes. Am J Ophthalmol 1982;93:777–786.

150. Aaberg TM, Blair CJ, Gass JDM. Macular holes. Am J Ophthalmol 1970;69:555.

151. Smiddy WE, Michels RG, Glaser BM, de Bustros S. Vitrectomy for impending macular holes. Am J Ophthalmol 1988;105:371–376.

152. Jost BF, Hutton WL, Fullet DG, et al. Vitrectomy in eyes at risk for macular hole formation. Ophthalmology 1990;97:843–847.

153. Kelly NE, Wendel RT. Vitrectomy surgery for idiopathic macular holes: results of a pilot study. Arch Ophthalmol 1991;109:654–659.

154. de Bustros S. Early stages of macular holes. To treat or not to treat? Arch Ophthalmol 1990;108:1085–1086.

155. Poser CM, Patsy DW, Scheinberg L, et al. New diagnostic criteria for multiple sclerosis: guidelines for research protocols. Ann Neurol 1983;13:277–231.

156. Gorelick PB. Clues to the mystery of multiple sclerosis. Postgrad Med 1898;85:125–134.

157. Ashworth B, Aspinall PA, Mitchell JD. Visual function in multiple sclerosis. Doc Ophthalmol 1990;73:209–224.

158. Vighetto A, Grochowicki M, Aimard G. Altitudinal hemianopsia in multiple sclerosis. Neuro-Ophthalmology 1991;11:25–27.

159. Keltner JL, Johnson CA, Spurr JO, Beck RW, and the Optic Neuritis Study Group. Baseline visual field profile of optic neuritis: the experience of the Optic Neuritis Treatment Trial. Arch Ophthalmol 1993;111:231–234.

160. Goodkin DE, Rudick RA, Ross JS. The use of brain magnetic resonance imaging in multiple sclerosis. Arch Neurol 1994;51:505–516.

161. Shahrokhi F, Chiappa KH, Young RR. Pattern shift visual evoked responses. Two hundred patients with optic neuritis and/or multiple sclerosis. Arch Neurol 1978;35:65–71.

162. Fukazawa T, Moriwaka F, Sugiyama K, et al. Cerebrospinal fluid IgG profiles and multiple sclerosis in Japan. Acta Neurol Scand 1993;88:178–183.

163. Nuland H, Naess A, Eidsvik S, et al. Effect of hyperbaric oxygen treatment on immunological parameters in multiple sclerosis. Acta Neurol Scand 1989;79:306–310.

164. Curtain BJ. Myopia: a review of its etiology, pathogenesis and treatment. Surv Ophthalmol 1970;15:1.

165. Sperduto RD, Seigel D, Roberts J, Rowland M. Prevalence of myopia in the United States. Arch Ophthalmol 1983;101:405.

166. Curtain BJ, Karlin DB. Axial length measurements of fundus changes of the myopic eye. Am J Ophthalmol 1971;71:42.

167. Hampton GR, Kohen D, Bird AC. Visual prognosis of disciform degeneration in myopia. Ophthalmology 1983;90:923.

168. Foressman B. A study of congenital nystagmus. Acta Otolaryngol 1964;57:427–428.

169. Smith DP. Diagnostic criteria in dominantly inherited juvenile optic atrophy: a report of three new families. Am J Optom Physiol Opt 1972;49:183–200.

170. Horoupian DS, Zucker DK, Moshe S, Peterson H. Behr syndrome: a clinicopathologic report. Neurology 1979;29:323–327.

171. Francois J. Hereditary degenerations of the optic nerve (hereditary optic atrophy). Int Ophthalmol Clin 1968;8:999–1054.

172. Wallace DC. A new manifestation of Leber's disease and a new

explanation for the agency responsible for its unusual pattern of inheritance. Brain 1970;93:121–132.

173. Krause AC, Hopkins WG. Ocular manifestations of histoplasmosis. Am J Ophthalmol 1951;34:564–566.

174. Gass JDM, Wilkinson CP. Follow-up study of presumed ocular histoplasmosis. Trans Am Acad Ophthalmol Otolaryngol 1972;76:672–693.

175. Smith RE, Ganley JP. An epidemiologic study of presumed ocular histoplasmosis. Trans Am Acad Ophthalmol Otolaryngol 1971;75:994–1005.

176. Fountain JA, Schlaegel TF Jr. Linear streaks of the equator in the presumed ocular histoplasmosis syndrome. Arch Ophthalmol 1981;99:246–248.

177. Bralry RE, Meredith TA, Aaberg TM, et al. The prevalence of HLA-B7 in presumed ocular histoplasmosis. Am J Ophthalmol 1978;85:859.

178. Macular Photocoagulation Study Group. Argon laser photocoagulation for ocular histoplasmosis: results of a randomized clinical trial. Arch Ophthalmol 1983;101:1347–1357.

179. Lewis ML, Schiffman JC. Long-term follow-up of the second eye in ocular histoplasmosis. Int Ophthalmol Clin 1983;23:125.

180. Archambault P, Gomolin JE. Incidence of retinopathy of prematurity among infants weighing 2000 g or less at birth. Can J Ophthalmol 1987;22:218–220.

181. Schulenburg WE, Prendiville A, Ohri R. Natural history of retinopathy of prematurity. Br J Ophthalmol 1987;71:837–843.

182. Tasman WS. The natural history of retinopathy of prematurity. Ophthalmology 1984;91:1499–1503.

183. Flynn JT, Bancalari E, Bachynski BN, et al. Retinopathy of prematurity. Diagnosis, severity, and natural history. Ophthalmology 1987;94:620–629.

184. Committee for the classification of ROP. An international classification of retinopathy of prematurity. II. The classification of retinal detachment. Arch Ophthalmol 1987;105:906–912.

185. Topilow HW, Ackerman AL. Cryotherapy for stage 3+ retinopathy of prematurity: visual and anatomic results. Ophthalmol Surg 1989;20:864–871.

186. Cryotherapy for Retinopathy of Prematurity Cooperative Group. Multicenter trial of cryotherapy for retinopathy of prematurity: one-year outcome: structure and function. Arch Ophthalmol 1990;108:1408–1416.

187. Greven C, Tasman W. Scleral buckling in stages 4B and 5 retinopathy of prematurity. Ophthalmology 1990;97:817–820.

188. Finer NN, Schindler RF, Peters KL, Grant GD. Vitamin E and retrolental fibroplasia: improved visual outcome with early vitamin E. Ophthalmology 1980;90:428.

189. Kretzer FL, Mehta RS, Johnson AT, et al. Vitamin E protects against retinopathy of prematurity through action on spindle cells. Nature 1984;309:793–795.

190. Zillis JD, de Juan E, Machamer R. Advanced retinopathy of prematurity: the anatomic and visual results of vitreous surgery. Ophthalmology 1990;98:821–826.

191. Merin S, Auerbach E. Retinitis pigmentosa. Surv Ophthalmol 1976;20:303–346.

192. Boughman JA, Conneally PM, Nance WE. Population genetic studies of retinitis pigmentosa. Am J Hum Genet 1980;32:223–235.

193. Jay M. Figures and fantasies. The frequencies of the different genetic forms of retinitis pigmentosa. Birth Defects 1982;18:167–173.

194. Jay M. On the heredity of retinitis pigmentosa. Br J Ophthalmol 1982;66:405.

195. Pruett RC. Retinitis pigmentosa: clinical observations and correlations. Trans Am Ophthalmol Soc 1983;81:693.

196. Pagon RA. Retinitis pigmentosa. Surv Ophthalmol 1987;33:137.

197. Biro I. Sectoral retinitis pigmentosa. Ophthalmologica 1944;107:149–157.

198. Batra DV. Bilateral symmetrical sectoral retinal pigmentation. Br J Ophthalmol 1966;50:734.

199. Joseph R. Unilateral retinitis pigmentosa. Br J Ophthalmol 1951;35:98.

200. Carr RE, Siegel IM. Unilateral retinitis pigmentosa. Arch Ophthalmol 1973;90:21–26.

201. Fishman GA, Kumar A, Joseph ME, et al. Usher's syndrome: ophthalmic and neuro-otologic findings suggesting genetic heterogeneity. Arch Ophthalmol 1983;101:1367.

202. Berson EL, Rosner B, Sandberg MA, et al. A randomized trial of vitamin A and vitamin E supplementation for retinitis pigmentosa. Arch Ophthalmol 1993;111:761–756.

203. Fishman GA, Maggiero JM, Fishman M. Foveal lesions seen in retinitis pigmentosa. Arch Ophthalmol 1978;95:625.

204. Pearlman JT. Mathematical models of retinitis pigmentosa: a study of the rate of progress in different genetic forms. Trans Am Ophthalmol Soc 1979;77:643–656.

205. Fishman GA. Fundus flavimaculatus: a clinical classification. Arch Ophthalmol 1976;94:2061.

206. Hadden OB, Gass JDM. Fundus flavimaculatus and Stargardt's disease. Am J Ophthalmol 1976;82:527.

207. Moloney JBM, Mooney DJ, O'Connor MA. Retinal function in Stargardt's disease and fundus flavimaculatus. Am J Ophthalmol 1983;96:57.

208. Anmarkrud N. Fundus fluorescein angiography in fundus flavimaculatus and Stargardt's disease. Acta Ophthalmol 1979;57:172.

209. Sabetes R, Pruett RC, Brockhurst RJ. Fulminant ocular toxoplasmosis. Am J Ophthalmol 1981;92:497.

210. Schlaegel TF Jr, Weber JC. The macula in ocular toxoplasmosis. Arch Ophthalmol 1984;102:697–698.

211. Krick JA, Remington JS. Current concepts in parasitology: toxoplasmosis in the adult—an overview. N Engl J Med 1978;298:550–553.

212. Eichenwald HF. A Study of Congenital Toxoplasmosis with Particular Emphasis on Clinical Manifestations, Sequelae and Therapy. In J Siim (ed), Human Toxoplasmosis. Copenhagen: Munksgaard, 1960;41–49.

213. Benson WE. Ocular toxoplasmosis and visual field defects. Am J Ophthalmol 1980;90:25–29.

214. Weiss MJ, Velazquez N, Hofeldt AJ. Serologic tests in the diagnosis of presumed toxoplasmic retinochoroiditis. Am J Ophthalmol 1990;109:407–411.

215. Lakhanpal V, Schocket SS, Nirankari VS. Clindamycin in the treatment of toxoplasmic retinochoroiditis. Am J Ophthalmol 1983;95:605–613.

216. Ghartey KN, Brockhurst RJ. Photocoagulation of active toxoplasmic retinochoroiditis. Am J Ophthalmol 1980;89:858–864.

CHAPTER SEVEN

Magnification Associated with Low Vision Systems

Alvin Byer

A basic property of magnification is that it is a ratio. A statement such as, "the magnification produced by this optical system is 4×," is meaningless unless one knows to what the magnified image is being compared. That is, four times bigger than what? Without knowing the original (unmagnified) image size to which the magnified image is being compared, nothing is known about the size of the magnified image. It is as though someone asked the size of a box and the answer was, "It's twice as large." One can only know how large the box is if it is compared to a box of known size. It is this basic principle that is probably responsible for the fact that optical magnification associated with lenses for both the normally sighted and the partially sighted populations is often found to be a confusing concept. If a magnifier in a catalog is advertised as a 4× magnifier, does that mean it will produce 4× magnification when it is used? Only under very specific conditions. So it is important to understand what this ratio is. But first, the ratio should be defined as to what it is not.

The first magnification concept that one usually meets in the study of optics is the ratio of the size of the image to the size of the object, usually called the *transverse magnification* (m_T). When the object space and image space are both air, it is given by the following equation:

$$m_T = \frac{\text{image size } (y')}{\text{object size } (y)} = \frac{\text{object vergence } (U)}{\text{image vergence } (V)} = \frac{\text{image distance } (v)}{\text{object distance } (u)}$$

When this concept is applied with the human eye as the optical system, the size of the image on the retina is being compared with the size of the object of regard. For example, when someone looks at a letter that subtends 5 minutes of arc at the eye, and the object is 6 m from the eye (often called a 6/6- or a 20/20-size letter), the size of the letter will be approximately 8.73 mm in height, and its conjugate image on the retina will be approximately 0.03 mm. The eye therefore is producing a transverse magnification of 0.03/8.73, or 0.00344×. Neither the absolute size of this retinal image nor the magnification that the eye is producing is of any interest in low vision. What is of interest is the *change* in the size of the retinal image that occurs when the eye views through a lens. So in the study of vision rehabilitation using various kinds of optical systems, it is the change in the retinal image that the optical system produces that is important, not the comparison of an image size to an object size. The comparison is between two image sizes: the one that has been magnified and the original. This comparison leads to the retinal image magnification (RIM):

$$RIM = \frac{\text{magnified retinal image size}}{\text{original retinal image size}} = \frac{y'_A}{y'_{UN}}$$

where y'_A = retinal image size with the magnifier (aided), and y'_{UN} = retinal image size without any magnification added (unaided).

Note. The terms *aided* and *unaided* do *not* correlate to *with* and *without lenses* to correct a refractive error. They refer to *with* and *without a magnifier*. The eye in which a retinal image is being magnified must be emmetropic, either naturally or corrected. It is pointless to magnify an image without first assuring that it is in focus on the retina.

COMPONENTS OF RETINAL IMAGE MAGNIFICATION

The RIM is the product of three factors, as shown by the following formula:

$$RIM = (RSM)(RDM)(LVM)$$

where RSM = relative size magnification, RDM = relative distance magnification, and LVM = lens vertex magnification.

Each of these is discussed in detail in sections that follow. For now, however, a brief introduction to the terms is in order. The meanings of RSM and RDM are almost self-explanatory. Both can be achieved without the use of a lens, whereas the LVM term, as the name implies, is magnification that depends on the kind of lens that is placed before the eye and its location. The term *angular magnification* is avoided because it is less specific; all three components given in the previous paragraph produce angular magnification, which in turn produces RIM. In practice, the depth of field impacts on the final RIM. It allows the use of magnifiers in ways that produce images on the retina that are usable and functional, although not in perfect focus. But for the purpose of this chapter, calculations of RIM always assume that the retinal image is in focus. Otherwise, there would be an infinite number of possible answers depending on the depth of field that accompanied each specific situation.

PRESCRIBED MAGNIFICATION VERSUS BY-PRODUCT MAGNIFICATION

The literature is anything but consistent in the modifiers that are placed in front of the term *magnification*. Magnification associated with vision can be divided into two classifications: One is specifically prescribed for a partially sighted person; the other occurs as a by-product of correcting a refractive error. The former (i.e., prescribed magnification) includes the RDM, RSM, and LVM factors. The latter, (i.e., by-product magnification) involves only the LVM factor, and in the context of prescribing spectacle lenses to correct an ametropia, is usually called *spectacle magnification* (SM). Optically, LVM and SM are the same quantity. Normally sighted patients wear relatively low-power corrective lenses at spectacle plane vertex distances that rarely exceed 15 mm, resulting in SMs on the order of 10–15%. Visually impaired patients use high-power lenses either at spectacle plane vertex distances or considerably longer. Higher-power lenses or longer vertex distances, or both, combine to produce higher magnifications, typically of magnitudes starting at approximately the 2× (100%) level. Because the area of interest here is the visually impaired patient, the lens magnification term in this chapter will be *LVM*. But optically, LVM and SM are the same quantity. The label *spectacle magnification* is historically associated with that which comes from correcting an ametropia; it is called *lens vertex magnification (LVM)* when it is specifically prescribed for a visually impaired patient.

THIN LENS MODEL OF THE EYE

The magnification that is of interest in this book is obviously associated with low vision, and in particular, how visual function can be enhanced by the use of magnification. For the purpose of discussing these magnification principles, the human eye will be represented by what is commonly referred to as the *thin lens model of the eye*, shown in Figure 7-1.

The total refracting power of the eye is represented by a thin lens. The axial length is coordinated with the thin lens power to make it emmetropic. The nodal point is at the intersection of the lens with the optical axis. This makes it convenient for the purpose of showing a ray trace of the retinal image because it can be done with a single ray, namely the nodal ray from the object point to its conjugate image point on the retina (Figure 7-2).

For an emmetropic eye, the retinal surface is the location of the secondary focal plane of the eye, (the F' plane). Parallel rays entering the eye will therefore result in a focused image on the retina. It is worth repeating that the image on the retina must be in focus before any magnification is prescribed. Otherwise a blurred image will be magnified, which will probably result in the need for more magnification than would otherwise be necessary.

RELATIVE DISTANCE MAGNIFICATION

RDM can be achieved without a lens, but more often than not, is achieved with the help of a lens (Figure 7-3). To begin with, no lens will be used to avoid the need to consider the LVM component; that factor will be considered in Relative Distance Magnification and Lens Vertex Magnification Combined. Note that object y at distance u_1 produces a conjugate image y'_1, but when the object is moved closer (to distance u_2), the retinal image increases to size y'_2. The increase in the size of the retinal image is the ratio of the two distances:

$$RDM = \frac{y'_2}{y'_1} = \frac{l(\tan\theta')}{l(\tan\theta)} = \frac{\dfrac{y}{u_2}}{\dfrac{y}{u_1}} = \frac{u_1}{u_2}$$

$$RDM = \frac{u_1}{u_2}$$

So if an object is initially held 50 cm from the eye, and the patient has sufficient accommodative amplitude to bring it in to 25 cm, 2× RIM will result.

RELATIVE SIZE MAGNIFICATION

RSM can be achieved by changing the size of the object while it remains stationary, and no lens is involved. An example of this magnification is the replacement of standard size text with a large-print edition. Figure 7-4 illustrates this concept.

The magnification of the image is simply the ratio of the enlarged size of the object to the original size:

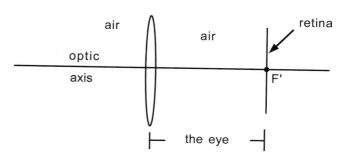

FIGURE 7-1.   **Thin lens model of the eye. (F' = secondary focal plane.)**

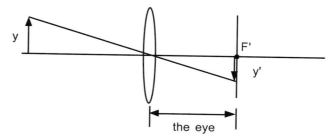

FIGURE 7-2.   **Retinal image ray trace. (y = object size; y' = retinal image size; F' = secondary focal point.)**

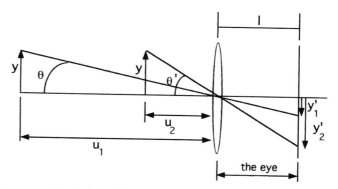

FIGURE 7-3.   **Relative distance magnification. (l = length; θ = angle subtended at eye by object at u_1; θ' = angle subtended at eye by object at u_2; y = object size; u_1 = original object distance; u_2 = new object distance; y'_1 = image size when object is at u_1; y'_2 = image size when object is at u_2.)**

$$RSM = \frac{y_2}{y_1}$$

Thus, when a 10-mm tall letter is replaced with a 20-mm tall letter, the retinal image is likewise doubled in size and the RSM = 2×.

Note. In all subsequent sections the RSM factor will be treated as unity, meaning that no change will be made in object size.

LENS VERTEX MAGNIFICATION

To examine the LVM uncontaminated by an RDM factor, the object must not be moved after the magnifier lens is added. Therefore the situation is one in which the patient, for exam-

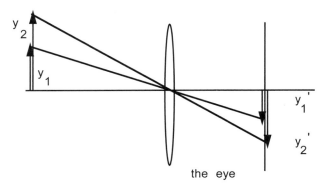

FIGURE 7-4.   **Relative size magnification. (y_1 = original object size; y_2 = new object size; y_1' = image size of object y_1; y_2' = image size of object y_2.)**

ple, looks at some text, has difficulty reading it, and enlists the aid of a handheld magnifier. If the object is to remain stationary, the magnifier location is constrained to be no further than one focal length from the object. (Any distance greater than one focal length results in an inverted and blurred image on the retina.) When the magnifier is added such that the object is between it and the magnifer's primary focal plane, a larger retinal image results (Figure 7-5A, B).

Figure 7-5A shows a retinal image, y', of object y produced by the eye alone. Figure 7-5B shows the same object at the same location, but this time a magnifier has been added. The magnifier produces virtual image y', which subtends a larger angle at the eye than the original object and so produces larger retinal image y". The ratio of image y" in Figure 7-5B to image y' in Figure 7-5A is the LVM. The fact that the object has changed in neither size nor location means that the relative distance and RSMs are both equal to unity. The magnitude of the LVM is given by the following formula[1]:

$$LVM = \frac{1 - dU}{1 - dV}$$

where d = vertex distance (always positive), U = object vergence incident at the lens, and V = image vergence leaving the lens.

Notice that if d is zero, which corresponds to a contact lens with the thin lens model, then LVM = 1, and there is no magnification benefit from the presence of the lens. Only for nonzero values of d will there be a nonunity LVM component. When a magnifier lens is held at the spectacle plane, the typical vertex distance will be approximately 12 mm. The contribution to the overall retinal magnification of an LVM factor with d values this small is clinically insignificant in low vision. Under these circumstances, the magnification will principally come from the relative distance factor. For example, the placement of a +10.00 D magnifier lens in the spectacle plane will enable the patient to move the object of regard to 10 cm, resulting in a significant amount of RDM. If the RDM that resulted was 4×, correction for the LVM factor would make the RIM 4.5×, a clinically insignificant difference. If there is some unusual circumstance that requires a more precise calculation, the LVM factor can always be calculated for whatever vertex distance applies.

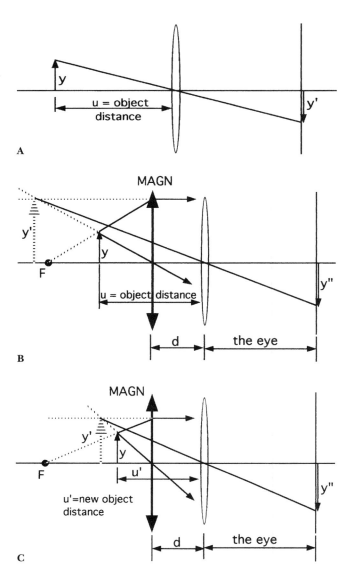

FIGURE 7-5.   **A. Retinal image size without the magnifier. (y = object size; y' = retinal image size.) B. Lens vertex magnification. (MAGN = magnifier; d = vertex distance; y = original object size; y' = virtual image size; F = primary focal point of magnifier; y" = magnified retinal image size.) C. Lens vertex magnification combined with relative distance magnification. (MAGN = magnifier; d = vertex distance; y = original object size; y' = virtual image size; F = primary focal point of magnifier; y" = magnified retinal image size.)**

RELATIVE DISTANCE MAGNIFICATION AND LENS VERTEX MAGNIFICATION COMBINED

Probably the most common method of providing magnification at near is the combination of RDM and LVM. When the print is unreadable with full accommodation or habitual spectacle lens add power, the need for some magnification is indicated. The patient would typically use a magnifier held at some distance from the spectacle plane, producing some LVM, and also move the object to the front focal plane of the magnifier or closer, producing some RDM. The final RIM is the product of these two components (Figure 7-5C):

$$RIM = (RDM)(LVM)$$

This chapter will show two approaches to the calculation of the RIM. The first one shown below is a little more involved but is more informative in that it keeps the RDM and LVM components intact so that one can see how much each is contributing to the total. As such, it has been labeled the *product formula*.

$$RIM = (RDM)(LVM)$$

$$RIM = \left(\frac{u_R}{u_{eye}}\right)\left(\frac{1-dU}{1-dV}\right) \quad \text{(the "product" formula)}$$

The LVM terms were defined in Lens Vertex Magnification; the RDM terms include the *unaided* (i.e., without the magnifier) *reading distance* (u_R) and the *aided* (i.e., with the magnifier) *reading distance* (u_{eye}), which is the distance from the object to the eye. The u_{eye} term is also the sum of object distance to lens plus lens distance to the eye.

Consider the following situation. For a reading distance of 40 cm, some combination of accommodation and add power equal to +2.50 D is needed. Assume that this patient can provide a maximum of +2.50 D of accommodation. Because of the existence of macular disease, however, he or she cannot read at 40 cm and elects to use a +10.00 D handheld magnifier.

First isolate the LVM component by assuming that the patient holds the magnifier one focal length from the object *and does not move the object*. This constraint forces the vertex distance (d) to be 30 cm. Parallel rays will be incident at the eye, thus requiring no accommodation (Figure 7-6). Calculation using the product formula is shown here. (Note: More details of this calculation are given in Appendix A.)

$$RIM = (RDM)(LVM)$$

$$= \left(\frac{u_R}{u_{eye}}\right)\left(\frac{1-dU}{1-dV}\right)$$

$$= \left(\frac{40}{40}\right)\left[\frac{1-(0.30)(-10)}{1-(0.30)(0)}\right] = (1)(4) = 4\times$$

Notice that all the magnification comes from the LVM factor because the object remained stationary and therefore RDM = 1.

More commonly, the placement of the magnifier will be followed by a movement of the object closer to the patient, adding an RDM factor. For example, suppose this patient held the magnifier 5 cm from the eye and then moved the object in to the same distance from the magnifier as before (i.e., 10 cm). What is the RIM now (Figure 7-7)?

$$RIM = (RDM)(LVM)$$

$$= \left(\frac{u_R}{u_{eye}}\right)\left(\frac{1-dU}{1-dV}\right)$$

$$= \left(\frac{40}{15}\right)\left[\frac{1-(0.05)(-10)}{1-(0.05)(-0)}\right]$$

$$= (2.67)\left(\frac{3}{2}\right) = 4\times$$

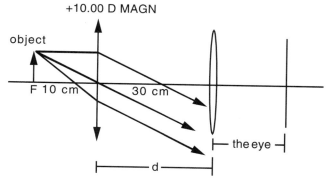

FIGURE 7-6.   **Lens vertex magnification without relative distance magnification. (MAGN = magnifier; F = primary focal point of magnifier.)**

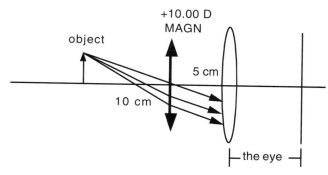

FIGURE 7-7.   **Lens vertex magnification with relative distance magnification. (MAGN = magnifier.)**

Using the component formula to calculate the RIM allows one to see how much magnification comes from the RDM and LVM factors. In the previous case, all the magnification was LVM. Here we see that now the RDM is responsible for most of the magnification (2.67×), whereas the 5-cm vertex distance contributes an LVM factor of 1.5×.

On the other hand, if the magnifier was held in the spectacle plane and the object of regard was again held one focal length from the lens (10 cm for a +10.00 D lens), what magnification would result?

$$RIM = (RDM)(LVM)$$

$$= \left(\frac{u_R}{u_{eye}}\right)\left(\frac{1-dU}{1-dV}\right)$$

$$= \left(\frac{40}{10}\right)(1)$$

$$= 4\times$$

The LVM factor becomes unity because the vertex distance d is treated as zero for magnifiers held in the spectacle plane. So all the magnification comes from the RDM component. Notice that the same magnification results in all three cases (4×), but the distribution shifted from all LVM in the first case, to all RDM in the last case. The reason that 4× resulted in all cases is that *the magnification is independent of the vertex distance for the special case in which the*

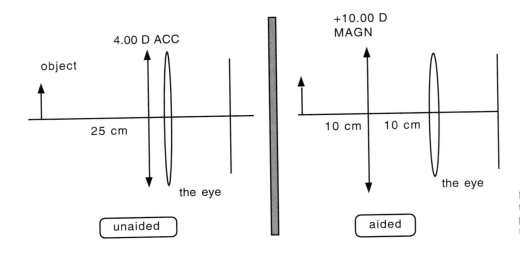

FIGURE 7-8. **The special magnification = D/4 case, where D = dioptric power of the magnifier. (MAGN = magnifier; ACC = accommodation.)**

object is held one focal length from the magnifier. Proof of this is provided in the ray trace schematic shown in Appendix B.

MAGNIFICATION IN TERMS OF THE EQUIVALENT POWER

Up to this point, the formula used for the RIM calculation has been the product of the RDM and the LVM so that the reader could see how these two components interact and also know the magnitude of each. It is the longer way to calculate the RIM, but it is more informative for the student of magnification. Once the topic is understood, and one simply wants the answer by the most expedient method, the use of the Gauss equivalent power formula is the method of choice.

Before proceeding to that calculation, the reader should examine Appendix B, which shows, using a ray trace, that the magnification is independent of the vertex distance when the object is held in the front focal plane of the lens. That is true whether the lens is a single thin lens or a thick system represented by an equivalent thin lens using gaussian optics. Furthermore, if the magnification is independent of the vertex distance, the simplest vertex distance can be used for calculation purposes, and that would be a vertex distance of zero. Under these circumstances, the LVM component in the product formula becomes unity and all the magnification comes from RDM. The relative distance component is simply the ratio of the unaided reference distance (u_R) to the aided distance (u_2), where the aided distance is one focal length (f_e) from the equivalent thin lens. The minus sign is added because in the usual sign convention, the reference distance will be negative.

$$RIM = \frac{u_1}{u_2} = \frac{u_R}{u_2} = \frac{u_R}{f_e} = -u_R D_e$$

where D_e is the standard gaussian equivalent power, given by the following:

$$D_e = D_1 + D_2 - dD_1D_2$$

So the RIM produced by any optical system can always be found from the product of the equivalent power and the

unaided (without magnifier) viewing distance, usually referred to as the *reference distance* (u_R).

$$RIM = (-u_R)(D_e)$$

For instance, in the previous illustration in which the patient used a +10.00 D magnifier at various vertex distances, in each case the only lens in the system was the magnifier, and the original viewing distance was 40 cm. So the magnification calculation using the Gauss formula is simply $-(-0.4) \times (10) = 4\times$ as was found when calculated using the component formula.

THE D/4 AND (D/4) + 1 FORMULAS

One can analyze the same problem another way and discover the origin of two magnification formulas that are often found in the older literature. The first says that the magnification is calculated from m = D/4, sometimes called the *effective magnification*. The second says the magnification is m = (D/4) + 1, sometimes called the *conventional magnification*. In each case, the symbol D represents the dioptric power of the magnifier. Both of these formulas are still in use by some vendors of magnifiers. Labels such as *effective* or *conventional* in front of the term *magnification* add nothing to the understanding of the topic and should be avoided. There is only one magnification that counts, and that is the enlargement of the retinal image size relative to its unaided size—that is, without any magnifier. That is why the term *RIM* has been adopted and is the only one used.

The m = D/4 formula is a special case that presupposes that the unaided reading distance is 25 cm and that the object of regard is held one focal length from the magnifier. Unless these conditions are met, the D/4 formula does not apply. What vertex distance should be used? Once again, the fact that the object is held one focal length from the lens enables one to use any vertex distance. So, for this calculation, a vertex distance of 10 cm will be arbitrarily chosen. The unaided and aided situations are shown in Figure 7-8. On the left, the object is held at the assumed 25-cm distance and so the eye must accommodate by 4.00 D. On the right, when the

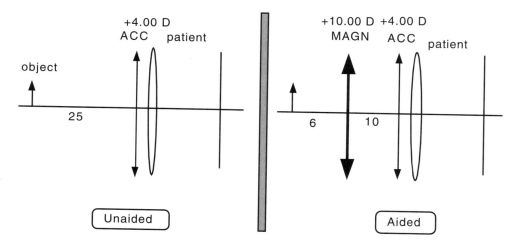

FIGURE 7-9. **The special magnification = (D/4) + 1 case, where D = dioptric power of the magnifier.** (ACC = accommodation; MAGN = magnifier.)

magnifier is used, the object is held in the front focal plane of the lens, which produces parallel rays out of the magnifier and into the eye, thus requiring no accommodation.

The object was originally at 25 cm. When the magnifier is used, the object is moved in to the front focal plane of the lens, which is 10 cm from the lens and 20 cm from the eye. The calculation of the magnification by the product formula follows:

$$RIM = (RDM)(LVM)$$
$$= \left(\frac{u_R}{u_{eye}}\right)\left(\frac{1-dU}{1-dV}\right)$$
$$= \left(\frac{25}{10+10}\right)\left[\frac{1-0.1(-10)}{1-0.1(0)}\right]$$
$$= \left(\frac{25}{20}\right)(2) = 2.5\times$$

If the Gauss formula is used, the result is

$$RIM = (-u_R)(D_e)$$
$$-(-0.25)(+10) = 2.5\times$$

If the formula m = D/4 is used, the result would be the correct answer of 2.5×. But it is important to notice the constraints on this formula. If the unaided distance had been any distance other than 25 cm or if the object was held closer than one focal length from the magnifier, the D/4 formula would not have produced the correct answer.

For example, what is the correct magnification if the unaided distance (the reference distance) had been 40 cm?

$$RIM = (RDM)(LVM)$$
$$= \left(\frac{u_R}{u_{eye}}\right)\left(\frac{1-dU}{1-dV}\right)$$
$$= \left(\frac{40}{10}\right)(1) = 4\times$$

Or by the Gauss method, RIM = −(−0.40)(10) = 4×.

Can the same +10.00 D magnifier, held at the same distance from the eye (at d = 10 cm) produce two different magnifications? That is what these two different answers

imply, but it is important to understand what these numbers mean. The two different numbers result from the aided retinal image in the first case being compared to an unaided image produced by an object 25 cm from the eye, whereas in the second case, the aided image is compared to an unaided image associated with an object at 40 cm. *But the final image size on the retina is the same in both cases.* To use another rather mundane analogy, if the length of a piece of lumber (A) is characterized as 2× and another (B) as 3×, A and B can be of the same length if A is twice as long as a 6-ft piece (its reference piece) and B is three times as long as a 4-ft piece (its reference piece). They are both 12 ft long.

On the other hand, if the m = (D/4) + 1 formula is applied to the +10.00 D lens, the result would be a magnification value of 3.5× instead of 2.5×. Where does this extra one unit of magnification come from? In the D/4 case, the patient was required to accommodate by 4.00 D when viewing without the magnifier. Then when the magnifier was used, the object was brought in to the front focal plane of the lens, resulting in parallel light leaving, and no accommodation being required. The argument can be made that if 4.00 D of accommodation is available when unaided, for consistency, the same amount of accommodation should be used with the magnifier. With this assumption, the before and after conditions are as shown in Figure 7-9 and the following calculation:

$$RIM = (RDM)(LVM)$$
$$= \left(\frac{u_R}{u_{eye}}\right)\left(\frac{1-dU}{1-dV}\right)$$
$$= \left(\frac{25}{6+10}\right)\left[\frac{1.0-(0.1)(-16.67)}{1.0-(0.1)(-6.67)}\right] = 2.5\times$$

Alternately, the calculation could be made from the equivalent power formula.

Note. In the u_{eye} term, the object must be 6 cm from the magnifier to create a virtual image at 25 cm from the eye that acts as the object for the +4.00 D accommodation lens. This concept is illustrated in Appendix A.

$$m = -u_R D_e = 0.25[10+4-(10)(4)(0.1)] = 2.5\times$$

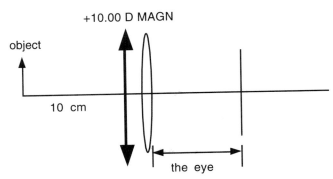

FIGURE 7-10.   **Viewing through the carrier. (MAGN = magnifier.)**

An answer of 2.5× is not the expected result. What is wrong? Where is the extra one unit of magnification that the (D/4) + 1 formula predicts? Once again, these off-the-shelf formulas only work under certain conditions. In this case, the condition that was violated was the vertex distance. The only way that 3.5× results when this magnifier is combined with 4.00 D of accommodation is when the vertex distance is zero. When d = 0, then the 4.00 D of plus from accommodation combines directly with the +10.00 D of the magnifier, yielding a total of +14.00 D. The object then must be moved in to the front focal plane of a +14.00 D lens, which is a distance of 7.14 cm. Then the magnification becomes as follows:

$$RIM = (RDM)(LVM)$$

$$= \left(\frac{u_R}{u_{eye}}\right)\left(\frac{1-dU}{1-dV}\right)$$

$$= \left(\frac{25}{7.14}\right)(1) = 3.5 \times$$

Or, alternately, $m = -u_R D_e = -(-0.25) \times 14 = 3.5\times$. So the m = (D/4) + 1 formula gives the correct answer only when the special conditions have been met. On the other hand, the RIM = RDM × LVM formula and the gaussian formula are totally general.

WHEN THE OBJECT IS NOT IN THE F PLANE OF THE LENS (u ≠ f)

When an object is held closer than one focal length (f) from the magnifier, causing diverging rays of light to be incident at the eye, a virtual image is created. There is therefore a need for some plus power at the eye either by accommodation or add power in a spectacle lens. This concept is important because virtually all stand magnifiers are designed with the distance from the plane of the reading material to the lens being less than one focal length. Two numerical examples follow.

Example 1
The patient is an absolute presbyope wearing bifocal spectacles with a 2.50 D add. Under these conditions, he is having trouble reading small print. He enlists the aid of a +10.00 D handheld magnifier. He holds the magnifier 10 cm from his eye. How much magnification is achieved?

First, one must realize that there are two ways that a bifocal wearer might use the magnifier in conjunction with his spectacles: (1) He or she could view through the carrier, or (2) he or she could view through the segment. Second, one must realize that once the dioptric power of the magnifier has been selected, there are two variables under the control of the patient—namely the vertex distance and the distance the object is from the magnifier.

Viewing Through the Carrier
In the presence of absolute presbyopia, viewing through the carrier requires the object to be held at the focal plane of the magnifier. If it is held farther away than one focal length, the image produced will be inverted and blurred; if held closer than one focal length, the image rays will be divergent and blurred because there is neither accommodation nor add power available.

When using a stand magnifier and viewing through the carrier, the choice of stand magnifiers is limited to those that produce a virtual image at relatively long distances from the lens. If the virtual image is far enough from the lens such that its incident negative vergence at the eye is not too great, then the amount of blur of the retinal image might be within the patient's depth of focus limitation. The retinal image will be out of focus but still usable. The blur of the retinal image under these conditions can be further reduced by holding the stand magnifier as far from the eye as possible.

If the patient wants to view through the carrier and achieve better focus than the stand magnifier produces, he or she must use a handheld magnifier. With a handheld magnifier, the patient can hold the reading material very close to the front focal plane of the lens, thus producing essentially parallel rays at the eye and assuring a focused retinal image. Under these circumstances, the magnification produced is independent of the vertex distance (see Appendix B), so the calculation of the magnification can be simplified by assuming a zero vertex distance. The result is simply the RDM ratio of 40 to 10, or 4×, as found in Lens Vertex Magnification. The optical setup is shown in Figure 7-10.

Viewing Through the Segment
A point that is often overlooked in the case of a patient with absolute presbyopia using a magnifier is that *the habitual add power determines the unaided (reference) distance*, and to calculate the magnification of the conjugate focused image on the retina, this is the reference distance that must be used. In other words, when this patient attempts to read by looking through the segment of the bifocals, there is only one distance from the eye that will be conjugate with the retina, and that is the front focal plane of the add power (40 cm for a +2.50 D add). Therefore, the reading material will only be in focus on the retina when held 40 cm from the eye. This establishes the reference distance, and no other number is correct for a reference distance (u_R) under these conditions.

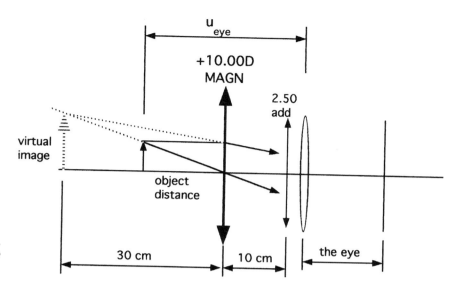

FIGURE 7-11. **Viewing through the segment.** (MAGN = magnifier; u = distance from lens to object; u_{eye} = distance from object to eye.)

$$RIM = (RDM)(LVM)$$
$$= \left(\frac{u_R}{u_{eye}}\right)\left(\frac{1 - dU}{1 - dV}\right)$$

It is worthwhile to review again what the u_{eye} term is because it now has to be calculated. It is the aided viewing distance: the distance from the object to the eye when the magnifier is in use. If the distance to the magnifier from the eye is known (assume 10 cm again), and if the distance of the object from the lens can be determined (u), then u can be added to the 10 cm to get the u_{eye} value. How is u found? The patient is looking through 2.50 D of plus add power. For the object to be seen clearly, the virtual image produced by the magnifier must be 40 cm from the eye. Because the lens is 10 cm from the eye, the virtual image must be 30 cm from the magnifier (see Figure 7-10).

It is now easy to find out how far the object-to-lens distance (u) is by simply using the standard object/image/power formula (Figure 7-11):

$$U + D = V$$

where U is the object vergence at the lens, D is the lens power, and V is the image vergence leaving the lens. The object vergence at the lens is the value being sought. The lens power is + 10.00 D, and the image vergence leaving the lens must be V = 1/v = −1/0.3 m = −3.33 D, where v is the image distance from the lens. This number must be negative because the rays are divergent and the image is virtual.

$$U + D = V$$
$$U + 10 = -3.33$$
$$U = -13.33 \text{ D}$$
$$u = \frac{100}{-13.33}$$
$$u = -7.50 \text{ cm}$$

The distance from the object to the eye (u_{eye}) is 7.50 cm + 10 cm, or 17.50 cm. At this point, the RDM factor is known (40/17.50 = 2.29×). The LVM component is

$$LVM = \frac{1 - dU}{1 - dV}$$
$$= \frac{1 - 0.1(-13.33)}{1 - 0.1(-3.33)}$$
$$= \frac{2.33}{1.33} = 1.75 \times$$

Therefore, the total magnification is

$$RIM = (RDM)(LVM)$$
$$(2.29)(1.75) = 4 \times$$

This approach shows where the magnification comes from. In this case, more comes from the RDM factor than the LVM factor. Be careful not to misconstrue the 4× result that was found again. The magnification for the case in which u < f will usually be different from the previous case in which u = f. The reason it came out to be the same here is due to the vertex distance, which, by coincidence, was chosen to be the same as the focal length of the magnifier. In Vertex Distance versus Magnifier Focal Length the more general situation in which the focal length of the magnifier and the vertex distance are different is shown.

The Gauss Solution
When the patient either accommodates or looks through a spectacle add power, the magnifier and accommodation/add power lens can be treated as a two-lens system, and the Gauss equivalent power formula can be used. The system in the following calculation is a +10.00 D lens (the magnifier) 10 cm from a +2.50 D lens (the add power). The standard equivalent power formula for two thin lenses in air is then applied:

$$D_e = D_1 + D_2 - (d)(D_1)(D_2)$$
$$= +10 + 2.50 - (0.1)(+10)(2.50)$$
$$= +10 \text{ D}$$

Once the equivalent power is known, that equivalent lens can be substituted for the two-lens system and the object of regard placed in the front focal plane of the equivalent lens, which in this case is 10 cm for a +10.00 D equivalent lens. The magnification can then be found from the product of the reference distance and the equivalent power.

$$RIM = (-u_R)(D_e)$$
$$RIM = (0.40)(10) = 4\times$$

Alternately, the magnification could be found by placing the equivalent lens at the eye and moving the object in to the F plane, which would be 10 cm. Then the RDM is calculated as the ratio of the two distances:

$$RIM = \frac{40}{10} = 4\times$$

Note. That the equivalent power came out to be the same as the magnifier power itself is again a quirk that the vertex distance and the magnifier focal length were equal. The section Vertex Distance versus Magnifier Focal Length discusses this in more detail.

Example 2

The patient is a 10 year old with 5.00 D of myopia and 10.00 D of accommodative amplitude. One way in which this case differs significantly from the absolute presbyope of Example 1 is in the value of u_R, the unaided (without any magnifier) reading distance. For the presbyope, there was no choice. For the image to be conjugate with the retina, the reading distance was constrained to the front focal plane of the 2.50 D add, or 40 cm. But for this younger myope, the accommodative amplitude and the myopia allow for many different possible unaided reading distances. For example, with the spectacles on and using 4.00 D of accommodation, the unaided reading distance would be 25 cm. With the spectacles off and using 3.00 D of accommodation, the excess plus power at the eye is +8.00 D, so the reading distance without any magnifier would be 12.5 cm. If a reduced Snellen acuity card is used, and the patient holds the card at the calibrated distance for this card (40 cm) with the spectacles on, the unaided reading distance would be 40 cm and the patient would accommodate by 2.50 D.

An infinite number of initial reading distances could be used by this patient depending on how much accommodation is used and whether the near acuity is measured with or without spectacles. For the purpose of this example, one situation will be arbitrarily selected and analyzed. A near reading card calibrated in the meter (M) system will be used. In this system, the overall size of the letter subtends 5 minutes of arc when held at its labeled distance. For example, the letters in the 1-M paragraph each subtend 5 minutes of arc when the card is held 1 m from the eye. It will further be assumed that the near acuity was measured with the spectacles on, and that 5.00 D of accommodation can be used for sustained reading. Under these conditions, the child will hold the card at 20 cm.

For the purpose of this example, it will be assumed that the smallest print the child can read is 3 M and that 1-M print is the desired goal. So at this point it is known that 3×

magnification is needed. To achieve 3× by RDM, the reading material must be moved in three times closer than 20 cm, to 6.67 cm. At 6.67 cm, the vergence at the eye is −15.00 D, so +15.00 D of plus power will be needed. If 5.00 D of accommodation can be sustained, this patient will need a +10.00 D add.

If the visual function necessitated that distance vision and near vision both be available for alternating from the blackboard to the notebook, a spectacle lens with −5.00 D carrier for distance and a 15.00 D add bifocal would provide the near vision without any accommodation. Any bifocal add power less than 15.00 D would have to be made up for by patient accommodation. If distance vision could be sacrificed, the spectacles could be removed, and a reading lens with +10.00 D would combine with the uncorrected myopia to achieve the total of +15.00 D needed at near, which is another option. The final decision as to which option to use is driven by each patient's individual needs.

The point being made here is that the magnification requirement at near for any given patient is dependent on the conditions under which the unaided (i.e., without magnifier) acuity at near was measured. Continuing from the preceding example, if the reading card was held at 40 cm, instead of obtaining a 3-M near acuity, the patient would only be able to see 6 M (twice as far away means it must be twice as big). Then with a 6-M starting point, to achieve 1 M as the desired result, 6× magnification would be needed. Using RDM only, six times closer than 40 cm is once again 6.67 cm, and therefore, the result is that again 15.00 D of plus power is needed. Without the knowledge of these optical principles, the 6× factor could lead one to reach for a magnifier labeled 6×, resulting in the selection of +24.00 D lens in a case in which only +15.00 D or +10.00 D is needed. And it is rarely advisable to prescribe any higher power lens than that which will accomplish the patient's visual needs.

A formal solution to this magnification calculation using the product formula follows. The assumption is that a single vision, near only, +10.00 D lens is prescribed as a spectacle mounted system. Then d = 0 and the second term becomes unity. All that is left is the relative distance term. The aided object distance will be 6.67 cm.

$$RIM = (RDM)(LVM)$$
$$= \left(\frac{u_R}{u_{eye}}\right)\left(\frac{1-dU}{1-dV}\right)$$
$$= \frac{u_R}{u_{eye}}$$

With a reference distance of 40 cm, the result is

$$RIM = \frac{40}{6.67} = 6\times$$

With a reference distance of 20 cm, the result is

$$RIM = \frac{20}{6.67} = 3\times$$

Once again, 3× and 6× sound like very different results, but the final image on the retina is the same. The differ-

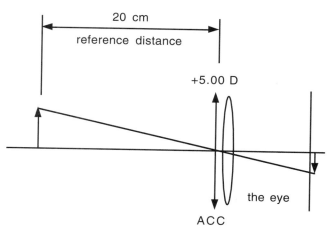

FIGURE 7-12. **Unaided conditions. (ACC = accommodation.)**

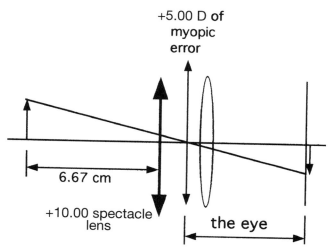

FIGURE 7-13. **Aided conditions.**

ent final magnification values arise from comparing the final retinal image size to different unaided retinal image sizes. Figures 7-12 and 7-13 show the unaided ($u_R = -20$) and aided conditions respectively.

Suppose a working distance of 6.67 cm was too close for writing in a notebook and that a vertex distance of 20 cm was needed. Instead of placing the plus power in the spectacle plane the recommendation was going to be a stand magnifier. Can any +15.00 D stand magnifier simply be used to achieve the desired 3× magnification? No. Each stand magnifier produces a virtual image at a distance from the eye that is a property of that particular stand magnifier, and that distance must be known. It is this distance, which, when added to the vertex distance, determines how much plus must be available at the eye either as accommodation or add power in a spectacle lens. Stand magnifier data is now available in the literature. This information together with the concept of the equivalent viewing distance (EVD) is what is needed to make this change.[2]

The EVD in this case is 6.67 cm because at this distance, the needed 3× magnification is achieved. It is achieved with an equivalent power of +15.00 D. So any optical system that provides +15.00 D of equivalent power will work. But now there is a two-lens system: the stand magnifier lens together with the plus power required at the eye from accommodation or add power. The vertex distance (20 cm) together with the stand magnifier virtual image location will determine the amount plus needed at the eye. Once that is known, the only unknown is the stand magnifier power, which can then be calculated from the Gauss equivalent power formula. This problem is summarized and worked out below. A diagram of the optical system is shown in Figure 7-14.

Given

- 3× needed to improve 3 M to 1 M.
- The 3 M was measured at 20 cm so a distance 3× closer is needed, which is 6.67 cm. This is the EVD.
- For a 6.67-cm EVD, 15.00 D of plus is needed. This is the equivalent power.

- A stand magnifier has been selected that produces a virtual image 20 cm from it.
- The vertex distance has been chosen to be 20 cm.

What power should this stand magnifier have to make this system work, and what plus power will be needed at the spectacle plane?

The first observation to make is that the virtual image is 40 cm from the eye (20 cm + 20 cm), and therefore +2.50 D is needed at the eye. In this case, that can be provided by the patient's accommodation. If the patient is a presbyope, add power in a spectacle lens would have to be provided. With that number known, the only unknown is the stand magnifier power.

$$D_e = D_1 + D_2 - (d)(D_1)(D_2)$$

where D_1 is the power of the magnifier; D_2 is any add power needed at the eye; and d is the vertex distance.

$$15 = D_1 + 2.50 - (0.2)(D_1)(2.50)$$
$$D_1 = 25 = \text{power needed in stand magnifier}$$

There is an important observation to be made here: The equivalent power of this two-plus-lens system turned out to be less than the power of the stand magnifier alone. That result is caused by the long vertex distance in comparison to the focal length of the stand magnifier. This topic is discussed in more detail in the next section.

VERTEX DISTANCE VERSUS MAGNIFIER FOCAL LENGTH

When a bifocal wearer uses a handheld magnifier, this constitutes a two-lens system. There are different ways in which this person might function, and different magnifications will ultimately result. The way to appreciate the various options and their impact on the magnification is to start with the equivalent power formula and then adapt

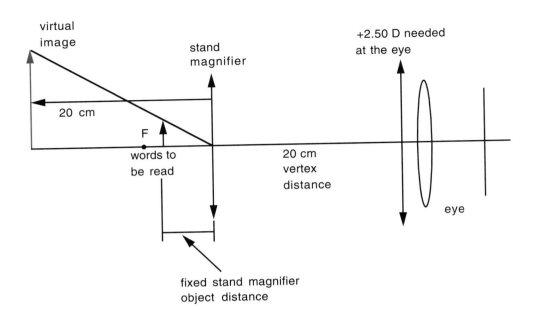

FIGURE 7-14. **The stand magnifier system. (F = primary focal plane of magnifier.)**

it to the patient situation. The equivalent power formula from gaussian optics is as follows.

$$D_e = D_1 + D_2 - (d)(D_1)(D_2)$$

For the situation examined here, the D_1 term is the magnifier, the D_2 term is the bifocal add power, and d is the vertex distance (magnifier to spectacle plane). The subscripts have been changed to reflect these quantities.

$$D_e = D_{mag} + D_{add} - (d)(D_{mag})(D_{add})$$

Next, factor out the add power from the last two terms and replace the magnifier power with its reciprocal, its focal length.

$$= D_{mag} + D_{add}\left[1 - d(D_{mag})\right]$$

$$= D_{mag} + D_{add}\left(1 - \frac{d}{f_{mag}}\right)$$

In this last form, the ratio of d to f is seen to have some interesting effects. First of all, when viewing through the carrier there is no add power and the second term goes to zero, making the equivalent power equal to the power of the magnifier alone. The system magnification now is simply the product of the reference distance and the equivalent power.

For example, assume the patient uses spectacles with a +2.50 D add power, but when using the magnifier, views through the carrier. The 2.50 add power means that the reference distance must be 40 cm. Then, if a +10.00 D magnifier is used, the magnification will be

$$RIM = (-u_R)(D_e) = (0.40)(10) = 4 \times$$

Another example may be seen when the patient views through the segment. Now the effect of the add power becomes dependent on the relationship between the focal length of the magnifier and the vertex distance. Consider first some special cases, e.g., the case in which d = 0, indicating that the user is holding the magnifier in contact with the spectacles (not the way a handheld magnifier is meant to be used). In this case, the second term in the bracket goes to zero, the full add power is added to the magnifier power, and the equivalent power is the sum, in this case +12.50 D. The magnification is increased as shown:

$$RIM = (-u_R)(D_e) = (0.40)(12.5) = 5 \times$$

This condition represents the maximum magnification achievable with this system. As the magnifier is moved farther from the spectacle plane, the equivalent power, and consequently the magnification, will decrease. The reason for this is that the second term in the bracket is negative, therefore any nonzero value for this term will be subtracted from the first term, with the net effect being that only a portion of the add power will combine with the magnifier power to give the equivalent power. For example, suppose this patient held the magnifier 5 cm from the spectacle plane. The results would be as follows:

$$D_e = D_{mag} + (D_{add})\left(1 - \frac{d}{f_{mag}}\right)$$

$$= +10 + (2.50)\left(1 - \frac{5}{10}\right)$$

$$= +11.25 \, D$$

$$RIM = (0.40)(11.25) = 4.5 \times$$

If the vertex distance is made even longer, for example, 10 cm (the transition point), which happens to be the magnifier focal length, the second term becomes unity, and the bracket goes to zero, the net effect being that there is no contribution from the add power. The equivalent power is simply the magnifier power alone. And worse yet, if the vertex distance is longer than the focal length, the add term becomes negative and the equivalent power is reduced below the value of the magnifier alone. The functional implication here is that it is pointless to have the patient view through a bifocal segment when the vertex distance is longer than the focal length of the magnifier. The magnification of the system becomes less than the power of the magnifier alone. So in most cases, when a bifocal wearer uses a handheld magnifier at a long vertex distance, if magnification is to be maximized, the patient should view through the carrier and hold the object of regard one focal length from the magnifier.

Conversely, viewing through the segment is usually preferred when the vertex distance is shorter than the focal length of the magnifier, assuming again that it is desired to maximize the magnification. The vertex distance that is equal to the focal length of the magnifier is called the *transition point* or *point of neutrality*. At this vertex distance, the effect of the add power is nullified and the patient may just as well view through the carrier because it is the larger and more accessible portion of the lens.

AFOCAL TELESCOPE

The product formula used in the previous discussions of magnification at near is applicable to distance viewing as well. When the particulars of telescopic viewing conditions are imposed on the product formula for RIM, the familiar afocal telescopic formula will result. Here is how this happens:

$$RIM = (RDM)(LVM)$$
$$= \left(\frac{u_R}{u_{eye}}\right)\left(\frac{1-dU}{1-dV}\right)$$

Consider the RDM term. It is the ratio of the unaided reference distance to the aided distance. When using a telescope, these distances are the same. For example, if one looks at the players on a football field without a telescope and then with a telescope, the viewing distance does not change. So, the first term becomes unity. The second term, the LVM, becomes the telescopic magnification based on the following analogy. Consider the optics of a spectacle lens–corrected hyperope. The hyperopic eye can be modeled as an emmetropic eye to which has been added a minus thin lens at the corneal surface. The minus lens represents the hyperopic error in the diagram in Figure 7-15.

The correct plus lens for this hyperopic eye is one that will receive parallel rays from a distant object and converge them onto the minus error lens, which renders them parallel for the emmetropic eye behind it. Parallel rays entering an emmetropic eye result in a focused image on the retina. Thus, the result consists of parallel rays in (to the correcting lens) together with parallel rays out (of the hyperopic error lens), which constitutes an afocal system. Such an afocal system is analogous to the emmetropic eye viewing through a telescope, in which the correcting lens is the objective and the error lens is the ocular. The magnification of an afocal telescope (m_{TS}) can be expressed in terms of

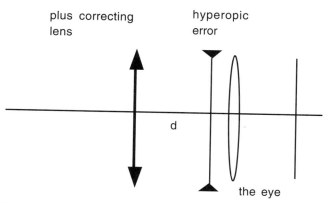

FIGURE 7-15.   **Model of corrected hyperopia. (d = vertex distance.)**

the objective lens power and the "tube length" (the vertex distance).

$$m_{TS} = \frac{1}{1 - dD_{obj}} \qquad \text{Equation A}$$

Now consider the LVM term in the product formula. The object vergence (U) in the numerator is zero for distant objects. Then from the U + D = V relationship, where if U = 0, then D = V, the final expression becomes the following:

$$RIM = \frac{1}{1 - dD} \qquad \text{Equation B}$$

Comparing equations A and B, it is apparent that the LVM term is the standard telescopic magnification formula with the spectacle lens power playing the role of the objective lens.

It then follows that any of the usual afocal telescopic magnification formulas, together with the tube length formula, can be used for analyzing the telescopic magnification. The following summarizes these formulas:

$$m_{TS} = RIM = 1 - dD_{oc} \qquad \text{Equation C}$$
$$m_{TS} = -\frac{D_{oc}}{D_{obj}} \qquad \text{Equation D}$$
$$d = f_{obj}' + f_{oc}'$$

where d = tube length, D_{oc} = power of the ocular, D_{obj} = power of the objective, f_{obj}' = secondary focal length of the objective, and f_{oc}' = secondary focal length of the ocular. When the telescope is used in its afocal configuration by an emmetrope (parallel rays in; parallel rays out), any of Equations A, C, or D can be used together with the tube length formula to calculate telescopic magnification (Figure 7-16).

For example, when viewing a distant object, an emmetrope using a Galilean telescope consisting of a −40.00 D ocular and a +10.00 D objective will have a retinal image size four times larger than when the same object is viewed directly without the telescope:

$$RIM = -\frac{D_{oc}}{D_{obj}} = \frac{-40}{-10} = 4\times$$

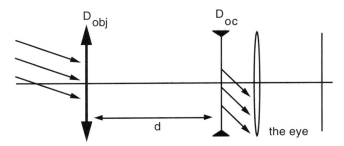

FIGURE 7-16.   **An afocal Galilean telescope. (D_{obj} = power of the objective lens; D_{oc} = power of the ocular lens; d = tube length.)**

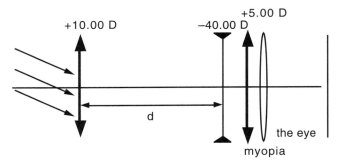

FIGURE 7-17.   **Galilean telescope used by an uncorrected myope. (d = tube length.)**

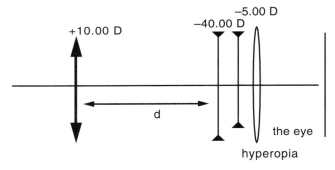

FIGURE 7-18.   **Galilean telescope used by an uncorrected hyperope. (d = tube length.)**

TELESCOPES USED BY UNCORRECTED SPHERICAL AMETROPES

The magnification formula expressed as the ratio of the lens powers is readily adaptable to other circumstances. For example, consider a Galilean telescope used by an uncorrected myope (Figure 7-17). The Galilean telescope has a negative ocular lens, and the uncorrected myope has a plus refractive error. The plus power of the myopia combines with the minus ocular lens to produce, in effect, an ocular of less minus power. It can be thought of as though 5.00 D of minus power of the ocular is used to correct the myopia, leaving only 35.00 D of minus for the telescope.

Note. These analyses ignore any effectivity corrections associated with the fact that the ocular lens is displaced some small distance from the corneal plane; correction for effectivity would have minimal effect on the answers.

The net –35.00 D ocular power results in a reduced magnification for the uncorrected myope using a Galilean telescope.

$$\mathrm{RIM} = -\frac{D_{oc}}{D_{obj}} = -\left(\frac{-35}{10}\right) = 3.5\times$$

If the uncorrected myope is to use the telescope and still have a focused image on the retina, the tube length must be adjusted. The afocal tube length is the sum of the focal lengths of the original system.

$$d = f_{obj}' + f_{oc}' = 10 + (-2.50) = 7.50 \text{ cm}$$

The –2.50-cm focal length of the –40.00 D ocular must now be replaced by the focal length of a –35.00 D ocular, which is –2.86 cm. When the –2.86-cm focal length is used to calculate the tube length, it is evident that the uncorrected myope will have to shorten the telescope.

$$d = f_{obj}' + f_{oc}' = 10 + (-2.86) = 7.14 \text{ cm}$$

A similar analysis for the uncorrected hyperope using a Galilean telescope will result in higher magnification and the need to lengthen the instrument. For example, consider a 5.00 D hyperope. When 5.00 D of minus power, representing the uncorrected hyperopia, is added to the ocular power, the new "ocular" power becomes –45.00 D. Once again, this can be thought of as though +5.00 D of power is extracted from the –40.00 D ocular to correct the hyperopia, leaving it as a –45.00 D ocular (Figure 7-18).

The magnification increase to 4.5× is as follows:

$$\mathrm{RIM} = -\frac{D_{oc}}{D_{obj}} = -\left(\frac{-45}{10}\right) = 4.5\times$$

A –45.00 D ocular has a focal length of –2.22 cm, so the new tube length calculation shows that the tube must be lengthened.

$$d = f_{obj}' + f_{oc}' = 10 + (-2.22) = 7.78 \text{ cm}$$

A similar analysis can be made for a Keplerian telescope (Figure 7-19).

The uncorrected myope, having a plus refractive error, causes the net ocular power to become +45.00 D and a magnification of 4.5× results (instead of the 4× for the afocal configuration). But the magnification for the uncorrected hyperope using the Keplerian telescope will be reduced to 3.5× because the hyperopic error is negative (–5.00 D), which when combined with the +40.00 D ocular, reduces it to +35.00 D.

The tube length must be shortened for the myope and lengthened for the hyperope. This is demonstrated in the following calculations. The afocal tube length for the Keplerian telescope is as follows:

$$d = f_{obj}' + f_{oc}' = 10 + 2.5 = 12.5 \text{ cm}$$

For use by the uncorrected 5.00 D myope, the system will consist of the +10.00 D objective, the focal length of which is 10 cm, and the net power ocular of +45.00 D, the focal length of which is 2.22 cm. The tube length must be shortened.

$$d = 10 + 2.22 = 12.22 \text{ cm}$$

For the uncorrected 5.00 D hyperope, the new ocular power is +40.00 D combined with −5.00 D for a net power of +35.00 D and a new ocular focal length of 2.86 cm. The uncorrected hyperope using a Keplerian telescope must increase the tube length.

$$d = 10 + 2.86 = 12.86 \text{ cm}$$

TELEMICROSCOPE

Telescopes can also be adapted for near viewing. One method is to add a plus lens (cap) to the objective. This creates a telemicroscope. For this analysis, a Keplerian telescope has been selected because of its larger field of view. Also, higher lens powers will be used to create telescopes with shorter tube lengths. Such a design better approximates what is often used for a spectacle-mounted system.

The parameters of the Keplerian telescope will be a +20.00 D objective with a +80.00 D ocular, giving a magnification of 4×. The afocal tube length calculation is shown here (Figure 7-20):

$$d = f_{obj}' + f_{oc}' = 5 + 1.25 = 6.25 \text{ cm}$$

Assume that the patient's best-corrected acuity at near is 4 M and that 1 M is judged to be what is needed. Thus, 4× magnification is required. In addition, the 4 M at near was found when the patient read through +2.50 D add spectacles and held the card at 40 cm. To achieve 4× magnification relative to 40 cm means moving the reading card four times closer to 10 cm, in turn requiring a total plus power of +10.00 D at the spectacle plane. The equivalent power is thus +10.00 D and the EVD is 10 cm.

A +10.00 D lens at the spectacle plane would be an option if a working distance of 10 cm was satisfactory. But in this case it is not. Perhaps the patient is an artist who requires a greater working distance to use tools or brushes. That is the reason the telemicroscope is being considered. When changing from one system to another, in this case from a simple plus lens at the spectacle plane to a telemicroscope, the +10.00 D of equivalent power must be maintained if the magnification is to remain constant.

It is further assumed that because this patient had been wearing +2.50 D add power, that 40 cm is the desired working distance. To summarize, a new system (telemicroscope) must produce 4× magnification at a working distance of 40 cm. Recall that the telescope that will be used has a tube length of 6.25 cm. This system might be designed in two ways. One option is to increase the working distance by the length of the tele-

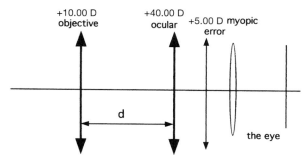

FIGURE 7-19. **Keplerian telescope used by an uncorrected myope. (d = tube length.)**

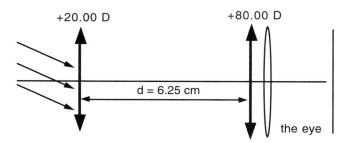

FIGURE 7-20. **Keplerian telescope in afocal configuration. (d = tube length.)**

scope to maintain a 40-cm working space. The other is to hold the working distance constant at 40 cm, which will reduce the working space by the length of the telescope (i.e., to 33.75 cm). The option to increase the working distance by the length of the telescope will be examined first (Figure 7-21).

If the working space is 40 cm, the object divergence at the objective lens is −2.50 D, so a +2.50 D cap will render those rays parallel for the afocal telescope behind it. Is the magnifying power of this two-element system still 4×? One way to confirm that is from basic principles—namely, that when there is a sequence of two optical systems, the total magnification of the system is the product of the individual magnifications. In this case a +2.50 D cap is combined with a 4× telescope. The magnifying power of the telescope itself is 4×. That means that the magnifying power of the cap must be unity in order that the product be 4×. Consider the cap situation.

Recall that the object of regard (when not using the telescope) was held at 40 cm because the patient was wearing a +2.50 D add power. Because the object is being held in the front focal plane of the cap, it makes no difference how far that system is from the eye. The magnification is independent of the vertex distance and is the product of the reference distance times the power of the cap (D_{cap}). Formally, it can be written as follows:

$$RIM = (RDM)(LVM)$$

$$= \left(-u_R D_{cap}\right)\left(m_{TS}\right)$$

$$= \left[-(-0.40)(2.50)\right](4\times) = 4\times$$

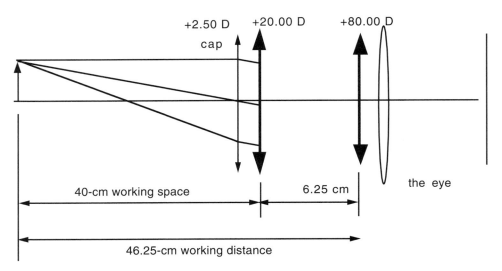

FIGURE 7-21. **Telemicroscope: increased working distance.**

On the other hand, if the 40-cm working distance is kept constant, the working space is reduced by the length of the telescope, changing the working space to 40 − 6.25 = 33.75 cm. At this distance, a slightly stronger cap is needed. The divergence at the objective lens from an object at 33.75 cm is approximately −3.00 D, so a +3.00 D cap is used. But now the telescopic magnification should be adjusted if the 4× is to be maintained (Figure 7-22).

Once again, the total magnification is the product of the cap magnification (m_{cap}) and the telescope magnification.

$$RIM = (m_{cap})(m_{TS})$$
$$= (-u_R D_{cap})(m_{TS})$$
$$= [(0.40)(3.00)](m_{TS})$$
$$= (1.2)(m_{TS}) = 4.8$$

In essence what has happened is that the stronger cap caused its magnification to increase from unity to 1.2×,

which produced a RIM of 4.8×. The telescope magnification would have to be reduced to 3.33× if the RIM is to remain constant at 4.00×. Of course in a clinical situation, this is not what would likely occur, because a 3.33× telescope would not be readily available, and the increase in the system magnification from 4.0× to 4.8× would probably be acceptable in most cases.

For completeness, this situation can be analyzed again using the equivalent power concept. Recall that the equivalent power was determined to be +10.00 D, so any system that satisfies this will meet the magnification requirements. For a telemicroscope, the equivalent power is related to the telescopic magnification and the dioptric power of the lens cap as follows[3]:

$$D_e = (D_{cap})(m_{TS})$$
$$10 = (3.00)(m_{TS})$$
$$m_{TS} = 3.33 \times$$

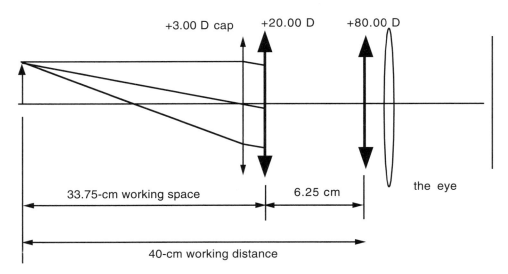

FIGURE 7-22. **Telemicroscope: decreased working space.**

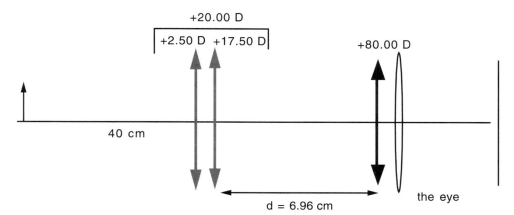

FIGURE 7-23. **Keplerian telescope adjusted for near. (d = tube length.)**

ADJUSTABLE TELESCOPE

Suppose the previous 40-cm working distance was to be achieved using an adjustable telescope. The simplest way to analyze this system is to treat it as though the +2.50 D of convergent power needed for the 40-cm working distance was taken from the objective lens, leaving the objective power reduced to +17.50 D. The +2.50 D taken from the objective will play the role of the cap, and the +17.50 D remaining becomes the new objective lens power of an afocal telescope behind it. The tube length will now have to be adjusted to re-establish the afocal property of the telescope. The new tube length is the sum of the focal lengths as usual, but with the objective power reduced to +17.50 D. The new tube length is d = f_{obj}' + f_{oc}' = 5.71 + 1.25 = 6.96 cm, where 5.71 cm is the focal length of a +17.50 D objective. The tube length must be increased (from 6.25 cm) to use it for near objects (Figure 7-23).

What is the effect on the magnification? The telescope is no longer a 4× system. The new magnification of the telescope can be found as the ratio of the ocular power to the new "objective" lens power.

$$RIM = -\frac{D_{oc}}{D_{obj}} = \frac{80}{17.50} = -4.57\times$$

Although a minus sign will always result when the basic magnification formula is applied to a Keplerian telescope (indicating the image is inverted), the Keplerian system will always have erecting prisms built in when it is designed for terrestrial use, as all low vision Keplerian telescopes are.

The same effect on magnification and tube length adjustment will occur when focusing for near, whether the telescope is Keplerian or Galilean, because both have plus objectives. When some of that plus power is treated as though it were a cap power, the net power left for the telescope objective is a lower plus number. When this lower power is used to calculate the magnification, the magnification will likewise be increased because the lower power is in the denominator. Similarly, the lower-power objective will have a longer focal length, so that when the tube

length is calculated, the result is that the tube length must increase to focus on a near object.

SELF-ASSESSMENT QUIZ

1. When using a magnifier to read, the reading material should be held
   (a) farther than one focal length from the magnifier.
   (b) closer than one focal length from the magnifier.
   (c) in the front focal plane of the magnifier.
   (d) a or c
   (e) b or c

2. When an object is maintained in the front focal plane of a plus lens, and the lens and object are moved closer to the eye, what is the effect on the RDM and LVM components of the total magnification?
   (a) both increase
   (b) both decrease
   (c) RDM increases and LVM decreases
   (d) RDM decreases and LVM increases
   (e) both remain constant

3. Patients A and B are both absolute presbyopes and have equal distance acuities. Patient A wears spectacles with 2.50 D add power; patient B wears spectacles with 4.00 D add power. They each view through the carrier portion of their spectacles while using a +10.00 D handheld magnifier. In each case, the object of regard is held in the F plane of the magnifier. Which of the following statements is correct?
   (a) Patient A will be able to read smaller print than patient B.
   (b) Patient B will be able to read smaller print than patient A.
   (c) Patient A will experience greater improvement in acuity than patient B.
   (d) Patient B will experience greater improvement in acuity than patient A.
   (e) Answers a and c are both correct.

4. A bifocal wearer uses a handheld magnifier. When viewing through the carrier, he or she holds the reading material in the F plane of the magnifier. When viewing through the segment, he or she holds the reading material closer than one focal length and achieves a focused image on the retina. Which of the following statements is true?
   (a) Greater magnification results if the individual views through the carrier.
   (b) Greater magnification results if the individual views through the segment.
   (c) The magnification will be the same whether viewing through the carrier or the segment.

5. What magnification is achieved by an absolute presbyope wearing spectacles with a prescription of $-2.75 + 1.50 \times 90$ with a 2.50 D add when he or she uses a +16.00 D handheld magnifier held at a distance of 10 cm from the spectacle plane and views through the carrier?
   (a) 3.2×
   (b) 4.2×
   (c) 5.0×
   (d) 6.4×
   (e) 8.0×

6. What magnification is achieved by an absolute presbyope wearing spectacles with a prescription of $+4.50 - 3.50 \times 180$ with a 3.00 D add when he or she uses a +20.00 D handheld magnifier held at a distance of 10 cm from the spectacle plane and views through the segment? Solve two ways: (1) using the product formula and (2) using the Gauss formula.
   (a) 3.33×
   (b) 4.33×
   (c) 5.67×
   (d) 6.33×
   (e) 6.67×

7. A corrected hyperope using a Keplerian telescope removes his or her spectacles and looks through the telescope again, adjusting it as required to obtain a focused image. What changes occur when the hyperope uses the telescope while uncorrected?
   (a) more magnification and a longer tube length
   (b) more magnification and a shorter tube length
   (c) less magnification and a shorter tube length
   (d) less magnification and a longer tube length
   (e) a shorter tube length with no change in magnification

8. A corrected myope using a Galilean telescope removes his or her spectacles and looks through the telescope again, adjusting it as required to obtain a focused image. What changes occur when the myope uses the telescope while uncorrected?
   (a) more magnification and a longer tube length
   (b) more magnification and a shorter tube length
   (c) less magnification and a shorter tube length
   (d) less magnification and a longer tube length
   (e) a shorter tube length with no change in magnification

Acknowledgment

The author acknowledges the assistance of Ian Bailey in the writing of this chapter. Dr. Bailey was generous with both his technical expertise and general editing skills, the result of which is an improved piece of work over the original version.

REFERENCES

1. Byer A. Theoretical Optics for Clinicians (4th ed). Philadelphia: Pennsylvania College of Optometry, 1996;293.
2. Bullimore MA, Bailey IL. Stand magnifiers: an evaluation of new optical aids from coil. Optom Vis Sci 1989;66:766–773.
3. Bailey IL. Principles of near vision telescopes. Optom Monthly 1981;Aug:32–34.

Appendix A

PRODUCT FORMULA

$$RIM = (RDM)(LVM)$$

$$= \left(\frac{u_R}{u_{eye}}\right)\left(\frac{1-dU}{1-dV}\right)$$

where RIM is the retinal image magnification, RDM is the relative distance magnification, and LVM = lens vertex magnification. This explanation relates to the problem diagrammed in Figure 7-6. Although this formula is more complicated to use than the equivalent power formula, it has the advantage of keeping the RDM and LVM factors separate. This enables one to know how much magnification derives from each factor. It combines the "before" situation in the u_R term with the "after" parameters in the other factors. The u_R term is a before factor because it is the reading distance used before (or without) any magnifier enters the picture; it is often called the *reference distance*.

When the magnifier is added, the after conditions apply. Specifically, u_{eye} is the distance from the reading card to the eye (which is the sum of the distance from the reading card to the magnifier) plus the vertex distance (d). The symbols U and V are the usual object and image vergences, respectively, at the magnifier.

The specific values for this problem are as follows:

1. The before distance (u_R) is 40 cm because the habitual bifocal add power is +2.50 D.
2. The after distance (u_{eye}) is also 40 cm because it is 10 cm from the reading card to the magnifier, plus a 30-cm vertex distance (d). The object location in this problem must be in the primary focal plane (F) of the magnifier, which for a +10.00 D lens is 10 cm.
3. The object vergence at the lens (U) is −10.00 D because the object is 10 cm from the magnifier.
4. The image vergence at the lens (V) is zero because an object in the F plane of a lens produces parallel light leaving the lens, which has a vergence of zero.

129

Appendix B

CONSTANT MAGNIFICATION FOR OBJECT AT PRIMARY FOCAL PLANE

The vertex distance (d) is a factor in the general magnification formula. In the special case in which the object is held in the front focal plane of the magnifier, however, the magnification becomes independent of the vertex distance. The easiest way to see this is by a ray trace (Figure 7B-1).

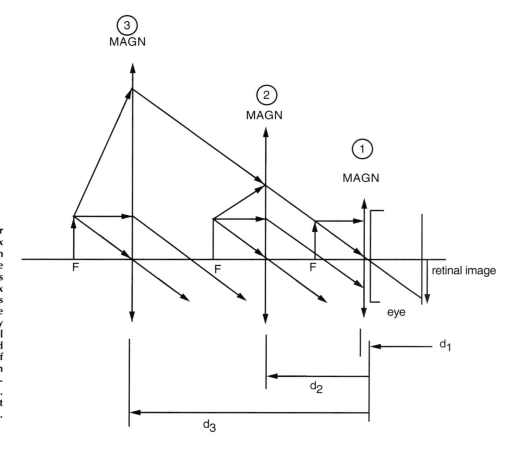

FIGURE 7B-1. **When the magnifier (MAGN) is in position 1, the vertex distance is zero (d_1). A nodal ray from the tip of the object traces out the retinal image. When the magnifier is moved out to position 2, the vertex distance becomes d_2. If the object is moved out also, and is still held in the F plane of the magnifier, the nodal ray leaving the magnifier will be parallel to the nodal ray of position 1 and therefore intersect the nodal point of the eye, making the same angle with the optic axis, and therefore will produce the same size retinal image. Position 3 illustrates the same effect at an even longer vertex distance (d_3). (F = primary focal point.)**

CHAPTER EIGHT

Low Vision Distance Systems I: Spectacles and Contact Lenses

Lee A. Hersh, Michael Spinell, and Jean Astorino

A common misconception in vision rehabilitation is that the use of a telescope is the only way to improve distance visual functioning for the visually impared. Although telescopes are often quite useful, other lenses and systems must be considered when prescribing for distance. The various options to consider are the following:

- Spectacles and contact lenses
- Absorptive lenses and coatings (see Chapter 13)
- Pinhole lenses (see Chapter 13)
- Telescopes (see Chapter 9)
- Field expanders and awareness systems for patients with extremely reduced peripheral fields (see Chapters 12 and 17)

An essential element in caring for patients with visual impairment is a low vision refraction. Correction of the patient's refractive error through conventional spectacles or contact lenses is frequently necessary. Certainly, some patients have moderate refractive errors, and their visual acuity does improve when wearing a prescription lens. These patients should be encouraged to do so. Contact lenses might seem a perfect choice for patients having a high refractive error, but this is not always so. For example, in high hyperopia or aphakia, or both, less magnification occurs with a contact lens than with a spectacle lens. Low vision patients typically rely on magnification, and therefore, they may function better in spectacles.

Two special needs may exist for the low vision patient wearing spectacle lenses: The first is the protection offered by a spectacle lens, and the other is correction of a high refractive error. Polycarbonate lenses are the most impact resistant. For this reason, a polycarbonate lens should be recommended for anyone who is at significant risk for eye injury, including monocular patients and those with hazardous occupations or hobbies. There is certainly a higher percentage of the better seeing eye being accidentally injured, because the better functioning eye lines up with the visual task. Other advantages of polycarbonate lenses are discussed in Prescribing for High Myopia, along with other lens materials and options.

Spectacle correction for low vision patients and for those with high refractive errors (4.00 D and above) will present potential problems in the way of image quality, cosmesis, weight, and lens thickness.[1] It is therefore important when prescribing for these patients to recommend specific characteristics, including frame size and shape, lens design, lens material, and special coatings or treatments. In general, the selected frame should be relatively round and not oversized so that the patient's interpupillary distance (IPD) is as close to the frame IPD as possible.[2] This results in little or no decentration when fabricating the spectacle lens.

SPECTACLE LENS CORRECTION

Aberration and Distortion

Naturally, providing the best quality optical image for the low vision patient with a refractive error is of ultimate importance. A thorough understanding of aberrations and distortions is therefore necessary.

Chromatic aberration is defined as a defocusing of the image due to the relationship between the refractive index of a lens material and wavelength of light.[3] An ophthalmic lens is actually a series of many prisms. In a minus lens, the prisms align apex to apex, and in a plus lens they are base to base. It is known that a prism bends visible light toward its base and that visible light consists of many different wavelengths. An ophthalmic lens will therefore bend, or refract, visible light to varying degrees and may result in slight image blur to the patient. Each lens material has a specific value representing the amount of chromatic aberration associated with its use, called the *Abbe*, or *nu value*.[3] An inverse relationship exists between this value and chromatic aberration such that a higher nu (Abbe) value represents less chromatic aberration, and thus better image quality. Chromatic aberration, therefore, depends on dioptric power and index of refraction of the lens. Choosing high-index lenses with a high Abbe will ensure good peripheral clarity with little to no chromatic aberration.

Another problem that occurs is spherical aberration. Spherical aberration relates to the fact that a spherical lens focuses light passing through its center later than light traveling through its periphery. Patients do not usually notice any degradation of image clarity, because the pupil acts as an aperture stop to block out the peripheral light rays. Spherical aberration can, however, become a problem to the patient with large, fixed, or distorted pupils.

Coma is an aberration similar to spherical aberration but results from a wide beam of light passing obliquely through an ophthalmic lens. This may, of course, produce a defocused optical image, but again is not typically interpreted by the patient due to the pupillary function. Marginal astigmatism also results from obliquely oriented light, but in this case the incident light is a narrow beam. This is significant because the patient may notice multiple image foci and report a blurred image.

Distortion differs from the aberrations mentioned in the preceding paragraphs in that the image in this case is not blurry, but rather, is changed in shape. Magnification differences (either enlargement or reduction) when comparing the periphery to the center of an ophthalmic lens are the cause of distortion. In barrel distortion, which happens with a concave lens, the image appears to bow outward. A convex lens produces pincushion distortion, in which the image seems to have an inward curvature.

The patient with low vision and high refractive error may be sensitive to the preceding problems, as he or she requires an image of good optical quality to obtain the best corrected visual acuity and function. Careful recommendations must be made regarding the various aberrations and distortion when constructing a pair of spectacles or contact lenses to minimize these possible problems for the patient with low vision.[1]

Prescribing for High Myopia

An important goal when prescribing for patients with high amounts of myopia is to reduce the edge thickness of the lenses. Lens material, lens design, and frame selection are important factors as well.

Selection of lens material is usually dependent on the index of refraction of the lens. The index of refraction is defined as the ratio of the velocity of light in a vacuum to the velocity of light in a given medium (air) at a given wavelength.[3] The higher the index of refraction of the lens material, the more efficient that material is in bending light and, therefore, the thinner the lens will be. Materials with higher indices of refraction are able to use flatter base curves to produce the same correcting power as that of crown glass (1.523 index of refraction) or CR-39 lenses (1.498 index of refraction). Flatter base curves produce less thickness at the lens periphery as well. Listed in Table 8-1 are the high-index material options currently available in high minus powers. High-index lenses should be recommended when prescribing for patients requiring prescriptions of –6.00 D and above.[4]

When prescribing high-index lenses, one must realize that chromatic aberration tends to increase. The increase is also dependent on lens power and how far the patient looks into the periphery of the lens. For example, a patient wearing a –5.00 D polycarbonate lens may lose one line of visual acuity (Snellen) when looking 10 mm off the optical axis of the lens; a patient wearing a –10.00 D lens may lose as much as two lines. High-index plastic lenses have less chromatic aberration than polycarbonate but are only as strong as CR-39 when comparing equivalent power and center thickness.[4] There is a direct relationship between lens power and chromatic aberration and an inverse relationship between the nu value and chromatic aberration. For example, as the power of the lens doubles and the nu value decreases by half, the amount of chromatic aberration will double. The patient will generally complain of a colored or "rainbow" pattern in the periphery of the lens as well as a decrease in image clarity with high amounts of chromatic aberration. Antireflective (AR) coatings are required to help reduce these problems.

Another concern when prescribing high-index lenses is the decrease in transmission of light through the lens. Table 8-2 shows that as the index of refraction increases, there is an increase in the light reflecting off the lens. AR coatings again decrease the amount of reflected light and thereby increase the amount of light entering the patient's pupil.[5]

TABLE 8-1
High-Index Lens Material Options

Material	Refractive Index	Availability	Concerns
Polycarbonate	1.586	To –12.00 D in strongest meridian	Chromatic aberration
High-index plastic	1.600	To –15.00 D	Chromatic aberration
High-index plastic	1.660	To –10.00 D	Chromatic aberration
High-Lite glass	1.700	To –20.00 D	Dense, heavy, poor impact resistance
Glass	1.800	To –24.00 D	15% lighter, 20% thinner than High-Lite

TABLE 8-2
Light Reflected from Lens Surfaces of Different Refractive Indices

Material	Refractive Index	Reflected Light (%)
CR-39	1.490	3.9
Crown glass	1.523	4.3
Polycarbonate	1.590	5.2
High-index plastic	1.660	6.2
High-index glass	1.800	8.2

After selecting the most appropriate lens material for the patient with high myopia, lens design should be considered to ensure maximum image quality (Figure 8-1). Any prescriptions above –15.00 D require special lens designs to provide optimal visual acuity and cosmesis. The current options are listed in Table 8-3.

Along with the lens design, frame selection is critical when prescribing for the patient with high myopia. Small, round frames minimize edge thickness most effectively, reduce aberrations and distortions, and allow for little or no decentration. Taking monocular PD measurements is critical. Frames with adjustable nosepads should be used because vertical frame alignment is especially crucial with higher-powered lenses. The vertex distance, which is typically 12 mm, should also be of some concern. For the high myope, a shorter vertex distance

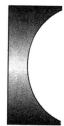 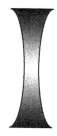 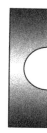 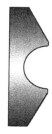

FIGURE 8-1. **Lens design options for a patient with high myopia.**

Full Field   Biconcave   Myodisc   Lenticular G

TABLE 8-3
Lens Design Options for High Myopia

Lens Design	Description
Biconcave	Both front and back surfaces are concave, reducing overall edge thickness.
Myodisc	Incorporates a small concave disc or bowl ground onto the back surface of a plano carrier; all power is concentrated in the 35- to 40-mm bowl portion (stronger power, smaller bowl).
Lenticular G	Has a bowl as well, but the carrier has a plus curve, resulting in a thinner edge than a plano carrier.
Blended myodisc	Has an aspheric curve (not usable) ground from the carrier portion to the bowl edge, reducing the edge of the bowl.

will reduce some of the minification effect of the spectacle lens.[6]

To maintain alignment with the eye's center of rotation, the rule of thumb is to drop the optical center 1 mm for every 2 degrees of pantoscopic tilt. Most frames have approximately 10 degrees of tilt; therefore, the optical center should be placed 5 mm below the patient's straight-ahead position.[7]

Polycarbonate lenses are substantially stronger than standard CR-39 spectacle lenses. They can therefore be ground to a center thickness of 1 mm and still pass the drop-ball test.[8] A thinner center translates into a thinner lens edge for a minus lens, and a thinner edge means a thinner center for a plus lens. The benefit is obvious; however, one must watch for lens warpage or distortions when center thickness is approximately 0.6 mm or less. If edge thickness is still very undesirable, edge treatments such as polishing, coating, or buffing may be recommended.[9]

Thus, when prescribing for high myopia, specifications for lens material, lens design, frame selection, coatings, edge treatments, and geometric measurements must be recommended for fabrication of the final spectacle correction.

Prescribing for High Hyperopia

As in prescribing for high myopia, the main concern when prescribing for high amounts of hyperopia is lens thickness. Reducing lens thickness will control other problems, such as weight, magnification, aberration, and distortion. The same lens materials used for high myopia are also options for high hyperopia and are available in approximately the same range of powers. The practitioner should again be aware of the potential problems of excessive reflections and the need for AR coating.

Lens design is crucial to the low vision patient with high amounts of hyperopia. Higher plus lenses are heavier and they may also have a decreased field of view caused by a ring scotoma. A ring scotoma, defined as a circular restriction in the peripheral visual field, is due to the prismatic effect of strong convex lenses. The ring scotoma will be larger with increasing lens power and size. Other factors affecting a ring scotoma include the following:

- A longer vertex distance reduces the size of the ring scotoma, but also moves it more centrally.
- Larger lens diameters move the ring scotoma toward the periphery.
- A smaller pupil size produces a larger ring scotoma.
- As lens thickness and, therefore, magnification increases, so does the size of the ring scotoma.
- Steeper base curves increase ring scotoma size.

The term *jack-in-the-box* refers to the fact that objects jump in and out of view as they move into and out of the area of the ring scotoma. Typically, this ring scotoma causes little problems at the normal reading distance of 40 cm or at distances of 20 ft and beyond. At intermediate ranges, however, patients may experience difficulty with mobility and eye-hand coordination. Patients may often feel disoriented and frustrated.

Marginal astigmatism is a considerable problem in convex lenses of greater power than +8.00 D. This aberration can reduce a patient's visual acuity and contrast sensitivity. To reduce or eliminate this aberration, an aspheric-designed lens should be prescribed.

Aspheric lenses are thinner and lighter than spherical lenses and produce less protrusion from the front of the frame. For example, a +6.00 D, 70 mm aspheric lens reduces center thickness by approximately 1 mm and edge thickness by 2 mm as compared to a spherical lens of equal power. This difference is clearly an advantage. Because aspheric lenses are flatter and have a shorter vertex distance, some patients may complain that their eyelashes touch the lenses. This is commonly called *lash crash*, and these patients are candidates for an aspheric lens with a steeper curve. Another potential concern with the aspheric lens design is that patients may initially feel disoriented.[10] Patients may be accustomed to a certain amount of undesired image magnification, which is reduced by the aspheric design. Objects may seem flatter as well, but these problems resolve with adaptation.

Concerning frame selection, the frame IPD should be as close to the patient's IPD as possible. Vertex distance should be small, and adjustable nosepads should be recommended to aid in vertical alignment. These factors are no different than those used for the patient with high myopia. The lens prescription should again include specifications for design, material, and coatings.

Prescribing High Add Powers

Many visually impaired patients obtain better reading performance with the addition of plus power over the distance correction. These patients differ from the typical presbyope in that achieving the necessary magnification often requires a very strong plus lens. The crucial measurement in recommending high add powers is the segment height. High-add bifocals should generally be fit higher than the standard bifocal.[6] The purpose for this is twofold. First, there will be less vertical prism induced because the visual axis through the segment will be closer to the distance optical center. Second, a higher segment will potentially enable the patient to view beneath it, aiding in mobility. Frame selection should be guided toward frames with adjustable nosepads that allow for minor adjustments to the segment height (Figure 8-2).

GLARE AND PHOTOPHOBIA

Glare and photophobia are two very common complaints of patients with low vision. Glare may refer to the condition in which a source of light is much brighter than the background environment. This type of glare is said to exist when the source light to background light is greater than a ratio of 3 to 1. Examples may be seen with an automobile headlight at night or the sun's reflection off of snow or water. These situations produce shiny glare, known as *disability glare,* which can interfere with a patient's visual functioning. Another type of glare that may be very bothersome to the low vision patient is discomfort glare. This type of glare can cause extreme asthenopic complaints from the patient, preventing him or her from spending any time outdoors. It may also present itself indoors when a patient is in a room with overhead fluorescent lights.

Disability glare and discomfort glare may occur individually or together. Visual function often improves by reducing glare and enhancing contrast. Several lens options are available for reducing glare, eliminating abnormal sensitivity to light, and improving contrast:

* Coatings and tints
* Polaroid filters
* Yellow or amber filters
* Photochromatic lenses

NoIR sun filters (NoIR Medical Technologies, South Lyon, MI), are commonly prescribed to visually impaired patients who have complaints of glare and photophobia when outdoors. These lenses filter 100% of the ultraviolet (UV) light while eliminating visible light from the sides and top as well. Many low vision patients find these lens filters an improvement over traditional sunglasses, as they are available in several light transmission levels. (See Chapter 13 section on NoIR Medical Technologies for more information.)

Ultraviolet Coating

Even though UV coatings do not eliminate glare or photophobic complaints, it is important to consider these lens coatings for patients, especially those who are visually impaired.

Much is still unknown regarding UV radiation. Radiation of wavelength between 200 and 400 nm is considered UV radiation. In patient care, two types of UV radiation are considered important: UVA and UVB. UVA has a wavelength ranging from 320 to 400 nm; UVB ranges from 290 to 320 nm.

UVB radiation increases the risk of developing cortical cataracts. UVA radiation may contribute to nuclear cataracts,

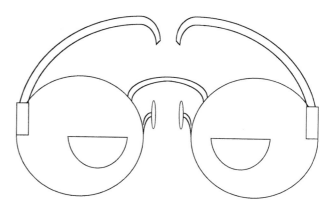

FIGURE 8-2. **In prescriptions for high add powers, a higher segment will enable the patient to have improved mobility by looking under the bifocal. Nosepads permit customized vertical frame adjustments.**

but the legitimacy of this is unclear. Cystoid macular edema is a common complication after cataract extraction. One hypothesis is that this problem is partially due to increased amounts of UVA reaching retinal tissue. However, most intraocular lens implants today have a UV absorber. Certain medications place patients at higher risk of ocular effects from UV exposure. These medications include oral contraceptives, some antibiotics, diuretics, and phenothiazines. Tints will reduce some UV radiation but only to the extent that overall illumination is limited. In other words, a tint that blocks 40% of ambient light will filter out 40% of the UV.

Most ophthalmic materials offer some inherent protection from UV with the exception of crown glass. CR-39 filters out radiation up to 350 nm; high-index plastics protect up to approximately 360 nm. Polycarbonate lenses have a UV filter combined with their scratch coating that screens out radiation up to 380 nm. It therefore seems that a UV protective coating is most critical for glass lenses. Many factors concerning the harmful effects of UV radiation are unclear; however, the general thinking is that patients at risk should have a UV protective coating recommended.

In an attempt to provide UV protection, contact lens manufacturers incorporate chemical additives, called *chromophores,* into the lens material. These chromophores, found in both soft and rigid gas-permeable (RGP) lenses, absorb UV radiation in the range of 200–370 nm, although the wavelength can vary depending on the lens power and thickness. There is not full protection of the sensitive areas of the eye from UV radiation, however, because soft lenses do not cover the sclera. RGP lenses do not fully cover the cornea, and the sclera is exposed as well. So again, UV protective spectacle lenses should be prescribed for patients spending time outdoors.

Antireflective Coating

An AR coating consists of three to six extremely thin layers of metal oxides that destructively interfere with light waves. Each layer is approximately 0.05 µ thick. The AR coating increases light transmission through the lens from 91% to 99.5% and eliminates front and rear surface reflections. Internal reflections, responsible for ghost images, are eliminated as well. As mentioned in Aberration and Distortion, AR coatings help reduce the chromatic aberration and intensive reflections found with use of higher-index lens materials and high-power designs. A clear, sharp image results, improving visual function. Cosmetic appeal is better, too, because the lenses appear invisible to the onlooker.[11] When recommending an AR coating on a tinted or photochromatic lens, the practitioner should be aware that the AR-coated tinted or photochromatic lens will appear lighter in color.

AR coatings are available in different forms with different application processes. Typically, the final layer of a multilayer AR coating is quartz. This layer has been responsible for complaints of debris and smudging in the past. Application of a top layer of silicone, however, presently eliminates these problems. This silicone coating also makes the lenses more scratch resistant. Patients with thick lenses, as sometimes happens in low vision, will benefit most. Moreover, AR coatings are helpful in reducing the effects of edge reflections from high-concave lenses. The ideal AR coating has an index of refraction equal to the square root of the index of the material being coated. Night drivers may also benefit, because glare from headlights lessens; windshield cleanliness and clarity of ocular media are factors here as well.

The practitioner should be aware of the many different brands of lens coatings and treatments. Occasionally, a compatibility problem exists, and lenses may crack or craze.[12] For example, a particular AR coating may not be able to bond with a scratch coating that is already on the lens. If the scratch coating is not stripped off, the AR coating may itself scratch off. Environmental factors may play a role as well because AR coatings are porous. It is therefore possible for foreign substances to penetrate the coating, causing it to peel off. Patients should be advised to clean their spectacles with warm water and a drop of mild liquid dish detergent and wipe them dry with a clean tissue.

Edge Coating

Edge coating refers to coating or "painting" the edge of a thick ophthalmic lens. This coating may minimize reflections even more when combined with an AR coating. Edge coating is available in one color or two or more colors to blend with a specific frame color. A flesh tone can also be painted on the inside lens edge to blend with the patient's facial skin color.

Polaroid Filters

Intense glare, as occurs from light reflected off horizontal surfaces, presents another problem. Patients will complain of an unpleasant sensation, temporary loss or blurring of vision, and ocular fatigue. Standard filters or tints do not reduce this type of glare because with a tint all levels of illumination decrease equally. Some low vision patients find tinted lenses more bothersome, as they often do not tolerate this overall reduction of background light. Polaroid filters are most helpful in controlling this type of glare problem.

Under normal conditions, light vibrates in all directions. When light reflects off of a shiny surface (i.e., snow, water, the surface of a car), the light becomes concentrated and thereby vibrates in a specific direction (horizontally). Polaroid filters, when properly placed (vertically) in front of the reflected light rays, filter out this problematic glare created by the specular reflection. This property is termed *plane polarization*.[13] When light is reflected at different angles, however, and not purely in a horizontal direction, the reflected light will be both polarized and nonpolarized and will therefore only be partially filtered or absorbed.

Plastic polarized spectacle lenses have the thin polarizer film molded within the spectacle lens 1–2 mm behind the front surface of the lens. This prevents the polarizer film from separating from the spectacle lens, a problem that had existed with the earlier forms of polarizing lenses. Polarized lenses are available in single-vision, bifocal, trifocal, and in several progressive lens designs. They can be fabricated in CR-39, crown glass, polycarbonate, photochromatic, and high-index lenses. When these lenses are dispensed, it is important for the practitioner to verify that the axis of polarization is vertical. To verify that the lens is correct, an uncut polarizing filter can be placed against the spectacle lens worn by the patient. If correct, the patient should report that the spectacle lens has become the darkest when the uncut polarizing filter is rotated to the horizontal position.

Tinted Lenses and Photochromatic Lenses

In some cases, normal levels of illumination may bother the low vision patient (discomfort glare). These patients are generally sensitive to scattering at the blue end of the visible spectrum, where wavelengths are less than 500 nm. Therefore, lenses that selectively absorb specific wavelengths of light are frequently necessary. Sometimes general tinted lenses are helpful. For example, yellow tinted lenses brighten the background on foggy, dark days and may improve reading performance and visual acuity through enhanced contrast. Brownish yellow tinted lenses, also known as *blue blockers*, may be used to eliminate outdoor glare and haze (blue end of the spectrum). They alter color perception, however. Lenses that produce an overall reduction in the intensity of all transmitted wavelengths of light are "neutral density filters" and are gray in color. A major advantage of a gray tinted lens is that it will not alter color perception, no matter how dark the tint is made. Gray lenses may not enhance contrast but are highly recommended for reduction of glare and photophobia outdoors.

Photochromic lenses change color when exposed to light. UV radiation is primarily responsible for this. Photochromic lenses are available in a variety of colors, with grays and browns the most popular for sun wear.

Photochromatic lenses do not have uniform color density. The color density will vary with the thickness of the lens so that a thicker lens will appear darker than a thinner lens. It is also important to note that the color density is dependent on the surrounding temperature. As the temperature becomes colder, the tint becomes darker.

Corning Photochromatic Filter (CPF) lenses are photochromatic lenses in four different spectral cutoff levels, manufactured by Corning Medical Optics (Elmira, NY). These glass lenses effectively relieve symptoms of glare discomfort and reduced vision due to light scattering. Contrast is enhanced, and adaptation time to changes in illumination is often aided as well. CPF filters eliminate virtually all of the UV and blue end of the visible spectrum. The CPF #450 lenses filter out approximately 96% of light of wavelength less than 450 nm. The #511, #527, and #550 lenses filter out approximately 98% of light below their respective cutoff values (see Chapter 13 for more information on CPF lenses).

Because many patients with low vision benefit from the use of a computer, consideration should be given to specially coated lenses that may possibly enhance contrast and reduce fatigue. One such coating, specifically designed for the computer user, consists of a 30% tint, a UV absorber, and an AR coating. This coating enhances contrast between the computer screen background and letter or picture colors. A gray tint for black and white screens, violet tint for green screens, and blue tint for amber screens may be recommended.[9]

CONTACT LENS CORRECTION

The fitting and wearing of contact lenses for a low vision patient is not a unique situation. Several situations exist in which the use of contact lenses may greatly benefit the patient with low vision. In some cases, a spectacle lens may not provide acceptable quality of vision because of aberrations, distortion, problems with image size, or other optical phenomenon. Therefore, contact lenses should be considered. Other times, the use of tinted or opaque lenses that reduce the amount of light entering the eye may be necessary. Contact lenses may also be used in conjunction with glasses, forming a unique telescopic system that affords a low vision patient greater magnification. Occasionally, a patient may require a therapeutic type of lens to enhance both vision and ocular health. This can occur with keratoconic corneas, postsurgical corneas, or on eyes that require scleral-type lenses. There are also cases in which color perception can be improved with the wearing of a contact lens.

In all of these instances, it is important to keep in mind certain fundamental ideas:

1. What is the actual problem?
2. What are the realistic goals of the patient?
3. What modalities exist to address the needs of the patient?

4. Where can one obtain these unique lens designs? (See Appendix A.)

The following discussion will describe many of these unique situations and options that are available to low vision patients. A thorough understanding of the basic differences between a spectacle lens and the equivalent-powered contact lens is needed before examining clinical applications. Four basic differences exist:

1. The effective power of a lens will vary as the correcting lens is brought closer to the eye. It follows that in myopia, the corrective power of a contact lens will be weaker than it would be with a spectacle lens. For a patient with hyperopia, a contact lens must be made stronger than a spectacle lens to correct the same eye.
2. Because the power of a contact lens is reduced over that of the spectacle lens in myopia (less minification), the patient will have a larger retinal image when the contact lens is worn (as compared to the retinal image size when the effective-powered spectacle lens is worn). The opposite effect occurs with hyperopia. A patient with high hyperopia wearing a contact lens will have a smaller retinal image size as compared to a patient wearing an effective-powered spectacle lens. However, this may be a disadvantage for a patient with low vision who may benefit from the magnification (larger retinal image) of a spectacle lens over the contact lens. For the monocular aphakic patient, who is unable to attain binocularity because of the increased magnification that a spectacle correction provides, a contact lens on the aphakic eye may solve this problem.
3. Just as the retinal image size changes when comparing a spectacle lens to a contact lens (for the same eye), so does the accommodative demand. When a patient with myopia switches from glasses to contact lenses, he or she has to accommodate more through the contact lens. When this patient has low vision and presbyopia, a higher add (in conjunction with the contact lenses) will be needed than if a bifocal was being used with a spectacle lens. Again, the opposite effect would occur for a patient exhibiting a high degree of hyperopia.
4. There are fewer aberrations as well as less distortion and a wider field of view with a contact lens as opposed to with an effective-powered spectacle lens. This factor is an important one to consider, particularly when dealing with high refractive errors. Elimination of the aberrations and distortion is dependent on the assumption that the contact lens maintains the appropriate movement, yet remains centered on the eye. When the contact lens remains centered on the eye, it provides another advantage over the high-prescription spectacle lens: elimination of induced base-in or base-out prism.

Prescribing for High Myopia

Patients who have progressive or pathologic myopia can often obtain good clinical results when fit with contact lenses. Factors 2 and 4 in the preceding section are influ-

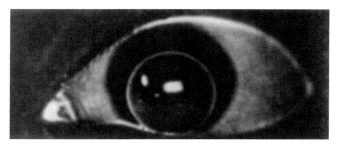

FIGURE 8-3. **A high plus lens positioning inferiorly. A modification in lens design is indicated, such as an increase in lens diameter or a minus edge lenticular carrier design.**

ential in this case. A major problem with very high minus contact lenses, however, is the peripheral edge. Specifically, the peripheral edge will be very thick and may create discomfort, increase the chances of physiologic upset, or encourage excessive superior lid grab. This excessive lid grab could displace the optical center of the lens, causing a degradation in vision. Obviously, some form of modification in lens design must be used.

Soft Lenses
Most soft lenses, including high-powered lenses, are usually considered stock lenses. Manufacturers typically incorporate specific design features to reduce the edge thickness by lenticularizing the anterior periphery of the lens. In doing this, an anterior optic zone or "cap" is simultaneously created. Because soft lenses are relatively large, any significant amount of lenticularization will result in a cap portion that could be too small, creating bothersome scattering of light. Light scattering may be even more problematic if the lens wearer has large pupils. "Customizing" the lens by increasing the size of the cap portion may appear to be a logical solution. Doing this, however, creates a thicker periphery, leading to problems of discomfort and physiologic upset. Most soft lens designs for high powers use anterior optic zones that are approximately 8.0 mm in size. If very thin lenses are used, the anterior optic zone may be larger.

Rigid Gas-Permeable Lenses
High minus RGP lenses may create similar comfort and physiologic problems. Often, a plus edge lenticular carrier is incorporated in the lens design to reduce the influence of the superior lid, which automatically creates an anterior optic zone or cap portion. In high minus prescriptions, it is sometimes beneficial to make the cap slightly smaller than the posterior optic zone. This adjustment makes the transition from the flat anterior curve of the cap portion to the carrier portion less abrupt. Of course, problems with flare could arise if the lens wearer has large pupils.

Prescribing for High Hyperopia

High-powered plus lenses are usually, though not always, associated with aphakia. Contact lenses for high plus cor-

rection provide a better optical system compared to an effective-powered spectacle lens. The main concern with a high-powered hyperopic contact lens is its weight. In the geriatric population, the superior lid typically loses some of its elasticity, resulting in less lid grab. This may allow the contact lens to drop inferiorly, which is undesirable. The contact lens design may be modified to solve this type of problem (Figure 8-3).

High plus lenses are relatively thick, and oxygen transmission through the central area is therefore reduced. With RGP lenses, central corneal edema may result, which is similar to that seen when polymethyl methylacrylate (PMMA) material was being used. With soft lenses, the cornea swells in a manner that causes folds in the deep stroma or in Descemet's membrane. These folds are referred to as *vertical striae*. If the edematous response is considered clinically significant, the practitioner must change to a material that will provide a greater potential for oxygen transmission. For RGP lenses, this would be a material with a higher dK, or permeability value. In the case of soft lenses, a material with a higher water content may be needed. These types of materials also have some disadvantages in that they are more prone to deposit formation and are less durable. Sometimes it may be necessary for the patient to reduce the amount of wearing time.

Although it may not seem important, some contact lenses are labeled in back vertex power (BVP), whereas others are labeled in front vertex power (FVP). In higher-powered lenses, clinically significant differences in power occur. Thus, it is very important to know how a given lens has been labeled. A lens that reads +15.00 D BVP will read lower in dioptric power if FVP is checked.

Regardless of contact lens type (RGP or soft) used, patients with monocular aphakia present some interesting problems due to large differences in retinal image size. This difference in retinal image size is called *aniseikonia*, and is approximately 10–12% when a contact lens is being worn by a monocular aphake. Some patients are able to fuse this size difference, but most cannot. For those low vision patients with fairly good acuity and the potential for binocular function, the following may be considered. The aphakic eye is prescribed a contact lens with more plus power than is required. This apparent "overplussing" can be compensated for by using a minus spectacle prescription. The theory in doing this is that the extra magnification caused by the overplussing of the contact lens will be *more than* compensated for by the minification of the minus lens at the spectacle plane. In a similar manner, if the better seeing eye is fit with a contact lens that has more minus power than required, the spectacle lens can be made in a compensatory plus power that will theoretically increase the image size and further improve one's ability to fuse.

Soft Lenses
Lens manufacturers usually incorporate lenticular changes in lens design for high-powered soft lenses. This type of design, as discussed in Soft Lenses under Prescribing for High Myopia, helps to avoid problems with lens thickness and weight. When performing the initial contact

lens evaluation, diagnostic lenses should be used that are within a few diopters of the anticipated power. This technique will minimize differences in overall lens performance and over-refraction between trial lens evaluation and final dispensed lenses. Patients commonly need more plus power than anticipated when considering only the refraction and effectivity. For example, an eye that refracts +14.00 D would appear to require a lens with a power of +17.00 D if effectivity alone was considered. Clinically, however, these eyes will not obtain maximum acuity with the +17.00 D contact lens. A stronger plus lens is often needed. This difference may be due to some flattening effect on the steep front curve of the contact lens when it is placed on the eye.

Rigid Gas-Permeable Lenses

High plus–powered RGP lenses can become rather thick and heavy as well, especially if the lens diameters approach 9.5 mm or larger. Consequently, most practitioners incorporate a minus edge lenticular carrier design to encourage lid grab. This lens type has become popularly known as the *Korb lens* or *Korb-type lens*, named after Dr. Donald Korb. The Polycon 9.5 mm–diameter lens is an example of this lens design. This lens usually positions superiorly and travels down with the superior lid during a blink. A well-fit lens will then move up with the superior lid as the blink is completed. These lenses are usually fit slightly flatter than the flat corneal curvature reading, facilitating superior lid grab and helping in achieving a good tear exchange during each blink. If the superior lid is not able to hold the lens, the practitioner can increase the lens diameter, change to a slightly flatter base curve, or flatten the anterior carrier radius by 0.2–0.4 mm.

Prescribing for High Astigmatism

High astigmatism, especially if it goes uncorrected during one's formative years, can cause amblyopia or reduced vision. Correction of this type of refractive error with a contact lens instead of a spectacle lens may provide advantages, again due to the better optical imagery. Although there are many soft lens manufacturers, there are relatively few who produce lenses that correct for high amounts of astigmatism. When prescribing a contact lens for even a small amount of astigmatism, it is imperative that the axis of the lens aligns properly with the axis of the astigmatic error of the eye. Otherwise, a resultant cylinder power is created that may cause a further reduction in vision.

If a patient has a significant amount of lenticular or physiologic astigmatism, a front toric lens may be needed. Front toric RGP lenses are probably one of the least used lens designs, as soft toric lenses frequently can be used instead. Assuming that a situation exists in which a front toric RGP lens is to be fit, however, it is again essential that the correcting cylinder aligns properly with the astigmatic refractive error. This alignment is usually done by adding prism or truncation to the lens design. Frequently, this still

results in a "swim" or rocking type of action during a blink, in which the lens becomes torqued nasally by the action of the lids. Many patients find this fluctuation in vision very annoying. The presence of the prism and truncation can also be bothersome to some patients. An interesting alternative to this design is to fit the patient with a basic RGP lens with an aspheric anterior surface that will hopefully provide a better optical image, therefore providing better acuity. This type of lens, often referred to as a *Panofocal lens* design, does not correct the residual cylinder. It simply reduces spherical aberration so the quality of vision is better.

High amounts of corneal astigmatism present both fitting and visual challenges. A spherical back curve RGP lens, when placed on a highly astigmatic cornea, often crashes down as it travels over the astigmatic "hump." Sometimes these lenses position inferiorly and are not picked up at all by the action of the superior lid. Nevertheless, visual, physiologic, and physical problems can occur. This situation is nicely addressed by using a back toric lens, in which individual consideration is given to each meridian of the cornea. The differences in indices between the lens material and the tear layer creates an induced cylinder. If not understood properly, however, this new power usually results in a great deal of confusion. The amount and location of this power is somewhat predictable, however, and practitioners may use this information in their fitting routines. Since the early 1990s, a special version of this lens design has become popular. This lens design uses ideas that Sarver presented in 1963.[14] He postulated that a great deal of the confusion regarding the optics of these lenses could be eliminated by grinding a cylinder on the front lens surface that canceled out the induced cylinder. This effect is relatively easy to achieve, because the amount of cylinder is a function of the differences in the two base curves of the lens multiplied by a constant. The axis of this cylinder is coincident with the axis of the flat corneal curvature. For example, suppose a lens has base curves of 42.00 D × 46.00 D, and the flat corneal curve is at axis 180. The amount of induced astigmatism can be determined by multiplying the amount of difference in base curves of the lens by a constant. Frequently, this constant is approximately 0.5. Consequently, using the "rule of one-half," it can be determined that 2.00 D of induced cylinder at axis 180 will be created by this combination of contact lens and tear lens. A laboratory can therefore grind a plus powered 2.00 D cylinder on the front curve at axis 180 to compensate for this induced cylinder. The end result is that the practitioner can then focus attention on the other aspects of the lens fit. These lenses are referred to as *spherical power effect* (SPE) lenses because they behave as spherical lenses on the eye. Usually, patients over-refract spherically or near spherically and obtain very good vision. Occasionally, a lens wearer will require a spherocylindrical overcorrection to obtain the best vision. This slight modification in lens design is then referred to as a *CPE lens*.

There are several different fitting techniques for fitting bitoric lenses. A very popular one is fitting the flat meridian of the cornea either "on K," or one-fourth

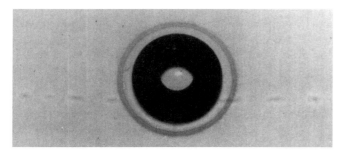

FIGURE 8-4.   **Opaque Iris lens with a clear 4-mm pupil.**

diopter flatter. The steep meridian is also fit flat by an amount relative to the amount of corneal toricity. As a guide, some practitioners undercorrect the steep meridian by approximately one-third of the corneal toricity. Thus, a cornea that measures 42.00 D × 45.00 D with the flat axis at 180 could have an initial lens with base curves of 42.00 D and 44.00 D. The steep meridian is determined by taking one-third of the 3.00 D difference between the two keratometric meridians and fitting the lens flatter by that amount (one-third of 3.00 D = 1.00 D; 1.00 D flatter than 45.00 D is 44.00 D). The amount of induced cylinder has been ground on the front curve of the lens. In this case, using the before-mentioned rule of one-half, the amount of induced cylinder is: 0.5 × 2.00 D or –1.00 D, at axis 180. Thus, a +1.00 D cylinder is ground on the front surface of the contact lens at axis 180, eliminating the induced cylinder.

Another advantage of using SPE lenses is that an excellent set of diagnostic lenses is readily available. These sets are usually designed with base curves that reflect a 2.00 D, 3.00 D, and 4.00 D difference between the two base curves. The actual fit is evaluated in the usual manner. Thus, lens movement, lens position, vision, and fluorescein pattern are assessed. If necessary, the appropriate lens design changes can then be made.

TINTED AND OPAQUE LENSES FOR LOW VISION PATIENTS

Prescribing for Albinism

Glare and photophobia are common complaints encountered in the low vision examination. These problems can be due to degenerative or congenital conditions. An example of a congenital problem producing photophobic complaints is seen in patients with albinism. These individuals frequently display a pendular nystagmoid movement of their eyes as they attempt to use their hypoplastic maculas. This type of movement may further reduce vision.

Contact lenses can be used to address a variety of problems that are experienced by patients with this condition. For one thing, vision may be improved with contact lenses because the nystagmoid movement is slowed. The actual reason for this is unclear. One theory is that the nystagmus

decreases due to a proprioceptor feedback mechanism that causes the eyes to move less. More probable, however, is that a contact lens provides a better optical system. These lenses can be prescribed to provide the proper visual correction and can also be tinted or made with an opaque periphery to aid in sensitivity to light. Some companies (i.e., Adventures in Color [Golden, CO], Custom Color Contacts [New York, NY]) will customize these tints so that a more precise amount of light absorption occurs. The practitioner must remember that if a tint is too dark, the lens may be helpful during bright daylight activities but could prove to be problematic at night or during reduced illumination activities.

Prescribing for Aniridia

A more dramatic form of photosensitivity problem occurs in patients with aniridia. Special contact lenses can be used to help these individuals as well.[15] Stock opaque artificial iris lenses, such as the Illusion lens from CIBA Vision (Duluth, GA), the Natural Touch lens from Cooper Vision (Fairport, NY), and the Wesley-Jessen (Des Plaines, IL) Opaque series, are all available. These lenses have approximately a 4-mm clear pupillary zone that can be tinted to further reduce the amount of light entering the eye. The pupillary zone may be clear or opaque (Figure 8-4). Lenses with a clear pupil can also be custom tinted by other companies such as Adventures in Color. Wesley-Jessen also has a special set of prosthetic lenses available for these situations. Some of their lenses have a double-dot matrix, which makes them even more opaque. They also have an underlying meshwork that can make them still more opaque. The pupillary zone can again be clear or opaque. The practitioner should keep in mind that patients with aniridia are already accustomed to their appearance. Any sudden change to a flamboyant color could prove to be too dramatic to the patient as well as to their acquaintances.

These special lenses are not always needed. Frequently, a good cosmetic and visual result can be obtained by using a simple dark brown or black donut-shaped iris simulation lens. These lenses usually have a 4-mm pupillary opening and provide an adequate reduction in the amount of light entering the eye. They are available from companies such as Adventures in Color, the Narcissus Eye Research Foundation (now part of the Wesley-Jessen Company), and Custom Color Contacts (New York, NY). The latter two companies also make custom lenses with artificial irides in many colors to help people with ocular disfigurements, whether they be monocular or binocular.

When fitting these lenses, it is always a good idea to have a good diagnostic lens available. This lens can be used to check for adequate lens movement and positioning, as well as to refine the final lens power required. A lens that moves too much is not only uncomfortable and creates a poor appearance but also produces visual disturbances because the visual axis may infringe on the iris/pupillary border.

The situation is further complicated if the practitioner decides to fit a pinhole lens. These lenses, sometimes referred to as "reduced aperture lenses," attempt to make use of depth of focus to improve visual acuity. The key to success is to align the pinhole properly with the visual axis. This alignment is difficult when fitting a spherical lens because it continuously rotates on the eye. Enlarging the pinhole increases the margin for error but reduces the overall effect of the pinhole. Designing the lens with a prism or with prism/truncation may help stabilize the lens but can cause lens awareness problems. Multiple pinholes have been tried with some degree of success. The design of these lenses is very challenging, however, because the practitioner cannot always predict the optimum location for all the holes.

Prescribing for Keratoconus

Keratoconus is a noninflammatory protrusion, or ectasia, of the cornea, which becomes thinner and distorted. It usually is bilateral, with one eye progressing ahead of the other. From the standpoint of this disorder, the most important consideration is that many times the cornea becomes so irregular that quality of vision cannot be improved with spectacle lenses. A contact lens provides immediate advantages because it acts as a "new" cornea or refracting surface. The corneal irregularities that create havoc with light rays entering the eye become more normalized by this new temporary ocular surface. The end result is that a better macular focus is obtained and vision dramatically improves. It is important to realize that sometimes objective acuity may not be dramatically better, but the patient subjectively appreciates much better visual function. This is often demonstrated during the early stages of the condition. As the condition advances, the apex of the cornea becomes more irregular, covering a greater area, and almost always starts to droop inferiorly. This often provides one of the extreme challenges to the practitioner who realizes that if a good positioning lens can be designed that moves sufficiently, vision can usually be quite adequate. There are times when scars interfere with the path of the light rays entering the eye such that optimum results are not always possible, although vision is still much better with contact lenses than with spectacles.

There are a number of approaches that practitioners use when fitting keratoconic patients. Some practitioners think that soft lenses have value because they may be less "traumatic" to the cornea. The fact that vision may not be as good, even if an overcorrection incorporating a significant amount of cylinder is used, is not regarded as a disadvantage. Other practitioners think that rigid lenses provide the best overall direction to follow.

Most practitioners who fit patients with keratoconus learn by their own experiences. It is important to realize and accept that these eyes have serious problems; therefore, many concepts used when fitting healthy eyes have to be modified. For example, it is extremely common for practitioners to notice certain corneal problems. Staining,

vertical striae, prominent nerves, and scarring are often seen with the biomicroscope, regardless of whether contact lenses have been worn. It takes some experience on the part of the practitioner to reach a comfort level when evaluating these patients.

Similar thinking must be practiced during the actual fitting and evaluating of the lenses. All practitioners strive for a well-centered lens that moves during the blink. They want a fluorescein pattern that reveals a somewhat aligned central pattern, with a good peripheral reservoir of tears that flushes in when the patient blinks. In reality, this is seldom seen with keratoconic eyes, except in the early stages of the condition when many variations in lens design are all clinically acceptable. As the condition progresses, the prudent practitioner must continuously redesign the lens to obtain the best results possible relative to the specific circumstances present. This invariably requires a great deal of flexibility on the part of the practitioner. Thus, the practitioner must be open minded to the variety of lens designs that are now available in gas-permeable materials rather than become dogmatic with one particular design.

For example, small lenses with relatively small optic zones were popular when PMMA material was the only material available. These lenses were usually positioned over the optic cap. They were sometimes flicked out of the eye by the lids during ocular excursions. As gas-permeable materials became available, larger lenses were used in the hope of gaining better coverage and stability with less concern for physiologic upset. Some designs, such as the Nicone lens (Lancaster, PA), advocated rather large diameters and optic zones in an attempt to have the bearing area on the healthier areas of the cornea. Some practitioners believed that a better cornea-lens relationship could be obtained by fitting a keratoconic eye with aspheric base curve designs. This aspheric base curve design has become even more practical with the availability of lenses with high eccentricity values. These lenses have curves that appear to be fit on the steep side. These lenses flatten out quickly in the paracentral and peripheral areas, however, where the keratoconic cornea may be much more regular or more typical of a normal cornea. It is important to have the optical center of the lens centered over the visual axis to obtain the best vision.

In clinical situations in which the lens does not position properly or excessive apical bearing is occurring, it is strongly suggested that alternative philosophies in lens design be attempted. However, this requires a large number of different diagnostic lenses with a variety of diameters and base curves. It may be difficult to try many different lenses on these patients during the same visit, especially if they do not have any prior experience with rigid lenses and tearing becomes a major factor. Even though it is frowned on, it may be helpful to use a topical anesthetic to facilitate the evaluation.

There are times, however, when all attempts to fit keratoconic patients with contact lenses result in poor lens position and stability, or the lenses are not tolerable to the patient. These patients should be considered for some form of keratoplasty.

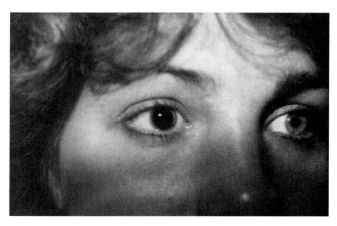

FIGURE 8-5.   **An X chrom lens on a light iris is very noticeable and resembles anisocoria.**

Prescribing for Loss of Color Vision

Occasionally, a contact lens can be used to enhance color perception. Approximately 8% of the male population and 0.5% of the female population have some form of color vision problem. Individuals who have anomalous trichromatism can match colors with red, green, and blue but require more of one color than normal. Dichromatism is the other form of color vision abnormality, whereby two colors are used to match all colors. These individuals have difficulty with red and green, while also experiencing a general reduction in brightness. In either case, color vision problems can be an everyday nuisance, as they may cause problems with activities of daily living.

Dr. Harry I. Zeltzer published a paper in 1971 describing a red or X chrom contact lens that transmitted light in the red zones from approximately 590 to 700 nm.[16] Even though this lens does not cure color vision conditions, it can enhance color perception or make things appear more "vivid." The lens is usually worn on the nondominant eye, though this is not always the case. Patients with anomalous trichromatism seem to achieve the best results with the X chrom lens. Patients with dichromatism, however, may find this lens helpful as well (Figure 8-5).

The mechanism of how this lens works is uncertain. It is theorized that binocular individuals, wearing one lens, send new and possibly confusing information to the brain. Through the process of retinal rivalry, information from each eye may be alternated such that a new perception of color discrimination is experienced by the individual.

These lenses are available in PMMA and in hydrogel materials as well, in which the central portion of the lens is dyed red. It is important that this red area be made large enough so that extraneous light from the periphery does not enter the pupil. There is the possibility that an RGP material can be specially dyed to the right color. It is important that the tint not be too dark, as insufficient transmission of light may adversely affect any benefit in color perception. Lens wearers using this type of lens usually accept about 0.50 D more plus power than expected.

Although many patients appreciate an improvement in color perception, only a few elect to order this lens. The practitioner should be aware that patients with light irides have apparent anisocoria when wearing the X chrom lens. The potential also exists for problems with dim illumination, such that scotopic function for low vision patients may be of concern.

CONTACT LENS TELESCOPIC SYSTEM

A contact lens may be used in the design of a Galilean telescopic system. The ocular, or eyepiece, is a high-powered concave contact lens and the objective is a lower-powered convex spectacle lens. The separation distance (d) between the contact lens and the spectacle lens is determined by the algebraic sum of the focal lengths (f_{obj} and f_{oc}) of the spectacle lens power and the contact lens power, respectively.

$$d = f_{obj} + f_{oc}$$

The total magnification (M) of the system can be determined by the ratio of the dioptric power of the contact lens (D_{oc}) to the dioptric power of the spectacle lens (D_{obj}).

Note. When the minus power of the contact lens combines with the negative sign in the magnification formula, it produces a positive magnification; the image is erect.

$$M = -D_{oc}/D_{obj}$$

A contact lens telescopic system produces a relatively large field of view as compared to an equivalent powered Galilean handheld or spectacle-mounted telescope. Practically speaking, however, the maximum amount of magnification that can be obtained with a contact lens telescopic system is approximately 1.8×. As seen in Table 8-4, if the system is made more powerful, the distance between the contact lens and spectacle lens becomes so great that the spectacle lens can no longer be worn on the nose.

Proper frame selection is very important for a contact lens telescopic system. Because the vertex distance increases with this system compared to a standard spectacle vertex distance, the nosepads should be quite long and adjustable to lift the spectacles up and out. This positioning allows the patient to fixate through the optical center of the spectacle lens in primary gaze. Also, when possible, the temples should be riding bow comfort cables, which provide stability and help prevent the spectacles from slipping down off the nose due to the weight of the spectacle and the increased vertex distance.

FITTING CONTACT LENSES ON POSTSURGICAL CORNEAS

During corneal transplantation, the trephination is typically made 0.25–0.50 mm smaller than the intended donor button. This insures good wound coaptation and reduces the chance of wound leakage. The actual procedure involves approximately 90% of the corneal thickness. The donor button is anchored with four cardinal sutures. Various techniques are used, including those involving continuous sutures, others involving interrupted sutures, and some using a combination of both. Interrupted sutures can be selectively modified after the operation to control astigmatism. Continuous sutures may be better to ensure wound healing and may be adjusted to control astigmatism as well. These are usually left in longer than interrupted sutures. Frequently, because of anisometropia and high amounts of residual astigmatism, a contact lens must be used postoperatively to obtain the best acuity. Soft lenses, various RGP designs, piggyback systems, and even scleral lenses are all considerations. The practitioner usually bases the final design on factors such as the corneal topography, the physiology of the graft, the anticipated power of the lens, and whether the patient is comfortable with a particular lens type. Any neovascularization, either due to pre-existing inflammation or from the actual healing process, must also be considered because hemorrhaging or graft rejection can occur. RGP lenses are advantageous in this case because they do not cover the entire cornea and therefore are less apt to clamp down in the periphery. This decreases the chance for propagation of the limbal vasculature. The practitioner must remember that the cornea has undergone dramatic changes in innervation and endothelial function. Thus, it is important to use a lens material and design that minimizes physiologic disturbance. Fluoropolymers providing good oxygen transmission and wettability, as well as good tear exchange, should be emphasized.

The topographic shape of the cornea makes fitting postoperative keratoplasty patients challenging. Traditional keratometric readings are helpful but do not relate the true situation. The availability of computerized topographic instruments has enabled the practitioner to have a better appreciation of the location of the apex and the asymmetric asphericity of the cornea and to determine whether the central area is protruding or sunken. Sometimes the transition area between central and peripheral areas is very abrupt, which may cause many contact lenses to decenter. A standard keratometer may "measure" a large amount of corneal cylinder, suggesting the need for a back toric lens. The midperiphery of this cornea may, however, be less astigmatic, so fluorescein pattern analysis is critical. Regardless of what lens design is used, careful attention must be given to any residual astigmatism so that refractive error is completely corrected. The contact lens should provide suitable wearing time, adequate comfort, and be physiologically tolerable to the eye.

Rigid Gas-Permeable Lenses

The introduction of fluorosilicone acrylate materials has enabled practitioners to design lenses with good oxygen

TABLE 8-4
Contact Lens Telescopic System

Contact Lens	Spectacle Lens	Vertex Distance (mm)	Magnification
−20.00	+10.00	50.0	2.00
	+12.00	33.4	1.67
	+14.00	21.5	1.43
	+15.00	16.7	1.34
−25.00	+12.00	43.4	2.09
	+14.00	31.5	1.79
	+16.00	22.5	1.57
	+18.00	15.6	1.39
−30.00	+16.00	29.1	1.88
	+18.00	22.2	1.67
	+20.00	16.6	1.50
	+21.00	14.3	1.43
−35.00	+18.00	27.0	1.95
	+20.00	21.4	1.75
	+22.00	16.9	1.59
	+24.00	13.1	1.46
−40.00	+18.00	30.6	2.23
	+20.00	25.0	2.00
	+22.00	20.5	1.82
	+24.00	16.7	1.67
	+25.00	15.0	1.60

transmission and good wettability. These contact lenses stay relatively clean and do not flex or warp as earlier lens materials often did.

The physiologic advantages of these lens materials allow designs with larger lens diameters than could be designed previously. These lenses, often with diameters of 9.2 mm or greater, help to obtain adequate positioning, good movement, good lid interaction, and good tear flushing action. The optic zone can also be made relatively large, although care must be taken not to cause paracentral binding and reduced tear exchange. Base curve determination is via trial and error, but a good initial lens has a base curve that is between one-third and one-half of the keratometric readings. Thus, a patient with a keratometric reading of 44.00 D × 50.00 D may have an initial lens with a base curve approximately 46.50 D. The final curve is determined by the practitioner after evaluating various factors, including lens movement and position, fluorescein pattern, and flushing action. Usually, a three-point or divided support philosophy is desired. Peripheral curves should be designed relative to the fluorescein pattern appearance.

Occasionally, the central corneal graft is flatter than the periphery of the host cornea. This situation is rather unique and usually cannot be addressed with conventional lens designs. Several lens manufacturers have developed unconventional RGP lenses to address these cases. These contact lenses have peripheral curve systems that are *steeper* than the base curve of the lens, thus allowing flat or plateau-like central corneas to be fit. The OK lens (Contex Laboratories, Sherman Oaks, CA), the NRK lens (Lancaster Contact Lens Company, Lancaster, PA), and the RK Bridge lens (Conforma Laboratories, Norfolk, VA) are examples of these lenses.

Usually, the practitioner selects a base curve that is close to the mean keratometric curvature. Therefore, in the preceding example, a lens with a base curve of 47.00 D should be used initially.

Various forms of ellipsoidal, or aspheric, back curve lenses are available as well for consideration. Diagnostic fitting requires a special set of lenses that many practitioners do not have readily available, however, especially in higher powers. The practitioner can always check with the lens manufacturer to see if loaner, or library lenses, are available.

Soft Lenses

Soft lenses, covering a relatively large area of the ocular surface, often provide better centration and positioning. Patients, of course, usually enjoy the immediate comfort of these lenses. However, one disadvantage is that residual astigmatism may reduce acuity unless a spectacle overcorrection is worn. This occasionally requires oblique cylinders, which may make adaptation difficult.

Soft lenses are available in a variety of materials with many different characteristics. A low-water-content, thin lens in a nonionic material is often a good choice. These lenses are typically manufactured in a manner that makes them easy to handle. They usually provide good oxygen supply to the cornea without attracting surface debris, as most of the high-water-content, ionic materials do.

Patients with hyperopia or aphakia should be fit with higher-water-content lenses in an attempt to allow the maximum amount of oxygen to reach the cornea. Regardless of which lens is tried, a careful analysis of lens movement and positioning is required so that any changes in diameter or base curve can be made. In some cases, the overrefraction may indicate the need for a spectacle lens with an astigmatic component. Occasionally, soft toric lenses may be used. The practitioner must again consider the effect of lens thickness, however, especially if a thin-zoned toric lens design is not used. Clinically, soft toric lenses may not provide the quality of vision that the patient desires. Therefore, their use has been somewhat limited.

Piggyback Designs

Because the main disadvantage of soft lenses is reduced visual acuity and disadvantages of RGP lenses include lack of stability and comfort, the possibility of combining the positive attributes of both could be of some interest.

The design of the underlying soft lens is based on the corneal topography and the anticipated refractive error. For example, if the graft is protruding, a thin soft lens with minus power can be used. If the graft is sunken, a plus lens is advised because it gives the RGP lens a steeper

anterior surface to rest on and helps reduce some of the anticipated plus correction as well. In any event, the underlying soft lens is given time to equilibrate and is then evaluated. A keratometric reading is taken over the soft lens that provides information regarding initial RGP base curve. Usually, a base curve is selected that is midway between the two keratometric meridians. A little extra soft lens movement is desired, because this is often minimized when the rigid lens is placed on it. Due to the overall thickness of this complex optical system, the practitioner must be very careful in assessing the postwear physiologic health of the eye.

SELF-ASSESSMENT QUESTIONS

1. Distance devices that may help the low vision patient include all of the following *except*
   (a) field awareness systems
   (b) spectacles or contact lenses
   (c) absorptive lenses and coatings
   (d) microscopes
   (e) pinhole lenses

2. Which of the following ophthalmic lens materials should be recommended for monocular patients?
   (a) crown glass
   (b) polycarbonate
   (c) high-index plastic
   (d) RGP contact lenses
   (e) all of the above

3. Chromatic aberrations and reflections may best be reduced by which of the following lens options?
   (a) ultraviolet protective coatings
   (b) tint
   (c) high-index material
   (d) antireflective coating
   (e) edge coating

4. Glare and photophobia are common, sometimes debilitating complaints with patients having low vision.
   True or False

5. Because a great deal is unclear regarding ultraviolet radiation, ultraviolet protective coatings should be prescribed infrequently.
   True or False

6. Which of the following should be recommended in the final spectacle prescription for the low vision patient having a high refractive error?
   (a) lens material
   (b) lens design
   (c) coatings or lens treatments
   (d) all of the above are correct
   (e) a and c

7. The most accurate way of describing the results of the X chrom lens is
   (a) All lens wearers are able to achieve what would be described as "normal" color vision.
   (b) Many lens wearers appear to appreciate an improvement in color perception and vividness.
   (c) Lens wearers must use these lenses binocularly to achieve any color vision improvement.
   (d) The lens wearer appreciates an improvement in color perception especially under dim illumination.
   (e) All of the above statements are true in regard to the wearing of an X chrom lens.

8. The best way of describing SPE lenses would be
   (a) They are special back toric lenses that have a front cylindrical power ground on them that cancels out the effects of the induced cylinder.
   (b) They are special back toric lenses that correct for the total amount of residual astigmatism that is created by the patient's own lens.
   (c) They are special back toric lenses that do not require a front cylinder because they are only used on patients who have no lenticular astigmatism.
   (d) They are front toric lenses that correct for the effects of residual astigmatism by masking the corneal astigmatism.
   (e) None of the above is correct.

9. Practitioners can help patients with aniridia by
   (a) using stock opaque lenses that are available from several lens manufacturers.
   (b) using custom opaque lenses that can have either artificial irides or an opaque "donut" on the surface.
   (c) using stock tinted lenses that are usually used for enhancing light-colored irides.
   (d) using the X chrom lens design because it acts as a sunglass-type lens.
   (e) a and b

10. When fitting patients with keratoconus, all of the below statements are true but one. Which statement does *not* accurately relate to keratoconus?

   (a) Keratoconus is usually a bilateral ectasia of the cornea with one eye progressing ahead of the other.
   (b) As the condition advances, the apex of the cornea usually starts to position inferiorly or inferior-temporally.
   (c) The prudent practitioner knows that once a suitable lens design is determined, it is seldom necessary to modify it.
   (d) The prudent practitioner is continuously trying to arrive at a lens design that positions well and has good flushing action and physiologic results.
   (e) The prudent practitioner knows that many times a variety of lens designs with differing lens size, base curve, optic zone, and back curve geometry may be required.

REFERENCES

1. Milder B, Rubin M. The Fine Art of Prescribing Glasses (2nd ed). Gainesville, FL: Triad Publishing, 1991.
2. Welling M. Frames for high-powered Rxs. Eyecare Business 1995;4:40.
3. Cline D, Hofstetter HW, Griffin JR. Dictionary of Visual Science (4th ed). Radnor, PA: Chilton Trade Book Publishing, 1989.
4. Lee G. Sorting out those confusing ophthalmic lens options. Optom Manage 1991;10:45–49.
5. Bruneni J. A guide to AR lens coatings. Eyecare Business 1995;9:52–56.
6. Welling M. Mastering frame measurements. Eyecare Business 1995;5:32–33.
7. Zaccaria D. Distance optical center placement on single vision lenses. Eyecare Business 1995;11:45–49.
8. Lee J. Polycarbonate protects you and your young patients. Rev Optom 1993;8:41–46.
9. Lee J. Straight talk about spectacle lens coatings. Optom Manage 1993;8:39–40.
10. Bruneni J. Asperics—the future of lens design. Eyecare Business 1995;9:65–70.
11. Woythaler R. A/R coatings: the perception of invisible lenses. Eye Quest 1995;3:29.
12. Jarratt T. Anti-reflection coating. Optical World 1991;12:8–12.
13. Zeidner J. Polarization and the challenge to reduce glare. Eye Quest 1995;5:24.
14. Sarver MA. A bitoric gas permeable hard contact lens with spherical power effect. J Am Optom Assoc 1985;56:184–189.
15. Wodak G. Soft artificial iris lenses. Contacto 1977;21:4.
16. Zelter H. The X-chrom lens. J Am Optom Assoc 1971;42:933.

Appendix A

MANUFACTURERS AND SUPPLIERS OF SPECIALTY CONTACT LENSES

Note. This information does not denote a complete list of manufacturers and suppliers in the United States.

Adventure in Colors
1511 Washington Ave.
Golden, CO 80401
(800) 537-2845
(303) 271-9644

Alden Optical
13295 Broadway
Alden, NY 14004
(800) 253-3669
(716) 937-9181

Custom Color Contacts
55 W. 49th St.
New York, NY 10020
(800) 598-2020
(212) 765-4444

Narcissus Eye Research Foundation
1850 Sullivan Ave., Ste. 500
Daly City, CA 94015
(415) 992-8924

Wesley-Jessen
333 E. Howard Ave.
Des Plaines, IL 60018
(800) 488-6859
(847) 294-3324

CHAPTER NINE

Low Vision Distance Systems II: Telescopes and Telemicroscopes

Douglas R. Williams

The telescope is an optical instrument used to magnify the apparent size of a distant object. Most telescopes used in low vision rehabilitation are of the refracting type—that is, a telescope that uses a converging lens as the objective. It is the only device that is available for improvement of the distance and intermediate resolution when the patient cannot move closer to the object and when the best conventional spectacle or contact lenses do not provide the needed resolution. A telescope can be used to amplify light, enabling faint distant *point sources* of light to be seen. Its use in low vision with *extended sources* of light, however, is to produce an image of a distant object that will subtend a larger visual angle than the object would subtend if viewed without the aid of the telescope (angular magnification).

In its simplest form, a telescope consists of two elements:

1. The objective lens is a positive or convergent lens and is positioned closest to the object. It is generally large in diameter and is used to collect a large quantity of light. The objective lens will be designated D_{obj} or D_1. Likewise, the dioptric power of the objective is designated by the same notations.

2. The *ocular* or *eyepiece* may be either a convergent (positive) or divergent (negative) lens depending on the type of telescope (Keplerian or Galilean, respectively). The ocular lens is the lens closest to the eye. It will be designated D_{oc} or D_2. Similarly, the dioptric power of the ocular is designated by these notations.

When the objective and ocular lenses are separated by a distance equal to the absolute values of their focal lengths, the system is said to be *afocal* or in "*normal adjustment.*" An afocal lens system produces only angular magnification. An afocal telescope has incident parallel rays of light from infinity emerge as parallel rays of light. Because the telescope is afocal, both the object and image are located at infinity. When a parallel ray bundle of light strikes the convergent objective lens, the image formed by the objective lens is located in the plane of the secondary focal point. In an afocal system, the ocular lens is positioned so that its primary focal point is located coincident with the image formed by the objective lens. If a negative lens (divergent system) is used for the ocular, then its primary focal point (a virtual point) is coincident with the secondary focal point of the objective lens, and an erect, virtual image is formed by the eyepiece. This type of telescope is called a *Galilean* or *Dutch* telescope (Figure 9-1). If a positive lens (convergent system) is used for the ocular lens, then its primary focal point is coincident with the secondary focal point of the objective lens and an inverted, real image is formed by the eyepiece lens. This type of telescope is known as a *Keplerian* or *astronomical* telescope (Figure 9-2). It should be noted that the above combinations (a positive objective and a positive ocular or a positive objective and a negative ocular) are the only possible ways of producing an afocal system using two lenses.

When discussing an afocal telescope, the terms *power* and *magnification* should not be confused. Although the term *power* strictly refers to dioptric power, the term is frequently used synonymously with the term *magnification*. These terms, however, are not synonymous. For example, an individual may say that a particular telescope has "4 power" when in reality it has "4× magnification." The equivalent power of an afocal telescope is zero. The magnification of an afocal telescope (M_{TS}) can be determined by the formula:

$$M_{TS} = - \frac{D_{oc}}{D_{obj}}$$

When telescopic systems are *focal*, they have a finite focal distance. The magnification produced by the portions of the telescopic system that make the system focal are primarily due to relative distance magnification. When a telescope is focused for intermediate or near, it is said to be *made focal* and the device is then referred to as a *telemicroscope, reading telescope, surgical telescope, telescopic loupe,* or *near-point telescope.*

GALILEAN TELESCOPE

The following is a summary of the important concepts of a Galilean telescope:

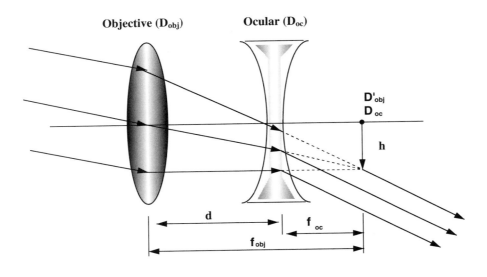

Objective (D_{obj})   Ocular (D_{oc})

D'_{obj}
D_{oc}

h

d f_{oc}

f_{obj}

FIGURE 9-1. **In a Galilean telescope, the primary focal point of the ocular lens (D_{oc}) is coincident with the secondary focal point of the objective lens (D'_{obj}) creating an erect, virtual image (h). The tube length (d) is equal to the sum of the focal lengths of the objective and ocular lenses ($f_{obj} + f_{oc}$).**

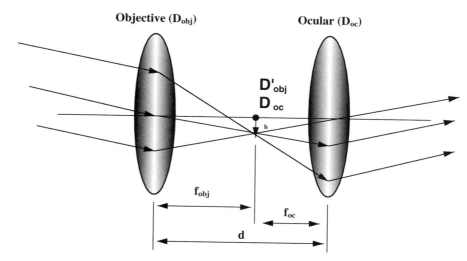

FIGURE 9-2. **In a Keplerian telescope, the primary focal point of the ocular lens (D_{oc}) is coincident with the secondary focal point of the objective lens (D'_{obj}) creating an inverted, real image (h). The tube length (d) is equal to the sum of the focal lengths of the objective and ocular lenses ($f_{obj} + f_{oc}$).**

1. The ocular lens (or eyepiece) is negative, and numerically its dioptric power is always stronger than the objective lens.
2. The magnification is given by a ratio of the ocular power to the objective power.

$$M_{TS} = -\frac{D_{oc}}{D_{obj}}$$

The magnification is positive, indicating that the image is erect or upright.

3. The length of the telescope (tube length) is equal to the algebraic sum of the focal lengths of the objective (f_{obj}) and ocular lenses (f_{oc}) ($d = f_{obj} + f_{oc}$). Because the eyepiece is negative, the length of the telescope is shorter when compared to a Keplerian telescope of comparable magnification and objective lens power.
4. The exit pupil of a Galilean telescope, which is the image of the objective lens as seen through the ocular lens, is virtual. It is usually located inside the telescope. The size and location of the exit pupil are important factors in determining the light transmission and field of view of the telescope.

Example

A telescope is composed of a +20.00 D objective lens and a −40.00 D ocular lens. The system is focused for infinity by an emmetropic patient. Determine the following:

1. The magnification of the telescope
2. The type of telescope
3. The tube length (lens separation) of the telescope

Answer:

1.

$$M = -\frac{D_{oc}}{D_{obj}}$$

$$= -\frac{(-40)}{20}$$

$$= 2 \times$$

The magnification is 2×.

2. Because the magnification is positive, one can conclude that the image is erect, and therefore, the telescope is a Galilean telescope.

3.

$$d = f_{obj} + f_{oc}$$

$$f_{obj} = \frac{100}{20} = 5.00\,\text{cm}$$

$$f_{oc} = \frac{100}{-40} = -2.50\,\text{cm}$$

$$d = 5.00 + (-2.50) = 2.50\,\text{cm}$$

The tube length is 2.50 cm.

KEPLERIAN TELESCOPE

The following is a summary of the important fundamental concepts in a Keplerian telescope:

1. The ocular lens (or eyepiece) is positive and numerically stronger than the power of the objective.
2. The magnification is given by a ratio of the ocular power to the objective power.

$$M_{TS} = -\frac{D_{oc}}{D_{obj}}$$

It is important to note that in the Keplerian telescope, both the objective and eyepiece are positive in power; thus, the magnification will always be *negative*. Negative magnification indicates that the image is inverted.

3. When the image remains inverted, the Keplerian telescope can also be called an *astronomical telescope*. Additional elements (usually prisms) must be added to the Keplerian telescope to make the final image upright. When this is done, the telescope can now be called a *terrestrial* telescope. Generally, *Keplerian* is used as the generic terminology, even though all Keplerian telescopes used in low vision are of the terrestrial type.

4. The length of the telescope is equal to the algebraic sum of the focal lengths of the objective and ocular lenses ($d = f_{obj} + f_{oc}$). Because both lenses are positive, the tube length is longer than a Galilean telescope of comparable magnification and objective lens power.
5. The exit pupil of a Keplerian telescope is real and is usually located behind the eyepiece (outside of the telescope) close to the patient's eye (entrance pupil).

Example
A telescope is composed of a +20.00 D objective lens and a +40.00 D ocular lens. The system is focused for infinity by an emmetropic patient. Determine the following:

1. The magnification of the telescope
2. The type of telescope
3. The tube length (lens separation) of the telescope

Answer:

1.
$$M = -\frac{D_{oc}}{D_{obj}}$$
$$= -\frac{40}{20}$$
$$= -2\times$$

The magnification is 2×. Negative magnification indicates that the image is inverted and may require an erecting system (prisms) to create an upright image. It does not imply minification.

2. Because the magnification is negative, one can conclude that the image is inverted and therefore the telescope is of Keplerian design.

3.
$$d = f_{obj} + f_{oc}$$
$$f_{obj} = \frac{100}{20} = 5.00 \text{ cm}$$
$$f_{oc} = \frac{100}{40} = 2.50 \text{ cm}$$
$$d = 5.00 + 2.50 = 7.50 \text{ cm}$$

The tube length is 7.50 cm.

The values that describe a telescope are the power of the objective and ocular lenses, the magnification, and the separation of the lenses. The relationships are the same for Keplerian and Galilean telescopes, allowing the same formulas to be applied to either, remembering that the magnification is always negative in a Keplerian system and positive in a Galilean system. Although the two basic types of telescopes used in low vision rehabilitation have some commonalties, there are many distinct differences. Table 9-1 summarizes some of the distinct characteristics of both types of telescopes; Table 9-2 presents the formula relationships that exist with these telescopes.

TABLE 9-1
Comparison of Galilean and Keplerian Telescopes

Characteristic	Keplerian	Galilean
Objective lens	Positive	Positive
Ocular lens	Positive	Negative
Eyepiece system	Always compound system	Simple lens system
Weight	Heavier	Lighter
Length (optical path)	Longer	Shorter
Exit pupil location	Outside system	Inside system
Magnification available	Low and high	Low
Effect of focusing for an uncorrected myope	Increased magnification	Decreased magnification
Effect of focusing for an uncorrected hyperope	Decreased magnification	Increased magnification
Field of view	Larger	Smaller
Image quality	Better	Poorer
Cost	Higher	Lower

TABLE 9-2
Formulas for Telescopic Systems*

Given:	Find			
	M	d (m)	D_{obj}	D_{oc}
M and d	—	—	$\frac{M-1}{Md}$	$\frac{1-M}{d}$
M and D_{obj}	—	$\frac{M-1}{D_{obj}M}$	—	$-D_{obj}M$
M and D_{oc}	—	$\frac{1-M}{D_{oc}}$	$\frac{-D_{oc}}{M}$	—
d and D_{obj}	$\frac{1}{1-dD_{obj}}$	—	—	$\frac{D_{obj}}{dD_{obj}-1}$
d and D_{oc}	$1-D_{oc}d$	—	$\frac{D_{oc}}{dD_{oc}-1}$	—
D_{oc} and D_{obj}	$\frac{-D_{oc}}{D_{obj}}$	$\frac{1}{D_{obj}}+\frac{1}{D_{oc}}$	—	—

*Given any two values, the other two can be calculated.
M = magnification; d = tube length (in meters); D_{obj} = dioptric power of the objective; D_{oc} = dioptric power of the ocular.

MIRROR TELESCOPES

A mirror telescope is an example of a reflecting telescope—that is, a telescope that uses a concave mirror as the objective. Although not currently available for patient care, mirror telescopes grew out of the first mirror telescope proposed by Dixon in 1785. Eschinardi had described a similar system approximately two centuries earlier.[1] In 1956, Feinbloom introduced the Mirrorscope. This mirror telescope used the Cassegrain principle, which uses a parabolic concave mirror to collect light from a distant object and a hyperbolic convex mirror to transmit the light back to an eyepiece. The Mirrorscope (Figure 9-3) was a compact design that focused for infinity and provided 3.5× magnification. A patient's refractive correction could be cemented to the back surface of the unit behind a 9.2-mm sight hole. The

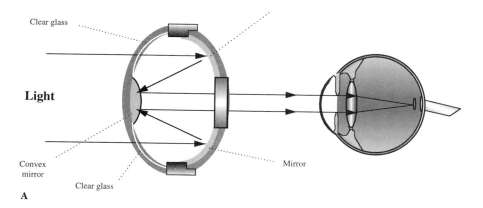

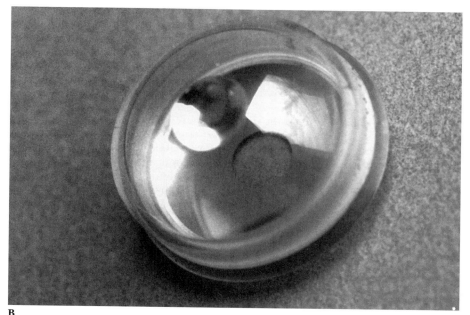

FIGURE 9-3. **A. The Feinbloom Mirrorscope positioned glass lenses and mirrors in a plastic housing. The tube length was 21 mm and it provided 3.5× magnification. The telescope provided a field of view of approximately 4 degrees and had a dark spot in the center caused by the convex mirror. B. Feinbloom's Mirrorscope.**

mirrorscope had a field of view of approximately 4 degrees and had a dark spot in the center caused by the convex mirror.[2]

CONTACT LENS TELESCOPE

As early as 1936, Dallos suggested the theoretical possibility of using a contact lens telescope that used a strong concave contact lens and a weaker convex lens worn in the spectacle plane.[3] It was not until 3 years later, however, that Bettman and McNair reported the successful fitting of a contact lens telescope on a patient with disciform macular degeneration.[4]

The principle of the contact lens telescope is relatively simple. The contact lens is fitted so that it compensates for any ametropia of the wearer along with incorporating the power of the ocular lens of the Galilean telescopic system. A convex spectacle lens is then positioned a given distance from the contact lens to create the objective lens of this telescopic system. Chapter 8 (see Table 8-4) provides infor-

mation on possible contact lens–spectacle lens combinations along with the magnification that can be obtained through a contact lens telescopic system. The advantages and disadvantages of the contact lens telescopic system are summarized in Table 9-3. As is shown, the disadvantages far outweigh the advantages. It is not surprising that Dallos revisited the problem in 1957 and indicated that the telescopic contact lens combination was not practical because the change in perspective for walking was more unpleasant than a lesser degree of visual acuity.

To minimize the disadvantages of the contact lens telescope, various systems have been designed to allow a simultaneous viewing of a magnified and unmagnified portion of the visual field. One of the first such systems was the Bivisual Contact Lens Telescope designed by Voss in 1958.[5] This system used a standard contact lens that contained a strong concave segment in the center (Figure 9-4). With this arrangement, when the patient desired to have the lens act as a telescopic system, spectacles could be put on, and the concave segment in the center of the lens could act as the ocular of the Galilean system. When the

TABLE 9-3
Advantages and Disadvantages of Contact Lens Telescopes*

Advantages
    Wide useable field of view
    Better cosmetic appearance
Disadvantages
    Limited range of magnification
    Contact lens movement causes apparent field movement
    Difficulty in adaptation due to parallax and head movements
    High powered convex spectacles are not cosmetically acceptable
    Precise maintenance of vertex distance (of spectacle) is required
    When a nonmagnified view is desired, the contact lens must be
        removed

*Versus spectacle-mounted telescopic system.

distance telescope was not desired, the spectacles could be removed, allowing normal corrected vision through the normal contact lens portion. The primary disadvantage of this type of system, however, is that the optical performance of both portions of the contact lens are compromised by the design.

In 1959, Filderman described the Telcon system.[6] This system had a small (2.50- to 3.50-mm) optic zone providing the desired high concave ocular power for the telescope. Around this small optic zone was an annular optical zone to correct the patient's ametropia. The center optic zone was made smaller than the daylight pupil size. Because of this arrangement, both the telescopic and refractive zones are before the pupil at the same time. The objective lens was a spectacle lens having a plano carrier onto which a central 10-mm segment with the desired positive power was cemented. This arrangement claimed to produce the desired magnified central image superimposed on a nonmagnified peripheral image, which aids in spatial orientation. The problems encountered with this system included comfort and the difficulty in maintaining the correct separation of the lenses. The practical limits of magnification are approximately 2×.

A self-contained contact lens telescopic lens was developed by Feinbloom in 1960.[7] This lens was called the *Miniscope* (Figure 9-5). The self-contained contact lens telescope attempted to eliminate the telescopic parallax and increase the field of view. The system was bulky, and it was difficult to precisely control the separation between the objective and ocular surfaces. Another major disadvantage was that the objective lens was relatively small (6.00 mm), which led to poor light-gathering abilities and a dim appearance of all objects in the visual field.

SPECIAL TELESCOPIC SYSTEMS FOR APHAKIA AND HIGH HYPEROPIA

Fonda described a method of obtaining magnification up to 4× by holding plus spheres in front of a patient with uncorrected aphakia, hyperopia, or dislocated lenses.[8] Patients with these uncorrected conditions may be considered to have the equivalent of a built-in eyepiece, with the power of the eyepiece equal to the refractive error at the cornea. The objective lens would then be the plus lens held away from the eye at a distance allowing its secondary focal point to be coincident with the primary focal point of the ocular component. Table 9-4 lists the magnification that may be achieved with handheld plus lenses of +3.00 D, +4.00 D, and +5.00 D held so that their secondary focal point will be coincident with the far point of the uncorrected hyperopic eye.

OPTICAL DESIGN OF TELESCOPIC SYSTEMS

The optical design of a telescopic system is a complex task. Many factors must be taken into consideration and compromises must be made to eliminate the greatest number of troublesome problems and incorporate the greatest number of desirable features into the system. It should be noted that different telescopic systems often have different design criteria. Some strive for a wide field, some strive for a lightweight unit, and still others are designed with cosmesis as the main design criteria.

From a practitioner's point of view the ideal telescope used for low vision would have the following features:

1. A wide field of view
2. Lightweight

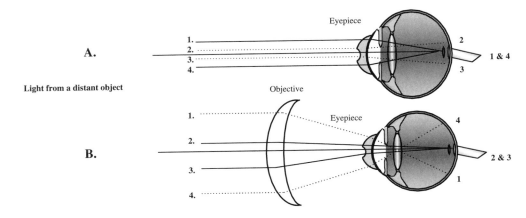

A.

Light from a distant object

B.

FIGURE 9-4. **The Voss Bivisual Contact Lens Telescope. A.** When used as a contact lens system, only the peripheral rays (1 and 4) come into focus on the retina. Rays that pass through the central region (2 and 3) do not come to a clear focus on the retina. **B.** When the contact lens is used in conjunction with a convex spectacle lens to form a telescope, central rays (2 and 3) form a magnified clear image on the retina. Peripheral rays (1 and 4) will be out of focus.

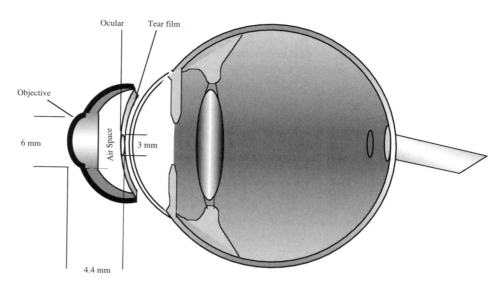

FIGURE 9-5. **The Miniscope provided 2× magnification. It was constructed as a doublet system with an air space between the objective and ocular lenses.**

3. Limited or no aberrations
4. Excellent light transmission
5. Effective retinal illuminance
6. Compactness
7. Low cost
8. Focusability (see section on focal telescopes)
9. Appropriate magnification (see section on determining the required magnification)

To date, no telescope can boast all of these features, and therefore, the patient and practitioner must decide which features are most important when evaluating available systems.

Field of View

In most cases, it is desirable to have as wide a field of view as possible when looking through a telescope. The field of view is usually limited by the size (diameter) of the objective lens, the magnification of the system, and the separa-tion of the objective and eyepiece. The vertex distance also plays an important part in the determination of the field of view.

The exit pupil of a telescope helps to define the field of view when comparing a Galilean telescope to a Keplerian telescope of equal magnification and equal objective lens diameter. The Keplerian telescope will provide the larger field of view because the exit pupil is located outside of the telescope, closer to the entrance pupil of the patient's eye. The distance of the telescope to the eye (vertex distance) must also be taken into account when determining the field of view of a telescope. In general, the shorter the distance a telescope sits from the eye, the greater the field of view.

The location and size of the exit pupil are very important considerations in the design and fitting of telescopes and are often sources of problems in establishing the best alignment with the patient's eye. When a patient uses a telescope with a small exit pupil that may be eccentrically positioned in reference to the patient's pupil, less light will reach the retina, and the field of view may appear to be reduced. A larger exit pupil, in many cases, will allow

TABLE 9-4
Uncorrected Aphakia and High Hyperopia Telescopic Systems

Objective Power →	+3.00 D		+4.00 D		+5.00 D	
Refraction at Cornea (D)	Distance from Eye (cm)	Magnification	Distance from Eye (cm)	Magnification	Distance from Eye (cm)	Magnification
+10.00	23.33	3.33×	15.00	2.50×	10.00	2.00×
+11.00	24.24	3.66×	15.91	2.75×	10.91	2.20×
+12.00	25.00	4.00×	16.66	3.00×	11.67	2.40×
+13.00	25.64	4.33×	17.30	3.25×	12.31	2.60×
+14.00	26.19	4.66×	17.85	3.50×	12.86	2.80×
+15.00	26.66	5.00×	18.33	3.75×	13.33	3.00×
+16.00	27.08	5.33×	18.75	4.00×	13.75	3.20×
+17.00	27.45	5.66×	19.11	4.25×	14.17	3.40×
+18.00	27.77	6.00×	19.40	4.50×	14.44	3.60×
+19.00	28.07	6.33×	19.73	4.75×	14.74	3.80×
+20.00	28.33	6.66×	20.00	5.00×	15.00	4.00×

the patient to view an object with more ease and better results.

The diameter size of the exit pupil can be determined by the following formula:

$$\text{Exit pupil (in mm)} = \frac{\text{Diameter of objective lens (in mm)}}{M_{TS}}$$

From a clinical perspective, the exit pupil of a telescope can be determined in a number of ways:

1. The diameter of the objective lens can be measured with a millimeter ruler, and this number can be divided by the magnification of the telescope, when known (sometimes written on the front or side of the telescope).
2. On most handheld telescopes, there are a few numbers written on the telescope (e.g., 8×35, 10×20, or 10×40). The first set of numbers (before the ×) indicates the magnification, whereas the second set indicates the diameter of the objective lens measured in millimeters. The 8 or 10 in these examples represents the magnification of the individual telescopes, whereas the 35, 20, and 40 represent the diameter of each objective lens measured in millimeters. Therefore, the exit pupil size can be determined in theses examples by dividing 35 by 8, or 20 by 10.
3. When holding a telescope a given distance from the eye and looking toward the eyepiece, a circle of light is seen. This circle of light is the exit pupil of the telescope and can be measured directly with a ruler. (It may be more difficult to visualize in a Galilean telescope, because the exit pupil is within the housing of the device.) The position of the exit pupil of a telescope can be judged by movement of the telescope's ocular lens back and forth and observing the apparent change in direction or parallax. For the Galilean telescope, with its internal virtual exit pupil, the parallax motion is a "with" motion. For the Keplerian design telescope, the exit pupil is located as a real image, external to the ocular with an "against" motion or parallax.

Example
Which of the following telescopes has the largest exit pupil?

1. 7×50
2. 8×35
3. 10×20
4. 10×40

Answer:

1. $\frac{50}{7}$ = 7.14 mm

2. $\frac{35}{8}$ = 4.38 mm

3. $\frac{20}{10}$ = 2.00 mm

4. $\frac{40}{10}$ = 4.00 mm

Therefore, the 7×50 has the largest exit pupil.

The Keplerian design also lends itself to the use of a field lens to increase the field of view. A field lens has a prismatic effect on rays of light that would normally miss the ocular lens, bending them so that they pass through the ocular. This lens, therefore, increases the useable field of view. The field lens, however, adds to the weight and cost of the telescopic design.

Weight

Good design dictates a telescope that is as lightweight as possible. This need indicates that either plastic lenses or mountings (housings) be used. If plastic lenses are used, the index of refraction is less than glass, and therefore the lenses would have to be made thicker, resulting in a heavier system. The weight of the telescopic system, however, is largely determined by the diameter of the objective lens. Thus, the larger the diameter, the heavier the telescope. When comparing Galilean to Keplerian telescopes of equal magnification, Keplerian telescopes tend to be heavier because they have a longer tube length (which adds weight), and more important, they require a mirror or prism system (to erect the image), which substantially adds to the weight.

Aberrations

With an increase in magnification, there is an increase in various aberrations. It is extremely difficult, if not impossible, to correct or eliminate these aberrations entirely. Chromatic aberration is produced when the colored rays that collectively make up ordinary light are bent unevenly as they pass through the various elements of the telescopic system. Chromatic aberrations may be effectively reduced with the use of cemented doublet objective and eyepiece lenses. If doublets are used, they must be balanced against each other and, in general, the chromatic dispersion of the objective lens must be lower than that of the eyepiece. Doublets add weight and expense to the optical design and the added weight and cost must be carefully considered. In simple lenses, chromatic aberrations can be reduced by selectively choosing different types of glass or plastic.

Spherical aberration is a minor problem, unlikely to be noticed by the average patient and largely controllable by limiting the size of the lenses. Astigmatism and curvature of field are largely a function of the power and refractive index of the objective and ocular lenses. Curvature of field in a telescope is exemplified when it is found to be impossible to bring both the center and the edge of the field into clear focus at the same time. When a telescope is said to have a *flat field*, the reference is to the relative absence of the curvature of field aberration.

Light Transmission

When light is traveling through a number of transparent media having different indices of refraction, the majority of light passes through; however, a small amount is reflected. This reflected light produces ghost images, haze, and glare. There is an approximate 4% loss of light at each uncoated optical surface, mostly due to reflected light. By applying antireflective coatings to the lenses, internal reflections can be reduced and light transmission increased. In the better telescopic systems, antireflective coatings are used to reduce the glare and scatter and increase the brilliance of the image. Because of the eye's sensitivity to yellow-green light (approximately 555 nm) and because it is the wavelength of maximum visibility, an antireflective coating designed for this wavelength is generally selected. Therefore, when the reflection for this wavelength is eliminated, reflections tend to increase toward the ends of the spectrum, producing a mixture of red and purple or a magenta color. Because of this effect, properly coated or color-corrected lenses have a purplish to purple-green reflective color. If the color coating appears too blue, the coating is too thick; if the coating appears straw-colored, the coating is too thin. In either case, loss of light will be the result.

Although the index of the coating material should be close to the square root of the index of refraction of the glass being coated, the color of the optically perfect coating will always be magenta-purple to purple-green. This color, however, is not always the most cosmetically acceptable color. To overcome the objectionable magenta color often encountered with higher-index lenses, the coating is applied thinly, compromising some light transmission for the more acceptable straw color. By holding the telescope in such a way that the reflection of an overhead fluorescent lamp can be seen, the color of the coating can be viewed. If no color is seen, it is apparent that the surface has not been coated. The hardness of the coating is also an important factor in both performance and durability. If the coating comes off with repeated cleaning, it is too soft.

Retinal Illuminance in Telescopes

The image brightness (retinal image illuminance) is important in prescribing telescopes. Many low vision patients have reduced sensitivity to light and require additional illumination to achieve a functional level. Telescopes reduce the brightness of extended sources of light because of the reflection of light off of the various optical lenses. As mentioned in the previous section, there is a loss of approximately 4% at each lens surface. Antireflective coatings may reduce the light loss but cannot eliminate it entirely.

The patient's pupil (eye-pupil) and the exit pupil of the telescope play an important role in determining how much light reaches the patient's retina. The retinal illuminance is proportional to the area of the exit pupil of the eye-telescopic system. When the telescope is used to view an object (extended source of light) and the exit pupil of the telescope is larger than or equal to eye-pupil of the viewer, the image brightness will appear to be just as bright as that observed by the naked eye. When the patient's pupil (eye-pupil) is smaller than the exit pupil of

the telescope, then the eye-pupil becomes the aperture stop or limiting factor on the amount of light that reaches the retina.

When the telescope is used to view a point source, such as a star or a pinhole, the image becomes bright, but not larger. When the telescope is used to view an extended object (when the source of light subtends a finite angle), the result is an enlarged image, but no increase in retinal illuminance. For extended sources, while the image is magnified, it is enlarged over a magnified area, so that the magnification exactly offsets the increase light-flux density resulting in no increase in image brightness compared to the unaided eye.

Example 1
A patient whose pupil size is 8 mm under normal lighting looks through the four telescopes below. Which telescope will appear to be the brightest?

1. 7×50
2. 8×35
3. 10×20
4. 10×40

Answer:

1. $\frac{50}{7} = 4.38$ mm

2. $\frac{35}{8} = 4.38$ mm

3. $\frac{20}{10} = 2.00$ mm

4. $\frac{40}{10} = 4.00$ mm

The 7×50 would appear to be the brightest, followed by the 8×35, then the 10×40, and the 10×20 (least bright).

Example 2
A patient whose pupil size is 4 mm under normal lighting looks through the four telescopes in Example 1. Which telescope will appear to be the brightest?

In this case, the 7×50, 8×35, and 10×40 will all appear equally bright to this patient and the 10×20 will appear to be the least bright.

Example 3
A patient whose pupil size is 2 mm under normal lighting looks through the four telescopes in Example 1. Which telescope will appear to be the brightest?

In this case, all of the telescopes will appear equally bright (or equally dark).

When the exit pupil of the telescope is smaller than the eye pupil, there will be a reduction in brightness as compared to the unaided eye (Table 9-5). This reduction can be calculated by a ratio of the square of the telescope's exit pupil diameter (EP) to the square of the eye-pupil diameter ($E_{eye}P$).

TABLE 9-5
Brightness Considerations for Extended Sources

When: exit pupil of telescope	is greater than	eye-pupil diameter	**Then**: eye pupil is filled with light
	Image brightness is same as unaided eye		
When: exit pupil of telescope	is equal to	eye-pupil diameter	**Then**: eye pupil is filled with light
	Image brightness is same as unaided eye		
When: exit pupil of telescope	is less than	eye-pupil diameter	**Then**: full eye pupil is not filled with light
	Reduction in image brightness		

$$\text{Reduction in brightness} = \frac{(EP)^2}{\left(E_{eye}P\right)^2}$$

Example 4

What percentage of decreased illumination will a patient have when he or she views through a 4×12 telescope as compared to his or her naked vision when his or her pupil size is 5 mm?

Answer:

$$\text{Reduction in brightness} = \frac{(EP \text{ of telescope})^2}{\left(E_{eye}P\right)^2}$$

$$= \frac{(3)^2}{(5)^2} = \frac{9}{25}$$

$$= 0.36$$

Thus, this telescope causes approximately a 36% reduction in illumination over that of the naked eye (not taking into consideration light lost from reflection off the lenses in this telescope).

Manufacturers may specify the light transmitting power of their telescopes by listing the *relative brightness* or *brightness index*. This term may also be referred to as the *relative light efficiency*. The relative light efficiency, relative brightness, or brightness index (on uncoated optics) is calculated by squaring the exit pupil diameter.

$$\text{Relative light efficiency} = (EP)^2$$

Thus, a 7×35 binocular has a relative light efficiency rating of 25. The relative light efficiency of a 15×60 binocular has a relative brightness of only 16, which is 36% less bright than the 7×35 binoculars. When antireflective coatings are used on the surface of the lenses, the numeric value of the relative light efficiency is increased 50%. Thus, an uncoated system with a relative light efficiency rating of 25 would have a rating of 37.5 when coated optics are used.

The problem with specifying the relative light efficiency is that it does not take into consideration how telescopic magnification performs in dim illumination or low light levels. A more accurate method of determining performance in dim illumination is by means of the *twilight factor*. The twilight factor is calculated by determining the square root of the product of the diameter of the objective lens (d_{obj}) and the magnification of the telescope (M_{TS}).

$$\text{Twilight factor} = \sqrt{d_{obj}M_{TS}}$$

For example, the 7×35 telescope has a twilight factor of 15.6, whereas the 15×60 telescope has a twilight factor of 30. What this means to the patient is that he or she will be able to see an object 30 yards away under dim illumination with the 15×60 telescope, whereas the object would have to be 15.6 yards away to be seen with the 7×35 telescope.

Another way to compare the performance in dim light is to multiply the magnification of the telescope times the diameter of the objective lens. The larger the number, the more detail the patient will see through the system in dim light. The performance of each telescope can then be compared by using Table 9-6.

Compactness and Expense

Galilean telescopes tend to be smaller in size and less expensive than Keplerian telescopes having equivalent magnification and the same power objective lens. Compactness is related to the tube length. Because the length of the telescope is equal to the algebraic sum of the focal lengths of the objective and ocular lenses ($d = f_{obj} + f_{oc}$), the Keplerian telescope is less compact because both lenses are positive. Keplerian telescopes are generally more costly because of the expense of incorporating erecting prisms or mirrors into the system. To make the Keplerian design more compact, additional mirrors and prisms would be needed, adding to the weight and expense of the system. Also adding to the cost of telescopic systems are the coatings applied to the optical elements.

ACCOMMODATION AND TELESCOPES

When telescopes are in normal adjustment (adjusted for viewing objects at optical infinity), parallel light strikes the

TABLE 9-6
Comparison Table for Telescopic Performance in Dim Illumination

$M_{TS} \times D_{obj}$	Per Performance or Use
0–100	Suited for use only in full daylight
100–150	Suited for general daytime use
150–200	Good for dark shade, dimly lit surroundings
200–250	Adequate for dusk, dawn
250–300	Good for dusk, dawn
300–400	Good for use in bright moonlight
400 or greater	Good for night use

D_{obj} = dioptric power of the objective; M_{TS} = magnification of an afocal telescope.

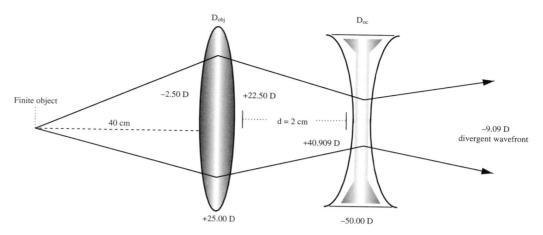

FIGURE 9-6. **Accommodation through an afocal Galilean telescope. A 2× Galilean telescope is used for viewing a finite object at 40-cm away. A divergent wavefront of −9.09 D will result, requiring accommodation to clear the image. (D_{obj} = objective lens; D_{oc} = ocular lens; d = tube length.)**

objective lens and exits the system with a vergence of zero. Because the light is brought to focus by the objective lens at the primary focal point of the ocular, the final image is located at infinity and no accommodation is required to view it. When an object is at a finite distance, however, the amount of accommodation required when viewing this object through a telescope is governed by the vergence of the final image at the ocular, not the vergence of the object at the objective lens.

Various approximations and suggestions have been made to calculate the amount of accommodation through a telescope. Most of these approximations state that the accommodation at the eyepiece (A_{oc}) of the telescope is

$$A_{oc} = M^2 U$$

(Approximate formula)

Thus, the accommodation at the ocular can be approximated by the product of the square of the magnification times object vergence at the objective lens (U). This formula is sometimes referred to as the *Sloan-Boeder approximation.*[9]

The total amount of accommodation required when a patient views an object closer than infinity through an afocal Galilean telescope can be determined by calculating the vergence at each refractive surface (Figure 9-6). Rather than doing this complex and long wavefront vergence analysis, the accommodation can be determined by a simple formula. If the Sloan-Boeder formula is used, a discrepancy exists when comparing the Sloan-Boeder results to the results derived by calculating the vergence at each refractive surface, as seen in Figure 9-6. In this particular example, the discrepancy is almost 1.00 D (A_{oc} = $[2]^2[-2.50]$ = −10.00 D). Freid is credited with the derivation of an exact formula that eliminates the discrepancies found when using the approximate formula.[10] The exact amount of accommodation through a telescope as stated by Freid is

$$A_{oc} = \frac{M^2 U}{1 - dMU}$$

If the Freid vergence amplification formula is used, with d being the tube length of the telescope measured in meters,

the amount of accommodation in the preceding example can be accurately calculated as the following:

$$A_{oc} = \frac{(2)^2(-2.50)}{1 - (0.02)(2)(-2.50)}$$

$$= \frac{-10}{1 - (-0.10)} = \frac{-10}{1.10} = -9.09 \text{ D}$$

The same Freid formula can be applied to a 2× Keplerian telescope with the same tube length of 2 cm. The Keplerian telescope, however, must be composed of a +75.00 D objective lens and a +150.00 D objective lens (to produce the same 2× magnification and maintain the 2-cm separation between lenses). Figure 9-7 depicts the wavefront vergence analysis at each refracting surface. Again, the patient is looking at an object 40 cm away when using the Keplerian telescope.

$$A_{oc} = \frac{(-2)^2(-2.50)}{1 - (0.02)(-2)(-2.50)}$$

$$= \frac{-10}{1 - (0.10)} = \frac{-10}{0.90} = -11.11 \text{ D}$$

It must be remembered that for Keplerian telescopes, the magnification sign is negative, indicating an inverted image. With the Sloan-Boeder formula, the resultant accommodation is

$$A_{oc} = M^2 U = (-2)^2(-2.50) = -10.00 \text{ D}$$

The difference between the Freid formula and the Sloan-Boeder formula is again approximately 1.00 D in this case example. It has been shown that the Sloan-Boeder formula will provide the closest approximation to the Freid formula when limited to Galilean telescopes of low power (2–4×) and when the objects being viewed are greater than approximately 3 m from the objective lens of the telescope.[10]

It should be noted that when Keplerian and Galilean telescopes have equal magnification and the same tube length, the Keplerian telescope will require the greater accommodation when both are used to view a near-point object.

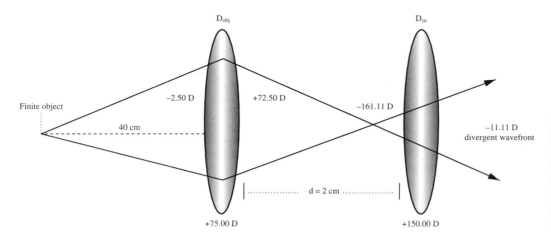

FIGURE 9-7. **Accommodation through an afocal Keplerian telescope: A 2× Keplerian telescope is used for viewing a finite object at 40 cm. A divergent wavefront of –11.11 D will result, requiring accommodation to clear the image. (D_{obj} = objective lens; D_{oc} = ocular lens; d = tube length.)**

FOCAL TELESCOPES

Telescopes designed for distance vision can be adapted for intermediate or near use using three different methods. If an afocal telescope is not adapted by one of these three methods, then a greater accommodative demand will be placed on the patient as discussed in the previous section (vergence amplification formula). The three methods are

1. Increasing the power of the objective lens (D_{obj})
2. Decreasing the power of the ocular lens (D_{oc})
3. Increasing the separation (d) of the objective and ocular lenses

The main advantage of having a telescope for near work is that it will provide a relatively longer focal distance than will a microscopic system of equivalent power. The main disadvantage is a reduction of field. Near vision telescopes or telemicroscopes may be monocular or binocular, fixed in focus for a particular distance, or focusable.

Increasing the Power of the Objective Lens

When an afocal telescope is used to view near objects, there is a divergent wavefront that will strike the objective lens. If the divergent wavefront can be "neutralized" by an increase in power of the objective lens so that the focal point of this added convex lens is coincident with the object, then parallel bundles of light will enter the telescopic system. Increasing the power of the objective lens by adding a "reading cap" to the front of the telescope is probably the easiest way in which the telescopic system can be made focal. Therefore, the working distance of the near telescope is equal to the focal length of the reading cap or additional plus power added to the objective lens.

The equivalent power of the near telescope can be determined by multiplying the power of the reading addition or cap by the magnification of the telescope:

$$\text{Equivalent power} = \left(D_{cap}\right)\left(\left|M_{TS}\right|\right)$$

In this formula, M_{TS} is relative angular magnification of the telescope. Both Galilean and Keplerian telescopes produce relative angular magnification. Although the magnification is given in a Galilean telescope as positive and in a Keplerian telescope as negative, the minus sign associated with the Keplerian telescope only refers to the inversion of the image; it does not imply minification. As such, the absolute value of the relative angular magnification should be used when determining equivalent power. The equivalent power can also be calculated (second method) by using the formula for equivalent power and by having the new objective lens be equivalent to the original power of the lens plus the additional add (reading cap) power.

Example
What is the equivalent power of a 2× Galilean telescope consisting of a +25.00 D objective and a –50.00 D ocular that is focal for 20 cm?
Answer:
First method

$$D_{eq} = \left(D_{cap}\right)\left(M_{TS}\right)$$
$$= \left(+5.00\right)\left(2\times\right) = +10.00\ D$$

Second method

$$D_{eq} = \left(D_{cap} + D_{obj}\right) + \left(D_{oc}\right) - \left(d\right)\left(D_{cap} + D_{obj}\right)\left(D_{oc}\right)$$
$$= \left(+5.00 + 25.00\right) + \left(-50.00\right) - \left(0.02\right)\left(+30.00\right)\left(-50.00\right)$$
$$= \left(+30.00\right) + \left(-50.00\right) - \left(-30.00\right) = +10.00\ D$$

The preceding system is equivalent to +10.00 D and will therefore enable a patient to read the same size print as a +10.00 D reading lens (microscope). Although both systems are equivalent in power, the near telescope has a working distance of 20 cm (the focal point of the +5.00 D reading cap), and the microscope has a closer working distance of 10 cm. The working distance is increased by a factor equal to the magnification of the telescope when comparing a telescope with a reading cap to a microscopic lens of equivalent power. The depth of field is the same with the telemicroscope and the equivalent powered microscope; however, the field of view of the telemicroscope is smaller.

Decreasing the Power of the Ocular Lens (Eyepiece)

Looking at the example in the previous section, if no reading cap (or change in the total power of the objective lens) was added to the telescope, the object at 20 cm would be totally blurred when looking through the 2× telescope. The reason for this blur is that a divergent wavefront would emerge from the eyepiece and a significant amount of accommodation would be required to clear the image. In this case, the required amount of accommodation could be eliminated by changing the power of the ocular lens. The amount of plus that must be added to the eyepiece can be calculated directly from the vergence amplification formula derived by Freid to determine the amount of accommodation at the eyepiece:

Example

What additional power would have to be added to the eyepiece of a 2× Galilean telescope consisting of a +25.00 D objective lens and a –50.00 D ocular lens that is focal for 20 cm?

Answer:

$$A_{oc} = \frac{M^2 U}{1 - dMU}$$

$$= \frac{(2)^2(-5.00)}{1-(0.02)(2)(-5.00)}$$

$$= \frac{-20}{1-(-0.2)} = \frac{-20}{1.2} = -16.67\ D$$

Thus, the power of the ocular would need to be changed by adding +16.67 D to neutralize the divergent wavefront, enabling the patient to see the object clearly at 20 cm.

It is interesting to note that when additional plus is added to the ocular lens of an afocal telescopic system to make the system focal, the equivalent power of the system (D_{eq}) is now given by the following equation:

$$D_{eq} = \frac{D_{add}\ (\text{at eyepiece})}{|M_{TS}|}$$

Thus, in the preceding example, if +16.67 D was added to the eyepiece, +8.34 D would be the equivalent power. This could also be determined by using the longer formula for equivalent power:

where the modified $D_{oc} = \text{eyepiece}(-50.00) + D_{add\ at\ eyepiece}(+16.67)$

$$D_{eq} = (D_{obj}) + (D_{oc} + D_{add}) - (d)(D_{obj})(D_{oc} + D_{add})$$

$$= (+25.00) + (-50.00 + 16.67) - (0.02)(+25.00)(-50.00 + 16.67)$$

$$= (+25.00) + (-33.33) - (-16.67) = +8.34\ D$$

The *anterior focal length* (f_V) of the add-to-the-ocular telescopic *system* can be derived from Freid's formula and is given by

$$f_V = (M_{TS})(d) + (M_{TS})^2 (f'_{add\ to\ ocular})$$

where $f'_{add\ to\ ocular}$ = focal length of the added power to the ocular lens. Note. In this formula, due to usual sign convention, both the anterior focal length of the add-to-the-ocular telescopic system and focal length of the add at the ocular will be negative quantities and demand that the magnification be taken as a positive quantity for Galilean systems and as a negative quantity for Keplerian systems.

In the same example

$$f_V = (2)(2) + (2)^2(-6)$$

$$= (4) + (-24) = -20.00\ cm$$

Thus, when the telescopic system is made focal by adding plus to the ocular lens, the system would have an equivalent power of +8.34 D and an anterior focal length of approximately 20 cm.

In a Keplerian telescope of the same magnification with a 2-cm tube length (+75.00 D objective and a +150.00 D ocular), viewing an object at 20 cm, the final vergence emerging from the eyepiece is –25.00 D. The power of the ocular lens (+150.00 D) would have to be increased by this amount. The equivalent power can be derived by the following equation:

$$D_{eq} = \frac{D_{add}(\text{at eyepiece})}{|M_{TS}|}$$

$$= \frac{25.00}{2} = +12.50\ D$$

The anterior focal length of the focal system is given by

$$f_V = (-2)(2) + (-2)^2(-4)$$

$$= -20.00\ cm$$

Increasing the Separation Between the Objective and Ocular Lenses

Both the Galilean and Keplerian telescope can be made focal by increasing the tube length or separation of the lens elements. In the example of the 2× Galilean telescope consisting of a +25.00 D and a –50.00 D eyepiece, with an afocal separation of 2 cm, the separation of objective and ocular lenses would have to be increased to 3 cm to make the telemicroscope focal for 20 cm. To determine the final tube length, the formula $d = f_{obj} + f_{oc}$ can be used. In this case, when the object is 20 cm from the telescope, light rays leave the object and strike the objective lens of the telescope with a vergence of –5.00 D. In essence, the –5.00 D combines with the +25.00 D objective lens to produce a resultant +20.00 D (+25.00 D + [–5.00 D] = +20.00 D). Therefore, the Galilean telescope would appear to now be composed of a –50.00 D ocular lens and a +20.00 D objective lens. The focal length of these two lenses would be (–)2 cm and 5 cm, respectively. By increasing the separation of the ocular and objective lens from 2 cm (the telescope is set for infinity) to 3 cm, an emmetropic patient will now clearly view an object located 20 cm from the front of the telescope.

Of the three methods used to make a telescope focal, the addition of a reading cap to the objective lens is by far the most common. This method is followed by "focusing" the telescope by increasing the length of the telescope or increasing the separation. Although theoretically possible, rarely is the power of the ocular lens changed to make a focal system.

A study by Jose and Morse[11] suggested that reading caps should be used for both Galilean and Keplerian systems when the near-point working distances are approximately 20 cm or less. If focusing is used (changing the length) for these same working distances (20 cm or less), there appears to be approximately a 20% loss of field when compared to using a reading cap.

CORRECTING A PATIENT'S REFRACTIVE ERROR

As described in the preceding sections, there are three ways in which a distance (afocal) telescope can be made focal. These same methods can be used to provide a correction for a patient's refractive error. Chapter 7 describes the methods of correction at the ocular lens and modification of the tube length; however, it does not discuss a change made at the objective lens. Even though a patient's refractive correction can be made at the objective lens, it is the least desirable method and from a clinical perspective, it is not worth the effort of determining the appropriate lens cap (using the vergence amplification formula) to fit over the objective lens of an afocal telescope. It is, however, important to be familiar with the relationships that exist between an afocal telescope and the correction of a patient's refractive error.

1. When possible, it is best to correct a patient's refractive error by incorporating the correction directly into the ocular lens or as a lens cap at the eyepiece of a Galilean or Keplerian telescope. When using this method, the total magnification of the system remains the same and no adjustment of the tube length of an afocal telescope has to be made to view an object at infinity.
2. When altering the tube length for the correction of myopia, the tube length must be made shorter for both the Galilean and Keplerian telescope. When altering the tube length, however, the myopic patient obtains less magnification with a Galilean telescope and achieves greater magnification with a Keplerian telescope (as compared to correcting the refractive error at the ocular lens of an afocal telescope).
3. The opposite effect occurs when the hyperopic patient has his or her refractive error corrected by altering the tube length of a Galilean or Keplerian telescope. The tube length must be made longer for both telescopes. The hyperope obtains more magnification with a Galilean telescope and achieves less magnification when focusing a Keplerian telescope (as compared to correcting the refractive error at the ocular lens of an afocal telescope).
4. If, for some reason, the objective lens is changed to correct for a patient's refractive error, the myopic patient would receive less magnification with a Galilean telescope and more with a Keplerian telescope. Again, the

opposite would occur with a correction at the objective lens for a hyperopic patient.

Woo[12] has suggested that the focusable telescope can be used to determine the refractive state of the patient. Using the technique of lengthening the telescope, a "fogging" is created similar to the fogging used by automatic refractors. The patient then focuses the telescope while viewing a distance target, and the refractive error is determined by the length at which the telescope lenses are separated. A shorter length than the "normal adjustment" (emmetropia) would indicate myopia, whereas a longer length than the normal adjustment, would indicate hyperopia. Woo reported that instrument accommodation does not seem to affect the results of the telescopic optometer refraction and, in fact, would counter some of the effects of vergence amplification.[13]

PRESCRIBING A TELESCOPE

Before any telescopic device can be properly prescribed, the goals and needs of the patient must be determined. A task analysis should be done and a prescribing strategy formulated to answer some basic questions in the determination of how much magnification and which type of telescope to prescribe. Only after these questions are answered and the task analysis has been completed will the practitioner be in a position to properly prescribe a low vision telescopic system.

Determining the Required Magnification

The tenet of prescribing a telescope is that the telescope will provide an increase in the retinal image size (proportional to the magnification provided) that provides the appropriate resolution. It is recommended that the magnification be as low as possible to adequately meet the needs and goals of the patient. Prescribing too much telescopic magnification will increase the inherent limitations of field and lessen the optical quality imposed by aberrations associated with the higher magnifications.

The amount of magnification generally depends on the patient's best visual acuity and the target acuity (acuity that is needed for the patient to attain his or her visual goal or concern at distance). The amount of magnification needed can be determined by the following formula:

$$M_{TS} = \frac{BVA}{TA}$$

where BVA is the best visual acuity, and TA is the target acuity.

The target acuity for most visual goals at distance is generally 20/40 or 20/50. It is assumed that a patient who attains 20/40 or 20/50 can accomplish a variety of his or her visual goals, such as reading street signs, watching television, and even driving a car (see Chapter 15).

Example 1

What telescopic magnification would be needed for a patient to see a street sign 20 ft away when the letter size is "normal size" and the patient's best corrected acuity is 20/200?

Answer: In this case, it is assumed that "normal size" is 20/40, and therefore a 5× telescope would be initially evaluated.

$$M_{TS} = \frac{200}{40} = 5\times$$

Example 2

A patient desires improved distance vision to be able to monitor the activities of children at play in her backyard. The patient's best-corrected acuity with conventional lenses is 10/100. An assumption is made that 20/50 acuity is needed for the task. What telescopic magnification should be selected as a starting magnification?

Answer: First 10/100 must be converted to a 20-ft equivalent acuity: 10/100 = 20/200 equivalent. Then, using the formula M_{TS} = BVA/TA, it is determined that a 4× telescope is required.

$$M_{TS} = \frac{200}{50} = 4\times$$

The calculated amount of magnification should be evaluated with the patient. Only by actual performance with the telescope can it be determined whether the task can be achieved. As stated, the practitioner should recommend the least amount of magnification that allows the patient to achieve his or her goal. When a patient requires a large amount of magnification (greater than 6×) or for those who have never experienced looking through a telescope, it is highly recommended that the practitioner begin the evaluation with telescopes of lower magnification. Once the patient has demonstrated some proficiency in using the devices, the practitioner can then demonstrate telescopes of higher magnification. For patients who experience difficulty when looking through the telescope or who may require greater amounts of magnification than what was initially predicted, the following factors may be responsible:

1. The telescope may be improperly focused.
2. The telescope may be misaligned with the patient's eye.
3. The patient may have poor localization skills when using the telescope.
4. The telescope may be causing too much of a reduction in brightness or loss of light reaching the retina.
5. The telescope may be too close to or too far away from the patient's eye.

If any of the preceding factors are the reason for the poorer than predicted acuity, they can be corrected by making appropriate changes to the telescope or by providing instruction on how to properly use the telescope. In certain cases, the telescope may have to be made more powerful than what was originally predicted for the patient to achieve his or her visual goal.

It is not uncommon for a patient's visual concerns to be at distances of 10 ft (3 m) or closer. As discussed in Accommodation and Telescopes, when telescopes are used to view objects closer than infinity, a great deal of accommodation is sometimes required by the patient. Because of the potential high demands placed on accommodation, the practical limit of a fixed focus afocal telescope is usually considered to be 3×. When greater magnification or a closer working distance than 10 ft is required, focusable telescopes should be used.

Binocular versus Monocular Telescopes

In general, the telescope is prescribed monocularly for the better seeing eye. Many low vision patients do not have binocular vision, and therefore monocular prescribing is predominate. Nonetheless, binocular prescribing is possible but should have the requisite of the patient having approximately the same acuity in each eye and demonstrating some degree of binocularity (see Chapter 3). The binocular telescopes should be of the same power and perfectly aligned so that their axes converge and meet at the target being viewed. Both Galilean and Keplerian telescopes are available as monocular or binocular systems.

Occasionally, it is possible to prescribe two telescopes of different magnifications for two different tasks, allowing alternate fixation between both eyes. This is termed *biocular use*, rather than *binocular use*. For example, if a patient wanted to see a baseball game, he or she may elect to use a low-powered telescope to obtain a larger field of view, thereby taking in more of the field with one eye. When the patient wanted to see more detail of a batter or pitcher, however, he or she will then have to use a telescope with higher magnification with the other eye.

If binocular systems are prescribed for near use, a determination of a fixed working distance is needed so that the telemicroscopes will converge at the point of fixation. If there is a need for change of fixation to various near distances, a focusable monocular system, not confined by the restraints of binocular convergence, may be more appropriate.

To achieve multiple foci with monocular systems, either multiple caps can be used on fixed focus afocal telescopic units or focusable monocular telescopic units can be used.

Handheld versus Spectacle-Mounted Telescopes

Telescopes can be either handheld or spectacle mounted (Figure 9-8). Handheld and spectacle-mounted telescopes may be of either the Galilean or Keplerian design. If the device is going to be used for temporary or occasional use, a handheld telescope is preferable. If the task is to be long term or involve prolonged viewing, a spectacle-mounted telescopic device may be more suitable. For viewing the blackboard in a classroom, a handheld monocular may suffice; however, if the patient wants his or her hands to be free for writing, a spectacle-mounted device would be indicated. Handheld uses may include reading street signs, determining addresses on buildings, ascertaining the color of a traffic light, viewing scenery, observing children at play, or enjoying a sporting event. Handheld telescopic

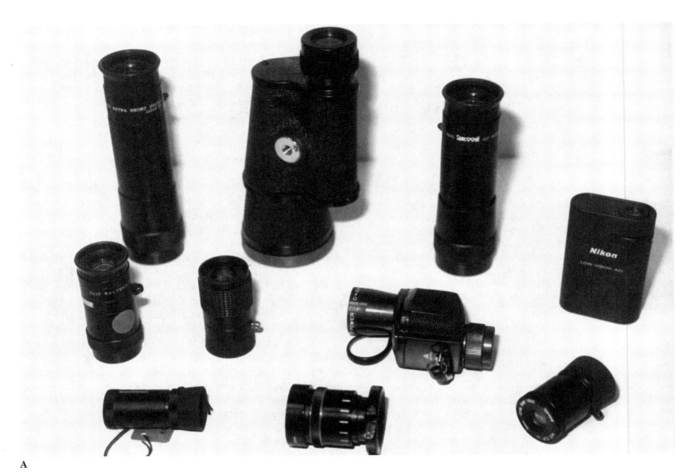

A

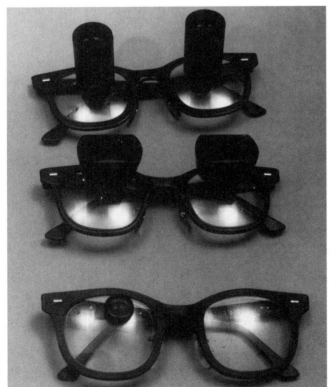

B

FIGURE 9-8. **Various manufacturers make a wide range of hand-held and spectacle-mounted telescopes. They can be monocular or binocular and of Galilean or Keplerian design. A. Handheld telescopes. B. Spectacle-mounted telescopes.**

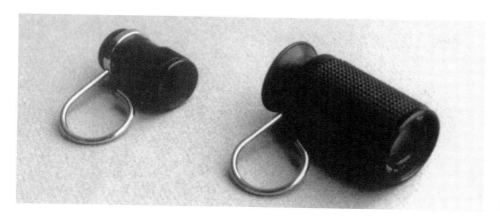

FIGURE 9-9. **Finger-ring telescopes.**

units often come with cords or straps, allowing them to be conveniently carried around the neck when not being used.

In large part, the availability, durability, weight, clarity of optics, illumination, and field of view govern the decision as to which is the best handheld telescope to prescribe. If the unit is to be used for distance tasks as well as near tasks, it is advisable to prescribe a focusable unit. The Keplerian models will boast a better field over comparable Galilean systems. As the magnification increases, the field decreases, and therefore, patients requiring 4× magnification or greater would benefit more from Keplerian systems. Above 10× in magnification, handheld telescopes may need to be supported by a stand or tripod to hold the unit steady.

A particularly useful item in prescribing handheld monocular telescopes is the finger-ring telescope. The telescope is attached to a small ring that is worn on the hand. The telescope can then be cupped in the hand and held covertly while the palm is braced against the forehead (Figure 9-9).

Spectacle-mounted telescopes may be used for some of the same activities as handheld telescopes but are generally involved with activities that demand more prolonged viewing (e.g., watching television or a movie) or for which the patient's hands need to be free (e.g., driving). There are a number of options available to the practitioner if a spectacle-mounted telescope is considered. A clip-on telescope can be secured directly to a patient's frame and may be considered one type of spectacle-mounted telescope (Figure 9-10A). Some clip-on telescopes allow the telescope to be flipped up out of the patient's line of sight when it is not being used and flipped back down when it needs to be used (Figure 9-10B). The following are some advantages of clip-on telescopes:

1. Can be easily removed when not desired.
2. Allows hands-free use of a telescope.
3. Offers a less expensive alternative to the spectacle attachment of a telescope.
4. Easily allows for a patient's spectacle correction to be incorporated into a spectacle-mounted telescope.
5. In many cases, the telescope can be removed from the clip-on system and be used as a handheld telescope as well.

The disadvantages of a clip-on telescope include the following:

1. The possibility of scratching the spectacle lenses that the clip-on rests on
2. The mechanical difficulties encountered in clipping it to a particular spectacle correction (particularly high myopic or hyperopic prescriptions)
3. Determining the correct position and maintaining the proper alignment on the frame
4. The additional weight common to many clip-on devices
5. Reduction of the field of view due to the exit pupil being placed far from the eye when the telescope is clipped on the front of the spectacles

In general, the term *spectacle mounted* usually refers to telescopic devices that are placed into ophthalmic correction lenses called *carrier lenses*. The position of the telescope is custom fabricated for the patient. When the telescope is positioned in the center of the carrier lens, it is said to be in the *full-diameter* or *full-field* position. In this position, the telescope is lined up with the patient's line of sight; therefore, the patient is looking through the telescope, for the most part, full time. The full-field position is designed for distance tasks that are performed while the patient is stationary, such as watching television. It is important to note that any form of mobility with this type of telescopic design is not indicated. When the telescopic unit is positioned superiorly within the frame, the term *bioptic* is used. This term was coined by Designs for Vision, Inc. (Ronkonkoma, NY) to describe their miniature Galilean telescopes, which were prescribed for driving. The term has now become more generic and describes a telescopic system mounted in the upper portion of the carrier lens, which allows viewing under the telescope (through the carrier lens) when the telescopic magnification is not required. When the telescope is mounted in the lower position of the carrier lens (similar to a bifocal), the telescope is said to be in the *reading* or *surgical* position. As the name implies, a telescope mounted in this position would be used for near-point tasks. Other positioning can be used with telescopic units to accommodate eccentric fixation, special head postures, facial disfigurements, and unique working distances.

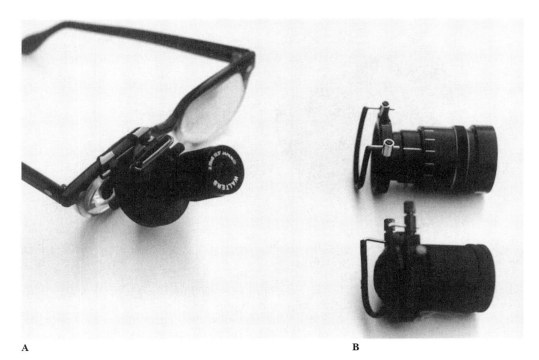

A   **B**

FIGURE 9-10. The clip-on monocular telescope allows for the temporary attachment to a spectacle frame. This telescope provides hands-free viewing and a less expensive alternative to a permanently attached telescope. A. A clip-on/flip-up attachment. B. Clip-on attachments.

A *trioptic* is a specially designed system in which a superiorly placed telescopic system is combined with an inferiorly mounted microscopic or telemicroscopic system (Figure 9-11). It is designed to meet the needs of the patient who requires both distance magnification and near magnification in the same spectacle. This telescopic system can be either Galilean or Keplerian.

Appendixes A–C have descriptions of commonly prescribed handheld and spectacle-mounted telescopic systems and telemicroscopic systems.

VERIFICATION OF TELESCOPIC DEVICES

The process of inspection and verification before dispensing a low vision telescopic device is an integral part of low vision care. It is not prudent to accept the manufacturer's description of products or custom designed systems as being accurate. Stock devices should be verified as well to determine what is actually being dispensed, because not all distributors, manufacturers, and suppliers use a universal terminology or adhere to the same standards.

Visual inspection of the device is an important part of the verification process. There should be a clean appearance to the device. If focusable, the telescope should turn smoothly and be capable of focusing at the expected distances. The telescope should be checked for loose lenses or prisms within the housing.

If the telescope is a custom made, spectacle-mounted device, there should be no glue residue on the carrier lenses or telescope housing. The carrier lenses and telescopic lenses should have no chips or defects in them. The telescope should be secure and not wobble in the carrier

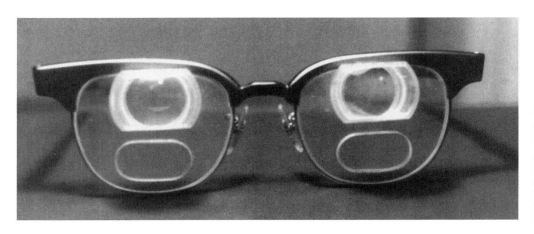

FIGURE 9-11. A *trioptic* is a specially designed system incorporating three optical systems. This trioptic, created by Designs for Vision, Inc. (Ronkonkoma, NY), consists of a superior-mounted telescope with an inferiorly mounted microscopic or telemicroscopic system mounted in a spectacle carrier lens.

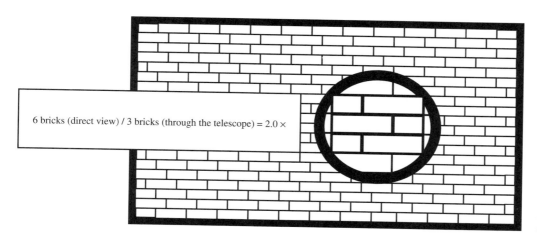

6 bricks (direct view) / 3 bricks (through the telescope) = 2.0 ×

FIGURE 9-12. **The magnification of a telescope can be estimated by using the comparison method. The telescope is held in front of one eye, spotting an object with a repeating pattern (e.g., brick wall, picket fence), while the fellow eye views the same unmagnified object. By comparing one image to the other the magnification can be determined.**

lens. The telescope should be positioned in the carrier lens at the recommended angle and interpupillary distance. The proper angle of the telescope can be verified with a protractor.

Verification of the Magnification of an Afocal Telescope

The magnification of a telescopic device can be verified in a number of ways. Probably the simplest way would be one of comparison. The comparison method involves spotting a distant object through the telescope in front of one eye and, while keeping the fellow eye open, superimposing the magnified view through the telescope over the nonmagnified view in the fellow eye (Figure 9-12). It helps if the distant target being viewed is a repeating pattern, such as a brick wall, so the comparison of the size of the magnified and unmagnified view can be easily determined. The comparison method is not very accurate, but it works reasonably well for a quick and rough estimation. When evaluating the

magnification of telescopes above 8×, it is sometimes easier to compare when the telescope is reversed (looking through the objective lens) and the unaided view is compared to the minified view.

A second method to determine the magnification of a telescopic device involves an actual measurement of both the diameter of the objective lens (d_{obj}) and the exit pupil of the telescope (Figure 9-13). As discussed in Optical Design of Telescopic Systems, their sizes are in a ratio equal to the magnification:

$$M_{TS} = \frac{d_{obj}}{EP}$$

A ruler or scale can be held in the plane of the exit pupil to measure the diameter of the exit pupil. The Galilean design, however, does not permit the ruler to be placed internally, so the ruler should be held above and in a location that approximates the exit pupil plane. Obviously, the accuracy of determining the magnification of a

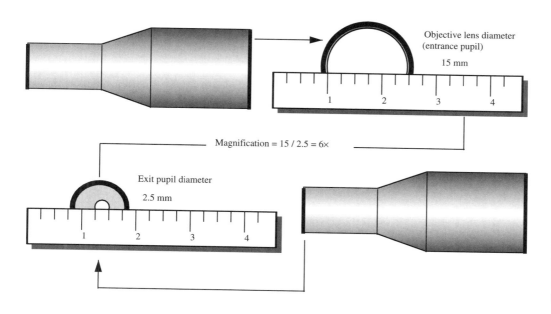

Objective lens diameter
(entrance pupil)

15 mm

Magnification = 15 / 2.5 = 6×

Exit pupil diameter

2.5 mm

FIGURE 9-13. **The magnification of a telescope can be determined from the ratio of the diameter of the objective lens to the diameter of the exit pupil.**

telescope will depend on how precisely these initial measurements are taken. Greater accuracy can be obtained on Keplerian systems in which the ruler can be positioned in the plane of the exit pupil.

A third method of determining the magnification of an afocal telescope uses the principle of vergence amplification. It was shown that vergence amplification was defined by Freid's formula as the following:

$$A_{oc} = \frac{M^2 U}{1 - dMU}$$

Magnification of Galilean telescopes may be measured by using vergence amplification. These telescopes have single-element lenses and contain no prisms or inversion systems, making the optical path length relatively short and the positions of the principal planes relatively easy to determine. Galilean telescopes also have the advantage of having a short tube length, enabling them to fit into the space between the lens stop and telescopic observation system of a lensometer.

The principle in using this formula for the determination of the magnification lies with the fact that when an afocal Galilean telescope (with no corrective lens incorporated into the ocular) is placed in a lensometer, a dioptric power of zero should be read. In other words, when the equivalent power is zero, it demonstrates that parallel light rays enter the telescope and parallel light rays exit the telescope.

If a lens of known value alters the entering vergence of light into the telescope, then the emergent vergence can be read in the lensometer and the difference in value determined. Knowing this difference and the length of the telescope, the vergence amplification formula can be applied to determine the magnification.

The procedure to determine the magnification is as follows:

1. The unknown telescope is positioned in the lensometer with the ocular lens against the lens stop (objective lens facing the practitioner).
2. If the Galilean telescope is focusable, it should be focused for infinity or adjusted to give a back vertex power reading of zero when in the lensometer.
3. Without removing the telescope from the lensometer, a trial lens of +1.00 D is held against the objective lens (or as close to it as possible).
4. The lensometer is then focused to obtain the new back vertex reading with the +1.00 D lens in place.
5. The telescope is removed from the lensometer and its tube length is measured.
6. The magnification can then be calculated by the following formula:

$$M = \frac{-\left[(A_{oc})(d)\right] + \sqrt{\left[(A_{oc})(d)\right]^2 - 4(A_{oc})}}{2}$$

where Aoc = the change in vergence at the eyepiece and d = the tube length of the telescope in meters.

Alternatively, the magnification can also be determined easily by using Table 9-7.

1. When a Galilean telescope of unknown magnification is placed in the lensometer, the reading is zero (assuming no refractive error).
2. When a +1.00 D trial lens is held against the objective lens of the telescope, a reading of +5.00 D is obtained (a change of 5.00 D).
3. The telescope is removed from the lensometer and the tube length is measured to be 16 mm.
4. By using the table, the magnification is determined to be closest to 2.20× (between 2.20× and 2.19×).

It is important to note that with the vergence amplification method, a high degree of accuracy can be obtained. Even with rather large inaccuracies in the measurement of the telescopic tube length or the measurement of the emerging vergence, there is little change in the effect of the magnification. It is, however, of utmost importance that the entering vergence be accurately known; therefore, a verified +1.00 D trial lens should be used for the procedure.

To determine the magnification of an unknown Keplerian telescope, Bailey has described a simple in-office method requiring little in the way of equipment and requiring few calculations.[14] In Bailey's method, a plastic or glass plate of known thickness and known refractive index is constructed so that one side of the test plate has vertical, equally spaced parallel lines and the other side has horizontal, equally spaced parallel lines. This test plate is then positioned between the exit pupil and the ocular lens of the telescope. It represents the two axially located points, which can act as a target in image space. Their conjugates are imaged into object space where (because of reversibility of light direction) two images are formed by the objective lens. The lateral magnification can be determined by the following:

$$M = \sqrt{\frac{I_{sep}}{\left(\dfrac{t}{n}\right)}}$$

where M is the lateral magnification, I_{sep} is the image separation, t is the thickness of the test plate target, and n is the index of the material (generally Plexiglas: n = 1.49).

Example

A piece of Plexiglas that is 4 mm thick and has a vertical grid on the front surface and a horizontal grid on the back surface is placed between the exit pupil and ocular lens of a Keplerian telescope. A light source placed very close to the Plexiglas illuminates its horizontal and vertical lines through the telescope and focuses onto a moveable screen. The distance of separation between the focused vertical and horizontal images is 200 mm. What is the magnification of this telescope (Figure 9-14)?

Answer. The example can be worked out in the following manner:

TABLE 9-7
Magnification of Galilean Telescopes

Change in Back Vertex Power when +1.00 D Added	Length of Telescopic system (mm)																		
	10	15	20	25	30	35	40	45	50	55	60	65	70	75	80	85	90	95	100
1	1.00	0.99	0.99	0.99	0.99	0.98	0.98	0.98	0.98	0.98	0.97	0.97	0.97	0.96	0.96	0.96	0.96	0.95	0.95
2	1.39	1.39	1.39	1.39	1.38	1.38	1.37	1.37	1.36	1.36	1.36	1.35	1.35	1.34	1.34	1.33	1.33	1.32	1.32
3	1.72	1.71	1.70	1.69	1.69	1.68	1.67	1.67	1.66	1.65	1.64	1.64	1.63	1.62	1.62	1.61	1.60	1.60	1.59
4	1.98	1.97	1.96	1.95	1.94	1.93	1.92	1.91	1.90	1.89	1.88	1.87	1.86	1.86	1.85	1.84	1.83	1.82	1.81
5	2.21	2.20	2.19	2.17	2.16	2.15	2.14	2.13	2.11	2.10	2.09	2.08	2.07	2.06	2.04	2.03	2.02	2.01	2.00
6	2.42	2.40	2.39	2.38	2.36	2.35	2.33	2.32	2.30	2.29	2.28	2.26	2.25	2.23	2.22	2.21	2.19	2.18	2.17
7	2.61	2.59	2.58	2.56	2.54	2.53	2.51	2.49	2.48	2.46	2.44	2.43	2.41	2.40	2.38	2.36	2.35	2.33	2.32
8	2.79	2.77	2.75	2.73	2.71	2.69	2.67	2.65	2.64	2.62	2.60	2.58	2.56	2.54	2.53	2.51	2.49	2.47	2.46
9	2.96	2.93	2.91	2.89	2.87	2.85	2.83	2.80	2.78	2.76	2.74	2.72	2.70	2.68	2.66	2.64	2.62	2.60	2.58
10	3.11	3.09	3.06	3.04	3.02	2.99	2.97	2.94	2.92	2.90	2.88	2.85	2.83	2.81	2.79	2.77	2.74	2.72	2.70
11	3.26	3.23	3.21	3.18	3.16	3.13	3.10	3.08	3.05	3.03	3.00	2.98	2.95	2.93	2.91	2.88	2.86	2.84	2.81
12	3.40	3.38	3.35	3.32	3.29	3.26	3.23	3.20	3.17	3.15	3.12	3.10	3.07	3.04	3.02	2.99	2.97	2.94	2.92
13	3.54	3.51	3.47	3.44	3.42	3.39	3.35	3.32	3.30	3.27	3.24	3.21	3.18	3.15	3.12	3.10	3.07	3.04	3.01
14	3.67	3.64	3.60	3.57	3.54	3.50	3.47	3.44	3.41	3.38	3.35	3.31	3.28	3.25	3.22	3.19	3.16	3.14	3.11
15	3.80	3.76	3.72	3.69	3.65	3.62	3.58	3.55	3.52	3.48	3.45	3.42	3.38	3.35	3.32	3.29	3.26	3.23	3.19
16	3.92	3.88	3.84	3.80	3.77	3.72	3.69	3.66	3.62	3.58	3.55	3.51	3.48	3.44	3.41	3.38	3.34	3.31	3.28
17	4.04	4.00	3.96	3.92	3.88	3.84	3.80	3.76	3.72	3.68	3.64	3.61	3.57	3.53	3.50	3.46	3.43	3.39	3.36
18	4.15	4.11	4.07	4.02	3.98	3.94	3.90	3.86	3.82	3.77	3.74	3.70	3.66	3.62	3.58	3.55	3.51	3.47	3.44
19	4.26	4.22	4.17	4.13	4.08	4.04	4.00	3.95	3.91	3.87	3.83	3.78	3.74	3.70	3.66	3.63	3.59	3.55	3.51
20	4.37	4.32	4.28	4.23	4.18	4.14	4.09	4.04	4.00	3.96	3.91	3.87	3.83	3.78	3.74	3.70	3.66	3.62	3.58
21	4.48	4.42	4.38	4.33	4.28	4.23	4.18	4.14	4.09	4.04	4.00	3.95	3.91	3.86	3.82	3.78	3.73	3.69	3.65
22	4.58	4.53	4.48	4.42	4.37	4.32	4.27	4.22	4.17	4.12	4.08	4.03	3.98	3.93	3.89	3.85	3.80	3.76	3.72
23	4.68	4.63	4.57	4.52	4.46	4.41	4.36	4.31	4.26	4.20	4.16	4.11	4.06	4.01	3.96	3.92	3.87	3.83	3.78
24	4.78	4.72	4.66	4.61	4.55	4.50	4.44	4.39	4.34	4.28	4.23	4.18	4.13	4.08	4.03	3.98	3.94	3.89	3.84
25	4.88	4.81	4.76	4.70	4.64	4.58	4.52	4.47	4.41	4.36	4.31	4.25	4.20	4.15	4.10	4.05	4.00	3.95	3.90

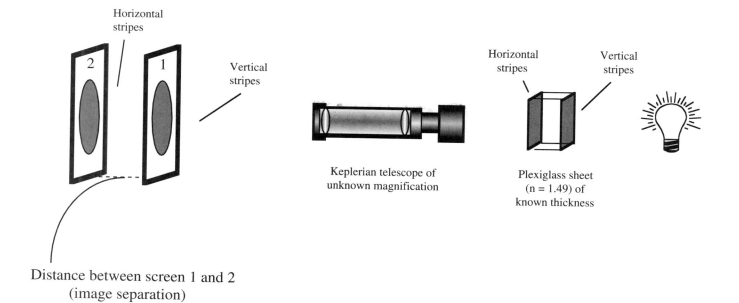

Horizontal stripes

Vertical stripes

Distance between screen 1 and 2
(image separation)

Keplerian telescope of unknown magnification

Horizontal stripes

Vertical stripes

Plexiglass sheet (n = 1.49) of known thickness

FIGURE 9-14.   A system used for measuring the magnification of a Keplerian telescope.

1. $\dfrac{t}{n} = \dfrac{4}{1.49} = 2.68$

2. $I_{sep} = 200$

3. $\dfrac{I_{sep}}{\left(\dfrac{t}{n}\right)} = \dfrac{200}{2.68} = 74.63$

4. $M = \sqrt{\dfrac{I_{sep}}{\left(\dfrac{t}{n}\right)}} = \sqrt{74.63} = 8.64\times$

Verification of a Prescription in an Afocal Telescope

The telescope should be placed in the lensometer so that the ocular lens is against the lens stop. The telescope must be positioned in the lensometer so that the center of the target is in the center of the field. The target will appear minified because the telescope is reversed. The prescription can be read directly from the lensometer as any spectacle lens would be read. This method can only be used to verify the back vertex power of a low-powered Galilean telescope, generally below 4×.

INSTRUCTION IN THE USE OF TELESCOPIC SYSTEMS

Success with a telescopic device is most likely to occur if the system has been selected carefully, keeping the patient's goals and needs in mind. Similarly, the patient's pathology, refractive error, acuity, fields, age, and motor skills should have also been taken into account. It is equally important that proper instruction in the use of a telescope be provided so that the patient is able to realize the full potential of the device.

Most patients have used binoculars at some point in their lives. Thus, they have some degree of familiarity with the concept of a telescope. This may make the task of instruction easier. The practitioner must be aware, however, that not all patients truly understand the concepts of "clear" and "blurry." This may be especially true of patients with congenital visual impairments.

Preparing for Instruction

In preparing for instruction with a distance device, the practitioner should select materials that are consistent with the patient's goals. Factors to be considered in selecting instructional materials include contrast, color(s), size of target, distance from the patient, and figure-ground considerations. Ideally, the instructional area and materials should be visually simple and uncluttered. A dimmer switch should be available on the overhead lighting so that light levels can be adjusted accordingly. Of course, the instructional area should also be quiet and free of distractions. Once the patient has mastered activities in a controlled environment, it is highly recommended that the patient be presented

with real environmental situations such as watching television and reading street signs, house numbers, and bus numbers (assuming that these are some of the patient's goals).

The ideal sequence for instruction should be as follows: Move from simple targets to more complex ones; move from static activities (target stationary) to dynamic ones. Instruction and practice sessions should be kept short and success oriented.

Instructional Sequence

Telescope instruction should begin with the introduction of the telescope and its parts: eyepiece, objective lens, focusing ring. Allow the patient to handle the telescope (without viewing through it) and to focus it all the way in and out. This exercise gives the patient a feel for the telescope and allows him or her to know what to expect when he or she is viewing through it. The patient should be instructed to only view through the telescope while sitting or standing still. In addition, the patient should be encouraged to describe what he or she is seeing through the telescope throughout the instructional session. This gives the practitioner information about the patient's proficiency with the device and some clues for troubleshooting if problems arise.

One important note: Once the patient begins viewing through the telescope, he or she may be so busy processing the visual input that auditory input from the practitioner may be ignored. Thus, concepts should be explained to the patient before he or she begins viewing through the telescope or when he or she is taking a break.

If the patient is using a handheld telescope, he or she should be encouraged to tuck it into the V made by the thumb and forefinger of the right hand (if using telescope with the right eye) or the left hand (if using the telescope with the left eye). The eyepiece should be placed flush with the edge of the thumb and forefinger so that the patient does not injure his or her eye when attempting to view through it. When the telescope is brought up to the eye, the thumb or forefinger should be rested against the face for stability. If the telescope has a collapsible eye cup, it should be folded down when held against a patient's spectacles to allow as wide a field of view as possible. For patients not wearing glasses, the eye cup should be left extended or unfolded. If using a clip-on telescope, the patient should be educated about how to mount and remove the clip-on unit from his or her spectacles. Some clip-on units involve small screws that can easily be dropped and lost. Thus, the patient should be seated at a desk or table when mounting or removing the clip-on unit. On some clip-on units, the telescope can easily be removed and used as a handheld telescope by screwing on an eye cup. This option should be discussed with the patient, as many can benefit from it.

There are a number of steps or procedures a patient should master to be considered proficient in the use of a telescope. Some of these procedures will be accomplished in a very short time, whereas others may require some time and persistence on the part of the patient. The following steps or procedures are recommended when instructing a patient to use a telescope:

1. Localization
2. Focusing
3. Spotting
4. Tracing
5. Tracking
6. Scanning

It is also important to provide a summary of the important points that were discussed during the instructional period. These points can be written down, preferably in large print, for the patient to refer to when needed. A sample of written instructions for a handheld telescope and a spectacle mounted telescope are found in Appendix D and Appendix E, respectively.

Localization

The first step in using a telescope is localization of the target—that is, finding the target and being sure the target, telescope, and eye are aligned. Most patients can successfully spot their target without the telescope, which makes the telescope use much easier. In such cases, the patient should be instructed to view the target unaided and then to keep viewing it while a handheld telescope is brought up to the eye. If using a mounted telescopic system (bioptic mount), the target should first be localized through the carrier lens and then the patient's head should be dropped to bring the target into view with the telescope. A head strap is often useful in stabilizing the spectacle and telescope; it also increases patient comfort by taking some of the device's weight off his or her nose. Patients may benefit from closing or patching his or her other eye. A clip-on telescope can sometimes slide out of position on the spectacles; patients should be aware that this can be a problem and should be taught to slide the unit back into place so that alignment is restored. Patients should be encouraged to think about the best viewing position for any given target and to move to that ideal position if at all possible. Normally, the best viewing position is perpendicular to the target.

Alignment of the target should be verified by asking the patient if the image is fully circular. If he or she reports a half-moon shaped image, then the telescope is not, in fact, properly aligned. A handheld telescope should be removed from the patient's eye and then brought into position again by the patient to obtain proper alignment. A mounted system may need some adjustment of the telescopic position or the nosepads.

The patient should sit or stand while viewing through the telescope. He or she should be encouraged to describe what is seen when looking through the telescope. Verbal feedback during instruction is encouraged. If the patient is seated when using a handheld telescope, his or her elbow may be rested on a table to aid stability. When standing, the patient may steady the telescope by holding his or her upper arm against his or her body or by supporting the elbow of the arm holding the device with the opposite palm. Leaning against a wall may also provide additional support and stability.

Focusing

Once the patient has mastered localization techniques, instruction should proceed to focusing the telescope. The patient must understand how the telescope focuses. He or she should also be informed about the range of focus of the telescope (e.g., from infinity to 12 in.). Initially, the telescope should be focused for the patient. When the telescope is in focus, the patient should view the target. The telescope should then be taken out of focus so that the patient can see the difference between "in focus" and "out-of-focus" positions. A patient should practice focusing on targets that are located at various distances. The patient should experiment on the closest and furthest distance that the telescope can be focused. Glasses should be worn while focusing the telescope if there is a refractive error. Patients who use the telescope without glasses and use the telescope to compensate for their refractive error can be asked if a target is in focus by having them describe the target. If the target is accurately identified, it is assumed that the telescope is in focus. When focusing the telescope, the patient should be encouraged to experience blurring on either side of the clear focus of the telescope. This will insure that the clearest focus will be obtained. On binocular systems, each telescope should be focused independently of the other. This can be accomplished by closing the eye behind the telescope not being focused.

If the concept of focusing the telescope is difficult to achieve for a patient, two alternatives exist. An autofocus telescope could be recommended, which obviously would eliminate any focusing problems for the patient. The other alternative would be for a patient who requires only one fixed distance (e.g., 8 ft when watching television), to make a marking on the telescope that would indicate the desired focus. If the telescope goes out of focus, it simply should be rotated in one direction or the other until the markings are realigned.

Spotting

The term *spotting* is used to describe the result of localization and focusing. It is the process of finding a target without benefit of the telescope, positioning the telescope so that it is aligned between the eye and the target, and focusing the telescope until the image is as clear as possible. Alignment is as important as focusing, and instructional exercises should emphasize both.

Tracing

Tracing is a skill that must be mastered after proficiency in spotting. It involves the following of a stationary line in the environment. Positional lines in the environment, such as telephone poles, telephone wires, streets, and curbs, will act as targets for a patient to obtain good tracing skills. The patient should move his or her head smoothly and slowly when tracing. This motion will allow him or her to maintain his or her orientation to the environment.

Tracking

Tracking is a slightly more advanced skill than is tracing, as it involves moving the head and telescope smoothly while following a moving target. Instruction in tracking should start preferably with the patient seated and observing a target that is perpendicular to the straight-ahead direction and moving at a constant rate. Simple targets should be introduced first and have high contrast and no figure-ground confusion. As this tracking skill is mastered, diagonal movements and movements toward the patient and away from the patient should be introduced. The target can be made smaller, and reversal of direction and curved paths can be introduced as well as different rates of movement.

Losing sight of the target is not unusual when patients first begin tracking activities. Patients should be encouraged to find the target again, unaided or through the carrier, and then resume tracking.

If the distance between the target and the patient changes, then the telescope will need to be refocused while the patient is tracking the target. Such an activity should not be used for practice until the patient has demonstrated good initial tracking skills.

Scanning

Scanning is generally the most difficult skill to master in the hierarchy of telescopic skills, but it is one of the most valuable. *Scanning* is using an organized search pattern to locate a target that cannot be located without the use of the telescope.

For scanning to be effective, the patient must first develop a concept of an environmental reference point or use some objects in the environment to define his or her location (e.g., scanning the area between two telephone poles). Kinesthetic awareness should be used to define how much to turn the body so scanning patterns will be approximately equal on either side of the body. Scanning is then performed in a grid pattern. For example, when targets are found in a vertical plane (e.g., street signs), the patient must scan horizontally to find the pole and then vertically up the pole until he or she finds the sign itself. In the same way, targets in the horizontal plane can be found by initially searching vertically.

Scanning can begin indoors with simple tasks such as finding printed sentences on a chalkboard. The patient should be encouraged to find the beginning of the sentence or paragraph and move across the first line to the end. He or she must then learn to retrace the first line and then drop down to continue the same pattern on the next line.

As scanning skills are mastered, the instruction can graduate to the outdoor environment. The technique that needs the most attention is the ability to overlap the scanning paths completely. Failure to develop a systematic scanning sequence may lead to the patient not finding the intended target. When tracking or scanning, patients may complain of discomfort due to the movement of the image. The patient should be reminded that the telescope magnifies both image size and motion and, therefore, he or she should be advised to move his or her head smoothly and slowly.

Most patients can master the techniques of localization, focusing, spotting, tracing, tracking, and scanning within one or two practice sessions. These skills, however, should be continuously practiced so that the fullest potential of the telescope will be realized. Written instructions in large type or audiotaped instructions may be helpful to remind the patient how to use the telescope. If home practice sessions are scheduled, they should be short and success oriented. Practice sessions should be frequent (several times a day) and patients should be encouraged to obtain help and feedback from relatives, friends, or coworkers during practice. If difficulty is encountered, the hierarchy of skills can be broken down into simpler components so that skills can be learned one at a time. If the patient is a child, the parents should observe the instruction so that they may assist with the practice sessions at home. Additional help may be offered if the patient has difficulty in developing the needed skills by working with a lower magnification telescope and when skills have been mastered, reintroducing the higher power.

TELEMICROSCOPES

Theoretically, any telescope can be made focal. The modifications that can be made to alter an afocal telescopic system and convert it into a focal system were discussed in Focal Telescopes. The main advantage of prescribing a telemicroscopic system over an equivalent-powered microscope is one of providing a longer working distance. It is important to note that the depth of field of a telescope (variation in the object distance that can be tolerable without incurring an objectionable lack of sharpness or blur) will be the same as the equivalent-powered microscope or reading addition.[15]

Telescopes that are focused for distances closer than infinity have an equivalent power. It should be noted, however, that a telescope does not provide the same magnification when used with a reading cap to focus as when its length is increased to focus at near. The equivalent power of a focused telescope is greater than the equivalent power of a telescope focused for the same distance with a reading cap. When an afocal telescope is focused for a close working distance and made to be focal, some of the power of the objective lens is "borrowed" from the objective, resulting in a weaker objective lens and a longer tube length (Figure 9-15). The formula for equivalent power can be used to clarify the concept of "borrowed power."

$$D_{eq} = \left(D_{cap} + D_{obj}\right) + \left(D_{oc}\right) - \left(d\right)\left(D_{cap} + D_{obj}\right)\left(D_{oc}\right)$$

The telemicroscope can be considered to be made up of an afocal telescope and an added reading cap. When the telescope is "focused" by increasing the separation of the objective and eyepiece lenses, however, and a cap is not actually used, the same dioptric power can be considered to have been "borrowed" from the objective lens to act as a reading cap, making the system focal. The "borrowed power" is equal to the reciprocal of the focal distance of the telemicroscope. The new tube length is equal to the algebraic sum of the focal lengths of the remaining objective power and ocular lens.

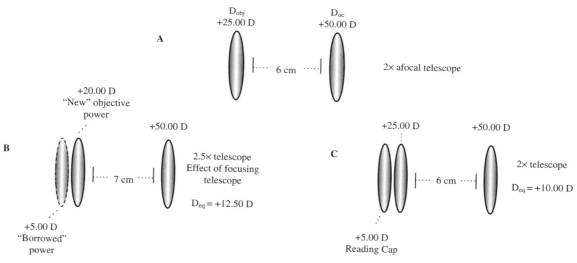

FIGURE 9-15.   **The effect of focusing a telescope versus adding a reading cap. A. 2× Keplerian telescope in afocal position. B. Keplerian telescope that has been focused to 20 cm by "borrowing" +5.00 D from the objective lens (D_{obj}), thus creating a stronger telescope (2.5×) and a total equivalent power (D_{eq}) of +12.50 D. C. 2× Keplerian system with a +5.00 D reading cap maintains the magnification of 2× while still focusing at 20 cm but only has a total equivalent power of +10.00 D. (D_{oc} = ocular lens.)**

Example 1

What is the equivalent power of a focusable telescope composed of a –50.00 D ocular and +25.00 D objective focused for 20.00 cm?

Answer. The example can be worked out in the following manner:

1. To focus this telescope, the equivalent of +5.00 D must be borrowed from the objective lens to focus at 20.00 cm. This results in the "new" objective lens being +20.00 D and the tube length being 3 cm.

$$\frac{100\ \text{cm}}{20\ \text{cm}} = 5.00\ \text{D}$$

2. Here, D_{cap} is the borrowed power (+5.00 D).

$$D_{eq} = \left(D_{cap} + D_{obj}\right) + \left(D_{oc}\right) - (d)\left(D_{cap} + D_{obj}\right)\left(D_{oc}\right)$$
$$= (5.00 + 20.00) + (-50.00) - (0.03)(5.00 + 20.00)(-50.00)$$
$$= -25.00 + 37.50 = +12.50\ \text{D}$$

or

$$D_{eq} = \left(\left|M_{TS}\right|\right)\left(D_{cap}\right)$$
$$D_{eq} = -\left(-\frac{50}{20}\right)(5.00)$$
$$D_{eq} = (2.5\times)(5.00) = +12.50\ \text{D}$$

Example 2

What is the equivalent power of a telescope composed of a –50.00 D ocular and a +25.00 D objective focused for 20 cm with a +5.00 D reading cap?

Answer. The example can be worked out in the following manner:

1. The objective lens remains +25.00 D and therefore the tube length remains at 2 cm.
2. The D_{cap} is given as +5.00 D.

$$D_{eq} = \left(D_{cap} = D_{obj}\right) + \left(D_{oc}\right) - (d)\left(D_{cap} + D_{obj}\right)\left(D_{oc}\right)$$
$$= (5.00 + 25.00) + (-50.00) - (0.02)(5.00 + 25.00)(-50.00)$$
$$= -20.00 + 30.00 = +10.00\ \text{D}$$

Specification of Telemicroscopic Magnification

There is often confusion in specifying the magnification of a telemicroscope. The total magnification of a system involves a comparison of retinal image sizes. In Chapter 7, Byer calls this the *retinal image magnification* or *RIM*. If 25 cm is chosen as a reference distance, then the magnification of a telescopic reading cap can be calculated in the traditional manner as $M_{25} = D/4$. The traditional magnification rating for the telemicroscope is a comparison between the apparent angular size of the image seen through the optical system as compared to the apparent angular size of the object viewed directly by the eye (with no optical device) from a distance of 25 cm ("least distance of distinct vision"). If, however, 40 cm is chosen as the reference distance, then the magnification of the reading cap is given by $M_{40} = D/2.5$.

The total magnification of a telemicroscope is the product of the telescope's magnification times the magnification of the reading cap (relative to some reference distance). If a telemicroscope consisting of the 2× telescope combined with the +5.00 D cap is examined, it can be seen that the total magnification (with a reference distance of 25 cm) is 2.5×, the product of the telescope (2×) times the magnification of the cap (+5.00/4 = 1.25×). If a reference distance of 40 cm is used, then the total magnification for that same system would be rated as 4×, the product of the telescope (2×) times the magnification of the cap (+5.00/2.5 = 2×).

As seen by the preceding examples, a telemicroscope can be assigned many different total magnifications, depending on the reference distances. Often the reference distance is not provided, making it difficult if not impossible to compare telemicroscopic systems rated in total magnification only. Therefore, when comparing one telemicroscope to another, it is always best to compare them in equivalent power when possible.

Example 1
Which telemicroscope is the most powerful?

A. 2× telescope with a +4.00 D reading cap
B. 4× telescope with a +2.00 D reading cap

Answer: When comparing these two systems, the equivalent power $D_{eq} = D_{cap} \times |M_{TS}|$ of each system can be compared. The equivalent power of telemicroscope A is +8.00 D (4×2) and the equivalent power of telemicroscope B is +8.00 D (4×2). Therefore, both systems have equal equivalent power and will provide the same magnified retinal image size. (The difference between the two telemicroscopes is that telemicroscope A will focus at 25 cm while telemicroscope B will focus at 50 cm.)

Example 2
A patient has a best corrected near acuity of 0.33/4 M and desires to read the newspaper, which is found to be 1-M print. What reading caps would be required for a 2.2× and a 3× telescope to accomplish this task and what is the total magnification of each system?

Answer. The example can be worked out in the following manner:

1. Determine what magnification would be needed to reach the goal acuity (see Chapter 10).

$$\text{Magnification needed} = \frac{\text{Reference size}}{\text{Goal size}}$$
$$= \frac{4\,M}{1\,M}$$
$$= 4\times$$

2. Determine the equivalent power for this amount of magnification.

$$D_{eq} = \frac{\text{Magnification}}{\text{Reference distance}}$$
$$= \frac{4}{0.33}$$
$$= +12.12\,D$$

This demonstrates what lens is needed in the spectacle plane to reach the desired acuity. Once the equivalent power is determined, the telescope and reading cap combinations can be determined.

3. (a) With a 2.2× telescope

$$D_{eq}\,(\text{of the telemicroscope}) = \left(|M_{TS}|\right)\left(D_{cap}\right)$$
$$+12.12\,D = \left(|2.2\times|\right)\left(D_{cap}\right)$$
$$\text{Reading cap} = +5.51\,D$$
$$\text{Total magnification} = \left(|2.2\times|\right)\left(\frac{5.51}{3.03}\right) = 4\times$$

(b) With a 3.0× telescope

$$D_{eq}\,(\text{of the telemicroscope}) = \left(|M_{TS}|\right)\left(D_{cap}\right)$$
$$+12.12\,D = \left(|3.0\times|\right)\left(D_{cap}\right)$$
$$\text{Reading cap} = +4.04\,D$$
$$\text{Total magnification} = \left(|3.0\times|\right)\left(\frac{4.04}{3.03}\right) = 4\times$$

Telemicroscopic Field of View

The linear field of view of a telemicroscope (expressed in centimeters) is equal to the afocal telescopic field of view (expressed in degrees) when objects are viewed through the telescope at 57 cm.[16] To determine the approximate field of view (in centimeters) of a telemicroscope focused at a particular distance, the angular field of view (in degrees) of the afocal telescope is multiplied by the quotient of the viewing distance (in centimeters) divided by 57. Thus, a 2.5× telescope with a 12-degree field focused at 40 cm will have a linear field of view of 8.42 cm (12[40/57]).

Telemicroscopic Depth of Field

The depth of field is the change in distance over which an object can be moved without incurring blur. As stated in the discussion on focal telescopes, there is no advantage or gain in the depth of field over comparable equivalent-powered microscopes or spectacle adds when using a telemicroscope. A formula for the depth of field of a lens system basically states that the range of movement, or the depth of field, varies inversely with the square of the equivalent power of the system.[15] Because the equivalent power of a telemicroscopic system is the power of the reading cap times the telescopic magnification, the depth of field of a 2× telescope with a +6.00 D reading cap and a 6× telescope with a +2.00 D reading cap would be equivalent.

When prescribing telemicroscopes, an attempt should be made to prescribe the lowest equivalent power with the weakest telescope and weakest reading cap consistent with the goals of the patient. Prescribing the weakest equivalent power will maximize the depth of field, and using the lowest telescopic magnification will maximize the field of view. Providing the low-power cap will enable a longer working distance. It is always best, however, to demonstrate the effect of working distance and field to the patient, and based on performance, decide which factors dictate the best prescribing option.

Prescribing Binocular Telemicroscopic Systems

If a binocular system is prescribed, the telemicroscopes will need to be angled in or converged to the near focal

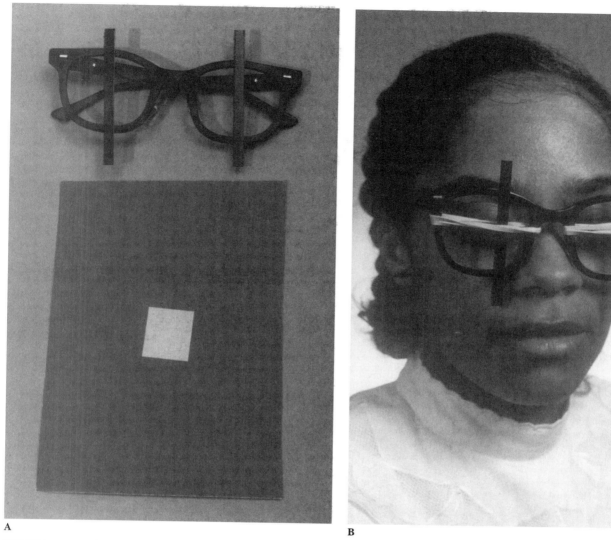

A   B

FIGURE 9-16.   A. The Englemann method for measurement of the functional interpupillary distance (IPD) uses complementary colored anaglyphs (red celluloid strips) on the frame and a red card with a centered green square held at the proper working distance. B. The binocular functional IPD is the distance from the corresponding point on one strip to the corresponding point on the fellow strip. The monocular functional IPD is measured from the center of the strip to the center of the bridge of the frame. The functional near IPD taken by this method, in many cases, will be different than that taken in the customary manner with an IPD ruler.

point for which they are designed. Failure to allow for the convergence of the binocular units will cause diplopia. Each telemicroscopic unit must be decentered inward to the monocular interpupillary distance (IPD) measurement when the patient is converged to the near focal point. Englemann has described a method of accurately measuring the IPD for the near telemicroscopic units.[17] Englemann's method involves the use of red celluloid plastic anaglyph strips that are placed vertically in front of the eyes (Figure 9-16). The patient is instructed to hold a card with a red background and a green fixation square in the center at the distance in which the telemicroscope would be focused. The red plastic celluloid strip is then carefully moved to a position on the spectacle frame at which the line of sight passes through the red strip and thus, the center green target (of the card being viewed) is perceived to be dark or black in color. The procedure is repeated for the other eye. When both eyes are used with the celluloid strips in the proper position on the spectacles, the center of the red card appears to have a black square (instead of a green square). The IPD is then measured from a corresponding point of one celluloid strip to a corresponding point of the other strip.

The IPD can also be determined with the use of a pupillometer. In some cases, however, the telemicroscope requires a closer working distance than the pupillometer is able to measure, and therefore measurement with the Englemann unit becomes necessary.

SELF-ASSESSMENT QUESTIONS

1. The telescope that produces an erect image is the
   - (a) Dutch telescope
   - (b) Keplerian telescope
   - (c) astronomical telescope
   - (d) all of the above
   - (e) b and c

2. What is the tube length of a telescope when the ocular lens is –75.00 D and the objective lens is +30.00 D?
   - (a) 1.33 cm
   - (b) 2.00 cm
   - (c) 3.33 cm
   - (d) 4.00 cm
   - (e) 4.66 cm

3. What is the dioptric power of the ocular lens of a telescope when its tube length is 3.00 cm and the objective lens is +25.00 D?
   - (a) +50.00 D
   - (b) +100.00 D
   - (c) –50.00 D
   - (d) –75.00 D
   - (e) –100.00 D

4. A patient who is able to read with a +24.00 D microscope would prefer to hold his or her reading material at a greater distance. The practitioner decides to prescribe a telemicroscope to accomplish this task. What power cap would be required for a 4× telescope to provide the equivalent power of the patient's microscopic lens?
   - (a) +2.00 D
   - (b) +4.00 D
   - (c) +6.00 D
   - (d) +8.00 D
   - (e) +12.00 D

5. What is the magnification when a 16.00 D hyperope holds a +3.00 D lens in front of his eye so that the lens' secondary focal point is coincident with the far point of the patient's uncorrected hyperopic eye?
   - (a) 3.66×
   - (b) 5.33×
   - (c) 8.14×
   - (d) 12.62×
   - (e) 19×

6. Which telescope(s) would appear to be the brightest to a patient having a 5-mm pupil? Telescope 1 = 3×10; telescope 2 = 3×16; telescope 3 = 4×20.
   - (a) telescope 1
   - (b) telescope 2
   - (c) telescope 3
   - (d) telescopes 1 and 2 will equally appear to be the brightest
   - (e) telescopes 2 and 3 will equally appear to be the brightest

7. What telescopic magnification would be required for a patient whose best visual acuity is 10/120 to see a movie where the estimated needed acuity is 20/40?
   - (a) 12×
   - (b) 6×
   - (c) 3×
   - (d) 2×
   - (e) none of the above

8. When a patient who is wearing his or her best spectacle correction looks through a 4× telescope, an acuity of 20/80 is obtained. What is the expected acuity (through the spectacle correction) when the telescope is removed?
   - (a) 10/10
   - (b) 10/20
   - (c) 10/40
   - (d) 10/80
   - (e) 10/160

9. When instructing a patient on how to properly use a telescope, which of the following statements is *incorrect*?
   - (a) The patient should be instructed with simple targets initially followed by more complex ones.
   - (b) Instruction and practice sessions should be kept short and success oriented.
   - (c) Instruction should begin in the real environment where the patient plans to use the telescope.
   - (d) Instruction should begin with static activities and then move on to dynamic ones.
   - (e) The practitioner or instructor should select materials to be used during instruction that are consistent with the patient's goals.

10. What is the approximate linear field of a 3× telemicroscope when the field of the telescope is 10 degrees and the system is focused for 40 cm?
    - (a) 5.00 cm
    - (b) 6.00 cm
    - (c) 7.00 cm
    - (d) 8.00 cm
    - (e) 10.00 cm

REFERENCES

1. von Rohr M. Zeitschrift fur Instrumentenkunde. Berlin: Springer, 1940.
2. Bier N. Correction of Subnormal Vision. London: Butterworths, 1960;56–58.
3. Dallos J. Contact glasses, the "invisible" spectacles. Arch Ophthalmol 1936;15:617–623.
4. Bettman JW, McNair GS. Contact-lens telescopic system. Am J Ophthalmol 1938;22:27–33.
5. Mandell RB. Contact Lens Practice: Basic and Advanced. Springfield, IL: Thomas, 1965;372–373.
6. Filderman IP. Clinical procedure for adapting the telcon lens. J Am Optom Assoc 1959;30:561–562.
7. Isen A. Feinbloom Miniscope Contact Lens. In PR Hayes (ed), Encyclopedia of Contact Lens Practice (Vol III, Suppl 13). Appendix B, Recent Developments. South Bend, IN: International Optics Publishing Corp., 1961;53–55.

8. Fonda G. Management of the Patient with Subnormal Vision (2nd ed). St. Louis: Mosby, 1970;49–52.
9. Sloan LL. Optical magnification for subnormal vision: historical survey. JOSA 1972;62:162–168.
10. Freid AN. Telescopes, light vergence, and accommodation. Am J Optom Physiol Optics 1977;54:365–373.
11. Jose R, Morse SE. Telescopes: to cap or not to cap. Rehabil Optom 1983;1:9–11.
12. Woo G. Use of low magnification telescopes as optometers in low vision. Optom Monthly 1978;69:529–533.
13. Woo G. Clinical dialogue. Optom Monthly 1978:69:117–120.
14. Bailey IL. Measuring the magnifying power of Keplerian telescopes. Appl Optics 1978:17:3520–3521.
15. Spitzberg LA, Qi M. Depth of field of plus lenses and reading telescopes. Optom Vis Sci 1994;71:115–119.
16. Musick JE. Clinical Strategies for the Visually Impaired Computer User. In RG Cole, BP Rosenthal (eds), Remediation and Management of Low Vision. St. Louis: Mosby, 1996;219–220.
17. Englemann O. Subjective pupillary measurement. Optom Weekly 1961;52:1908–1910.

Commonly Prescribed Handheld Telescopes

Manufacturer and Distributor*	Magnification	Field (degrees)	Type	Exit Pupil (mm)	Close Focus Distance (cm)
Eschenbach 2.75×9	2.80×	12.5	K	2.90	15.00
Eschenbach 3×23 clip-on	3.00×	9.5	G	7.66	70.00
Eschenbach 4×10	4.20×	10.0	K	2.50	20.00
Eschenbach 4×12	4.00×	12.5	K	3.00	20.00
Eschenbach 6×17	6.00×	10.5	K	2.83	25.00
Eschenbach 8×20	8.00×	6.5	K	2.50	30.00
Eschenbach 8×30	8.00×	8.5	K	3.75	52.00
Keeler 2.8× Panfocal	2.80×	12.5	K	2.86	16.00
Keeler 4.2× Panfocal	4.20×	12.5	K	2.86	20.00
Keeler 6.0× Panfocal	6.00×	10.0	K	2.67	35.00
Keeler 8.25× Panfocal	8.25×	7.0	K	2.42	30.00
Nikon 6×15	6.00×	7.5	K	2.50	300.00
Selsi 2.5× (#227B)	2.50×	20.5	G	9.20	100.00
Selsi 2.8× (#229B)	2.80×	16.0	G	9.29	200.00
Selsi 4×12 (#170)	4.00×	12.5	K	3.00	18.00
Selsi 6×16 (#167)	6.00×	9.3	K	2.67	23.00
Selsi 6×30 (#150)	6.00×	7.5	K	5.00	300.00
Selsi 7×25 (#168)	7.00×	10.0	K	3.57	38.00
Selsi 7×35 (#152)	7.00×	6.5	K	5.00	260.00
Selsi 8×20 (#163)	8.00×	7.0	K	2.50	27.00
Selsi 10×30 (#166)	10.00×	6.5	K	2.50	84.00
Selsi 6×18/8×24 (#162)	6.00×/8.00×	9.3/6.9	K	3.00	200.00/300.00
Specwell 2×8	2.00×	11.0	K	4.00	10.00
Specwell 2.75×8	2.75×	12.5	K	2.90	14.00
Specwell 3×9	3.00×	11.5	K	3.00	22.00
Specwell 4×10	4.00×	9.5	K	2.50	22.00
Specwell 4×12	4.00×	12.5	K	3.00	20.00
Specwell 6×16	6.00×	10.0	K	2.65	26.00
Specwell 7×25	7.00×	10.0	K	3.57	50.00
Specwell 8×20	8.00×	7.0	K	2.50	30.00
Specwell 8×20 (rubberized)	8.00×	7.0	K	2.50	30.00
Specwell 8×30	8.00×	8.5	K	3.75	60.00
Specwell 8×30 (rubberized)	8.00×	8.5	K	3.75	60.00
Specwell 10×20	10.00×	6.0	K	2.00	40.00
Specwell 10×30	10.00×	6.0	K	3.00	70.00
Specwell 10×30 (rubberized)	10.00×	6.0	K	3.00	70.00
Walters 2×8	2.00×	12.5	K	4.00	14.00
Walters 2.2× Mini	2.20×	9.0	G	5.70	12 ft
Walters 2.3×40	2.30×	25.0	G	17.40	4 ft
Walters 2.75×8	2.75×	12.5	K	2.90	14.00
Walters 3× Mini (3×0)	3.00×	10.0	G	6.66	12 ft fixed
Walters 3×20	3.00×	8.0	K	6.66	25.00
Walters 4×10	4.00×	8.5	K	2.50	16.50
Walters 4×12	4.00×	12.5	K	3.00	17.70
Walters 6×16	6.00×	10.0	K	2.66	25.00
Walters 6×16 (rubberized)	6.00×	10.0	K	2.66	25.00
Walters 7×25	7.00×	10.0	K	3.57	54.60
Walters 7×5 (folding)	7.00×	8.0	K	3.57	10 ft
Walters 8×20	8.00×	7.0	K	2.50	26.70
Walters 8×20 (rubberized)	8.00×	7.0	K	2.50	26.70
Walters 8×21	8.00×	6.5	K	2.63	29.80
Walters 8×30 (rubberized)	8.00×	8.5	K	3.75	49.50
Walters 8×50	8.00×	7.5	K	6.25	183.00
Walters 10×20	10.00×	6.0	K	2.00	38.10
Walters 10×22 (rubberized)	10.00×	5.7	K	2.20	83.80
Walters 10×25	10.00×	5.2	K	2.50	38.10
Walters 10×30 (rubberized)	10.00×	6.5	K	3.00	83.82
Walters 14×20	14.00×	3.5	K	1.42	43.18
Walters 20×50	20.00×	3.0	K	2.50	5 ft

K = Keplerian; G = Galilean.
*Manufacturers and distributors: Eschenbach Optik of America, Inc. (Ridgefield, CT); Keeler Instruments, Inc. (Broomall, PA); Nikon Optics (Melville, NY); Selsi Company, Inc. (Carlstadt, NJ); Specwell Corp. (Tokyo, Japan); Walters (Agoura Hills, CA).

Appendix B

COMMONLY PRESCRIBED HEADBORNE AND SPECTACLE-MOUNTED TELESCOPES

Beecher Research Company (Schaumburg, IL)

Mirage Telescopic Spectacles
These lightweight binoculars consist of a Keplerian system using mirrors to reduce the bulk of the conventional prism binocular. The 1-mm-thick mirrors are optically coated and, along with high-index lenses, provide a wide field of view and excellent light transmission in a headborne binocular system. The binoculars are designed with a "butterfly" hinge that enables changes in the pupillary distance (Figure B-1). Currently, there are six magnifications available and the units may be prescribed in either a binocular or monocular form. The Mirage telescopes have reading caps available for near applications (except for the 3× telescope) (Table B-1). Lenses to correct for refractive error that can be placed over the eyepiece are also available.

C.O.I.L. Combined Optical Industries, Ltd. (Elk Grove Village, IL)

COIL Spectacle Binocular
The COIL Spectacle Binocular is a headborne 2× adjustable telescope. The unit consists of a pair of molded plastic 40-mm-round objective lenses that are joined in a one-piece, moveable plastic front carrier (Figure B-2). The objective lenses are aspheric in design and approximately +11.50 D in power. The ocular lenses (28-mm diameter) are high-minus (approximately –23.00 D), plano-concave lenses mounted into a fixed, one-piece plastic holder. A dial on each temple of the frame allows forward and back adjustment of the objective lenses from the afocal separation. Maximum sepa-

ration of the lenses approaches 50 mm while minimum separation approximates 26 mm. The system can be ordered with light gray–tinted objective lenses or clear objective lenses. Table B-2 lists the specifications for the unit.

Designs for Vision, Inc. (Ronkonkoma, NY)

Full-Diameter Telescopes
Five Galilean "standard" and two "wide-angle" Galilean systems (Figure B-3) are manufactured with the specifications in Table B-3.

These full-diameter Galilean telescopes are constructed of glass lenses mounted in plastic housings. The telescope is mounted in a plastic carrier lens. Corrective lenses for refractive errors may be incorporated into the telescopic eyepieces. The wide-angle designs have larger objective lenses. Although the field of the 2.2× full-diameter system and the 2.2× full-diameter wide-angle both have the same

TABLE B-1
Specifications of the Mirage Telescopic Spectacles (Keplerian)*

Magnification	Objective Lens Diameter (mm)	Field (degrees)	Exit Pupil (mm)	Focus Range
3×	25	15.0	8.33	Infinity to 2 ft
4×	20	15.0	5.00	Infinity to 3.5 ft
5.5×	25	12.0	4.54	Infinity to 6 ft
7×	30	9.5	4.28	Infinity to 8 ft
8×	28	8.5	3.50	Infinity to 11 ft
10×	35	6.0	3.50	Infinity to 20 ft

*Available from Beecher Research Company, Schaumburg, IL.

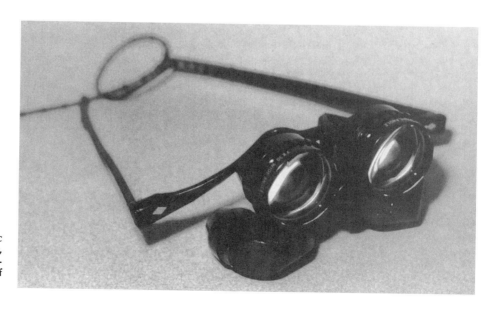

FIGURE B-1. **The Mirage Telescopic Spectacle (Beecher Research Company, Schaumburg, IL) is available as a monocular or binocular system in a number of magnifications.**

TABLE B-2
Specifications of the COIL Spectacle Binocular (Galilean)*

Magnification	Field (degrees)	Exit Pupil (mm)	Focus Range
2×	21.7	11 mm	Infinity to 1 m

*Available from C.O.I.L. Combined Optical Industries, Ltd., Elk Grove Village, IL.

field of view (16 degrees), the 2.2× wide-angle has a larger objective lens, thus providing a larger exit pupil, allowing for a less critical positioning of the unit as well as enabling more light to exit the telescope. The success of the 2.2× wide-angle telescope spurred the development of the 3.0× wide-angle system. The 3.0× wide-angle unit uses two meniscus lenses for the objective and a cemented doublet for the ocular, increasing the field of view over the standard 3.0×. The housings of the full diameter telescopes can be ordered in clear or black. The black housing is preferable to reduce reflections and improve optical performance. Reading caps are available for all systems, allowing near focus in a telemicroscopic design.

Bioptic (Nonfocusable) Galilean Telescopes

The standard bioptic Galilean telescopes are smaller than their full-diameter counterparts, with the exception of the 3.0× and 4.0× standard telescopes, which are identical to the full diameter systems. There are also two wide-angle bioptic systems (Figure B-4). When mounted in the "bioptic" position, the telescope is out of the way for various activities in which constant telescopic viewing is not needed. Table B-4 lists the specifications of the nonfocusable Galilean telescopes.

If the telescope is placed in the bioptic position, it must be angled up from the straight-ahead position so that it will be angled straight ahead when the patient lowers his or her head to use the telescope. The standard angle of inclination recommended by the manufacturer is 10 degrees up, however, any angle can be ordered. Generally, the tele-

scope is positioned as high as possible in the vertical dimension of the frame and horizontally decentered to the patient's interpupillary distance. Because some carrier lens is needed between the top of the lens and the top of the telescopic housing, approximately 3 mm is allowed to prevent cracking of the carrier lens. The center of the telescopic ocular lens is, therefore, 9 mm below the top of the carrier lens. As a general rule, for each millimeter above the patient's straight ahead line of sight that the telescope is located, the telescope must be angled up 2 degrees. The angle of inclination is also relative to the normal pantoscopic tilt of the spectacle frame. The standard drilling positions for all the Designs for Vision, Inc. telescopes is shown on the Low Vision Drilling Chart (Figure B-5). The patient's refractive correction can be incorporated into any of the telescopes and into the carrier lenses. The telescope is positioned as close to the eye as possible to provide as large a field of view as possible. The telescopic lens housings can be either clear or black. Reading caps are available for any of the bioptic systems allowing focus at near point.

Spiral Focus Galilean telescopes

The Spiral Focus Galilean telescopes (Figure B-6) allow for focusability, which the standard Galilean telescopes do not offer. The spiral action of the systems alters the tube length to provide a focal system. All the systems have the capacity to focus to 12 in. (30.5 cm). Table B-5 lists the specifications of these telescopes.

These units can be fitted in either a full-diameter or bioptic position. Due to the fact that the diameter of the oculars vary in size with this type of telescope, there is no standard bioptic mounting position. It will vary with each telescopic magnification system. Corrective lenses can be incorporated into the telescopes. Only a black housing is available.

Micro Spiral Galilean Telescopes (Clear View)

Originally introduced to the profession in late 1989, the micro spiral Galilean telescope was designed as a miniature focusable telescope. The first designs of the micro spiral telescopes, called Clear View I lenses, had three

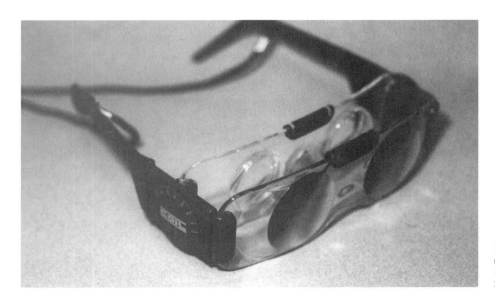

FIGURE B-2. **The COIL Spectacle Binocular (C.O.I.L. Combined Optical Industries, Ltd., Elk Grove Village, IL) is a headborne 2× telescope.**

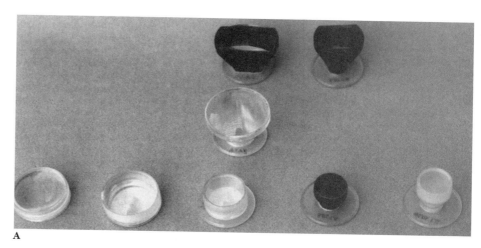

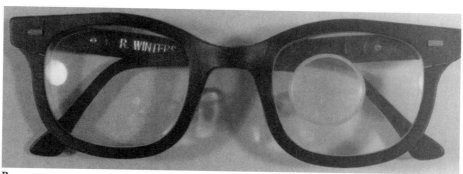

FIGURE B-3.   A. The Designs for Vision, Inc. full-diameter Galilean telescopes (Ronkonkoma, NY) are available in powers of 1.3×, 1.7×, 2.2×, 3.0×, and 4.0× (lower row). The 2.2× and 3.0× are also available in wide angle rectangular models (upper row). Wide-angle, full-diameter Galilean telescopes are available in 2.2× and 3.0×. The 2.2× is shown here (middle row). B. A 3.0× full-diameter Galilean telescope mounted in a spectacle "carrier" lens.

powers, 2.2×, 3.3×, and 4.0×. Shortly after the initial introduction, three additional powers of the series were introduced: 2.7×, 5.0×, and 6.0×, and at the same time the 3.3× and 4.0× were redesigned with a shorter barrel length. The Clear View I lenses had a 7-mm objective lens diameter and a 5-mm ocular lens diameter with the overall length varying from 9 mm to 13 mm. All of the telescopes focused from infinity to 25 cm. The Clear View I was further modified with larger lens diameters, the objective lens was increased to 11 mm, and the ocular lens was increased to 8 mm. With the introduction of these slightly larger diameters, the Clear View I design became known as the Clear View II design (Figure B-7). Table B-6 lists the current specifications of the Clear View II systems.

One of the difficulties in fitting the Clear View telescopic system is that, due to its small lens diameter and the Galilean design, the field of view is small and the exit pupil is therefore extremely small and difficult to align in the higher powers. Hoeft designed a special fitting frame for the Clear View I telescopic systems that allowed for a horizontal movement of the system in the frame to achieve a precise alignment.[1] The special fitting frame can also be used on the newer Clear View II telescopic units.

A unique feature of the Clear View system is that the telescope is mounted to the carrier lens in an adjustable collet pivot ring locking system. The pivot ring acts as a ball-in-socket joint that allows small micro-adjustments in

TABLE B-3
Specifications of Full-Diameter Designs for Vision* Galilean Telescopes

Telescope	Magnification	Objective Lens Size (mm)	Field (degrees)
Full diameter	1.3×	20.0	18
Full diameter	1.7×	35.0	28
Full diameter	2.2×	25.4	16
Full diameter	3.0×	20.0	8
Full diameter	4.0×	20.0	6
Wide-angle full diameter	2.2×	33.0	16
Wide-angle full diameter	3.0×	33.0	11

*Available from Designs for Vision, Inc., Ronkonkoma, NY.

TABLE B-4
Specifications of Bioptic Designs for Vision* Nonfocusable Galilean Telescopes

Telescope	Magnification	Objective Lens Diameter (mm)	Field (degrees)
Bioptic	1.7×	23.3×15.1	18
Bioptic (Model I)	2.2×	23.3×15.1	16
Bioptic (Model II)	2.2×	12.7	11
Bioptic	3.0×	20.0	8
Bioptic	4.0×	20.0	6
Wide-angle bioptic	2.2×	33.0×20.0	16
Wide-angle bioptic	3.0×	33.0×20.0	11

*Available from Designs for Vision, Inc., Ronkonkoma, NY.

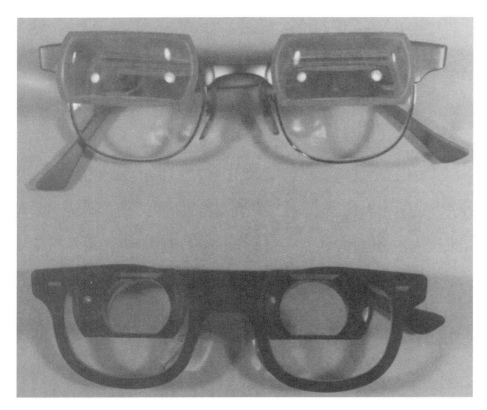

FIGURE B-4. **The upper device shows the Designs for Vision, Inc. 2.2× wide-angle Galilean bioptic (Ronkonkoma, NY) with a "clear housing" whereas the lower device demonstrates a 3.0× wide-angle Galilean bioptic with a "black housing."**

Distance Telescopes

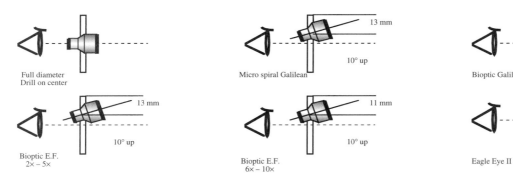

Full diameter
Drill on center

Micro spiral Galilean   13 mm   10° up

Bioptic Galilean   9 mm   10° up

Bioptic E.F.
2× – 5×   13 mm   10° up

Bioptic E.F.
6× – 10×   11 mm   10° up

Eagle Eye II   11 mm   10° up

Reading Telescopes

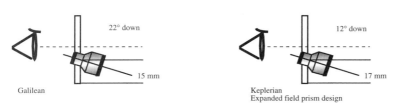

Galilean   22° down   15 mm

Keplerian
Expanded field prism design   12° down   17 mm

FIGURE B-5.   **The Designs for Vision, Inc. telescopic drilling chart (Ronkonkoma, NY). (E.F. = expanded field.)**

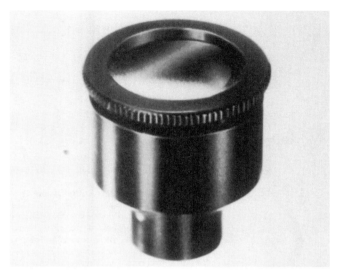

FIGURE B-6. **The Spiral Focus Galilean telescope (Designs for Vision, Inc., [DVI], Ronkonkoma, NY) allows for focusability that the standard DVI Galilean telescopes do not offer.**

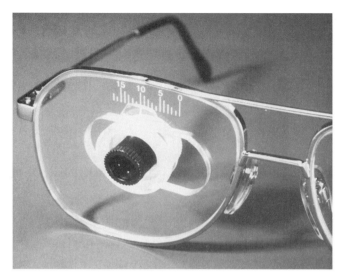

FIGURE B-7. **The Clear View II telescope (Designs for Vision, Inc., Ronkonkoma, NY) in its special fitting trial frame.**

TABLE B-5
**Specifications of the Designs for Vision*
Spiral Focus Galilean Telescopes**

Magnification	Objective Lens Diameter (mm)	Field (degrees)
1.7×	25.4	20
2.2×	15.9	11
3.0×	20.0	8
4.0×	20.0	6

*Available from Designs for Vision, Inc., Ronkonkoma, NY.

TABLE B-6
Specifications of the Clear View II Galilean Systems*

Magnification	Objective Lens Size (mm)	Field (degrees)
2.2×	11	7.0
2.7×	11	8.5
3.3×	11	5.7
4.0×	11	5.2
5.0×	11	4.5
6.0×	11	3.5

*Available from Designs for Vision, Inc., Ronkonkoma, NY.

the alignment of the system. Depending on the magnification of the unit, the pivot-ring collet allows up to a 30-degree axis tilt. When a corrective lens incorporating cylinder is placed into the telescope, there is a white line to indicate the axis alignment.

Although the Clear View lens is small enough to be positioned anywhere in the frame, Hoeft recommends that if the bioptic superior position is used, the optical axis of the system should be positioned 6 to 9 mm above the pupil.

Expanded-Field Spiral Focus Telescopes
The spiral focus spectacle-mounted telescopes are Keplerian in design and are manufactured with black housings only. The telescopes can be placed in any position or at any angle in the carrier lens; however, a full-diameter or bioptic position mounting is the most commonly prescribed. All of the telescopes are capable of having a patient's prescription incorporated into the system and allow a close focus to approximately 25 cm (Figure B-8).

If the bioptic position is chosen, it is again recommended that 3 mm be allowed between the top of the carrier lens and the top rim of the ocular. Although the standard inclination angle is 10 degrees up, there is a difference in the lower-powered expanded field units and

the higher-powered expanded-field units in the drilling positions as is illustrated in the drilling diagrams (see Figure B-5). The 2.0×, 3.0×, 4.0×, and 5.0× expanded-field units have their optical centers placed 13 mm from the top of the carrier in the standard bioptic position, whereas the higher powers of the 6.0×, 7.0×, 8.0×, and 10.0× units are drilled so that the optical center is located only 11 mm from the top of the carrier in the standard position. The lower-powered units have 18-mm-diameter oculars while the higher powers have smaller 14-mm-diameter oculars.

Table B-7 lists the specifications of the Expanded-Field Spiral Focus telescopes.

Honey Bee Lens Telescope
The Honey Bee lens grew out of the development of what was called the *Multi-Directional lens* described by Feinbloom in 1960.[2] Introduced in 1982 by Feinbloom and Brilliant, the Honey Bee lens is a spectacle-mounted, triple telescopic, Galilean system that gives the patient the largest visual field available in the respective powers of 3.0× and 4.0×. The lateral telescopes have thick base-in prisms mounted on their objective lenses (Figure B-9A, B). The purpose of the lateral prisms is to shift the fields of the right and left telescopes in such a manner that the fields

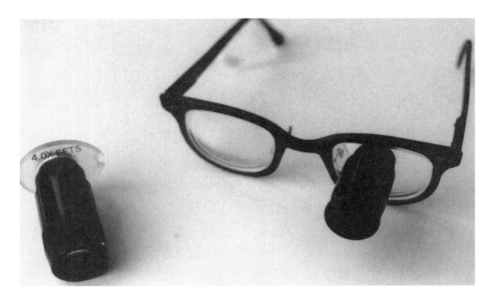

FIGURE B-8.   **The Designs for Vision, Inc. Expanded-Field Spiral Focus Keplerian telescopic series (Ronkonkoma, NY) are available in a number of magnifications. Shown here is the 3× monocular system mounted in a Yeoman frame and a 4× system mounted in a trial ring (which can be placed in a standard trial frame).**

of the three telescopes become merged into a larger continuous field. There is an area of blindness (scotoma area) that exists between the fields of the lateral and central telescopic fields (Figure B-9C). As described by Feinbloom,[2] the Multi-Directional lens (the possible forerunner to the Honey Bee lens) seemed designed for a rotating eye: "While the eye is alternating fixation from one system to the other in its panoramic gaze, the images through the other two systems are also registering on the retina to give increased information as to detail, position, and movement in the other directions." The Honey Bee telescope is designed to be used in a bioptic position. Correction lenses cannot be incorporated into this telescope. Table B-8 lists the specifications for the Honey Bee telescope.

Bailey has questioned the benefits of the Honey Bee lens, even though it provides a wider field.[3] In general, Galilean telescopes do not have the image brightness and image clarity across their fields as do the Keplerian designs. So although the absolute field may be larger in the Honey Bee, the field of view, which by convention is defined as the field of at least one-half illumination (50% vignetting zone) may not be as useable. Substantial chromatic aberration is also introduced by the base-in prisms in the lateral objective lenses.

Eagle Eye II Telescope

The Eagle Eye II telescopic system is a Galilean telescope that is especially designed to address the cosmetic issues plus allow for maximum fitting adjustability (Figure B-10). The telescope is exactly the same optical design as the 2.2× Model II bioptic telescope, but is mounted into a unique ball-in-socket housing on the back surface of the carrier lens. This ball-in-socket housing allows the practitioner to easily align the optical axis of the telescope to the visual axis of the patient. Corrective lenses can be incorporated into the telescope. Table B-9 lists the specifications of this unit.

TABLE B-7
Specifications of the Expanded-Field Spiral Focus Telescopes*

Magnification	Objective Lens Diameter (mm)	Field (degrees)
2×	14.0	18.0
3×	14.0	14.0
4×	21.3	9.0
5×	21.3	8.0
6×	21.3	6.5
7×	21.3	5.0
8×	21.3	4.0
10×	21.3	2.5

*Available from Designs for Vision, Inc., Ronkonkoma, NY.

Edwards Optical Corporation (Virginia Beach, VA)

Bi-Level Telemicroscopic Apparatus

The Bi-Level Telemicroscopic Apparatus (BITA) is a miniature, focusable, Galilean telescope that has a unique patented bi-level positioning system that is mounted in a tinted carrier (Figure B-11). This spectacle-mounted telescope was designed originally for cosmesis. It gains additional advantage, however, in that the telescope is positioned and angled in the carrier lens so that the patient's line of sight is slightly below the miniaturized telescope, allowing both a magnified and unmagnified view of the same distance object simultaneously. The proximity of the two views allows for the perception of the object in the field without loss of peripheral field, depth perception, or spatial orientation.[4]

Currently, three different objective diameter sizes are available. The sizes are shown in Table B-10, which also lists the specifications of the telescopes.

There are a number of different methods for determining the position of the BITA unit in the frame to achieve a bilevel position. One method has the patient fixate on a distant object while the practitioner uses a felt-tip marker to

FIGURE B-9. The Honey Bee lens (Designs for Vision, Inc., Ronkonkoma, NY) is a Galilean telescope available in 3× and 4× magnifications. A. Front view of the Honey Bee telescope. B. Rear view of the Honey Bee telescope. C. The field properties of the Honey Bee telescope.

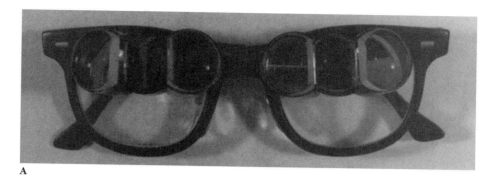

A

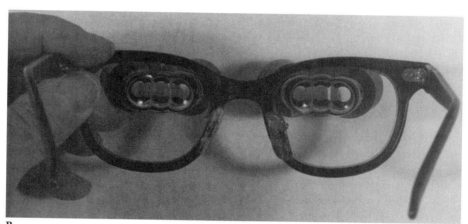

B

Honey Bee lens — without prisms

Honey Bee lens — with prisms

C

TABLE B-8
Specifications for the Honey Bee Galilean Telescope*

Magnification	Objective Lens Diameter (mm)	Field (degrees)
3×	48.9×20	24
4×	53.5×20	18

*Available from Designs for Vision, Inc., Ronkonkoma, NY.

TABLE B-9
Specifications of the Eagle Eye II Galilean Telescope*

Magnification	Objective Lens Diameter (mm)	Field (degrees)
2.2×	12.7	11

*Available from Designs for Vision, Inc., Ronkonkoma, NY.

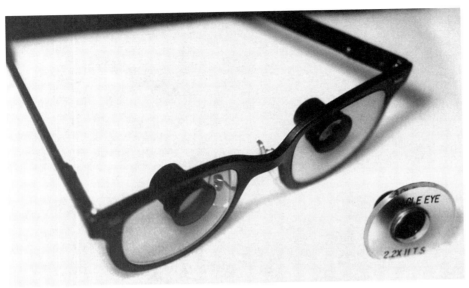

A

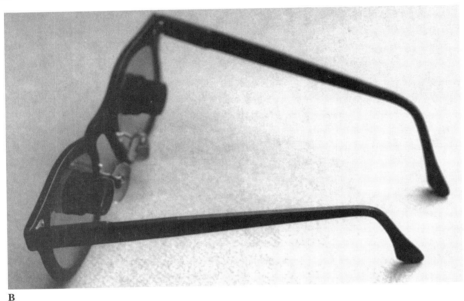

B

FIGURE B-10.   **The 2.2× Eagle Eye II telescopic system (Designs for Vision, Inc., Ronkonkoma, NY) showing the ball-in-socket housing that allows for adjustment in alignment. A. Front view. B. Rear view.**

dot the approximate location of the center of the pupil of the patient's dominant eye. This dotted position is used as a starting reference point in placing a strip of opaque tape, with a small hole in it centered over the dot. The tape can be moved on the carrier lens to fine-tune the position, so that the center of the hole is perfectly lined up with the patient's line of sight while looking at a distant target. If binocular units are being prescribed, the measurements can be made on each eye independently so that the final perspective will be one fused hole when viewing the distant target. Variations on this "tape method" of alignment include using a pupillometer and small filter dots, which can adhere to the carrier lens. These dots are initially placed according to the pupillometer reading and then moved (vertically or horizontally) to align with the patient's line of sight while he or she is fixating on a distant object. These positions, indicated by the alignment techniques, will

determine the exact position of the line of sight. The laboratory technician will take this information and drill the hole for the bilevel position between 3 mm and 5 mm above these marked positions. To determine how much the frame is angled, Edwards Optical recommends using the perpendicular reference indicator, which is a small protractor measuring device that can easily attach to the temple of the frame. A reading is taken while the patient is actually wearing the frame, and this information is sent along with the line of sight position to the laboratory.

Eschenbach Optik of America, Inc. (Ridgefield, CT)

Spectacle-Mounted Telescopes
Eschenbach has two fixed-focus Galilean 2.2× telescopes that are available with reading caps, and two focusable

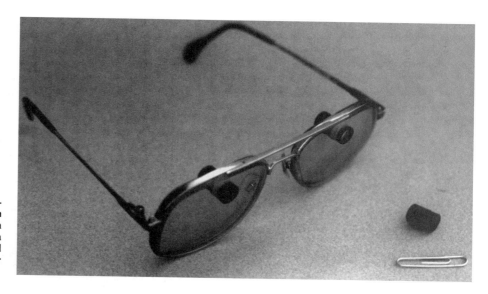

FIGURE B-11.   A 4×, ⅜-in. binocular Bi-Level Telemicroscopic Apparatus system (Edwards Optical Corporation, Virginia Beach, VA) is mounted in a frame while a 3×, ⅜-in. system is shown in foreground (compared to the size of a small paper clip).

Galilean telescopes in powers of 3.0× and 4.0×. The fixed-focus telescopes are available in two models: Model 1621-1, which is the 2.2×23 having a 16-degree field of view; and Model 1621, a 2.2×23 telescope that has a 14-degree field of view (Figure B-12A). Reading caps can be supplied over the base afocal fixed-focus distance units to make the systems focal for near. The focusable Galilean units include the 3.0×23 (Model 1633-3), which has a 9.5-degree field of view; and the 4×23 (Model 1633-4), which has a 7.5-degree field of view (Figure B-12B). The focusable Galilean units are capable of focusing as close as 71 cm (28 in.). The telescopes can be placed in spectacle lenses and mounted into frames via a specialized mounting kit available from the manufacturer. A patient's refractive correction can be incorporated into the eyepiece of the telescopes.

Eschenbach also manufactures one fixed-focus and four focusable Keplerian models. All of the Keplerian telescopic units are capable of spectacle mounting using the same methods described for Galilean units. Table B-11 lists the specifications for both types of systems.

Headborne Galilean Telescopic Systems

Eschenbach manufactures two Galilean binocular telescopic units in magnifications for 3× and 4×. These systems are ideal for watching television as they are spectacle mounted, lightweight, and come in a special frame that features an adjustable bridge and an adjustable bar for the pupillary distance. The pupillary distance range is from 54 mm to 74 mm (Figure B-13). The 3.0× system is also available as a clip-on monocular (Model 1635) (see Appendix A). Table B-12 lists the specifications of the binocular telescopic systems.

Keeler Instruments, Inc. (Broomall, PA)

Spectacle-Mounted Telescopes

Keeler Instruments, Inc. manufactures spectacle-mounted telescopes that can be mounted to a frame via a threaded

sleeve that has been cemented to the front surface of a corrective carrier lens. The telescope is then screwed into the threaded sleeve (Figure B-14). The threaded sleeves can be ordered as angled, which allows the telescope to be positioned upward. The smaller 2.8× and 4.2× Panfocal telescopes (see Appendix A) can be used as either hand-held monoculars or be spectacle mounted by the method just mentioned. Table B-13 lists the specifications of the Keeler spectacle-mounted telescopes.

The Multi-Cap Telescope from Keeler is a series within the Keeler Vision Enhancement System that is designed to provide a focus at varying working distances (Figure B-15). The distance system is a 1.75× Galilean unit. This telescope can be spectacle mounted by use of the threaded sleeve. The caps attach to the front of the telescope and provide

TABLE B-10
Specifications of the Bi-Level Telemicroscopic Apparatus (Galilean)*

Magnification	Objective Lens Diameter	Field (degrees)
2.5×	⁵⁄₁₆ in.	9.0
3.0×	⁵⁄₁₆ in.	8.0
3.3×	⁵⁄₁₆ in.	7.0
4.0×	⁵⁄₁₆ in.	6.0
5.0×	⁵⁄₁₆ in.	4.5
6.0×	⁵⁄₁₆ in.	4.0
2.5×	⅜ in.	9.0
3.0×	⅜ in.	8.5
3.3×	⅜ in.	8.5
4.0×	⅜ in.	8.0
5.0×	⅜ in.	6.0
6.0×	⅜ in.	5.5
2.5×	½ in.	10.5
3.0×	½ in.	9.0
3.3×	½ in.	8.5
4.0×	½ in.	8.5
5.0×	½ in.	7.0
6.0×	½ in.	6.5

*Available from Edwards Optical Corporation, Virginia Beach, VA.

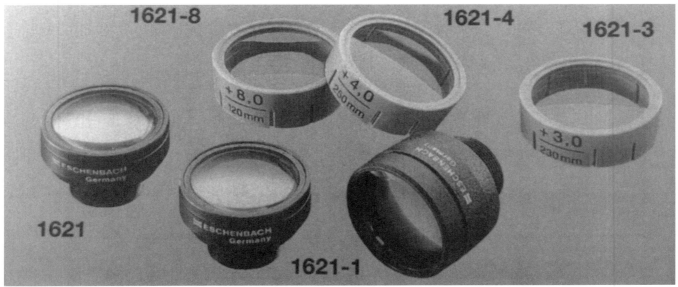

A

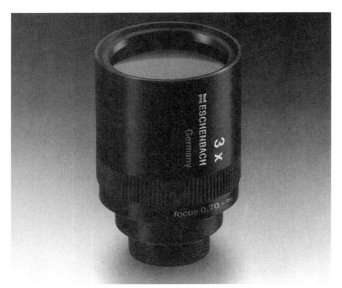

B

FIGURE B-12. **A. The Eschenbach model 1621 is a 2.2×23 Galilean telescope (Eschenbach Optik of America, Inc., Ridgefield, CT). The 1621-1 model is also a Galilean telescope; however, it has a slightly larger field. As shown, reading caps are also available. B. Focusable Galilean telescopes include the 3.0×23 (Model 1633-3) and 4.0×23 (Model 1633-4).**

TABLE B-11.
Specifications for the Eschenbach Spectacle-Mounted Telescopes*

Magnification	Catalogue No.	Field (degrees)	Exit Pupil (mm)	Type	Focal Distance
2.2×	1621	14.0	10.45	G	Afocal
2.2×	1621-1	16.0	10.45	G	Afocal
3.0×	1633-3	9.5	7.60	G	Infinity to 71 cm
4.0×	1633-4	7.5	5.80	G	Infinity to 71 cm
3.1×	1672-5	12.5	7.42	K	71 cm
2.8×	1672-1	12.5	2.90	K	Infinity to 15 cm
4.2×	1672-2	10.0	2.50	K	Infinity to 20 cm
4.2×	1672-3	12.5	3.00	K	Infinity to 20 cm
6.0×	1672-4	10.5	2.66	K	Infinity to 25 cm

G = Galilean; K = Keplerian.
*Available from Eschenbach Optik of America, Inc., Ridgefield, CT.

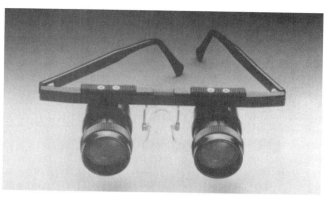

FIGURE B-13.   The Eschenbach binocular Galilean system is available in two magnifications, 3× and 4×. (Courtesy of Eschenbach Optik of America, Inc., Ridgefield, CT.)

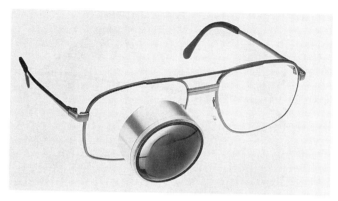

FIGURE B-14.   Keeler telescopes can be mounted to a spectacle lens via a threaded sleeve that is mounted to the front surface of the lens. Shown here is the Rapid Focus Telescope (LVA-50-1). (Courtesy of Keeler Instruments, Inc., Broomall, PA.)

near viewing. Each cap has two lenses, a fixed +0.50 D lens for viewing television at 2 m, and a flip-down lens for reading, which varies from +4.00 D to +9.00 D. The intermediate cap consists of a +1.00 D lens for viewing at 1 m and a +1.00 D, flip-down lens for 50 cm (two +1.00 D lenses combined). When the caps are used together, the caps and telescope combination has the total magnification designated as the lens cap.

M-Tech Optics Corporation (Royal Oak, MI)

Panavex Telescopes
The Panavex telescopic systems are focusable Galilean telescopes in design (Figure B-16). They use one mirror

and one right angle prism to deviate the light path. Currently, there are three magnifications available with the parameters listed in Table B-14.

Note that all systems use the same objective lens. The objective is an achromatic hyperconvex lens. The eyepiece is composed of a double concave lens. Antireflective coatings are placed on the objective and ocular lenses, as well as the mirror, and the surface (hypotenuse) of the prism. Spherical refractive errors from +10.00 D to −10.00 D may be corrected for with focusing of the telescope.

The near focus is achieved with the use of a precision cam lever. This provides forward movement of the objective achromatic lens, allowing the afocal system to become focal to approximately 12 in. (30.5 cm).

TABLE B-12
Specifications of the Eschenbach Headborne Galilean Telescopic Systems*

Magnification	Catalogue No.	Field (degrees)	Exit Pupil (mm)	Focus Range
3×	1634-3	9.0	7.66	Infinity to 70 cm
4×	1634-4	7.5	5.75	Infinity to 70 cm

*Available from Eschenbach Optik of America, Inc., Ridgefield, CT.

TABLE B-13
Specifications of the Keeler Spectacle-Mounted Telescopes*

Description	Catalogue No.	Magnification	Field (degrees)	Type	Near Focus
Rapid Focus Telescope	LVA-S0-1	1.9×	23	G	42 cm
Multi-Cap Telescope	LVA-S1-1	1.75×	20	G	infinity
"TV" Cap/"Flip-Down" Cap					
+0.50 D/+4.00 D	LVA-S1-2	2.00×	—	—	22.2 cm/200 cm
+0.50 D/+6.50 D	LVA-S1-3	3.00×	—	—	14.3 cm/200 cm
+0.50 D/+9.00 D	LVA-S1-4	4.00×	—	—	10.5 cm/200 cm
+1.00 D/+1.00 D	LVA-S1-1+1	0.875×	—	—	50.00 cm/100 cm

G = Galilean.
*Available from Keeler Instruments, Inc., Broomall, PA.

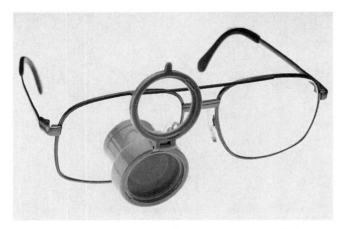

FIGURE B-15.   The Multi-Cap Telescope (LVA-51-1) is designed to provide focus at varying working distances. The distance system is a 1.75× Galilean telescope. (Courtesy of Keeler Instruments, Inc., Broomall, PA.)

Nikon Optics (Melville, NY)

Spectacle-Mounted Telescopes
Nikon has designed its main telescopic unit as a 2× system that is available in either a metal housing (Main Testing lens) or a plastic housing (Main Personal lens). The only difference between these two units is that the plastic Main Personal lens weighs less and has a slightly larger field of view (Figure B-17).

Testing is done with the 2× focusable metal telescope. Small spherical errors can be compensated for by adjustment of the length of the telescope. Astigmatic correction can be added behind the ocular lens if necessary with −1.00, −2.00, −3.00, or −4.00 D cylinder caps. Reading caps can be added for near viewing if desired. Caps are available in +6.00, +8.00, +10.00, +12.00, and +16.00 D. Caps

TABLE B-14
Specifications of the Panavex Galilean Telescopic Systems*

Magnification	Tube Length (mm)	Objective	Eyepiece	Field (degrees)
2.5×	18.0	+33.33 D	−83.33 D	21.75
3.3×	20.9	+33.33 D	−110.05 D	14.46
4.0×	22.5	+33.33 D	−133.3 D	11.16

*Available from M-Tech Optics Corporation, Royal Oak, MI.

are rated with effective magnification (M = D/4) and are labeled as the total magnification when combined with the 2× main telescopic unit (e.g., [2×] [+8.00/4] = 4×). Thus, the +8.00 D cap is labeled 4×.

When testing with the 2× main testing metal system has been completed, the final prescription is available for the patient in a 2× plastic system, with or without near reading caps. Tables B-15 and B-16 list the available specifications.

Ocutech, Inc. (Chapel Hill, NC)

Horizontal Light Path Vision Enhancing System
The Horizontal Light Path Vision Enhancing System (HLP-VES) is a Keplerian telescope that appears as if it were a horizontal periscope lying across the top of a spectacle frame (Figure B-18). The optics of the HLP-VES include a right-angle prism, an achromatic doublet objective (which is moveable to focus the system), a roof-penta-prism, and a Kellner two-lens, three-element eyepiece. The telescope has the ability to correct for refractive errors from +12.00 D to −12.00 D by focusing the telescope. For patients with higher prescriptions or astigmatism, a correction can be incorporated at the eyepiece of the telescope.

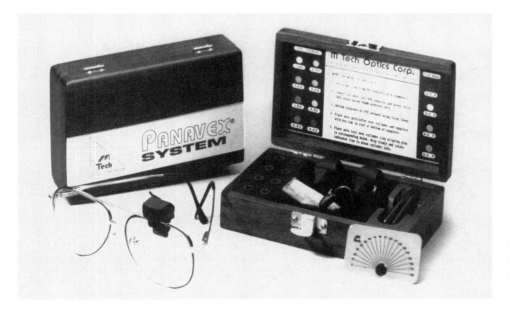

FIGURE B-16.   The Panavex system is a focusable Galilean telescope designed as a periscopic device. It is available in three magnifications. (Courtesy of M-Tech Optics Corporation, Royal Oak, MI.)

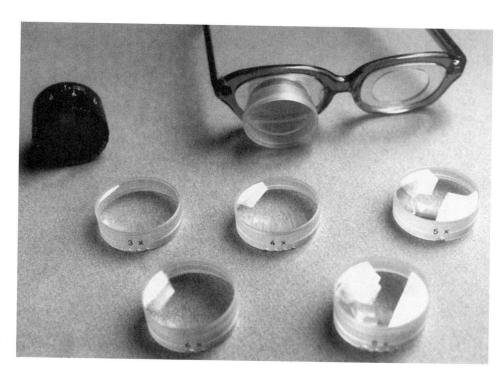

FIGURE B-17. **The Nikon 2× Main Testing/Main Personal telescopic system (Nikon Optics, Melville, NY) with reading caps.**

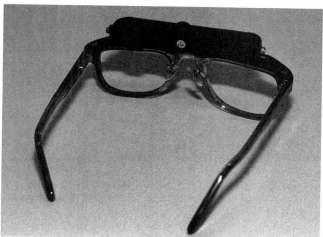

FIGURE B-18. **The rear view of the Horizontal Light Path Vision Enhancing System (Ocutech, Inc., Chapel Hill, NC). This Keplerian telescope lies across the top of the spectacle frame.**

TABLE B-15
Specifications of the Nikon Spectacle-Mounted Telescopes*

Telescope	Field (degrees)
2× Main Testing Telescope (metal)	17.2
2× Main Personal Telescope (plastic)	20.0

*Available from Nikon Optics, Melville, NY.

TABLE B-16
Specifications for Reading Caps for the Nikon Spectacle-Mounted Telescopes*

Reading Cap (D)	Magnification with 2× Telescope	Working Distance (cm)	Field of View (mm)
+6.00	3×	16.60	56
+8.00	4×	12.50	42
+10.00	5×	10.00	34
+12.00	6×	8.33	28
+16.00	8×	6.25	21

*Available from Nikon Optics, Melville, NY.

TABLE B-17
Specifications of the Horizontal Light Path Vision Enhancing System (Keplerian)*

Magnification	Field (degrees)	Focus Range
3×	11.5	Infinity to 18.0 cm
4×	10.0	Infinity to 30.5 cm
6×	8.0	Infinity to 30.5 cm

*Available through Ocutech, Inc., Chapel Hill, NC.

One of the design principles of the HLP-VES was to produce a cosmetically acceptable system that did not protrude forward and reduced the weight of the system. The HLP-VES distributes the weight over the top of the eyeglass frame and balances the entire weight of the unit. Three magnifications are available and the specifications are listed in Table B-17.

The HLP-VES unit is designed for in-office testing, fitting, and dispensing. The pupillary distance is adjusted by sliding the telescope to the right or left on the special mounting bracket attached to the frame. The desired position is then set by tightening the set screws. The angle

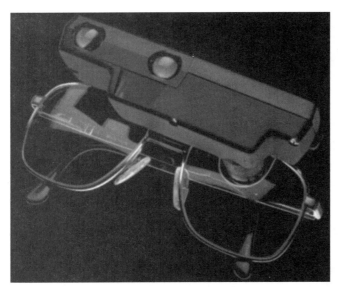

FIGURE B-19.   **The VES-AF system is available in 4× magnification and provides continuous focus from infinity to 12 in. The battery pack, which is the size of a cigarette pack, is not shown in this photo.** (Courtesy of Ocutech, Inc., Chapel Hill, NC.)

of inclination of the telescope and the vertex distance can be controlled by loosening the screws at each end of the telescopic unit, which is also attached to the mounting bracket. The telescope is a monocular system only. The telescope is simply flipped over if testing or fitting of the other eye is desired.

The telescope can be mounted in the standard bioptic position or, by using an alternate mounting bracket, can be mounted in a lower, full-diameter position. Pediatric frame styles are also available.

Vision Enhancing System–Autofocus
In 1996, Ocutech, Inc. introduced the Vision Enhancing System–Autofocus (VES-AF) bioptic spectacle-mounted telescope (Figure B-19). The autofocus or self-focusing system may address the difficulties of manual focusing devices. The visually impaired population often have difficulty focusing a

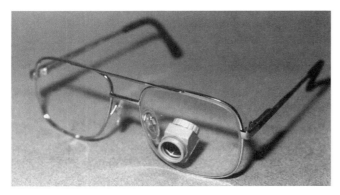

FIGURE B-21.   **The Behind-the-Lens telescope (Optical Designs, Inc., Houston, TX) is available in magnifications of 3× and 4×. Typically, the objective lens sits flush with the front surface of the carrier lens and is positioned in the bifocal position.**

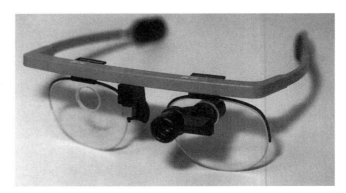

FIGURE B-20.   **The Vision Enhancing System Mini Telescope (Ocutech, Inc., Chapel Hill, NC) is available in 3× magnification and is shown here in its special fitting trial frame.**

telescopic device. When the telescope is used for near objects, the focusing demands are greater and constant refocusing is necessary. For these reasons, the autofocus may increase the acceptance of the telescope for both occupational and avocational use.

The VES-AF uses an infrared system that emits an invisible infrared beam of light that reflects off of the object being viewed and onto a detector on the front of the telescope. The automatic range finder (system software) determines the distance of the object from the patient and conveys this information to the motor, which moves the focusing lens to the appropriate position of focus.

The VES-AF provides a continuous focus from infinity to 12 in. and is exactly the same unit as the 4.0× HLP-VES unit. The telescope is not interchangeable as the HLP-VES, and therefore, when ordering the VES-AF, the eye being prescribed for must be specified. Its system features a focus sample rate of more than 30 times per second with a focus speed of less than one-third of a second between any two points. The focusable unit is powered by a rechargeable nicad battery pack. The battery is capable of 12 hours of continuous use. The telescope has a weight of 2.5 oz and the battery pack has a weight of 4 oz.

Vision Enhancing System–Mini
The VES-Mini is a miniature 3.0× Keplerian telescope with a 15-degree field of view. The unit is focusable to 12 in. (30.5 cm) and can compensate for refractive errors from +12.00 D to –12.00 D. The units may be fitted monocularly or binocularly and reading caps and filters are available as accessory items (Figure B-20).

Optical Designs, Inc. (Houston, TX)

Behind-the-Lens Telescope
The Behind-the-Lens (BTL) telescopic unit was developed to address the cosmetic objections that many patients have concerning spectacle-mounted telescopes.[5, 6] The original placement of the system was behind the spectacle carrier lens in an inferior or inferior temporal position. Typically, the objective lens was fit flush with the front surface of the carrier lens (Figure B-21). This telescope is of Keplerian

TABLE B-18
Specifications of the Behind-the-Lens Telescope*

Magnification	Field (degrees)	Focus Range
3.30×	9	Infinity to 25 cm
4.25×	9	Infinity to 30 cm

*Available from Optical Designs, Inc., Houston, TX.

design with the eyepiece consisting of a biaspheric lens. The objective lens is an achromatic doublet. Table B-18 lists the specifications for this telescope.

The finished system has the telescope mounted 15 mm temporal and 10 mm inferior from the patient's pupil center when looking straight ahead. This inferior temporal position of the telescope required the patient to make a 36-degree rotation of the eye to look through the telescope to see what is straight ahead (or in the direction that the nose is pointing). Currently, a simple inferior fitting position is recommended, requiring no lateral head movement. The eyepiece is focusable to correct for a patient's refractive error between −17.00 D and +50.00 D. Only a pupillary distance is necessary to fit the BTL telescope. The fitting kit comes with two frames with plano lenses that are drilled to fit all pupillary distances.

For patients with reduced peripheral fields (e.g., retinitis pigmentosa) either telescope can be reversed in the hole of the carrier lens so that the patient is looking through the objective lens rather then the ocular lens. This reversal can be accomplished because the housing for both the objective and ocular lenses is the same size. When looking through the reversed telescope, the patient

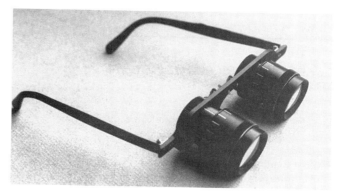

FIGURE B-22.   **The Selsi Sportglass (Sensi Company, Inc., Midland Park, NJ) is a binocular headborne Galilean telescope that is available in two magnifications, 2.5× and 2.8×.**

is able to obtain an apparent increase in his or her visual field of view (through minification).

Selsi Company, Inc., (Midland Park, NJ)

Sport Spectacles
Selsi Company is a distributor for both a 2.5× and a 2.8× Galilean, headborne, binocular spectacles (Sport Glasses) (Figure B-22). These units have a limited pupillary distance adjustment and a small range of refractive error correction from +2.00 D to −8.00 D (Table B-19).

TABLE B-19
Specification of the Selsi Sport Spectacles (Galilean)*

Magnification	Objective Lens Diameter (mm)	Field (degrees)	Exit Pupil (mm)	Range of Focus
2.5×	23	20.5	9.20	Infinity to 100 cm
2.8×	26	16.0	9.29	Infinity to 200 cm

*Available from Selsi Company, Inc., Midland Park, NJ.

REFERENCES

1. Hoeft WW. The Microspiral Galilean Telescope. In BP Rosenthal, RG Cole (eds), A Structured Approach to Low Vision Care. Philadelphia: Lippincott, 1991;490–494.
2. Feinbloom W. A new multi-directional lens for the aid of the partially blind. J N Y Optom Assoc 1961;39:8–11.
3. Bailey IL. The Honey Bee lens: a study of its field properties. Optom Monthly 1982;73:275–278.
4. Williams DR. The Bi-Level Telemicroscopic Apparatus (BITA). In BP Rosenthal, RG Cole (eds), A Structured Approach to Low Vision Care. Philadelphia: Lippincott, 1991;495–503.
5. Rosenthal BP, Hoeft WW. A Functional Approach to the Fitting of Spectacle Mounted Telescopic Systems. In RG Cole, BP Rosenthal (eds), Remediation and Management of Low Vision. St. Louis: Mosby, 1996;267–278.
6. Spitzberg L, Jose R, Kuether C. Behind the lens telescope: a new concept in bioptics. Optom Vis Sci 1989;66:616–620.

COMMONLY PRESCRIBED SPECTACLE-MOUNTED TELEMICROSCOPES

Designs for Vision, Inc. (Ronkonkoma, NY)

Near Telescopic Systems
Theoretically, any of the Designs for Vision telescopes can be modified to be a telemicroscope. All of the bioptic or full-field telescopes can be modified with the addition of a reading cap to the front objective lens. In addition, in the spiral focus Galilean and spiral focus expanded-field telescopes of Keplerian design, a near focus can be achieved by lengthening the tube length of the telescope.

There are, however, a few systems that have been designed as "reading" or "surgical" telescopes for special applications. Designs for Vision manufactures three reading telescopes of the Galilean design. They are listed as 2.5×, 3.5×, and 4.5× (Figure C-1). The telescopes are composed of the standard bioptic telescope (Model I). The telescopic objectives of these bioptic models have been altered to increase the objective power. Any working distance can be ordered for these telescopes. The manufacturer has listed the power as 2.5×, 3.5×, and 4.5× when in fact, however, the afocal telescopic portion uses the 2.2×, 3.0×, and 4.0× afocal systems, which are then modified by increasing the power of the objective lens for the needed near focal distance.

These Galilean telemicroscopes are generally mounted low in the carrier lens, with the standard position of the optical center of the ocular lens being 15 mm above the bottom of the carrier lens and the standard angle of declination being 22 degrees below the horizontal plane (see Figure B-5). If these units are fit binocularly, they must be converged and collimated for the working distance for which they are prescribed. The Englemann method is recommended to determine the near functional interpupillary distance.

Reading telemicroscopes have also been designed using the Keplerian telescopes ranging in magnification from 2.5× to 10.0×. The magnification in these telemicroscopes is listed as 2.5×, 3.5×, 4.5×, 6×, 8×, and 10×, when in reality, the 2×, 3.0×, 4.0×, 6×, 8×, 10× units are the telescopic components (Figure C-2). These systems, also known as *Expanded-Field Prism Design Reading Telescopes*, can be prescribed either monocularly or binocularly. The telescopes are mounted in the standard position with the optical center of the eyepiece 17 mm above the bottom of the carrier lens with an angle of declination of 12 degrees (see Figure B-5).

Eschenbach Optik of America, Inc., (Ridgefield, CT)

Near Telescopic Systems
Eschenbach Keplerian telemicroscopes are available in powers of 2.8×, 4.2×, or 6.0× as focusable units or the fixed-focus Keplerian 3.1× (Model 1672-5) with the addition of reading caps. Reading caps (Series 1621) fit over the 23-mm objective lens and range from +3.00 D up to +16.00 D. The Keplerian focusable 4.2× model is available in two objective diameters, either 10 mm or 12 mm. The 1625 mounting kit is used for binocular prescribing of the Keplerian models. The Keplerian units, which are focusable, can be binocularly mounted into spectacle frames with the use of convergence adaptors preset for 20 cm, 25 cm, or 33 cm working distances.

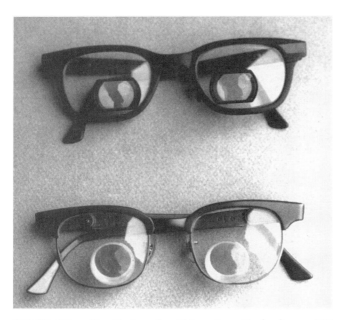

FIGURE C-1. **The Designs for Vision, Inc. (Ronkonkoma, NY) Galilean reading telescopes are available in 2.5×, 3.5×, and 4.5×. The upper system shown is a 2.5× (rectangular shape only in 2.5×) reading telescope with a "black housing," and the lower system is a 3.5× reading telescope with a "clear housing."**

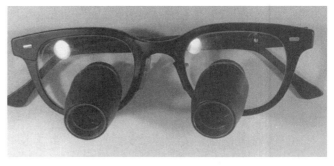

FIGURE C-2. **The Designs for Vision, Inc. (Ronkonkoma, NY) Keplerian reading telescopes are available in magnifications that range from 2.5× through 10×. Note the tube length of the Keplerian telescopes as compared to the Galilean systems seen in Figure C-1.**

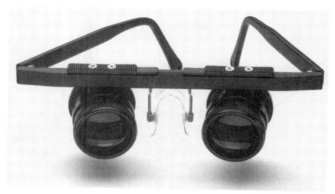

FIGURE C-3.   The Eschenbach Galilean telemicroscopes are available in magnifications of 2.5×, 3.0×, and 4.0×. They are premounted in a frame that allows for adjustment of the interpupillary distance. Note the similarity to the Eschenbach binocular telescope in Figure B-13, except that the telemicroscope has the telescopes converged for binocular near use.

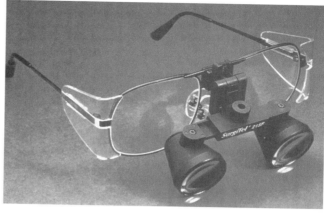

FIGURE C-4.   SurgiTel telemicroscopic systems are Galilean in design and range in magnification from 2.15× to 5.00×. (Courtesy of General Scientific Corporation, Ann Arbor, MI.)

TABLE C-1
Specifications for the Eschenbach Galilean Near Telescopic Systems*

Magnification	Model No.	Field (degrees)	Working Distance (cm)
2.5×	1636-2	15.0	7.5 to 35
3.0×	1636-3	12.5	4.5 to 20
4.0×	1636-4	8.0	3.5 to 25

*Available from Eschenbach Optik of America, Inc., Ridgefield, CT.

Galilean telemicroscopes from Eschenbach can consist of either the fixed-focus Galilean 2.2× (Models 1621 and 1621-1) with attached reading caps or the focusable Galilean units (1633 series) in powers of 3.0× and 4.0×. Units can be either monocular or binocular. The binocular near Galilean units in magnifications of 2.5×, 3.0×, and 4.0× (Model 1636 series) (Figure C-3) are premounted into a special frame that allows for the adjustment of the interpupillary distance. The units are preconverged and focusable with the specifications in Table C-1.

General Scientific Corporation (Ann Arbor, MI)

SurgiTel Magnification Systems
These telemicroscopic systems are Galilean in design (Figure C-4). They are small, lightweight, ergonomically designed systems in magnifications of 2.15×, 2.75×, 3.50×, and 5.0×. These magnifications refer to the telescopic *afocal* portion of the system.

The SurgiTel telemicroscopes are available in either a frame-mounted or headborne style. The system offers a pivotal adjustment for a flip-up feature and the ability to change the viewing angle of the scopes. In addition, the SurgiTel telemicroscope has sealed optics that allow for easier disinfecting (wiping with disinfectant and rinsing under running water). Table C-2 lists the SurgiTel specifications.

Heine USA, Ltd. (Dover, NH)

Near Binocular Loupes
Heine manufactures both Galilean and Keplerian binocular telescopic loupes (Figure C-5). The Galilean models

TABLE C-2
Specifications for the SurgiTel Galilean Telemicroscopes*

"Afocal" Telescopic Magnification	Total System Magnification (M25)	Model No.	Depth of Field (cm)	Working Distance (cm)
2.15×	1.70×	215N	24.0–46.2	31.6
2.15×	1.36×	215F	28.6–62.8	39.4
2.75×	2.22×	275N	25.0–40.4	30.9
2.75×	1.72×	275F	31.2–55.3	40.0
3.50×	2.95×	350N	25.2–36.2	29.7
3.50×	2.46×	350M	29.7–44.5	35.6
3.50×	2.18×	350F	33.1–51.2	40.2
5.00×	4.19×	500N	25.9–35.2	29.8
5.00×	3.50×	500M	30.6–42.7	35.6
5.00×	2.95×	500F	35.8–51.6	42.3

*Available from General Scientific Corporation, Ann Arbor, MI.

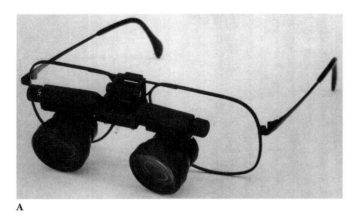

A

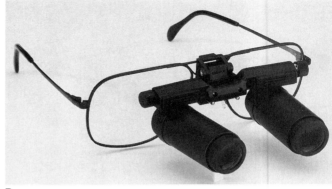

B

FIGURE C-5.   **Heine manufactures both Galilean (A) and Keplerian (B) binocular telemicroscopes that can be clipped on to most ophthalmic frames. (Courtesy of Heine USA Ltd., Dover, NH.)**

TABLE C-3
Specifications of the Heine Binocular Loupes*

Magnification	Model No.	Field (degrees)	Working Distance (cm)	Type
2.0×	c-00.32.111	13	42	G
2.5×	c-00.32.112	12	34	G
3.5×	c-00.32.113	9	42	K
4.0×	c-00.32.114	8	34	K
6.0×	c-00.32.115	7	34	K

G = Galilean; K = Keplerian.
*Available from Heine USA, Ltd., Dover, NH.

are available in 2.0× and 2.5× magnifications, and the Keplerian models are available in 3.5×, 4.0×, and 6.0× magnifications. A unique feature of the Heine binocular loupe is that the complete binocular loupe is available in a clip-on form that will fit most ophthalmic frames. The Universal Clip has an adjustable interpupillary distance from 50 mm to 70 mm. Table C-3 lists the specifications of the Heine binocular loupes.

Keeler Instruments, Inc. (Broomall, PA)

Near Telescopic Systems
In addition to the Multi-Cap Telescope discussed in Appendix B (see Figure B-15), Keeler also manufactures a Full-Field Near Telescope (LVA-22) that can be mounted monocularly using a threaded sleeve attachment. The magnifications range from 1.6× to 8.0×. Binocular forms are available in magnifications of 1.6×, 2×, and 3× for which the units may be fitted into special angled threaded sleeves for preset distances set to the proper convergence (Figure C-6). Table C-4 lists the specifications of the LVA-22 telemicroscopes.

Keeler also manufacturers the "Bar-Type" Near Telescope (LVA-21). With this near telescopic system, the working distance is constant and fixed at 15.5 cm. The magnification

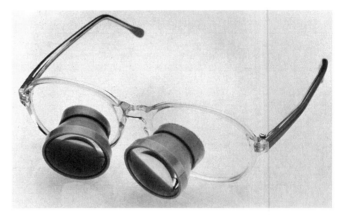

FIGURE C-6.   **The Keeler LVA-22 can be used binocularly by using specially designed, angled, treaded sleeves that are glued to the front surface of the carrier lens. (Courtesy of Keeler Instruments, Inc., Broomall, PA.)**

TABLE C-4
Specifications for the Keeler LVA-22 Telemicroscopes*

Magnification	Model No.	Field (cm)	Type	Working Distance (cm)
1.6×	LVA-22-1	12.0	G	21.5
2.0×	LVA-22-2	10.0	G	18.6
3.0×	LVA-22-3	6.5	G	14.0
4.0×	LVA-22-4	5.0	G	11.0
5.0×	LVA-22-5	4.0	G	9.5
6.0×	LVA-22-6	3.0	G	8.5
8.0×	LVA-22-7	2.2	G	7.0

G = Galilean.
*Available from Keeler Instruments, Inc., Broomall, PA.

varies from 2× through 5×. These units can be fit monocularly or binocularly using the glued-on threaded sleeve or a specially designed pupillary distance (PD) bar, which in turn attaches to a special frame. There are four sizes of PD bars that are preset and converged to the 15.5-cm working distance. Table C-5 lists the specifications of the LVA-21 series.

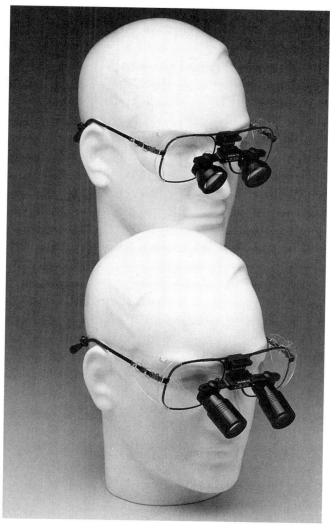

FIGURE C-7. **Keeler manufactures the Galilean Binocular Surgical Loupe (upper figure) and the Panoramic Binocular Keplerian Surgical Loupe (lower figure) in a number of magnifications. (Courtesy of Keeler Instruments, Inc., Broomall, PA.)**

TABLE C-5
Specifications for Keeler LVA-21 Bar-Type Near Telescope*

Magnification	Model No.	Field (cm)	Type	Working Distance (cm)
2×	LVA-21-1	9.0	G	15.5
3×	LVA-21-2	6.0	G	15.5
4×	LVA-21-3	3.5	G	15.5
5×	LVA-21-4	2.2	G	15.5

G = Galilean.
*Available from Keeler Instruments, Inc., Broomall, PA.

TABLE C-6
Specifications of the Keeler Keplerian Panoramic Loupes*

Magnification	Field (cm)	Working Distance (cm)
2.5×	8.5	34
2.5×	11.6	42
2.5×	12.2	46
2.5×	13.0	50
3.5×	6.6	34
3.5×	8.1	42
3.5×	8.9	46
3.5×	9.7	50
4.5×	4.2	34
4.5×	6.0	42
4.5×	6.6	46
4.5×	7.2	50
5.5×	3.8	34
5.5×	5.0	42
5.5×	5.5	46
5.5×	6.0	50

*Available from Keeler Instruments, Inc., Broomall, PA.

Panoramic Loupes

Keeler Panoramic Loupes are binocular, prefocused, telemicroscopic spectacles in Keplerian design that are secured to a lightweight frame (Figure C-7). The loupes have a total of five lenses in combination with a roof prism that provides distortion-free image resolution and edge-to-edge clarity in a lightweight system. There is an adjustable PD bar that allows the loupes to be accurately aligned for binocular vision. The bar may be flipped up out of the way when the loupe is not needed. Because the loupes are not mounted directly to the spectacle lenses, the patient's correction can be easily changed at any time. Table C-6 lists the specifications of these loupes.

Surgical Galilean Loupes

The Keeler Galilean Surgical Loupe is available in magnification of 2.5×. The system is made of a doublet objective lens and a high-power concave ocular lens designed to provide optimum field of view and image quality. It is available in four working distances (see Figure C-7). Table C-7 lists the specifications.

Nikon, Inc. (Melville, NY)

In addition to the afocal 2× Personal Lens telescopic unit that is available with attachable reading caps (see Appendix B), Nikon also manufactures three telemicroscopic units not requiring caps. The telescope is an afocal system having 1.3× magnification. By incorporating additional power into the objective lens, three different working distances are produced (along with the different magnifications). Table C-8 lists the specifications of the units.

Optical Designs, Inc. (Houston, TX)

T ● ● Specs

T ● ● Specs is a Galilean bifocal telescopic system. The objective lens is termed the *segment* and measures 25 mm

TABLE C-7
Specifications of the Keeler Galilean Surgical Loupe*

Magnification	Field (cm)	Working Distance (cm)
2.5×	9.0	34
2.5×	13.0	42
2.5×	14.0	46
2.5×	15.0	50

*Available from Keeler Instruments, Inc., Broomall, PA.

TABLE C-8
Specifications of the Nikon Main Near View Lens*

Magnification	Field of View (cm)	Working Distance (cm)
2×	11.3	17.0
3×	8.9	11.1
4×	5.8	8.5

*Available from Nikon, Inc., Melville, NY.

TABLE C-9
Specifications of the Galilean T • • Specs[a]

Equivalent Power	Field of View (cm)	Working Distance[b] (cm)	Working Space[c] (cm)
+4.00 D	13	43.9	42.5
+5.00 D	11	35.4	34.0
+6.00 D	9	29.7	28.3
+8.00 D	6	22.7	21.3

[a]Available from Optical Designs, Inc., Houston, TX.
[b]Working distance = distance from the spectacle plane to the object.
[c]Working space = distance from the front of the lens (in this case, telemicroscope) to the object.

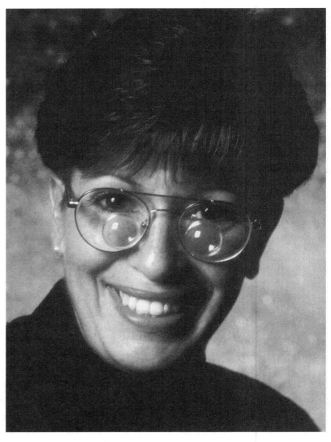

FIGURE C-8.   **T • • Specs is a Galilean bifocal telemicroscopic system available in four equivalent powers. (Courtesy of Optical Designs, Inc., Houston, TX.)**

in diameter. It is made by an injection-molded plastic process to form an aspheric objective button that also forms the housing, thereby maintaining the segment at a preset distance from the carrier lens. The ocular component of the telescope is contained on the carrier as an aspheric minus lens (Figure C-8).

The afocal telescope provides 1.8× magnification with a 17-degree field of view. By varying the objective lens component of the telescope along with the length of the housing, the telescope can be made focal at four different predetermined focal lengths. Thus, there are four focal caps. The caps are labeled with the total equivalent power of the telemicroscopic system. It must be remembered that with this system, the cap designation provides the total equivalent power of the system rather than the dioptric component of only the cap.

A prescription can be placed in the carrier lens. The telemicroscope can be monocular or binocular. It can be centered or decentered as any bifocal, and it can be placed in various positions on the carrier lens. Table C-9 lists the specifications of the units.

Optical Technology (Maitland, FL)

Oculus Loupe
The Oculus Loupe distributed by Optical Technology (Franel Optical Supply Co.) is a Galilean telemicroscope. The loupe is a 1.8× telemicroscope that is attached to an ophthalmic frame (52/20) (Figure C-9). The system focuses at 40 cm; however, with the addition of another cap (+3.75 D), the magnification is increased, thereby resulting in a decreased working distance. Table C-10 lists the specifications of the Oculus Loupe.

Orascoptic Research, Inc. (Madison, WI)

Orascoptic Loupes
These Galilean telemicroscopic loupes are available in three magnifications: 2.00×, 2.35×, and 2.60× (Figure C-10). There are two working distances that are available in each of the three magnifications. Table C-11 lists the specifications of the Orascoptic Loupes.

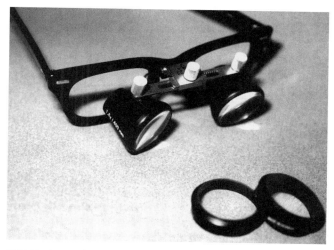

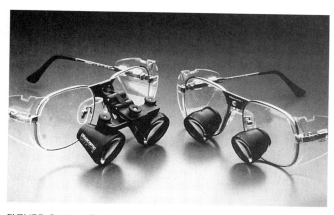

FIGURE C-10.   The Orascoptic telemicroscopes of Galilean design can be permanently attached to the carrier lens (right) or can be attached with a flip-up design (left). (Courtesy of Orascoptic Research, Inc., Madison, WI.)

FIGURE C-9.   The Oculus Loupe (Ocular Technology, Maitland, FL) is a binocular Galilean telemicroscope that focuses at 40 cm. With the addition of binocular caps, the magnification is increased while the working distance is decreased to 16 cm.

TABLE C-10
Specifications of the Oculus Loupe (Galilean)*

Description	Magnification	Working Distance (cm)
1.8× with no cap	1.8×	40
1.8× with 2.5× cap (+3.75)	4.5×	16

*Available from Optical Technology, Maitland, FL.

TABLE C-11
Specifications of the Orascoptic Loupes (Galilean)*

Magnification	Field of View (degrees)	Depth of Field (cm)	Working Distance (cm)
2.00×	19.3	30–43	36.8
2.00×	19.3	38–53	44.7
2.35×	13.6	30–43	36.8
2.35×	13.6	38–53	44.7
2.60×	15.5	30–43	36.8
2.60×	15.5	38–53	44.7

*Available from Orascoptic Research, Inc., Madison, WI.

Appendix D

YOUR HANDHELD TELESCOPE

Patient: _____   Date: _____

Your low vision device is called a *handheld telescope.* Telescopes can be handheld, clip-on, or mounted onto glasses. A telescope will help you to see things better at distance. The magnification of your telescope is _____ × (makes objects appear _____ times bigger).

You will be initially using your telescope for the following: _____
_____
_____

Use the telescope with your _____ eye. The other eye may be covered with a patch. The purpose of the patch is to allow you to concentrate on what you are seeing with the telescope. Patching will not harm your eyes. If you have a binocular telescope you will be using both eyes.

DO NOT TRY TO WALK AROUND WHILE LOOKING THROUGH YOUR TELESCOPE. YOU CAN EASILY TRIP AND FALL IF YOU DO SO.

Start by locating the object you wish to see without looking through the telescope. Make a V with the forefinger and thumb of your _____ hand. Put the telescope into the point of the V. The rubber eye cup, attached to your telescope, can be brought up to your eye, with the telescope pointed toward the target you wish to view. As you hold the telescope, rest your thumb or forefinger against your face. This technique will steady the device and block out the surrounding light. Hold the telescope as close to your eye or glasses as possible. Turn the focusing ring of your telescope with your _____ hand until the image is as clear as possible. The image should be circular if the telescope is properly aligned with your eye. To further steady the telescope, brace your elbow against your body or hold your elbow with your free hand. Move your head and telescope together when scanning to see an entire object or moving target. Always move slowly, because the telescope makes things appear to pass by quickly. If the distance between you and the object changes, you may need to refocus. If there seems to be a problem with lighting or glare, try repositioning yourself.

Practice for approximately 5–10 minutes several times a day in the beginning. Remember that some eye strain, muscle tightness, and possibly even a headache may occur. These symptoms are occurring because you are exercising your eyes in a new way. If these symptoms persist, you may want to contact Dr. _____.

Remember, learning to use your handheld telescope may take some time, practice, and patience.

Care of your telescope: Clean your telescope with a clean, damp, lint-free cloth. **Do not** clean your telescope with chemicals or immerse it in water.

If you have any questions, please feel free to call your low vision doctor at _____.

Specific Instructions:
_____
_____
_____

Appendix E

YOUR SPECTACLE-MOUNTED TELESCOPE

Patient: _____ Date: _____

Your low vision device is called a *spectacle-mounted telescope*. Telescopes can be either handheld, clip-on, or mounted onto glasses. A telescope will help you to see things better at distance. The magnification of your telescope is _____ × (makes objects appear _____ times bigger).

You will be initially using your telescope for the following: _____
_____
_____

Use the telescope with your _____ eye. The other eye may be covered with a patch. The purpose of the patch is to allow you to concentrate on what you are seeing with the telescope. Patching will not harm your eyes. If you have a binocular telescope you will be using both eyes.

DO NOT TRY TO WALK AROUND WHILE LOOKING THROUGH YOUR TELESCOPE. YOU CAN EASILY TRIP AND FALL IF YOU DO SO.

Locate the object you wish to see by raising the glasses or your chin and looking underneath the telescope. Keep looking at the object while you lower your chin or the glasses and look through the telescope to see the object clearly. You may have to turn the focusing ring with your _____ hand until the image is as clear as possible. (If you have a binocular telescope, focus one eye at a time while the other eye is closed.) Move your head and telescope together when scanning to see the entire object or moving target. Always move slowly, because the telescope makes things appear to pass by quickly. If the distance between you and the object changes, you may need to refocus. If there seems to be a problem with lighting or glare, try repositioning yourself.

If you are using your telescope for near tasks, you will need to adjust the focus for this closer distance by making the barrel of your telescope longer. If you have been given a reading cap, first make the barrel of your telescope as short as possible, then place the reading cap on the end of your telescope before beginning to read. To avoid back or neck strain, hold your reading material in a vertical position. A reading stand or clipboard may help you keep the material flat and steady and at the proper distance. Folding a newspaper into quarter sections or magazines in half can also help keep the reading material steady and at the proper focus for your telescope. To keep the image clear, it is crucial that you maintain a consistent distance between yourself and the page. To locate your place in the reading material, place your finger where you wish to start reading, then look through the telescope to find your finger to begin reading. Adjust your light to properly illuminate your reading material.

Practice for approximately 5–10 minutes several times a day in the beginning. Remember that some eye strain, muscle tightness, and possibly even a headache may occur. These symptoms are occurring because you are exercising your eyes in a new way. If these symptoms persist you may want to contact Dr. _____.

Remember, learning to use your spectacle-mounted telescope may take some time, practice, and patience.

If your frame or telescope goes out of alignment or breaks, do not try to adjust or repair it. Please call your doctor to schedule an appointment for the adjustment or repair of your telescopic system.

Care of your telescope: Clean your telescope with a clean, damp, lint-free cloth. **Do not** clean your telescope with chemicals or immerse it in water.

If you have any questions, please feel free to call your low vision doctor at _____.

Specific Instructions:
_____
_____
_____

Appendix F

TIPS FOR THE PATIENT USING A TELEMICROSCOPE

The following suggestions can be given to enhance success when prescribing a telemicroscope:

1. Relax. Be seated comfortably in an upright position before you begin reading.
2. Put reading material on a reading stand or clipboard. To keep the image clear, it is crucial that you maintain the same exact distance between yourself and the material. The ability to keep a consistent distance is the advantage of using a reading stand instead of a clipboard.
3. Position your light on the reading material while keeping in mind how close you will be to the page.
4. If you have been given a reading cap for your telescope, first make the barrel as short as possible. Then place the reading cap on the end of your telescope before beginning to read. To use the telescope for near without a reading cap, all you need to do is adjust the focus by making the telescope barrel longer.
5. To locate your place on the page, put your finger where you wish to start reading. Then look through the telescope, find your finger, and begin reading.
6. Adjust your light to better illuminate your reading material. Avoid putting your head between the light source and reading material because this will cause a shadow on the page.
7. While reading a paragraph of print it may be helpful to look quickly back across the same line you just finished reading. Then drop down to the next line. This will prevent you from losing your place while reading.
8. Use plenty of short practice sessions: 5 minutes or less, three to four times per day in the beginning. Increase your reading time when you experience less eye strain and when you can read more comfortably.
9. Remember that some items will be easier to read than others. Ease of reading depends on print size, lighting, color, spacing, and style.
10. Clean the telescope regularly with a soft, damp, lint-free cloth. *Do not* immerse it in water or wear it in the rain because condensation may develop, resulting in internal fogging. Avoid exposure to extremes in temperature and protect telescopes by always storing them in the box when not in use.

CHAPTER TEN

Low Vision Near Systems I: Microscopes and Magnifiers

Tracy Matchinski,
Richard L. Brilliant, and
Maryellen Bednarski

There is a specific process to solving a patient's near visual concerns. Initially, the patient's goals must be explored and defined. A patient's goals may encompass activities of daily living or educational, vocational, and recreational tasks. The next step in the process is determining the patient's functional vision. This includes assessment of many modalities, such as visual acuity (VA), visual fields, contrast sensitivity, oculomotor skills, eccentric viewing (if appropriate), binocular function, and photosensitivity. After the evaluation of the preceding factors, magnification may be introduced to create a large enough retinal image size to enable the patient with low vision better visual recognition. Finally, the patient's skill in using the devices, as well as the advantages and disadvantages of the various devices, is considered to determine the most appropriate magnification device or system.

There are a number of near magnification devices available. Telemicroscopes and electronic magnification systems are discussed in Chapters 9 and 11, respectively. This chapter focuses on microscopes, handheld magnifiers, and stand magnifiers. It is important to note that all of the preceding systems and devices can be interchanged when the *equivalent power* of each device is the same. By evaluating systems with the same equivalent power, the practitioner can provide the patient a number of choices in an attempt to solve his or her near visual concern(s) (Table 10-1).

PREDICTING NEAR MAGNIFICATION

When addressing a low vision patient's near goals, a trial and error approach will only frustrate and tire both the patient and practitioner. It is therefore recommended that the practitioner calculate a "target" point for determining the proper amount of magnification required by the patient. Undermagnification will not provide the proper resolution, whereas overmagnification may cause a number of disadvantages, such as a reduced field, a reduced depth of focus, and a reduced working distance. It is important to note that magnification calculations take place only after a patient's refractive error has been fully corrected. Uncorrected myopia or hyperopia will cause discrepancies in the expected results. Uncorrected astigmatism may distort the magnified image.

Near goals should be investigated before calculating magnification. Many patients want to read; however, this goal must be fully explored. For example, a patient's reading needs may range from spotting tasks involved in activities of daily living (e.g., reading daily mail, medicine bottles, thermostats, ingredients on food packages) to extended reading, such as reading newspapers or textbooks. A general starting point, or "target" acuity is 8-point, 20/50 reduced Snellen, or 1.0 M (meter system) print size. This is the approximate size of newspaper and magazine print. When a patient brings specific reading material to the examination, and the print size is unknown, the "rule of 1,000" can help determine the acuity demand of the material. This rule can be applied as follows:

TABLE 10-1
Comparison of Systems with the Same Equivalent Power

System	Equivalent Power	Distance
+20.00 D Microscope	+20.00 D	5 cm (microscope to object)
4× Telescope and +5.00 D reading cap	+20.00 D	20 cm (cap to object)
5× Telescope and +4.00 D reading cap	+20.00 D	25 cm (cap to object)
2× Telescope and +10.00 D reading cap	+20.00 D	10 cm (cap to object)
+20.00 D Handheld magnifier (object held at focal point)	+20.00 D	Variable (magnifier to eye) 5 cm (magnifier to object)
+28.00 D Stand magnifier and +2.50 D bifocal	+20.00 D	15 cm (magnifier to eye)
Closed-circuit television (CCTV) 2-mm print projected to 20 mm on monitor screen (while using a +2.00 D add)	+20.00 D	50 cm (eye to monitor screen)
CCTV 3-mm print projected to 15 mm on monitor screen (while using a +4.00 D add)	+20.00 D	25 cm (eye to monitor screen)

1. The number of letters and spaces in 1 in. of the text is counted. Taking the average of several inches is recommended.
2. By dividing the preceding number into 1,000, the resulting number will be the reduced Snellen denominator equivalent of the print size. (If using the point system, 144 is used instead of 1,000.)

Example
What is the reduced Snellen equivalent of a patient's textbook print when 25 letters and spaces are counted in a 1-in. line of text?
Answer:

$$1,000/25 = 40$$

Thus, 40 is the Snellen denominator and therefore the reduced Snellen acuity size of this text material is 20/40.

METHODS OF DETERMINING THE APPROPRIATE NEAR MAGNIFICATION

Several methods can be used to determine the amount of magnification or equivalent power for near:

1. Lebensohn's "reciprocal of vision" rule calculates the needed magnification by using the patient's best corrected distance acuity and a near "target" acuity. By dividing the denominator of the *distance* Snellen fraction by the denominator of the *near* Snellen fraction of the estimated target acuity, the required magnification is obtained. To convert the resultant magnifi-

cation to diopters, the magnification number can be multiplied by 4 (from the formula M = D/4).

Example 1

A patient's best distance VA is 20/200. How much magnification would be required for this patient to read print that is equivalent in size to 20/50 reduced Snellen?

Answer: Distance VA is 20/200. "Target" VA is 20/50 (newspaper print). Therefore, 200/50 = 4.

The required magnification is 4× or +16.00 D (M = D/4).

2. Kestenbaum's rule also uses distance acuity to predict near magnification. Using the Snellen fraction of best corrected distance acuity, the denominator is divided by the numerator to obtain the dioptric power needed to achieve 1 M or 20/50 reduced Snellen.

Example 2

A patient's best distance VA is 20/160. How much magnification would be required for this patient to read newsprint (equivalent to 20/50 reduced Snellen)?

Answer: Distance VA is 20/160. Therefore, 160/20 = 8.

The required dioptric power is +8.00 D or the required magnification is 2× (M = D/4) to read 20/50 print.

It is not recommended that distance VA be used to predict near magnification because there are many variables that prevent a true correlation between distance and near acuities. For example, through accommodation, pupillary constriction, and better lighting, many patients with low vision demonstrate better near acuity. The size and location of a patient's retinal scotoma, as well as corneal or lens opacifications may also cause a poor correlation between distance and near visual acuities. Two good examples may be seen with a posterior subcapsular cataract, which in many cases produces poorer near vision than distance vision, whereas a nuclear cataract may produce poorer distance vision and possibly better near vision by the increased myopia secondary to nuclear sclerosis.

3. Near magnification can also be determined by using a simple ratio comparing near VA to a target acuity. This method involves the following steps:
   a. The patient's best near acuity (BNA) is determined with a single character acuity card and the testing distance (TD) is recorded. Any distance can be used, but it must be recorded along with the optotype (i.e., 0.17/2 M, 0.33/1.6 M, 0.37/5 M).
   b. A target near acuity (TNA) is determined (relative to what the patient would like to see) and a ratio is set up (BNA/TNA = TD/?).
   c. The unknown number (?) is the new reading distance that the reading material must be brought to to obtain the appropriate magnification (relative distance magnification).
   d. The reciprocal of this new reading distance (?) will provide the practitioner with the power of the lens required to read the target acuity.

Example 3

What lens power would be required for a patient to read 1 M when the patient's best VA is 0.40/4 M?

Answer:

$$\frac{4\,M}{1\,M} = \frac{40\,cm}{?\,cm}$$

$$4(?) = 40$$

$$? = 10\,cm$$

$$\frac{100}{10} = +10.00\,D$$

Therefore, +10.00 D would be needed for this patient to read 1 M. He or she would have to hold the reading material at 10 cm (assuming no refractive error and no accommodation).

Example 4

What lens power would be required for a patient to read 0.8 M when best VA is 0.24/3 M?

Answer:

$$\frac{3\,M}{0.8\,M} = \frac{24\,cm}{?\,cm}$$

$$3.75(?) = 24$$

$$? = 6.40\,cm$$

$$\frac{100\,cm}{6.4\,cm} = +15.63\,D$$

Therefore, +15.63 D would be required for this patient to read 0.8 M. He would have to hold the reading material at 6.40 cm (assuming no refractive error and no accommodation).

It should be noted that 1 M is generally considered the target point for near acuity, because 1 M is the size of most print (e.g., newspaper, magazine). There is, however, a difference between VA and reading acuity. Most reading material is comfortably above the VA and contrast threshold of normally sighted readers. When evaluating near vision systems for patients with low vision, an attempt should be made to provide enough magnification so that the patient can read his or her goal materials with some measure of comfort and fluency. When calculating the near magnification, 1 M can be used as a starting point, keeping in mind that, in practice, the patient may require more magnification than the preceding formulas initially predict to achieve a measure of comfort and fluency in reading.

FINE-TUNING THE READING LENS

Once the predicted reading lens is determined, it must then be evaluated to see if it meets the needs of the patient. The reading material used should no longer be near acuity test cards, which have been found to have an average of 93.1% contrast, but rather practical material, such as a newspaper, which has been found to have an

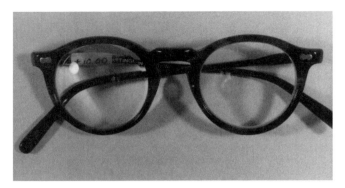

FIGURE 10-1.   **A +10.00 D full-diameter aspheric microscope OD.**

average contrast of 65.4%.[1] Some tips for refining the reading lens include the following:

1. The patient's reading rate should be evaluated. Is the patient reading fluently or experiencing difficulty? Reading efficiency decreases as the resolution limit is approached. Difficulty in reading may suggest a need for more magnification or a patient's poor reading skills.
2. The patient's reading skills should be evaluated. How many years have passed since the patient visually read a newspaper, magazine, and so forth? Was he or she an avid reader?
3. The practitioner should note how changes in illumination affect the patient's reading rate. Proper lighting may reduce the amount of the initial predicted magnification.
4. The practitioner should evaluate whether the patient does better monocularly or binocularly. Some patients may perform better when occluding the poorer seeing eye.
5. The patient's input should be solicited. Is he or she pleased with the reading performance provided by a given reading lens? Does he or she think it will enable him or her to meet his or her reading goals?

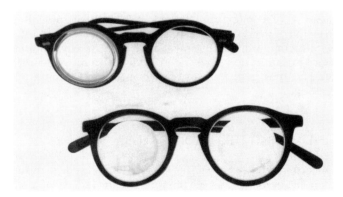

FIGURE 10-2.   **A +24.00 D aspheric lenticular microscope surrounded by a plano carrier lens OU (lower spectacle). The upper spectacle is a +24.00 D ClearImage II (Designs for Vision, Inc., Ronkonkoma, NY) doublet microscope OD.**

MICROSCOPES

A low vision microscope can be described as a *spectacle-mounted convex lens*. Microscopes enable the patient to take advantage of the principle of relative distance magnification. As a patient brings the reading material closer, an increased retinal image size is produced. The microscope does not produce the increased retinal image; rather it acts as a converging system to neutralize the diverging rays created by the close proximity of the reading material. Parallel rays of light will leave the convex lens and form an enlarged focused image on the retina without the need for accommodation. The microscopic lens itself will produce a small amount of magnification; however, this magnification is so small in relation to the relative distance magnification that it is considered negligible for practical or clinical purposes.

Lens Options

When considering a microscope, there are four basic options available: full-field, half-eye, bifocal, or loupe. The following outline summarizes each option.

1. *Full-field microscopes* are mounted in conventional frames at a normal vertex distance. Of the different microscopic choices available, the full-field offers the largest field of view. Several lens designs are available:
   a. *Spherical* lenses have the same power in all meridians. They can be prescribed in a biconvex or planoconvex form. Cylindrical correction can be incorporated. As these lenses are prescribed in higher powers, oblique astigmatism (marginal astigmatism) and curvature of field begin to distort the image. Therefore, this lens design should be used only for powers up to approximately +8.00 D.
   b. *Aspheric* lens design is used to minimize peripheral aberrations. Aspheric lenses have ellipsoidal surfaces—that is, the convexity (or power) of the lens is progressively reduced toward the periphery. The two types of aspheric lenses are full-diameter and lenticular designs. Cylindrical correction can be incorporated into both designs. Full-diameter aspheric lenses are appropriate in powers from +10.00 to +20.00 D (Figure 10-1). The aspheric lenticular design is an aspheric lens on a plano base (Figure 10-2). This design has the advantages of less weight and decreased thickness, with the disadvantage of smaller field of view. The aspheric lenticular lens generally has an optical zone diameter of 30–40 mm surrounded by the plano carrier lens. It has the characteristic "fried egg" appearance. This lens is appropriate for powers from +10.00 to +48.00 D.
   c. *Doublet*. A doublet lens is a combination of two convex lenses separated by an air space (Figure 10-3). These lenses may be of spherical or aspheric design and can be made of glass or plastic. The doublet design provides high amounts of magnification with

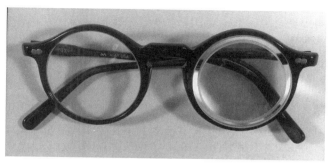

FIGURE 10-3. **A +32.00 D ClearImage II (Designs for Vision, Inc., Ronkonkoma, NY) doublet microscope OS.**

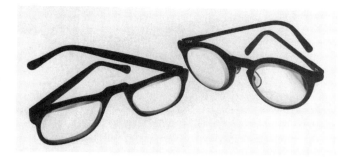

A

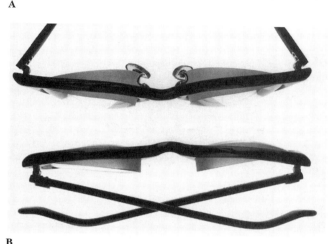

B

FIGURE 10-4. **A. Half-eye (left) and full-diameter frames incorporating +8.00 D lenses with 10 prism diopter base in in each lens. The base-in prisms aid in maintaining binocularity. B. Superior view of both frames demonstrating the base-in prism.**

minimal spherical aberration, coma, oblique astigmatism, and curvature of field in the peripheral area of the lens. Cylindrical correction can be incorporated as well. Doublet lenses can be found in magnifications ranging from 2× to 20×. The doublet lens is especially useful in magnifications of 5× and above.

2. *Half-eye microscopes* are convex lenses mounted in a half-eye frame worn at a normal to slightly longer vertex distance. The greatest advantage of half-eye microscopes is unobstructed distance viewing. *Classic half-eye microscopes* are convex spherical lenses with base-in prism designed for binocularity. Standard available powers run up to +12.00 D. The usual amount of prism incorporated into each lens is equal to the power of the microscope plus two additional prism diopters. For example, a +10.00 D half-eye would have 12.00 D of base-in prism before each eye (Figure 10-4). Any of the lens designs described under full-field microscopes can be cut to fit half-eye frames; however, base-in prism would not be incorporated because for all practical purposes, a patient cannot maintain binocularity when reading at a distance closer than 8 cm.

3. *Bifocal microscopes* are mounted in conventional frames at a normal vertex distance. Although the segment can be placed at the conventional height, it is commonly set slightly higher. The height depends on the patient's needs and the power of the bifocal. In special cases, depending on hobbies or vocational demands, a bifocal may be mounted in the superior position. There are several types of bifocals available.
   a. *One-piece molded plastic bifocals*: Flat-top segments are available up to +6.00 D and round segments up to +20.00 D.
   b. *Aspheric executive bifocals* are available up to +32.00 D. The bifocal segment is ground with elliptical curves to minimize distortions. These bifocals, available through Designs for Vision, Inc. (Ronkonkoma, NY) do not incorporate cylinder into the bifocal. The cylinder is limited to the distance portion of the lens.
   c. *Ben Franklin bifocals*: The Ben Franklin design uses two separate lenses that are cut in half, cemented together, and fit into a frame. The top can be the distance or an intermediate prescription and the bottom is the microscope. The microscopic bifocal, manufactured by Designs for Vision, can have a total gross power up to +20.00 D in any meridian, with cylinder (Figure 10-5). If cylinder is not needed, a Ben Franklin bifocal can be made up to +48.00 D through Tech Optics International (Freeport, NY). This laboratory also has binocular adds available in strengths of +4.00, +5.00, +6.00, +8.00, and +10.00 D with appropriate base-in prism incorporated.
   d. *Doublet bifocals*: Designs for Vision has also designed a doublet bifocal ranging in power from +8.00 D to +40.00 D. These doublets are composed of two planoconvex lenses with the convex sides facing away from the patient's eyes. They are available in two styles, type E (13×23 mm) and type R (19×25 mm) and appear somewhat similar to a flat-top bifocal (Figure 10-6).
   e. *Self-applied bifocal*: The self-applied bifocal allows the practitioner to apply the bifocal lens to a patient's prescription lens. This bifocal has the advantage of being placed in any position on a patient's spectacles. It also has the flexibility of being readily replaced or repositioned by the practitioner at any time. These lenses are lightweight and available in powers from +8.00 D to +40.00 D, through Unilens

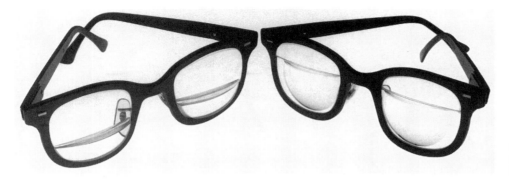

FIGURE 10-5. **Ben Franklin bifocals manufactured by Designs for Vision, Inc. (Ronkonkoma, NY).**

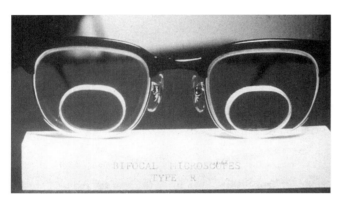

FIGURE 10-6. **Type R bifocal microscope is a 25-mm bifocal (19-mm high) manufactured by Designs for Vision, Inc. (Ronkonkoma, NY).**

Corp. (Largo, FL) or Eschenbach Optik of America (Ridgefield, CT) (Figures 10-7 and 10-8). Keeler Instruments, Inc. (Broomall, PA) also makes a bifocal segment that can be screwed into a threaded hole in a spectacle lens or a threaded sleeve that is attached to the front surface of a spectacle lens. These bifocal segments are interchangeable in power and are available from +8.00 D to +60.00 D (Figure 10-9).

4. *Loupes* are a variation of a microscope that allows for a slightly extended working distance. *Working distance* is defined as the distance from the spectacle plane to the reading material. *Working space* is the distance from the front of the optical device to the reading material (usually the focal length of the lens).[2, 3] Loupes increase the working distance by extending the lens in front of the spectacle plane. As the extension increases, the field of view decreases. Loupes can be mounted several ways. Many of these loupes have the ability to flip up, which allows for unobstructed distance viewing. Loupes can be binocular in powers up to +10.00 D and are available in monocular form in powers up to +32.00 D. *Headborne loupes* are supported by a strap around the patient's head (Figure 10-10). *Clip-on loupes* are secured to either the temple, bridge, or along the top of the frame directly above the patient's eye. These are sometimes referred to as *jeweler's loupes* (Figure 10-11).

5. A *contact lens microscope* can also be considered as an option.[4] The working distance of the contact lens

microscope would be closer than when using an equivalent powered microscopic spectacle. Two advantages exist with the contact lens microscope system: cosmesis and field of view. Binocularity may be applicable for those patients who demonstrate the ability to use both eyes together and who require a low powered lens. The major problem with a binocular system is that the patient would have to remove the lenses when he or she was not reading, which is certainly a major inconvenience. A monovision system may be another alternative, but would only be appropriate for a patient in whom the monocular blur would not cause a safety risk with mobility.

Advantages and Disadvantages of a Microscope

Like any low vision device, the microscope has a number of advantages and disadvantages. These advantages and disadvantages must be considered when prescribing a microscope for a patient.

Advantages

1. May be the easiest to adjust to because microscopes are most familiar or conventional
2. Cosmetically appealing because of "normal" appearance
3. Largest field of view of any near device
4. May be used binocularly (powers up to +12.00 D) when appropriate
5. Allows both hands free
6. Good for patients with hand tremors or poor dexterity (reading stand may be recommended in conjunction with the microscope)
7. Useful for prolonged reading
8. May sometimes be used for writing tasks
9. Astigmatic correction can be incorporated in most lenses

Disadvantages

1. As lens power increases:
   a. Working distance decreases
   b. Depth of focus decreases
   c. Lighting becomes more critical
   d. Possibility of binocularity decreases

FIGURE 10-7. **A. A high-add bifocal can be easily applied to a patient's spectacle correction by use of a Uni-Vision bifocal (Unilens Corp., Largo, FL). The front surface of the spectacle lens should have a plano to +8.00 D base curve. The UniVision lens can be applied by use of a contact lens DMV suction cup after the paper ring has been removed, exposing adhesive on the lens. B. For maximum flexibility of bifocal lens positioning, the frame should have a minimum of 25 mm from the center of the patient's pupil to the bottom of the frame.**

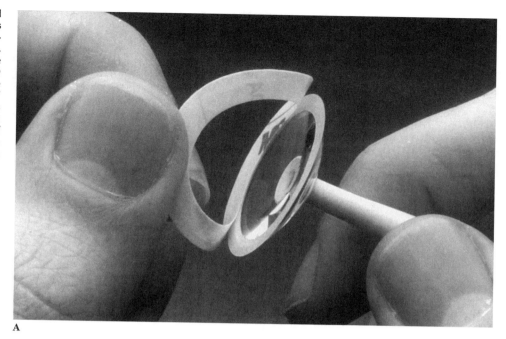

A

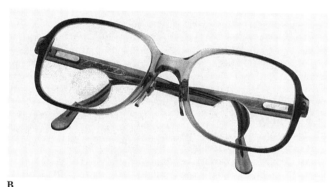

B

e. Lens distortions and aberrations increase
f. Field size decreases (lens diameter decreases)
g. Reduced reading speed generally occurs
2. When learning to use a microscope a patient should be warned of the following:
  a. Fatigue of neck, arm, and shoulder muscles
  b. Can cause nausea and dizziness
  c. Can cause eye fatigue
  d. May cause headaches in frontal or temporal areas, or both
  e. No mobility when wearing a full field microscope

Equivalent Power of a Microscope

When comparing one microscope to another, the *equivalent power* should be used. As a matter of fact, by knowing the equivalent power of a microscope, its predicted performance can be compared to any other optical system (e.g., magnifier, telemicroscope, closed-circuit television [CCTV]) with the same equivalent power. A major disad-

vantage of using equivalent power for a microscopic lens, however, is that it is not easily determined. An equivalent power cannot be determined by the use of a lensometer, with the exception of those microscopes that are planoconvex. With a planoconvex microscope, the equivalent power will be equal (or very close to being equal) to the front vertex power, and therefore, can be easily measured with the lensometer. Also, for some microscopic lenses that have a flat back surface power, the front vertex power will be close enough to be used clinically. Microscopic lenses that are biconvex or have a steep back surface, however, will show a fairly large difference between the front vertex power and the equivalent power (the front vertex power will provide a higher dioptric reading than the equivalent power). To determine the equivalent power in these lenses a method has been proposed by Bailey.[5] This procedure can easily be performed in an office and can provide the practitioner with the equivalent power of microscopes and magnifiers. This procedure will be discussed in the next section (Lens Verification).

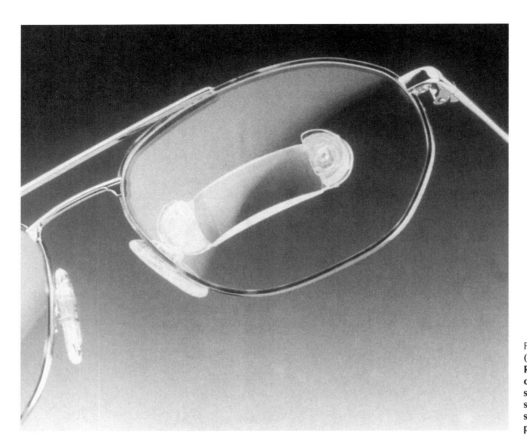

FIGURE 10-8. **The Eschenbach (Eschenbach Optik of America, Inc., Ridgefield, CT) aspheric bifocal lens can be placed on either the front surface or the rear surface of the spectacle lens. It is attached to the spectacle lens by use of adhesive pads.**

It is important to note that many manufacturers of microscopes and magnifiers do not provide the equivalent power of the system. In many cases, the dioptric power that is provided is the back vertex power of the lens. Therefore, it is important for the low vision practitioner to determine the front vertex power for those microscopic lenses previously discussed, or more accurately, to determine the equivalent power of all of the microscopic and magnifying lenses. By doing so, the practitioner can easily and accurately compare the advantages

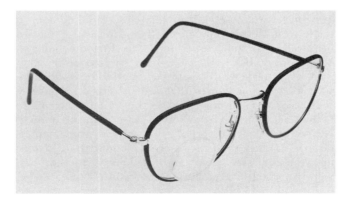

FIGURE 10-9. **The Keeler bifocal (LVA-12) is available in magnifications of 2×, 3×, 4×, 5×, 6×, 7×, 8×, 9×, and 15×. (Courtesy of Keeler Instruments, Inc., Broomall, PA.)**

and disadvantages of the various near magnification systems that produce the same retinal image size.

Lens Verification

An in-office technique to determine equivalent power is referred to as the *method of triangulation*. This method uses similar triangles to measure the equivalent focal length (f_{eq}) of the lens. Once the equivalent focal length is known, its inverse may be determined to arrive at the equivalent power (D_{eq}) of the near magnification lens. The method of triangulation involves the following:

1. An object is selected that has good contrast in relation to its background and can be measured accurately. For example, two penlights separated by a fixed distance can act as the object. Therefore, in this example, the object height (h) becomes the distance between the two penlights.

2. The object is placed at a fixed distance (l), greater than 3 m from the front surface of the lens. The distance must be at least 3 m to limit the divergent rays of light.

3. After the object's light rays pass through the lens, an image (h^1) will be created that must be clearly focused on a screen. The screen should be moved back and forth until a clear image is seen. The image on the screen is then measured. If two penlights were used,

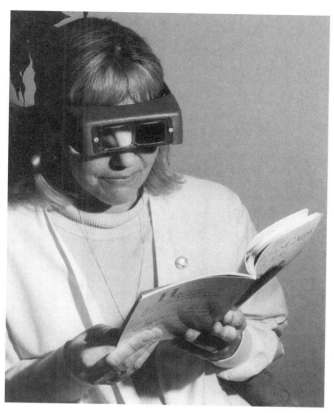

FIGURE 10-10. A binocular headborne loupe allows the patient to maintain a stereoscopic image with magnification. The large distance between the loupe and the patient's eyes enables the patient to wear a spectacle correction along with obtaining a greater working distance.

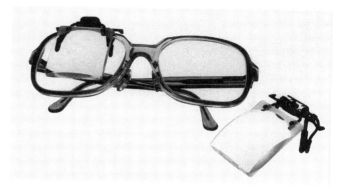

FIGURE 10-11. The COIL clip-on, flip-on loupe (C.O.I.L. Combined Optical Industries, Ltd., Elk Grove Village, IL) is available in three powers: +6.00, +10.00, and +15.00 D. It easily attaches to either eye of any frame.

$$\frac{1}{h} = \frac{l^1}{h^1}$$

$$l^1 = h^1\left(\frac{1}{h}\right)$$

$$l^1 = 6\left(\frac{4,000}{200}\right)$$

$$l^1 = 120 \text{ mm or } 12.0 \text{ cm}$$

$$l^1 = f_{eq} = 12.0 \text{ cm}$$

$$D_{eq} = \frac{1}{f_{eq}} = \frac{100}{12}$$

$$D_{eq} = +8.30 \text{ D}$$

then the separation of the two light images should be measured.

4. Once the object height (h) or object separation, object distance (l), and image height (h¹) or image separation are known, the image distance (l¹) can be calculated from the following formula:

$$\frac{1}{h} = \frac{l^1}{h^1}$$

The ratio of l to h is equal to the ratio of l¹ to h¹. The image distance, l¹, is the equivalent focal length of the lens. The inverse of the equivalent focal length will determine the equivalent power of the lens.

Example

Dr. Jones is attempting to determine the equivalent power of a patient's reading lens. When he positions two penlights 4 m from the front surface of the lens, he is able to focus the images (of the penlights) on a screen. The two penlights are separated from each other by a distance of 20 cm and their images are measured showing a separation of 6 mm. What is the equivalent power of this lens (Figure 10-12)?

Answer: All variables should be converted to the same units (in this case, mm). Therefore,

h = 20 cm (200mm); h¹ = 6mm; l = 4m (4,000mm) so,

Therefore, the equivalent power of the reading lens is +8.30 D.

There are several alternate methods of verification that provide an *estimate* of lens power. In these other methods, the lens being verified must be either planoconvex or have a back surface that is relatively flat so that its front vertex power will be fairly close to its equivalent power. These methods include the following:

1. *Hand neutralization*: A rough estimate is determined by using concave trial lenses to neutralize the against motion created by the convex lens of the microscope.

2. *Lens clock*: Lens clock readings from both surfaces can be taken and added together. This method results in only a rough approximation because the thickness of the lens is ignored.

3. *Lensometer*: The front vertex power is verified by placing the ocular surface of the microscope toward the individual neutralizing the lenses. This method provides the closest approximation of the equivalent power. The power of the convex lens may at times be beyond the range of the lensometer. If this occurs, a high-powered concave lens may be placed against the convex lens and the lens combination placed into the lensometer. This method is an approximation, as it ignores lens thickness and separation. Alternatively, a concave trial lens may be placed in

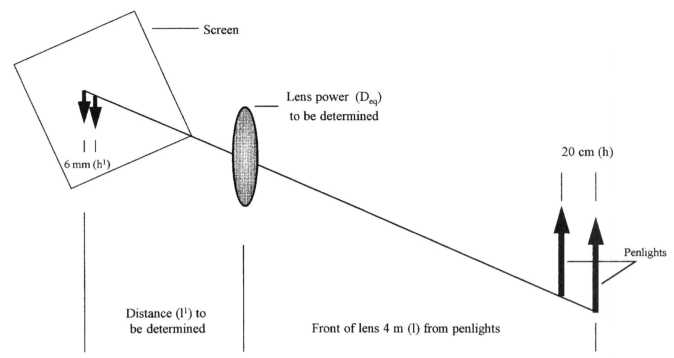

FIGURE 10-12.   **Determining the equivalent power of a convex lens. (h = object height; h¹ = image; l = fixed distance; l¹ = image distance.)**

the auxiliary cell of the lensometer to extend its range. The effective power of the added concave lens is determined by focusing the mires before it is placed in the lensometer. The effective power of the auxiliary concave lens will be less than its true power due to its distance away from the lens stop.

Prescribing Strategies

Once the dioptric power has been predicted to achieve a patient's target acuity, a low vision device must be used with the equivalent power to determine if it satisfies the patient's needs. Whether device selection involves microscopes or other near devices, the microscope is generally the first device introduced. This recommendation is based on three factors:

1. The microscope (reading spectacle lens) is generally the most familiar near device for the majority of patients.
2. The microscope is easier to use because the practitioner need only be initially concerned with the patient holding the reading material at the proper focal point and that the proper illumination is provided.
3. The microscope allows the practitioner to "fine-tune" the power of the lens easily by incorporating a patient's cylinder correction or adding (or subtracting) additional lens power.

Refractive Error
It is a logical deduction that the spherical component of a patient's refractive error will impact on the power of

the microscope. Myopia will allow for the use of a lower-powered microscopic lens while maintaining the correct amount of magnification, whereas hyperopia will create the need for a higher-powered lens. (The myopic refractive error can be subtracted from the microscope power whereas the hyperopic refractive error must be added to the microscope power.) It is important to note that the working distance must equal the focal distance of the prescribed microscope plus the patient's uncorrected refractive error. For example, when a +10.00 D microscope is required for a 6.00 D corrected myope, the patient can remove his or her habitual distance spectacle and use a +4.00 D reading lens. The total power in this case will be +10.00 D (i.e., +4.00 D from the lens and +6.00 D from the "uncorrected" myopic patient), with the reading material maintained at 10 cm. Another example would be a +4.00 D corrected hyperope who needs an add of +8.00 D to read at 12.5 cm. This patient can remove his or her distance spectacle and place a +12.00 D reading lens (microscope) on his or her face to obtain a total power of +8.00 D for reading (while still maintaining the 12.5 cm working distance).

Astigmatic error must also be considered. Some important factors that should be considered include acuity level, amount of astigmatism, and the total dioptric power required. In many cases, if there is a small amount of astigmatism in the distance prescription it can generally be ignored at near. Certainly, as the power of the microscope increases there will be less need for correcting small amounts of astigmatism. There are, however, a number of ways to deal with the cylindrical correction in a microscopic lens.

1. Use the spherical equivalent. This technique is also good for prefabricated microscopic lens designs.
2. If the amount of cylinder is less than half the denominator of the patient's best VA (BVA) at distance divided by 100, it can be ignored.

Example
BVA = 20/200

1. Half the denominator: 200/2 = 100
2. Divide by 100: 100/100 = 1.00

Answer: If cylinder for this patient is greater than 1.00 D, prescribe it. If cylinder for this patient is less than 1.00 D, ignore it.

3. Trial frame it. This technique is the best way to deal with cylinder. It takes relatively little time and allows for the patient's input.

Accommodation
Accommodation can also contribute to the final recommended power of a microscope. If both accommodation and a microscope are used together, the dioptric power of each must be added together to determine the total equivalent power being used. The working distance is set by the total dioptric power of this combined system. For example, if an emmetropic 15-year-old patient holds a book at 10 cm to read, it can be determined that he is using +10.00 D of accommodation. The length of time that this patient can sustain the accommodative efforts should be considered. If the patient reports asthenopic complaints, such as headaches, eye strain, or eye fatigue, then a reading lens may be required. The patient's amplitude of accommodation should be determined, or a trial frame can be used to determine maximum plus acceptance by the patient. In many cases with younger patients, the total dioptric power required (+10.00 D in this case) may be split between a microscopic lens and the patient's accommodative ability. Therefore, this patient may be prescribed a +5.00 D lens even though he continued to read at 10 cm. It is expected that this lens will eliminate his asthenopic complaints without forcing him to be "locked in" to the 10 cm reading distance that a +10.00 D lens would require.

Field of View
One of the biggest advantages of a microscope is its field of view. The closer the lens is held to the eye, the larger the field of view. Lens designs also affect field of view. As the power of the lens increases, the field of view decreases due to peripheral distortions. When more magnification is needed, the lens design prescribed should progress from spherical to aspheric to doublet. This progression will maximize field of view.

Monocular or Binocular Microscope
Microscopes are generally prescribed monocularly for the better seeing eye. The large majority of low vision patients have a visual impairment in which one eye has worse VA than the fellow eye. When acuities are less than 20/200 or the two eyes differ by more than two lines of acuity, there is less chance for binocularity. There are several tests to evaluate binocular vision, and these tests are discussed in Chapter 3. When a patient is monocular and using a microscope, an opaque patch is recommended for the poorer seeing eye to eliminate any possible interference or retinal rivalry between the two eyes.

Some patients will have equal or similar acuities in each eye. These patients do have potential for binocularity and may benefit from a binocular microscope. Advantages of a binocular microscope may include a larger and more complete field of view (cancellation of monocular scotomas if present), stereopsis, and depth of field; better acuity; and a psychological edge.[2] Disadvantages include increased weight and expense. The limiting factor of prescribing binocularly is the working distance of the microscopic system. The more powerful the microscope, the closer the reading material must be held and the higher the convergence demand. It is generally accepted that the limit for achieving binocularity with a microscope is no closer than an 8–10 cm working distance.

Convex lenses relieve the accommodative effort but not the convergence effort. To calculate the actual amount of convergence required, the following formula can be used[6]:

$$C = (IPD)\left(\frac{1}{w + h}\right)$$

where C = convergence demand expressed in prism diopters; IPD = (distance) interpupillary distance in centimeters; w = working distance, spectacle plane to object, in meters; and h = vertex distance from spectacle plane to the eye's center of rotation in meters (0.027 m is the standard value).

Example 1
A patient, whose IPD is 64 mm, is reading with a +8.00 D microscope. How much convergence is required for this patient to read with this microscopic lens?

Answer:

$$C = (IPD)\left(\frac{1}{w + h}\right)$$
$$= (6.4)\left(\frac{1}{0.125 + 0.027}\right)$$
$$= (6.4)(6.58) = 42.11 \text{ prism diopters}$$

This patient must generate 42.11 prism diopters of convergence to bifixate the near target (21.06 prism diopters per eye).

An estimation of convergence demand can be quickly determined by using meter angles. One meter angle is a unit of convergence approximately equivalent to 1.00 D of accommodation. The value of a meter angle is found by dividing the patient's working distance into 100. Meter angles are expressed in centimeters. When this value is multiplied by the IPD, also in centimeters, the result approximates the amount of convergence required in prism diopters.

$$C = (MA)(IPD)$$

where C = convergence demand in prism diopters; MA = meters angles (100/working distance); and IPD = (distance) interpupillary distance, in centimeters.

Example 2
A patient, whose IPD is 64 mm, is reading with a +8.00 D microscope. How much convergence is required for this patient to read with this microscopic lens (same example as example 1)?
    Answer:

$$C = (MA)(IPD)$$
$$= \left(\frac{100}{12.5}\right)(6.4)$$
$$= 51.20 \text{ prism diopters}$$

This patient must generate 51.20 prism diopters of convergence to bifixate the near target (25.60 prism diopters per eye).

Comparing results from both equations, it is found that determining convergence using meter angles overestimates the demand.[7] This is especially true with closer working distances and larger IPDs. Using either method, it becomes obvious that a tremendous amount of convergence is required.

To help relieve the large amounts of convergence needed, base-in prism is required. Prism relocates the image toward its apex, so with base-in prism, the images are directed out (or temporally), relieving convergence. This prism can be generated by decentering the lenses or grinding prism into the lenses. A Fresnel prism may also be used, but this type of prism often degrades the image and decreases contrast.

When decentering lenses to obtain the prismatic effect, the lenses first need to be decentered for the near IPD. A plus lens can be thought of as two prisms aligned base to base. (Conversely, a minus lens may be considered as two prisms aligned apex to apex.) If plus lenses are not decentered for near, the eye is not looking through the optical center. Rather, it is looking through the base-out portion, actually creating more convergence demand. Therefore, the lenses must first be decentered for the near IPD. Additional decentration can then create the base-in prism effect, helping to relieve some convergence demand.

To determine the near IPD when using a particular microscopic lens, the following formula, derived by similar triangles, can be used[8]:

$$NIPD = (IPD)\left(\frac{w}{w + h}\right)$$

where NIPD = (near) interpupillary distance, in millimeters; IPD = (distance) interpupillary distance, in millime-

ters; w = working distance (spectacle plane to object), in millimeters; and h = vertex distance from spectacle plane to eye's center of rotation, in millimeters (27 mm is the standard value used).

Example 3
A patient with a distance IPD of 64 mm requires the use of a +12.00 D microscope to read a textbook. The patient holds the textbook at a distance of 8.3 cm from the microscope. What is the patient's NIPD?
    Answer:

$$NIPD = (IPD)\left(\frac{w}{w + h}\right)$$
$$= (64)\left(\frac{83}{83 + 27}\right)$$
$$= 48.3 \text{ mm}$$

This patient's NIPD is 48.3 mm when looking at an object 8.3 cm from the spectacle plane. Therefore, to eliminate any additional convergence demand from the convex lenses themselves, the lenses must be decentered to a binocular NIPD of 48.3 mm. This adjustment, however, does not eliminate any convergence demand created by using both eyes to view an object at such a close distance. This convergence demand can be aided with base-in prism in each eye once the reading lenses have been properly decentered to the patient's NIPD.

Bailey[8] recommended a method for determining near optical center placement or a patient's NIPD. The lens should be decentered 1.5 mm for each diopter of add. If the distance PD is greater than 65 mm, decenter 1 mm further.

Example 4
A patient with an IPD of 62 mm requires the use of a +6.00 D microscope to read a textbook. What is the patient's NIPD?
    Answer:

$$6(1.5) = 9 \text{ mm}$$
$$62 - 9 = 53 \text{ mm}$$

Therefore, the near interpupillary distance would be 53 mm.

Example 5
A patient with an IPD of 67 mm requires the use of a +6.00 D microscope to read a textbook. What is the patient's NIPD?
    Answer:

$$6(1.5) = 9 \text{ mm}$$
$$9 + 1 = 10 \text{ mm}$$
$$67 - 10 = 57 \text{ mm}$$

Therefore, the NIPD would be 57 mm. Again, this method only determines the NIPD. To create base-in prism, more decentration would be necessary or prism can be ground into the lens.

Once the lens is decentered for a patient's NIPD, further decentration to create base-in prism can be determined through Prentice's rule:

$$P = (D)(d)$$

where P = lens-induced prismatic effect (base-in or base-out) depending on the lens (convex or concave) and the direction of decentration (temporally or nasally); D = power of lens, in diopters; d = distance from optical center, in centimeters.

Example 6

A practitioner would like to create 6 base-in prism for a patient using a +10.00 D microscope. How much decentration would be required to accomplish this, assuming that the lenses have already been decentered to the patient's NIPD?

Answer:

$$P = (D)(d)$$
$$d = \frac{P}{D}$$
$$d = \frac{6}{10}$$
$$d = 0.6 \text{ cm or 6 mm}$$

In this case, the lens would be decentered 6 mm nasally to obtain a base-in prismatic effect. Again, this value would be added to the amount of decentration for the patient's NIPD. The total amount of decentration possible is limited by the size of the lens blank.

Another approach to compensate for the high convergence demand was suggested by Fonda.[9] He recommended decentering 1 mm in each eye or grinding 1 base-in prism diopter in each eye for each diopter of add. For example, a +6.00 D microscope would need 6 base-in prism diopters per eye, or 12 base-in prism diopters total. Otherwise, each lens would have to be decentered 6 mm nasally.

A biocular system may also be considered. In this system, a lens is prescribed for each eye to be used alternately. No decentration or added prism is necessary. Both lenses would provide the full microscopic power, so the patient can switch from one eye to the other to help prolong reading time by preventing eye strain and fatigue. A patch would be worn on the lens not used at the time to prevent one eye from interfering with the other. Another option is to have a monovision system. One lens would have the full microscope power and the other lens would have the patient's distance correction or a correction for use at an intermediate distance. Biocular microscopic prescriptions would therefore be tailored to the patient's specific, individual needs.

Fitting and Dispensing

Microscopes are available prefabricated, or they may need to be specifically designed for the individual patient. Some considerations in frame selection include the following:

1. The selected frame should be sturdy with a minimal vertex distance, allowing the lens to be as close to the eye as possible.
2. A small eye size will minimize edge thickness and lens weight.
3. For a bifocal microscope, the frame should have adjustable nosepads.
4. Lightweight frames with wide bearing surfaces will aid in even distribution of weight.[7]
5. Temple joints should allow for adjustment of pantoscopic tilt.
6. Vertical and horizontal eye size of the frame should be close to the anatomic eye position. This sizing will allow for proper centration of the lens, close to the visual axis of the eye.
7. When fitting a bifocal microscope, the segment should be set higher than a conventional bifocal. It may be set as high as the lower pupil margin. This is recommended because higher power bifocals have lower optical centers within the segment. By raising the height, the patient can sight through the optical center without excessive eye movements.[10]
8. A monocular bifocal should never be decentered.[11]

The dispensing visit can be used to reinforce proper use and care of the microscope. Adjustments can also be made to correctly position the lens both for vertex distance and pantoscopic angle. Comfort of the frame must also be addressed. Headbands and jumbo nosepads may contribute to the comfort of the frame as well.

INSTRUCTION TECHNIQUES FOR NEAR DEVICES

This section details the approach to instruction with all near devices. It is followed by techniques specific to microscopes.

Instructing the patient in the proper use of his or her low vision device greatly enhances the likelihood of success with the device. Ideally, instruction should take place before dispensing the device, and sufficient time should be allowed. During instruction, the practitioner or instructor should demonstrate to the patient that the device can indeed be useful for meeting his or her near-point goals, and that lighting, filters, and reading stands can enhance comfort and endurance. The patient is more likely to leave the office with confidence that the device will indeed be of benefit. Having the patient's family members or friends present during instruction may help, as they can assist in home practice and in reinforcing proper use of the device.

Before the Instructional Session

A number of factors should be considered when preparing for instruction with the patient. First, the length of the instructional session will depend on time available and such factors as patient age and fatigue. Next, the sequence of instructional activities should be considered. Ideally, the instruction would begin using large-print materials of excellent quality and contrast among other features. Then one would work down to the patient's goal materials. Due to practical limitations, such as time and patient energy level, however, it is often best to start with materials similar to, or slightly larger than, the patient's goal size; if successful, one can then introduce the goal materials. If unsuccessful, one can move up in print size or quality and have the patient practice with these materials for a week or so before reintroducing goal materials. The session should be geared toward positive experiences and success, to enhance patient motivation. Third, the patient's needs should be kept in mind. The practitioner or instructor should plan to move quickly from one activity to another during the instructional session to avoid fatigue. Frequent breaks may help forestall fatigue; during breaks, the instructor can casually talk with the patient, but the device should be set aside during this time. The practitioner or instructor must guard against overwhelming the patient with too much information; it is best to be economical in one's choice of words. Simple explanations are best. Summarizing the findings of the session at its conclusion can be very helpful. It would be helpful to send home a written summary of the instructional findings as well, as patients may forget some of what they were taught. If this is not practical, the practitioner or instructor should send home written instructions for home practice and perhaps some practice materials as well. A general set of instructions for each type of device can be prepared and photocopied for distribution to patients (see Appendixes A, B, and C). These instructions can be written in large print, or an audiotape summarizing the instructions may be considered.

The instructional area should be carefully designed and organized as well. Materials should be organized and within easy reach of the instructor. The area should be quiet and comfortable in terms of temperature. Interruptions should be minimized. Seating should allow for patient comfort and good postural support. A variety of task lamps and bulbs should be easily accessible. The patient can evaluate different types of lamps, including incandescent, fluorescent, or combination incandescent and fluorescent. Bulbs should be available in different wattages also. Reading stands should be included in the instructional area, as they can greatly enhance postural comfort. Clipboards can also be used to keep lightweight reading material flat. Nonoptical materials of importance include occluders, typoscopes, and line markers to reduce glare and assist in keeping one's place. Colored acetate filters are often helpful in enhancing contrast and reducing glare as well. Other useful items include spectacle head straps for stability and writing aids, such as felt tip markers, bold-lined paper, large-print checks, and various templates (e.g., check-writing, signature, envelope, and letter-writing guides).

Finally, a wide variety of reading materials is helpful to ensure that one is prepared for diverse patient goals. Typical patient goals include reading newspapers, magazines, mail, textbooks, checkbooks, price tags, receipts, labels on prescription bottles, and food packaging labels. Sheet music, recipes, accounting or bookkeeping forms, computer printouts, bus or train schedules, and various forms of bills should also be included. Patients with unusual goals should be encouraged to bring samples of goal materials with them. This suggestion is also beneficial for the patient who does not speak English as his or her native language.

Practice materials of excellent quality should be provided to enable success. Factors impacting on quality of practice materials include print size, spacing, font style, contrast, and color. Practice materials should be available in high-contrast print of various sizes (e.g., 0.8 M, 1.0 M, 1.5 M, 2.0 M, and 3.0 M). Font style should be simple and spacing should be varied (double or triple spaced at the top of the practice page, single spaced at the bottom). Quillman exercises are useful practice materials. In each print size, the Quillman exercises include one page of single letters (upper case on top half, lower case on bottom), one page of two-letter words; one page of three-letter words; one page of four- and five-letter words; one page of longer words; and one page of double- or triple-spaced sentences. These exercises can be especially helpful for patients who need to practice eccentric viewing because the spacing and print size are controlled. Some short stories (one or two pages) can be produced in several print sizes and varied line spacing as well. As each of the practice materials is introduced, the print size should be described in comparison with materials that are familiar to the patient (e.g., "this is the size of newsprint").

The idea is to control the difficulty of the reading material so that patients can have success with the device. Some patients may not be able to reach their goals with a low vision device until they have mastered eccentric viewing, however. Eccentric viewing is a very difficult process, although new training techniques are currently being investigated (see Low Vision Instruction and Rehabilitation in Chapter 5). Other patients may never be able to reach their goals. For example, the best acuity with the device may still not allow the patient to read a regular (print size) newspaper; in such cases, a patient may need to consider reading large print newspapers (published on a weekly basis only) or using a radio reading service, in which the newspaper is read daily over the air.

In addition to the overall print quality of materials, the reading level should be considered as well. It is best to use materials that are below the patient's reading level (e.g., a patient with a tenth-grade reading level should be given reading material that is below the tenth-grade level). Thus, the patient is not overwhelmed by being forced to comprehend difficult material while also learning how to use the device.

Instructional Sequence

Once the patient is comfortably seated, the practitioner or instructor should clarify the patient's goals or visual concerns. Some patients may initially report very modest goals but realize during the instruction process that low vision devices may enable them to achieve other goals as well. Typical patient goals should be discussed by the practitioner or instructor, as this may elicit other desired tasks. For example, many patients do not think to mention reading price tags in grocery and department stores or reading a menu in a restaurant. If, however, this is mentioned in discussion, patients often indicate that they would like to do so. Naturally, this discussion may result in the need for an additional near or intermediate device, because devices are often goal specific (e.g., microscopes are better for long-term reading; illuminated handheld or stand magnifiers may work best in stores or restaurants).

The patient should be asked to describe his or her visual condition and its functional implications, to ensure that he or she adequately understands both. This discussion of the patient's ocular condition may lead into eccentric viewing instruction if appropriate. In many cases, the instructor can help the patient understand the concept and find a viewing position that is best for using a particular device. The patient should be encouraged to practice eccentric viewing at home to refine the viewing position. For example, if a 12 o'clock viewing position is found to be best, the patient must still experiment to learn how far above the target he or she must look to obtain the best image. Written instructions explaining the concept of eccentric viewing and suggestions for practice activities should also be provided.

Where eccentric viewing is concerned, the patient must consistently use the best retinal locus. Eccentric viewing instruction should be done with the better seeing eye while the other eye is patched. Eccentric viewing may be explained by asking the patient to think of the target (e.g., the instructor's nose) as being in the center of a clock face. The patient is then asked to hold his or her head still and to direct his or her gaze above the instructor's nose (i.e., toward 12 o'clock), below it (6 o'clock), to the left (9 o'clock), and to the right (3 o'clock). Other clock positions should also be explored. The goal is to find the clock position that provides the best overall image of the instructor's nose. If the clearest view is provided by looking up, toward the instructor's forehead, then 12 o'clock is the patient's best eccentric viewing position.

Generally, the best eccentric viewing position for viewing the instructor's nose is also the best position for reading. This position should be verified by asking the patient to use the appropriate add to view a single letter that is two to three times his or her threshold acuity (to minimize strain). The patient should be directed to look above, below, to the left, and to the right of the letter. The goal is to have the patient obtain the clearest view of the letter. Once this position is found, the patient should be urged to use it consistently while reading. Many patients find it helpful to fixate on the first word of each page using their best eccentric viewing position. Then they hold their head and eye still while scrolling the page before their eyes. This technique helps them to maintain their best eccentric viewing position. Once eccentric viewing has been discussed, the instruction can move on to the proper use of the device and its use for reading goal materials.

If a patient is struggling to find and maintain the best eccentric viewing position, it may be helpful to cut a hole in a clip-on patch that corresponds to the best eccentric

viewing position and then place the patch over the patient's eye. When the patient looks straight ahead while wearing this patch, he or she will be prevented from seeing anything. Repeated practice with the patch may "train" the patient's eye to use the best eccentric viewing position, even without any conscious awareness of the patient as to which eccentric viewing position is being used.

Patients should be encouraged to handle the devices and to explore them visually before attempting to use them. After the patient has a basic familiarity with the device, instruction can proceed into the area of visual skills while using the device. Skills to be addressed should include eccentric viewing, establishing and maintaining the correct focal distance and page orientation, localization, keeping one's place, speed and ease of reading, and eye and head movements.

To aid in establishing the correct focal distance with a microscope, patients are advised to bring the reading material up to their nose and then push it out until a clear focus is obtained. When using a microscope, patients should be instructed to hold their head and eyes still and scroll the material in front of them, similar to a typewriter carriage. When using a handheld magnifier, the magnifier should be laid on the page and then lifted until the best compromise between magnification and distortion has been achieved. The page can then be scrolled beneath the magnifier as the patient maintains the best eccentric viewing position.

Throughout the instructional session, patients should be asked to read all practice materials aloud so that the instructor can monitor their performance with the device. Before beginning to read in detail, patients are encouraged to scan an entire page to learn its format. To maintain orientation to the page, it may be helpful to have the patient move his or her hand down the edge of the page when proceeding from one line to the next. Localization skills should be verified by asking the patient to find specific targets on the page. For example, the patient may be asked to find and read the first sentence on a page, or the third word on the fourth line. If the patient is interested in reading mail, envelopes with return addresses should be included in the instructional materials. People tend to view return addresses first when picking up their mail, so patients are asked to read them along with letters and bills during the instructional session.

Although some patients have no trouble keeping their place when using a device, others may have difficulty and require assistance. A typoscope or line marker may be useful for this purpose. Patients are urged to read across a line and then to scan back along that same line before dropping down to the next line. If the patient immediately drops down to the next line when reaching the end of a line, he or she may miss the last few words of a paragraph and thus skip a line. When using a hand or stand magnifier, the typoscope may be cut and taped to the bottom of the device.

A patient's ocular history may provide a reason for a patient's poor attitude toward using a low vision device. If adventitiously visually impaired, the patient probably has well-established visual skills that require some modification (e.g., may be accustomed to a certain working distance and initially resist a closer one). In addition, he or she may expect to be able to read at greater speeds because he or she was able to do so before the onset of visual impairment. Patients should always be asked to comment on their performance with the device, and the instructor should provide some general feedback. Endurance should be addressed as well. Patients must be informed that although their device may enable them to read the goal materials, their acuity or contrast sensitivity reserves might not be what a fully sighted person's are. Therefore, patients may need frequent breaks or might need to spread their reading sessions over the course of the day. Patients should be advised that this is a common occurrence. Eccentric viewing may also require more concentration by the patient, thus slowing the reading speed. Timed readings are useful for tracking patient progress over the course of several visits. They may also be useful for comparing different devices or to allow students to evaluate a device's practicality for school materials and assignments. For example, it may be most efficient to use a microscope or magnifier to read materials, such as math books, but to use a CCTV or taped materials for other subject areas, such as novels for English class. The practitioner and instructor should be able to assist the student in choosing the best combination of devices to maximize visual efficiency. The idea of combining reading media (e.g., talking books) with various low vision devices should, in fact, be discussed with most patients.

As the patient works with the device, the practitioner or instructor should observe the types of reading errors that are made. Does the patient struggle only with longer words, unfamiliar words, or in one area of the page? Observations and their implications should be discussed with the patient. The patient may need to practice eccentric viewing if only longer or unfamiliar words are missed. Problems in a specific area of the page may indicate a scotoma, failure to maintain the proper working distance, or an eccentric viewing problem. If a patient consistently struggles to identify various words in a passage, it is appropriate to ask the patient if he or she can see all the letters in the words without difficulty. It may also be useful to ask him or her to spell out the words. If the patient spells them with ease but still cannot pronounce them, a reading problem may be indicated. If he or she struggles to spell them out, then practice with eccentric viewing or the need for more magnification may be indicated. When asked to spell out words, patients will many times freely admit that they have reading difficulties (e.g., "I never was a very good reader"). In such cases, the patient's goals usually match his or her reading skills (e.g., the patient's only goal is to read mail). Patients may also be concerned that near devices will hurt their eyes or make them worse because they experience headache, eyestrain, or fatigue. These concerns must be addressed; otherwise, the patient may discontinue use of the device. Patients should be encouraged to give plenty of feedback about the device. This feedback can be a good vehicle for discussion of various concepts. The practitioner or instructor should give reinforcing feedback throughout the session as well.

At some point during the instructional session, reading stands, lighting, and filters should be evaluated. It is often helpful to place two reading materials of different print quality, but similar size, side by side on a clipboard or reading stand. This demonstration reminds the patient that the quality of print material is highly variable from one item to the next. Various types of lighting can be introduced and the patient can be asked to choose the best one. Usually, the task lamp used should be a flexible-arm lamp, and patients are advised to position the lamp themselves to provide adequate lighting for viewing the material. The close working distance of many near devices prohibits typical table or floor lamps from providing enough light on the page; thus, flexible-arm lamps are recommended. After the best type of light has been determined, the wattage, and color of bulb (e.g., soft white, pastel) should be addressed by comparing several options. Patients should be encouraged to experiment at home to learn the best combination of task and room lighting and to evaluate natural light as compared to artificial light as well.

After lighting has been evaluated, filters of various colors or shades can be introduced. As in the lighting evaluation, it may be helpful to have two reading samples of different quality placed side by side. Using the preferred lighting, each filter can be placed over a portion of the samples. Patients are then asked if the filters enable them to read the material more easily, and if so, to determine the preferred color filter. Patients are encouraged to use filters at their discretion to maximize reading performance. For example, a student may use a filter only for reading photocopied material. For patients who do not respond well to filters but still experience significant glare, slipover sun lenses in lighter tints can be evaluated. The use of a visor may also be helpful.

During instruction, the patient's posture should be observed and suggestions for maximizing comfort should be made (e.g., use a chair with armrests while using a clipboard to hold the reading material). It is impractical to have a large number of reading stands in the instructional area, as this requires a good deal of space. Several stands should be demonstrated to the patient, however, to determine if one would be beneficial. Low vision product suppliers often carry several reading stands, and catalogs can be given to the patient at the end of the instructional session. Patient goals are important in selecting a reading stand. For example, textbooks will require a sturdier stand than magazines or mail. Portability should also be considered. A simple, noncumbersome stand is probably the best. The stand should be positioned so that the patient can read from the top to the bottom of the page without undue postural strain. Reading stands and proper positioning are especially important for patients with special concerns, such as arthritis, tremors, or paralysis (see Chapter 13 section on posture and comfort maintenance).

Writing concerns should be addressed during the near instructional session. Use of a felt-tip pen can be demonstrated because its bolder lines can be more easily read than those of a typical ball-point pen. To write evenly across a line, bold-lined or raised-line paper can be demonstrated. A letter-writing guide is another alternative. For check writing, bold-lined checks, large-print checks, and check-writing guides can be demonstrated. An envelope and signature guide should also be shown. If writing is a goal but the prescribed microscope has a working distance that prevents holding the pen between the microscope and the paper, then a lower power, half-eye spectacle may be appropriate. For completing writing tasks with any device, placing a lap desk on the patient's desk or table can prevent undue back and neck strain.

Safety concerns, care, and cleaning of the device should be discussed as well. Regarding safety, patients should be warned not to walk around while wearing a microscope. They should also be discouraged from looking through the microscope at any distant object for any period because this may cause nausea.

Finally, suggestions and instructions for home practice should be given. Several short practice sessions per day usually work very well. Patients should be advised to build their endurance slowly. Written practice materials and instructions may be very useful. Loaning a device for home practice is recommended, because it allows the patient to determine whether the device will truly meet his or her needs. After a period of successful usage at home, both the practitioner and the patient will feel confident about the recommendation of the device. A follow-up phone call, shortly after a device has been prescribed, can be useful for addressing any difficulties that may have arisen with the device. It also affords the patient an opportunity to discuss any concerns that were not previously addressed.

Techniques Specific to Microscopes

The previous section presented general information for instructing patients on how to successfully use near devices. This section concentrates on specific information for instructing a patient on how to properly use a microscope.

1. The practitioner or instructor should always be positive and provide appropriate encouragement.
2. It should never be assumed that patients know how to properly use the microscope.
3. Discuss the importance of maintaining the correct focal length.
   a. For lower-powered microscopes, the patient should bring the material closer until a clear focus is found.
   b. With higher-powered microscopes, patients should start with the material touching their nose and then push it away until it is in clear focus.
4. The patient's visual axis should be perpendicular to the lens surface, passing through the optical center, and also be perpendicular to the reading material.
5. Reading material should be flat to maintain the correct focal distance.
6. Material should be scrolled before the eye. If the patient moves his or her eye or head, or both, the focal distance changes, resulting in blur or distortion.

Problem Solving with Microscopes

If a patient is experiencing difficulty in using a microscope, the following information may be helpful.

Problem	Remedy
1. Material out of focus (Figure 10-13)	a. The proper working distance should be checked and reinforced; physically assisting the patient in maintaining the working distance may be required. The patient should be told to touch the reading material to his or her nose, then push it out until clear. A pipe cleaner or stiff cardboard can be taped to the temple of the microscope to reinforce the working distance.
	b. Material should be flat (sometimes bound material will curve upward toward the binding as the patient reads), a clipboard to hold the material flat may be recommended.
2. Postural fatigue	a. Reading stands should be investigated.
	b. Chairs with a firm back and arm support should be used.
3. Asthenopia	a. The practice or reading times should be initially shortened.
	b. Eccentric viewing should be reinforced and practiced.
	c. If a binocular system is used, the amount of prism or the need to be monocular should be investigated; if monocular, the poorer eye should be occluded.
	d. If a patient has an astigmatic correction in his or her distance spectacle lens, it may have to be evaluated for incorporation into the microscope.
4. Losing place while reading	a. The use of a typoscope or finger to mark his or her place should be reviewed, a systematic approach to scanning material should be reinforced (read across then back along same line, then drop down to the next line).
	b. Eccentric viewing should be practiced.
5. Double vision	a. The poorer eye should be occluded.
	b. If binocular, the near interpupillary distance of the patient and lenses should be checked.
	c. If binocular, the need for base-in prism or the amount of prism should be checked.
	d. If wearing a bifocal, it should be adjusted to ensure that the

Problem	Remedy
	patient is not looking through the edge of the bifocal lens.
6. Distortion	a. The orientation and position of the reading material should be checked.
	b. Lenses may need cleaning.
	c. Frame may have to be adjusted.
	d. Eye movements should be limited; remind the patient to scroll reading material before his or her eyes.
7. Glare	a. Direction of illumination should be changed or illumination source should be moved closer or further from the object.
	b. A typoscope may be recommended.
	c. Acetate filters may be recommended or a tinted filter may be worn over the microscope; a visor may also be of some help.
8. Dimness of reading material	a. Direction of illumination should be changed or illumination should be increased by bringing it closer to the object, or the light source should be increased.
	b. Shadows should be eliminated.
	c. Yellow acetate filter should be placed on the reading material to increase contrast.

HANDHELD MAGNIFIERS

A handheld magnifier is a convex lens that a patient holds by means of a handle at various distances from the specta-cle plane. Ideally, the near object is held at the focal distance of the magnifying lens. In this situation, the convex lens will neutralize the divergent rays from the near object and allow parallel rays (or zero vergence) to exit the magnifier and travel (parallel) to the eye. The handheld magnifier with the near object held at the focal length of the lens will create a magnified retinal image without the need for an add or accommodation. The patient's refractive error, however, must be fully corrected.

Handheld magnifiers use the principles of relative distance magnification and angular magnification. As the magnifier and object are brought closer to the eye (with the object held at the focal point of the lens), relative distance magnification increases and angular magnification decreases. If the magnifier and object are pushed further away from the eye, angular magnification increases and relative distance magnification decreases. In both cases, the total magnification, or retinal image size, remains constant as long as the object remains at the focal point of the magnifying lens.

Options

There are three common types of convex lens designs used in handheld magnifiers. Detailed explanations were covered in the microscope section under Lens Options.

1. *Spherical lenses* can be planoconvex or biconvex. They are generally available in powers ranging from +3.00 D to +14.00 D (Figure 10-14). These magnifiers may have large-diameter lenses, especially those with low dioptric powers. The planoconvex and biconvex magnifiers are the least expensive and quite often can be purchased at a local stationery or craft store.

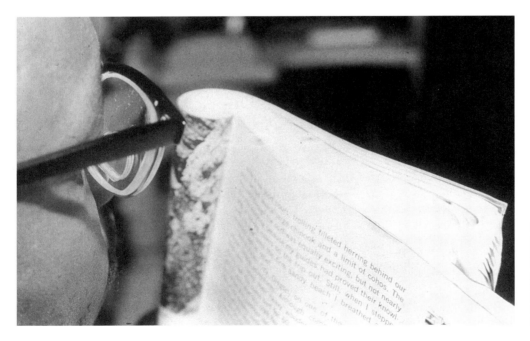

FIGURE 10-13. **When using a reading lens of high power, the focal distance is critical and must be properly maintained. If the reading material is not perfectly flat and at the correct focal length from the lens, the patient will report that the reading material appears to be in and out of focus.**

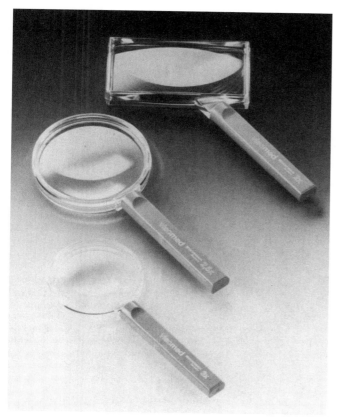

FIGURE 10-14. **Eschenbach spherical biconvex handheld magnifiers (Series 2614) are available in +3.90, +5.10, and +7.40 D. (Courtesy of Eschenbach Optik of America, Inc., Ridgefield, CT.)**

3. Patient familiarity and acceptance
4. Easy to prescribe
5. Widely available with many shapes and sizes
6. Allows for an extended working distance
7. Allows for head movement
8. No lens fabrication required
9. Binocularity possible in lower powers with large lens diameter
10. May be helpful for patients with reduced peripheral fields who require magnification at near
11. May be used with or without an add (equivalent power will vary, however)
12. Useful for quick spotting
13. Illumination available (halogen or incandescent)
14. May be helpful, in low powers, for patients wishing to write (e.g., writing signature, writing check)

Disadvantages

1. Requires a steady hand and coordination
2. Decreased field of view with increased working distance
3. Need to replace bulbs and batteries for illuminated magnifiers
4. Decreased reading speed (when compared to equivalent powered microscope)
5. Must be held parallel to the reading material to avoid print distortion
6. Increased distortion noted in the periphery of the lens of many handheld magnifiers as they are held further from the eye

Equivalent Power

The equivalent power of a handheld magnifier depends on how it is used. When the object (or reading material) is held at the focal point of the magnifying lens, parallel light will leave the lens and therefore the patient's best distance spectacle correction should be in place. The equivalent power in this situation is equal to the equivalent power of the magnifying lens itself. When the object is maintained at the focal point of the magnifying lens, the magnifier and object can be moved closer to or further away from the patient with the equivalent power (or retinal image size) remaining constant. In other words, the equivalent power or the total magnification of the system is independent of the distance from the magnifier to the spectacle plane as long as the object is held at the focal point of the magnifying lens.

When the object or reading material is held within the focal point of the handheld magnifier, divergent rays of light leave the lens. When this occurs, the emmetropic patient is forced to use some accommodation or an add to see the object clearly. When a handheld magnifier is used in combination with a patient's accommodation or add, the equivalent power can be determined from the following formula:

$$D_{eq} = D_1 + D_2 - (d)(D_1)(D_2)$$

where D_1 = dioptric power of the handheld magnifier; D_2 = dioptric power of the add, accommodation used, or

2. *Aspheric lenses* are the most commonly prescribed of the three options. They can be spherical on one surface and aspheric on the other, or biaspheric (Figure 10-15). They are generally available in powers ranging from +6.00 D to +40.00 D. When using a magnifier with an aspheric surface, the curved surface should face the patient and the flatter or spherical surface should face the object. When biaspheric, it does not matter which surface faces the patient.

3. *Aplanatic lenses* consist of two planoconvex lenses with the convex surfaces in contact with each other (doublet lens). They are generally available from +6.00 D to +40.00 D. This magnifier provides the least amount of image distortion from edge to edge (Figure 10-16). It is generally the most expensive of all of the handheld magnifiers.

Advantages and Disadvantages of a Handheld Magnifier

The advantages and disadvantages of a handheld magnifier must be considered before prescribing one for a patient.

Advantages

1. Portability
2. Relatively inexpensive

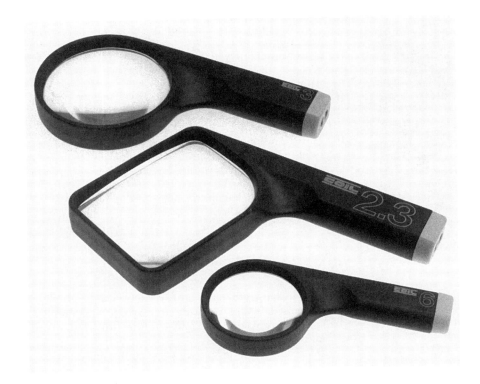

FIGURE 10-15. **COIL biaspheric handheld magnifiers (C.O.I.L. Combined Optical Industries, Ltd., Elk Grove Village, IL) are available in equivalent powers of +2.70, +5.00, + 7.60, +10.50, and +18.00 D. They are ergonomically designed to be easily used by both right-handed and left-handed patients.**

uncorrected myopic refractive error at the spectacle plane; and d = separation, in meters, between D_1 and D_2.

Example 1
An emmetropic patient is looking through both a +2.50 D bifocal and +10.00 D handheld magnifier to read the newspaper. What is the equivalent power when the magnifier is held against the bifocal?
   Answer:

$$D_{eq} = D_1 + D_2 - (d)(D_1)(D_2)$$
$$= 10.00 + 2.50 - (0)(10.00)(2.50)$$
$$= +12.50 \text{ D}$$

   When a handheld magnifier is held in contact with a bifocal, the D_{eq} will be at its maximum value for that particular combination of lenses.

Example 2
An emmetropic patient is looking through both a +2.50 D bifocal and a +10.00 D handheld magnifier to read the newspaper. What is the equivalent power when the magnifier is held 5 cm from the bifocal?
   Answer:

$$D_{eq} = D_1 + D_2 - (d)(D_1)(D_2)$$
$$= 10.00 + 2.50 - (0.05)(10.00)(2.50)$$
$$= +11.25 \text{ D}$$

   As the magnifier is moved away from the add, the equivalent power will decrease. In this case, however, (when the magnifier is held within one focal length of the add) the equivalent power is still greater (when

using the bifocal) than the power of the magnifying lens alone.

Example 3
An emmetropic patient is looking through both a +2.50 D bifocal and a +10.00 D handheld magnifier to read the newspaper. What is the equivalent power when the magnifier is 10 cm from the bifocal?
   Answer:

$$D_{eq} = D_1 + D_2 - (d)(D_1)(D_2)$$
$$= 10.00 + 2.50 - (0.10)(10.00)(2.50)$$
$$= +10.00 \text{ D}$$

   When the magnifier is held at its focal length from the add, the equivalent power is always equal to the equivalent power of the magnifier alone. This point is called the *neutral point,* or *transition point.* Therefore, in this situation it would not matter whether the patient looked through his or her distance spectacle correction with the magnifier (with the object held at the focal point of the magnifying lens) or looked through the bifocal with the magnifier (with the object held within a given distance of the focal point of the magnifier and the magnifier held one focal length from the bifocal). In both cases, the equivalent power would be equal to the power of the magnifying lens alone.

Example 4
An emmetropic patient is looking through both a +2.50 D bifocal and a +10.00 D handheld magnifier to read the newspaper. What is the equivalent power when the magnifier is held 20 cm from the bifocal?

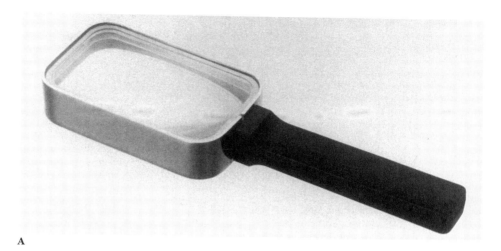

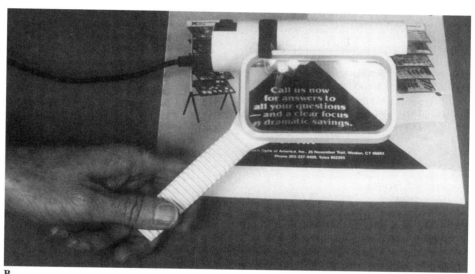

FIGURE 10-16. **A.** The Eschenbach rectangular aplanatic magnifier consists of two planoconvex lenses that allow for minimum distortion from edge to edge. Series 2465 and 2466 are available in powers of +5.60, +6.80, +7.40, +7.80, and +11.00 D. (Courtesy of Eschenbach Optik of America, Inc., Ridgefield, CT.) **B.** The Eschenbach aplanatic series 2666 is less expensive than series 2465 and 2466 and is available in powers of +6.80, +7.40, +11.30, and +14.00 D. This magnifier is also demonstrating an illuminated source that can be easily added (and removed) to many of the Eschenbach magnifying lens systems. (Courtesy of Eschenbach Optik of America, Inc., Ridgefield, CT.)

Answer:

$$D_{eq} = D_1 + D_2 - (d)(D_1)(D_2)$$
$$= 10.00 + 2.50 - (0.20)(10.00)(2.50)$$
$$= +7.50 \text{ D}$$

When the magnifier is held greater than one focal length from the bifocal, the equivalent power of the handheld magnifier and the add combined is actually less than the handheld magnifier alone. When the handheld magnifier is held further than one focal length from the add, there is a disadvantage to using the add. As the distance between the magnifier and the add increases by one focal length of the magnifier, the equivalent power decreases by the add power. In the preceding example, when the magnifier is held at 20 cm (transition point plus one focal length), D_{eq} decreases by +2.50 D. At 30 cm (transition point plus two focal lengths), the D_{eq} will decrease by +5.00 D.

Example 5

An emmetropic patient is looking through both a +2.50 D bifocal and a +10.00 D handheld magnifier to read the newspaper. What is the equivalent power when the magnifier is held 60 cm from the bifocal?

Answer:

$$D_{eq} = D_1 + D_2 - (d)(D_1)(D_2)$$
$$= 10.00 + 2.50 - (0.60)(10.00)(2.50)$$
$$= -2.50 \text{ D}$$

When a handheld magnifier is held at a distance greater than the focal length of the add that is being used with the magnifier, a reversed astronomic telescope is formed. The patient will see a small inverted image.

In summary, when a patient uses a handheld magnifier in conjunction with a bifocal (or the patient's accommodation or uncorrected myopia), the equivalent power can be less than, equal to, or greater than the magnifier alone, depending on how far the magnifier and object are held from the spectacle plane. The neutral point, or transition point, occurs when a handheld magnifier is held one focal length (of the magnifier) from the spectacle plane (bifocal). If the magnifier is held closer than one focal length, there is indeed an advantage to using the add. If the magnifier is held farther away than one focal length, however, there is a disadvantage in using the add, as the equivalent power will decrease. When the magnifier is held farther away than one focal length from the spectacle plane, the distance portion of the spectacles should be used. Patients should therefore be instructed to use either the add or their distance correction, depending on where they choose to hold the magnifier.

In situations in which the magnifier is not held at its focal length from the reading material, variable vergence can exit the magnifier. If the material is held within the magnifier's focal length, divergent rays will exit the lens. In this situation, an add or accommodation is then needed to clear the magnified image. Divergent rays of light exiting a magnifier, however, can also correct for myopia if the patient is not corrected with spectacle lenses (or contact lenses). Conversely, if the handheld magnifier is being held too far from the page, or farther away than the focal length, convergent rays of light will exit the lens. An uncorrected hyperope will capitalize on these convergent rays of light and therefore see a clear, magnified image. When reading material is held at a distance greater than the focal length of the magnifying lens, however, an emmetropic patient will see the reading material as being upside down or inverted.

Prescribing Strategies

Because a patient may have many different near demands, one magnifier may not solve all the visual concerns. A patient may therefore need several magnifiers to meet his or her needs. For example, a patient may need a high-powered magnifier for viewing information in a phone book, a weaker-powered illuminated magnifier for a restaurant menu, and a moderately powered pocket magnifier for checking price tags and labels while shopping. Patients should be encouraged to evaluate different magnifiers for different needs. Some variations to consider are the following:

1. *Power.* Amount of magnification needed for a particular task (Figure 10-17).
2. *Flexibility.* Some magnifiers have multiple lenses that can be used alone or in combination to create increased power (Figure 10-18); some handheld magnifiers can also be converted to stand magnifiers using folding legs.
3. *Shape.* Rectangular versus round. The patient should understand that power is the biggest controlling factor of shape. Rectangular magnifiers are found only in low-powered magnifiers.
4. *Size.* As the power of the magnifier increases, the overall diameter of the magnifier will get smaller.
5. *Illumination.* Some magnifiers are illuminated and others are not (Figure 10-19). For those magnifiers that are illuminated, the bulbs can be incandescent or halogen.

6. *Coating and tints.* Some magnifiers have antireflective coatings to increase light transmission and eliminate some lens aberrations, whereas other magnifiers have tints to help enhance contrast.

Field of View

Another important consideration with handheld magnifiers is the field of view. Factors affecting the field of view include lens power, lens size, and distance of the lens to the eye. As the power of the lens increases, lens diameter decreases to help minimize peripheral aberrations, which in turn results in a smaller field of view. The field is also affected by the separation between the eye and magnifier. This concept is represented in the following equation[11]:

$$W = (d)\left(\frac{f}{h}\right)$$

where W = linear width of the visible field; d = lens diameter; f = focal length of the magnifier; and h = distance from the lens to the eye. **Note.** All terms must be in the same measurement units.

Example 1
What is the linear field of view of a +8.00 D handheld magnifier with a 20 mm lens diameter when it is held 6.25 cm from the eye?
Answer:

$$W = (d)\left(\frac{f}{h}\right)$$
$$= (2)\left(\frac{12.5}{6.25}\right)$$
$$= 4 \text{ cm or } 40 \text{ mm}$$

If the magnifier is held at half its focal length from the eye, the field of view is twice the diameter of the lens.

Example 2
What is the linear field of view of a +8.00 D handheld magnifier with a 20 mm lens diameter when it is held 12.5 cm from the eye?
Answer:

$$W = (d)\left(\frac{f}{h}\right)$$
$$= (2)\left(\frac{12.5}{12.5}\right)$$
$$= 2 \text{ cm or } 20 \text{ mm}$$

If the magnifier is held one focal length from the eye, the field of view is equal to the diameter of the lens.

Example 3
What is the linear field of view of a +8.00 D handheld magnifier with a 20 mm lens diameter when it is held 25.0 cm from the eye?

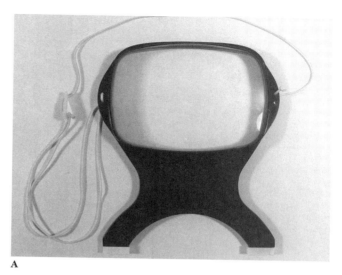

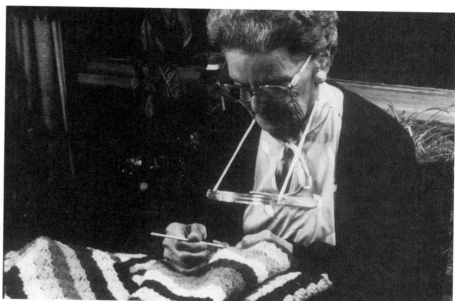

FIGURE 10-17. **A. Chest magnifiers vary slightly in shape and power (equivalent powers of approximately +2.50 D to +5.00 D in the main magnifying lens with a smaller lens of a higher power insert) with various manufacturers. All systems, however, allow for hands-free operation and are helpful with needlework or knitting. B. The cord supplied with the magnifier allows the patient to easily adjust the distance of the magnifier from her spectacle correction. The needlework is held at the correct focal distance from the magnifier. (Courtesy of Eschenbach Optik of America, Inc., Ridgefield, CT.)**

Answer:

$$W = (d)\left(\frac{f}{h}\right)$$
$$= (2)\left(\frac{12.5}{25.0}\right)$$
$$= 1 \text{ cm or } 10 \text{ mm}$$

If the magnifier is held two focal lengths from the eye, the field of view is reduced to half the diameter of the lens.

Example 4
What is the linear field of view of a +8.00 D handheld magnifier with a 20 mm lens diameter when it is held 40.0 cm from the eye?

Answer:

$$W = (d)\left(\frac{f}{h}\right)$$
$$= (2)\left(\frac{12.5}{40.0}\right)$$
$$= 0.6 \text{ cm or } 6 \text{ mm}$$

Therefore, the farther away the magnifier is held, the smaller the linear field of view.

In summary, as the distance from the magnifier to the eye is increased, the field of view of the handheld magnifier decreases. When the magnifier is held one focal length away from the eye, the field of view is equal to the diameter of the lens. When the magnifier is held at half the focal

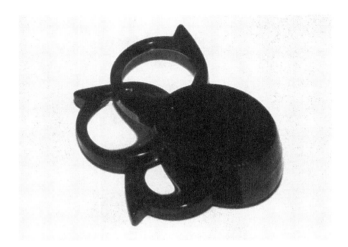

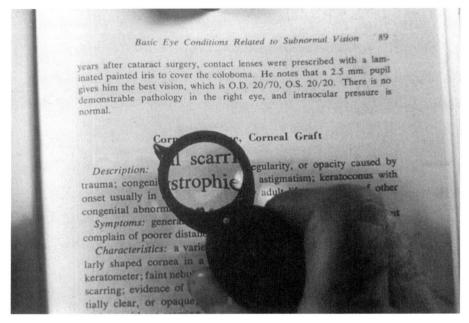

FIGURE 10-18. **This magnifier combines two or three lenses into a handheld magnifier that allows the patient the possibility of three or four magnifications in one device.**

length from the eye, the field of view is doubled, and when held two focal lengths from the eye, the field of view is half the diameter of the lens. It is not uncommon for a patient to start out holding the magnifier far from the spectacle plane; however, in most cases (especially when reading) he or she will gradually decrease this distance as the benefit of the increased field of view is realized.

Lens Verification

The equivalent power of a handheld magnifier may be estimated by the same methods detailed in the microscope section under Lens Verification. These methods include the method of triangulation, lens clock neutralization, hand neutralization, and lensometry. The method of triangulation is the most accurate. When using a lensometer, however, the most convex surface should be placed against the lens stop to obtain the most accurate reading.

Dispensing

Proper use and care of the device should be reviewed at the dispensing visit. If an illuminated handheld magnifier is being dispensed, the patient should be instructed on how to change the batteries and bulbs.

Instruction Techniques

The general approach to instruction with near devices can be found in the Instruction Techniques section under Microscopes. The following is a list of techniques specific to handheld magnifiers:

1. The practitioner or instructor should always be positive and provide appropriate encouragement.
2. It should never be assumed that the patient knows how to properly use the handheld magnifier.

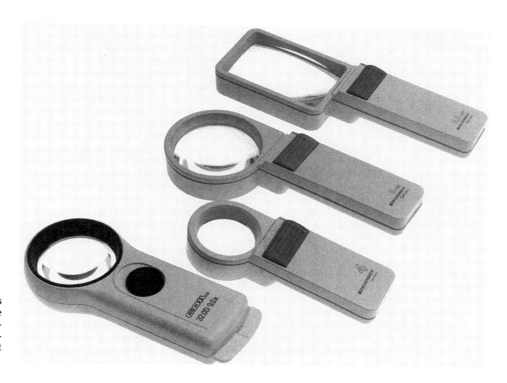

FIGURE 10-19. **Illuminated magnifiers are very useful to patients who require magnifications in poorly lit environments (e.g., reading a menu in a restaurant, reading a thermostat in a poorly lit room).**

3. To ensure the correct focal length, the patient should be instructed to lay the magnifier on the page and to slowly pull the magnifier away from the page until the clearest image is found.
4. The patient should be instructed to use the carrier or add, depending on the magnifier-to-eye distance of the handheld magnifier. Some patients will benefit from understanding the transition point concept.
5. The patient should be shown how the field of view increases as the lens and object are brought closer to the eye.
6. For illuminated magnifiers, the patient should be reminded to turn the light off when the device is not in use.
7. For nonilluminated magnifiers, the patient should be shown how to use direct illumination from a lamp without causing glare and reflections off of the magnifying lens.
8. The magnifier's lens should be held parallel to the reading material.
9. The magnifier's lens should be parallel to the spectacle plane, so the line of sight can be perpendicular to the lens.
10. The patient should be instructed to move his or her eye and the magnifier together as a unit.
11. To minimize peripheral distortions, the most curved side (convex side) of the magnifying lens should be held toward the patient's eye.

Problem Solving

Problems encountered by the patient using a handheld magnifier may require additional instruction. There are several problems that may have simple solutions.

Problem	Remedy
1. Material out of focus	a. Maintaining the proper focal distance should be stressed.
	b. The reading material must be kept stationary and flat.
	c. It should be determined if the patient is using his or her distance or near correction with magnifier.
2. Postural fatigue	a. The patient's arms and wrists should be braced.
	b. A reading stand may be suggested.
	c. A microscope or stand magnifier may be suggested instead of using the handheld magnifier.
3. Loses place while reading	a. A typoscope or finger to mark his or her place may be suggested.
	b. Instruction in scanning may be recommended.
	c. Instruction in eccentric viewing may be recommended.
4. Distortion	a. The magnifier and object should be moved closer to the patient's eye.
	b. The magnifier must be held parallel to the object; the patient should be looking through the center of magnifying lens.
	c. The most convex surface of the magnifier must be facing the patient's eye.
	d. The object should be held slightly inside the focal length of the magnifier (the patient may have to use an add or some accommodation).
	e. A better quality magnifier of equivalent power may have to be considered (e.g., aplanatic).

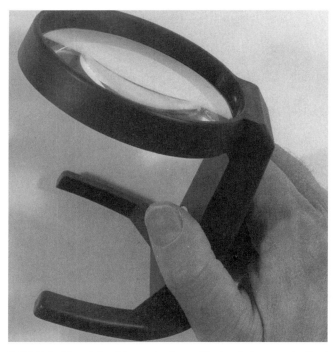

FIGURE 10-20.   **A fixed-focus stand magnifier has its lens set at a fixed distance from its base.**

Problem	Remedy
	f. The patient may be lifting the magnifier too far from the page: the proper distance between the magnifier and object should be reinforced.
5. Small field of view	a. The magnifier and object should be moved closer to the eye.
	b. May consider another magnifier of equivalent power with a larger lens diameter.
	c. May consider an aplanatic magnifier.
6. Inverted image	a. Object or reading material is being held outside of the focal length of the magnifier, and the patient should bring the object closer to the magnifier.
7. Reflections off lens surface	a. An illuminated magnifier may be considered.
	b. The direction of the external light source may have to be changed.
	c. Handheld magnifier may have to be repositioned.
	d. Magnifier with antireflective coating may be considered.
8. Glare	a. The position of the light source should be changed.
	b. The illumination should be decreased.
	c. A typoscope should be evaluated.
	d. Filters should be evaluated.
	e. Tinted magnifier may be considered.
	f. Handheld magnifier may have to be repositioned.
9. Dimness of reading	a. Illuminated magnifier should be used.
	b. The direction of the light source should be changed.
	c. The light intensity should be increased.
	d. Yellow tint or yellow filter may increase contrast, making reading material less dim or less faint.

STAND MAGNIFIERS

As with handheld magnifiers, stand magnifiers are familiar devices. They are appropriate for both extended reading and quick spotting tasks. A stand magnifier is a convex lens that is mounted at a fixed distance from the reading material. The patient is not required to hold the magnifier; rather, it is supported by legs or a housing that "stands" on the reading material. Total magnification of a stand magnifier results from relative distance magnification and angular magnification by the lens. There are two types of stand magnifiers: variable focus and fixed focus. Focusable stand magnifiers have lenses that can be adjusted closer to or farther away from the reading material. Focusing can compensate for uncorrected refractive error or accommodative demand of the stand magnifier.

A fixed-focus stand magnifier has its lens set at a fixed distance from the base (Figure 10-20). In most cases, the distance from the reading material to the lens is slightly less than the focal length of the lens. (There are a small number of stand magnifiers that are manufactured to stand at the focal length of the convex lens. The COIL "blue line" [C.O.I.L. Combined Optical Industries, Ltd., Elk Grove Village, IL] is the most common example.) By positioning the material within the focal length, there is a decrease in peripheral lens distortions. A fixed-focus stand magnifier (with the object held within the focal length of the lens) creates an erect, virtual image located at a finite distance behind the magnifier. When a convex lens is mounted within its focal length, it cannot neutralize all of the divergent rays of light created by the reading material. Therefore, divergent rays will exit the stand magnifier and require an add or accommodation to see the image clearly.

Options

As occurs with handheld magnifiers and microscopes, stand magnifiers are available in several lens designs.

1. *Spherical lenses* can be planoconvex or biconvex. They are available in powers from approximately +5.00 D to +24.00 D. A bar magnifier is a variation of a stand magnifier (Figure 10-21). It is a planoconvex lens with a cylindrical component that only magnifies in the vertical meridian. The availability of a bar magnifier is limited to low powers of +2.00 D to +3.50 D.
2. *Aspheric lenses* can be spherical on one surface and aspheric on the other or biaspheric. The majority of

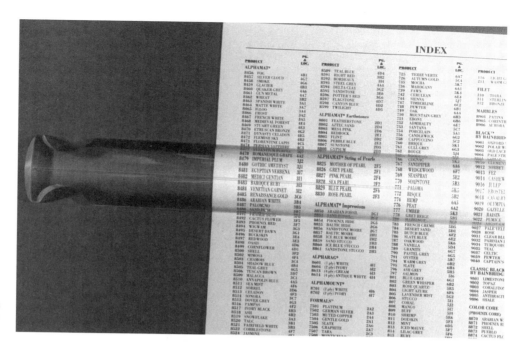

FIGURE 10-21.   **A bar magnifier is available in low powers and magnifies only in the vertical direction.**

stand magnifiers are made with aspheric lens design. Powers range from +7.00 D to +40.00 D for aspheric and from +20.00 D to +60.00 D for bispheric designs.

3. *Aplanatic lenses* consist of two planoconvex lenses with their convex surfaces in contact. They are available from approximately +20.00 D to +40.00 D.

Advantages and Disadvantages of a Stand Magnifier

The advantages and disadvantages of a stand magnifier must be considered before prescribing one for a patient.

Advantages

1. Extended working distance
2. Some designs may be useful for writing (Figure 10-22)
3. Portability
4. Relatively inexpensive
5. Good for patients with tremors or poor motor control because of its stable base
6. Good for specific detailed tasks, such as hobbies (e.g., stamp collecting, coin collecting)
7. Large range of powers available
8. Available with or without an illumination source (Figure 10-23)

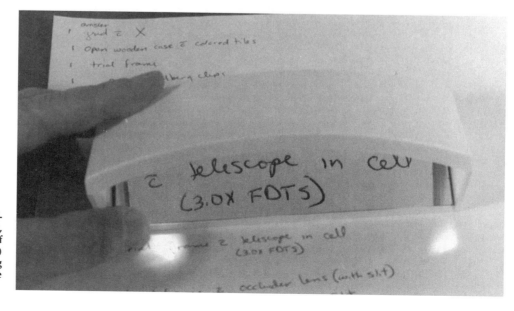

FIGURE 10-22.   **The Mirror magnifier (Optical Designs, Inc., Houston, TX) provides the equivalent power of +13.30 D with a reading field (width) of 5 in. It is convenient for writing because the system magnifies the material directly in front of it.**

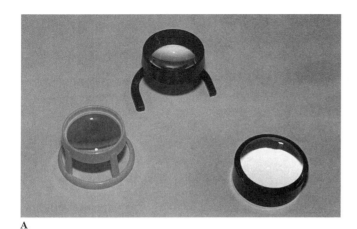

A

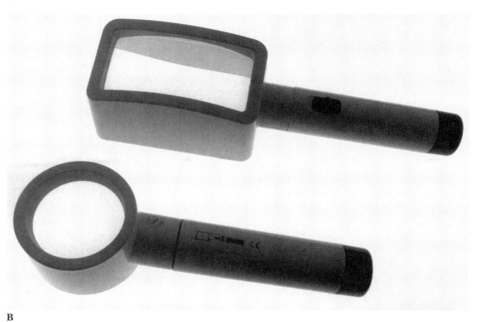

B

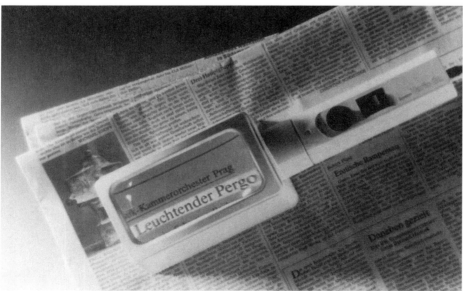

C

FIGURE 10-23. **Stand magnifiers are available in various shapes and sizes. They are also available with and without an illumination source. A. Fixed-stand magnifiers with no illumination. B. Fixed-stand magnifiers with an illumination source attached. C. The Highlighter is an illuminated stand magnifier (Series 1588-04) in which the entire field under the magnifying head is illuminated; however, it also has an orientation line that is brighter and therefore highlights one line of print at a time. (B and C courtesy of Eschenbach Optik of America, Inc., Ridgefield, CT.)**

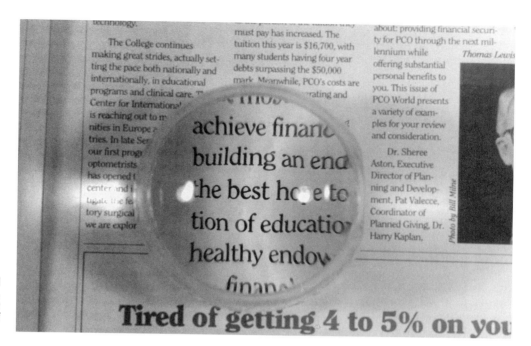

FIGURE 10-24. **The Jupiter stand magnifier (The Lighthouse, Inc., Long Island City, NY) has a clear housing that allows illumination of the reading material.**

9. May be helpful for patients with constricted fields who require magnification for near tasks

Disadvantages

1. Accommodation or add needed (for most fixed-focus stands)
2. Decreased field of view (as compared to an equivalent-powered microscope)
3. Lens aberrations induced if line of sight is not perpendicular to the lens optical center
4. Bulky, cumbersome
5. Some are heavy, especially those with batteries
6. May create posture and fatigue problems
7. Must determine equivalent power of most systems (manufacturer's labels overestimate magnification)
8. Difficulty maintaining proper illumination unless the magnifier has an illumination source or clear housing (Figure 10-24)

Equivalent Power

As previously mentioned in the introductory paragraph of the stand magnifier section, in most cases the distance from the base of a stand magnifier to its lens is less than the focal length of the lens. The printed material held at the base of the stand will produce an erect, virtual image at a finite distance behind the base, which requires that the patient use accommodation or an add to see the image clearly. To determine the equivalent power of the stand magnifier, the practitioner must first determine the proper add (or accommodation) that is required to see the image clearly and the distance that the stand magnifier's lens is held from the spectacle plane. Once these are determined, the equivalent power can be calculated by the familiar formula:

$$D_{eq} = D_1 + D_2 - (d)(D_1)(D_2)$$

where D_1 = the dioptric power of the lens of the stand magnifier; D_2 = the dioptric power of the add, accommodation, or patient's uncorrected myopia; and d = distance separation, in meters, of the lens of a stand magnifier to the spectacle plane (i.e., bifocal).

Example 1

A +20.00 D stand magnifier is placed on a newspaper and the lens of the magnifier is permanently fixed at 4 cm from the base of the stand. If the lens of the stand magnifier is 20 cm from the patient's spectacle plane, what power bifocal would be required for this patient to see the magnified image of the newspaper clearly?

Answer (Figure 10-25): The print at 4 cm from the magnifying lens will have a vergence of –25.00 D at the lens. The +20.00 D lens will neutralize 20.00 D of the 25.00 D of divergence, thereby allowing 5.00 D of divergence to exit the lens. The 5.00 D of divergence will create a virtual image located 20 cm behind the lens. Therefore, if the virtual image is 20 cm from the lens, and the lens is 20 cm from the patient's spectacle plane, then the virtual image is 40 cm from the patient's spectacle plane. For a patient with absolute presbyopia to see this image clearly, he or she would require a +2.50 D add.

Example 2

A +20.00 D stand magnifier is placed on a newspaper and the lens of the magnifier is permanently fixed at 4 cm from the base of the stand. If the patient is wearing a +3.00 D bifocal, how far away must the lens of the stand magnifier be (from the bifocal) for this patient to see the magnified image of the newspaper clearly?

Distance from spectacle plane to virtual image must be determined

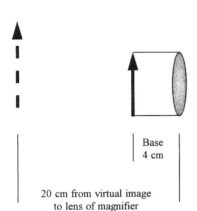

Base
4 cm

20 cm from virtual image
to lens of magnifier

20 cm from spectacle plane
to lens of magnifier

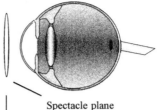

Spectacle plane
(Add to be determined)

FIGURE 10-25.   **A +20.00 D stand magnifier used 20 cm from a patient's bifocal spectacle correction.**

Answer (Figure 10-26): The print at 4 cm from the magnifying lens will have a vergence of −25.00 D at the lens. The +20.00 D lens will neutralize 20.00 D of the 25.00 D of divergence, thereby allowing 5.00 D of divergence to exit the lens. The 5.00 D of divergence will create a virtual image located 20 cm behind the lens. If the patient is wearing a +3.00 D bifocal, the virtual image must be 33.33 cm from the bifocal to be seen clearly. Because the virtual image is 20 cm from the lens, and the virtual image is 33.33 cm from the patient's bifocal, then the lens of the magnifier must be 13.33 cm from the patient's bifocal.

From the preceding examples, one can see that a bifocal (add) or accommodation is required when using a fixed stand magnifier, in which the base is closer than the focal length of the lens. The power of the bifocal (or accommodation) will have an effect on the equivalent power of a stand magnifier–bifocal system. The same stand magnifier can be used with different adds, resulting in a number of different equivalent powers, and therefore, different magnifications (different retinal image sizes).

Example 3

A +20.00 D stand magnifier is placed on a newspaper and the lens of the magnifier is permanently fixed at 4 cm from the base of the stand. If the lens of the stand magnifier is 20 cm from the patient's spectacle plane, what is the equivalent power of this stand magnifier–bifocal system, assuming that the patient is an absolute presbyope?

Answer: From Example 1, it was determined that a +2.50 D bifocal is required. By using the formula $D_{eq} = D_1 + D_2 − (d)(D_1)(D_2)$, the equivalent power is

$$D_{eq} = +20.00 + (+2.50) − (0.20)(+20.00)(+2.50)$$
$$D_{eq} = +12.50 \text{ D}$$

Example 4

A +20.00 D stand magnifier is placed on a newspaper and the lens of the magnifier is permanently fixed at 4 cm from the base of the stand. If the patient is wearing a +3.00 D bifocal, what is the equivalent power of this stand magnifier–bifocal system?

33.3 cm from spectacle plane to virtual image

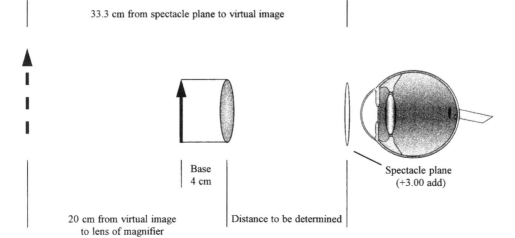

Base
4 cm

20 cm from virtual image
to lens of magnifier

Distance to be determined

Spectacle plane
(+3.00 add)

FIGURE 10–26.   **A +20.00 D stand magnifier used in conjunction with a +3.00 D bifocal.**

Answer: From Example 2, it was determined that a distance of 13.33 cm is required between the lens of the stand magnifier and the +3.00 D bifocal. By using the formula $D_{eq} = D_1 + D_2 - (d)(D_1)(D_2)$, the equivalent power is

$$D_{eq} = +20.00 + (+3.00) - (0.13)(+20.00)(+3.00)$$

$$D_{eq} = +15.20\ D$$

Thus, if a +20.00 D stand magnifier provides the needed magnification when used at 13.33 cm, it will be underpowered if used at 20 cm. Therefore, a higher-powered stand magnifier is needed at the greater working distance. The importance of determining the equivalent power is therefore apparent.

A second, perhaps simpler method to determine D_{eq} can be found in the following equation:

$$D_{eq} = (D_2)(ER)$$

where D_2 = the patient's bifocal or accommodation and ER = the enlargement ratio, and is defined as the increased image size as compared to the size of the object. This is also known as *transverse magnification, lateral magnification,* or as the *multacc factor* (multiply by accommodation).[12] The enlargement ratio can be defined by the following equation:

$$ER = \frac{L' - D_1}{L'}$$

where D_1 = dioptric power of the lens of the stand magnifier and L' = image vergence out of D_1; it is a negative value because it represents divergence.

Example 5

A +20.00 D stand magnifier is placed on a newspaper and the lens of the magnifier is permanently fixed at 4 cm from the base of the stand. If the lens of the stand magnifier is 20 cm from the patient's spectacle plane, what is the equivalent power of this stand magnifier assuming that the patient is an absolute presbyope?

Answer: From Example 1, it was determined that the image vergence from the +20.00 D lens was –5.00 D. By using the preceding two formulas, the equivalent power can easily be determined.

1.
$$ER = \frac{L' - D_1}{L'}$$
$$ER = \frac{(-5.00) - (+20.00)}{-5.00} = 5\times$$

2.
$$D_{eq} = (D_2)(ER)$$
$$D_{eq} = (+2.50)(5) = +12.50\ D$$

This is the same result as calculated using the equivalent power equation. Both ER and L' are constant for a given fixed-focus stand magnifier and a given object-to-lens distance (4 cm in this case). The resultant equivalent diopters

(D_{eq}) will therefore be dependent on the add or amount of accommodation used.

Focusable stand magnifiers may have variable vergence exiting the lens. The stand magnifier can be focused so that parallel light, or zero vergence, exits the lens. In this case, when the reading material is held at the correct focal length of the lens, the equivalent power of the stand magnifier is equal to the equivalent power of the lens itself. Other times, the magnifier may be adjusted to create vergence to compensate for an uncorrected refractive error.

Prescribing Strategies

As occurs with handheld magnifiers, patients may have goals requiring more than one stand magnifier. Different stand magnifiers may be shown to the patient in an attempt to meet as many near goals as possible. Some variations to demonstrate to the patient include

1. *Power.* Amount of magnification needed for a particular task.
2. *Flexibility.* Some stand magnifiers can also be converted to handheld magnifiers by folding the legs; some stand magnifiers are focusable; the type of base will vary with the magnifier—some are open on the bottom for writing.
3. *Shape.* Rectangular versus round; the patient should understand that power is the biggest controlling factor of shape. Rectangular magnifiers are found only in low-powered magnifiers.
4. *Size.* As the power of the magnifier increases, the overall diameter of the magnifier decreases to reduce peripheral distortions.
5. *Illumination.* Some magnifiers are illuminated and others are not. For magnifiers that are illuminated, some may be battery-operated, whereas others have to be plugged into an electrical outlet. There are also a few magnifiers that when plugged into an electrical outlet have a rheostat to vary the illumination. And finally, for those magnifiers that are illuminated, the bulbs can vary from incandescent to halogen to the new generation of compact (energy-saving) fluorescent.
6. *Coating and tints.* Some magnifiers have antireflective coatings to increase light transmission and eliminate some lens aberrations, whereas other magnifiers have tints to help enhance contrast.

Refractive Error

A variable focus stand magnifier can be used to compensate for uncorrected refractive error. If the lens is moved closer to the page, light rays will leave with divergence, thus correcting for myopia. When the lens is moved farther out from the page, converging light rays will exit, correcting for hyperopia. A fixed-focus stand magnifier (with the base shorter than the focal length of the lens) will require the patient to be fully corrected and use a bifocal if presbyopic.

Accommodation

As discussed in the equivalent power section, accommodation or an add is needed to neutralize the divergent rays leaving most fixed-focus stand magnifiers. This creates a flexible system for the pre-presbyope. Patients with the ability to vary their accommodation can therefore vary the equivalent power of their system. To increase magnification, the patient can bring the magnifier closer to his or her eye, stimulating more accommodation. There is a maximum amount, or limit, of magnification that a particular magnifier can offer. Conversely, absolute presbyopes do not have this flexibility. This second group of patients will typically use their magnifier at one distance as determined by the power of their add. Some other options include the use of trifocals or progressive addition lenses. Progressive addition lenses offer the patient a range of add powers, allowing different viewing distances from the stand magnifier, as well as variability in the equivalent power.

Typical adds that are used with fixed-focus stand magnifiers range from +2.50 D to +4.00 D. An add can be prescribed specifically for use with a magnifier, but the magnifier is usually recommended based on the patient's habitual add.

Field of View

Field of view depends on the power of the lens and the distance the lens is held from the eye. The equation reviewed under the section on field of view in the handheld magnifier section assumes that the reading material is at the focal length of the lens. This is not the case for most fixed-focus stand magnifiers. The same concept applies, however. As the eye to lens distance increases, the field of view decreases. Patients who may initially choose a handheld or stand magnifier because of the extended working distance may find themselves bringing their magnifiers closer to increase their field of view.

Instruction Techniques

The general approach to instruction with near devices can be found in the instruction techniques section under the section on microscopes. The following is a list of techniques specific to stand magnifiers:

1. The practitioner or instructor should always be positive and provide appropriate encouragement.
2. It should never be assumed that the patient knows how to properly use the stand magnifier.
3. The presbyopic patient should be told of the need to use his or her add while using the magnifier.
4. The patient should be instructed to let the stand magnifier rest on the reading material. The magnifier can simply slide along the page. Some patients will lift the magnifier slightly off of the page to obtain a clearer image or more magnification.

5. The patient should be instructed to move his or her eyes and the magnifier together as a unit.
6. The patient should be reminded to turn off the illumination source when finished using the magnifier.
7. The patient should be instructed to properly position external lighting sources to avoid casting shadows by the magnifier's legs and reflections from the magnifier's lens surface.
8. The patient should be reminded that his or her line of sight must pass perpendicular to the magnifier's optical center to limit distortions.

Problem Solving

Some patient difficulties may have simple solutions. Otherwise, further rehabilitation instruction is recommended. Some troubleshooting tips include the following:

Problem	Remedy
1. Material out of focus	a. The power of the add or the magnifier should be modified.
	b. The distance between the magnifier and the patient's eye may require modification.
2. Postural fatigue	a. Reading stands should be considered.
	b. Chairs with a back and arm support should be considered.
3. Asthenopia	a. Initial reading times should be decreased.
	b. Eccentric viewing should be practiced.
	c. The bifocal may have to be increased.
	d. The magnification of magnifier-bifocal system may have to be increased.
4. Loses place while reading	a. A typoscope can be taped to the base of the magnifier.
	b. A systematic approach to scanning the material may have to be demonstrated.
	c. Eccentric viewing should be reviewed and practiced.
5. Distortion	a. Patient should be instructed to look through the center of the magnifying lens.
	b. Magnifier must be held parallel to material.
	c. The patient should bring the magnifier closer to his or her eye (increase in bifocal may be required).
6. Small field of view	a. The magnifier should be moved closer to patient's eye.
	b. Another stand magnifier of equivalent power with a larger diameter lens may be considered.
	c. A microscope of equivalent power should be considered.
7. Pulling magnifier off page	a. The power of the stand magnifier should be increased

b. The power of the bifocal should be increased.

8. Reflection off lens surface
   a. A self-illuminated magnifier should be considered.
   b. The position of the external light source should be readjusted.
   c. The magnifier should be repositioned.
   d. A magnifier with an antireflective coating or a tint should be recommended.

9. Glare
   a. A magnifier with an antireflective coating or a tint should be recommended.
   b. A typoscope should be demonstrated.
   c. A filter over the reading material should be demonstrated.
   d. Illumination level and position should be addressed.

10. Dimness of reading material
    a. A self-illuminated magnifier should be demonstrated.
    b. The external illumination level and position of the light source should be investigated.
    c. A yellow tint or filter may be demonstrated to increase contrast.

SELF-ASSESSMENT QUESTIONS

1. A student, who is visually impaired, presents for an examination and reports that he is having problems reading his textbook, which he has brought to the examination. You pick one typical page from the book and count 72 letters and spaces in a 3-in. line of text. What is the equivalent point size of this print?
   (a) 2 point
   (b) 4 point
   (c) 6 point
   (d) 8 point
   (e) 12 point

2. A patient's best distance visual acuity is measured at 10/180. What power reading lens would be required for this patient to read 8-point type (assuming the patient is an emmetropic 85 year old)?
   (a) +7.25 D
   (b) +18.00 D
   (c) +23.50 D
   (d) +26.00 D
   (e) +32.00 D

3. When a patient requires a cylindrical correction in his or her distance prescription, the same amount of cylinder has to be incorporated into his or her microscope. True or False

4. What power lens would be required to allow a patient to read 0.6-M print when his or her best near acuity is 0.25/3 M with the present prescription of planosphere/+4.00 OU?

(a) +3.00 D
(b) +12.50 D
(c) +18.00 D
(d) +20.00 D
(e) +25.00 D

5. Bifocal lenses are not available in a higher power than +6.00 D. True or False

6. How much binocular convergence is required by a patient when he or she is reading with a +6.00 D lens and his or her distance IPD is 65 mm?
   (a) 33.47 prism diopters
   (b) 46.78 prism diopters
   (c) 48.00 prism diopters
   (d) 53.26 prism diopters
   (e) 58.00 prism diopters

7. To help relieve large amounts of convergence when reading with a microscope, base-in prism is required. True or False

8. What is the equivalent power when a +20.00 D hand-held magnifier is used in combination with a +3.00 D bifocal? The 72-year-old patient is holding the magnifier 10 cm from the bifocal and is able to see the print clearly.
   (a) +14.00 D
   (b) +17.00 D
   (c) +20.00 D
   (d) +21.50 D
   (e) +23.00 D

9. A patient complains that the reading material appears distorted when looking through a handheld magnifier. Which of the following may be responsible for this complaint?
   (a) The patient may be holding the reading material farther than the focal length of the magnifying lens.
   (b) The magnifying lens may be held at an incorrect angle to the reading material.
   (c) The magnifying lens may be of poor quality.
   (d) a and b
   (e) a, b, and c

10. What power bifocal would be required when an 80-year-old patient is using a +24.00 D fixed focus stand magnifier that is 10.8 cm from his spectacle lenses? The base of the magnifier is resting on the reading material, 3.3 cm from the lens.
    (a) +10.00 D
    (b) +6.00 D
    (c) +5.50 D
    (d) +4.75 D
    (e) +3.75 D

REFERENCES

1. Cohen J. Contrast of common near point reading materials. J Vis Rehabil 1993;7:2–4.

2. Mehr EB, Fried AN. Low Vision Care. Chicago: Professional Press, 1975;107, 139.
3. Jose RT (ed). Treatment Options: Understanding Low Vision. New York: American Foundation for the Blind, 1983;226–229.
4. Eldred KB. Use of contact lenses as a microscope. J Vis Rehabil 1989;3:23–28.
5. Bailey IL. Verifying near vision magnifiers—part 2. Optom Monthly 1981;72:34–38.
6. Nowakowski R. Primary Low Vision Care. Norwalk, CT: Appleton & Lange, 1994;162.
7. Williams D. An evaluation of the optical characteristics of prismatic half-eye spectacles for the low vision patient. J Vis Rehabil 1991;5:21–35.
8. Bailey IL. Centering high addition spectacle lenses. Optom Monthly 1979;70:523–527.
9. Fonda GE. Management of Low Vision. New York: Thieme–Stratton, 1981;136–140.
10. Faye E. Clinical Low Vision. Boston: Little, Brown, 1984;165.
11. Bailey IL. Magnification for near vision. Optom Monthly 1980;71:119–122.
12. Bailey IL. The use of fixed focus stand magnifiers. Optom Monthly 1981;72:37–39.

Appendix A

TIPS FOR THE PATIENT USING A MICROSCOPE

The following information provides tips and techniques that can be given to the patient who is using a microscope.

1. Be seated comfortably before you start reading.
2. Put reading material on a clipboard or reading stand.
3. Adjust your lighting while keeping in mind how close you will be to the reading material.
4. Put your reading glasses (microscope) on. Touch your nose with the reading material and then slowly move the material away until the letters on the page come into focus.
5. Readjust your lighting to ensure that no shadows are on the material.
6. Remember to view through the center of the lens. Remind yourself to move your chin down toward your chest if you are accustomed to looking through a bifocal.
7. While reading, hold your head and eye still, and move the clipboard left to right in front of your eye. The material must be parallel to the lenses in your glasses.
8. Use plenty of short practice sessions: 5 minutes or less, three or four times a day in the beginning. Increase your reading time when you experience less eye strain and when you can read more comfortably.
9. Remember that some items will be easier to read than others. Ease of reading depends on print size, color, spacing, style, contrast, and paper quality.
10. Clean reading glasses regularly with a clean, damp, lint-free cloth. Keep them in their case when not in use.

Note. Do not walk with these glasses on. They are only for reading.

Appendix B

TIPS FOR THE PATIENT USING A HANDHELD MAGNIFIER

The following information provides tips and techniques that can be given to the patient who will be using a handheld magnifier.

1. Be seated comfortably before you start reading.
2. Put reading material on a clipboard or reading stand so that you are facing the material while seated upright in a chair. This will prevent you from bending over and creating a shadow on the reading material.
3. Adjust your lighting to properly illuminate your reading material if a light is not built into your magnifier.
4. To determine how far away to hold the magnifier from the reading material, place your magnifier on the reading material. Slowly bring it away from the material until the words on the page come into focus.
5. Readjust your lighting to ensure that no shadows are on the material and no reflections are on the magnifier's surface.
6. Hold the reading material parallel to the magnifier.
7. Remember to view through the center of the magnifier. Hold your reading material in an upright position so that you are not bending over to read.
8. Use plenty of short practice sessions: 5 minutes or less, three or four times a day in the beginning. Increase your reading time when you experience less eye strain and when you can read more comfortably.
9. Remember that some items will be easier to read than others. Ease of reading depends on print size, color, spacing, style, contrast, and paper quality.
10. Clean your magnifier regularly with a clean, damp, lint-free cloth. Keep it in a case when not in use.

Appendix C

TIPS FOR THE PATIENT USING A STAND MAGNIFIER

The following information provides tips and techniques that can be given to the patient who will be using a stand magnifier.

1. Be seated comfortably before you start reading.
2. Adjust your light so that it is close to the print to avoid reflected glare from the lens.
3. Place the stand magnifier on the page to ensure that the print is automatically in focus.
4. If you wear bifocals, look through the bifocal (bottom portion of lens) while using the stand magnifier. If you have a COIL "blue line" (C.O.I.L. Combined Optical Industries, Ltd., Elk Grove Village, IL) stand magnifier, look through the distance part of the spectacle lens (upper portion of lens).
5. Look through the center of the magnifier.
6. Readjust your lighting to ensure that no shadows are on the material and reflected glare is not present on the magnifying lens.
7. Use plenty of short practice sessions: 5 minutes or less, three or four times a day in the beginning. Increase your reading time when you experience less eye strain and when you can read more comfortably.
8. Remember that some items will be easier to read than others. Ease of reading depends on print size, color, spacing, style, contrast, and paper quality.
9. Clean the stand magnifier regularly with a clean, damp, lint-free cloth.

CHAPTER ELEVEN

Low Vision Near Systems II: Electronic Magnification Systems

Laurel A. Tucker and
Richard L. Brilliant

The most commonly recognized electronic magnification system for reading and writing used by visually impaired children, youth, and adults is the closed-circuit television (CCTV) system. A CCTV system incorporates both projection magnification and relative distance magnification. A CCTV permits the low vision patient to visually access printed or handwritten material and a multiplicity of other objects by means of a magnified image projected onto a monitor screen.

A number of new electronic systems have been developed that may revolutionize the field of low vision. These systems feature a binocular, head-mounted display that uses liquid crystal display (LCD) technology along with charged coupled device (CCD) miniature cameras. Using computer generated software, these systems have the ability to provide visual enhancement at distance, intermediate, and near. Two such systems are now commercially available. They are known as the *Low Vision Enhancement System* (LVES) and *V-max* (Enhanced Vision Systems, Costa Mesa, CA) and are described later in this chapter. In addition, a listing of manufacturers and suppliers of electronic magnification systems is provided in Appendix A.

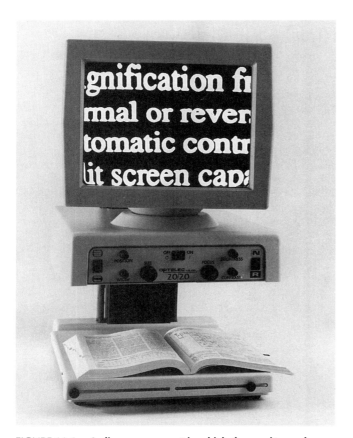

FIGURE 11-1.   **In-line arrangement in which the monitor and camera are aligned in a single unit. The moveable platform (X-Y table) has control knobs (or a lever), which appear in this figure as two knobs on the front edge of the table. These knobs allow the table to be locked in place or to provide tension control when moving the table for near activities, such as reading. (Courtesy of Optelec, Westford, MA.)**

CLOSED-CIRCUIT TELEVISION

The standard CCTV consists of three major components: camera, monitor, and moveable reading platform. The video camera that transmits a "live" image is focusable with a zoom lens and aperture. Most CCTV systems made in 1989 or later use a CCD camera. The apparent advancements of the CCD are enhanced image contrast, brightness, and clarity of images; less "ghosting" of letters on the monitor when the text is moved, increased depth of field, and no "burn-in" of images when reading material is left under the camera for an extended time.

A monitor serves as the screen onto which the enlarged print image is projected. Many systems available today have monitors dedicated solely to the reading system. At the time of evaluation and purchase, the patient determines the monitor size appropriate for personal use, need, and placement in the space available. The smaller (12-in. and 14-in.) dedicated monitors can be arranged "in-line," an arrangement in which the monitor and camera are configured in a single vertical line above the reading material (Figure 11-1). The 19-in. (and larger) monitors are generally placed in a side-by-side configuration with the camera unit (Figure 11-2). The dedicated monitors have height adjustments for positioning the screen at a comfortable eye-level view.

A moveable platform or X-Y table sits on a flat table or desk (see Figure 11-1). The material to be read or written on is placed on the platform, which is designed to be positioned underneath the camera. The X-Y table or platform glides horizontally (left and right) and vertically (up and down) on a fixed frame when manipulated by hand. The movement of the X-Y platform can be loosened or tightened with a tension control or friction brake. Margin stops, similar to margins set on a typewriter, may be manually set by use of two screws on the front edge of the platform. Some companies sell a separate automated viewing table (X-Y table) for hands-free viewing of reading materials. Automated viewing tables and automatic-focus cameras have been developed to reduce hand manipulation by the patient. They are ideal for typing or word processing, and for those with poor motor skills or limited range of motion or hand tremors.

Additional Closed-Circuit Television Features

The majority of CCTV systems are accompanied by a built-in or attached illumination source. Reflected glare may be reduced with the adjustment of manual controls for brightness, contrast, color, and image polarity. Unwanted incoming light may be controlled by using an antiglare screen, tilting the monitor, adapting room lighting, or placing the monitor in a location in which natural and artificial light does not reflect off the equipment surface.

An additional feature available on many CCTV systems is a "window." With manual controls the patient can bring onto the screen an electronically enhanced curtain or window that blocks out portions of the screen. This feature allows the patient to isolate one line or a section of the

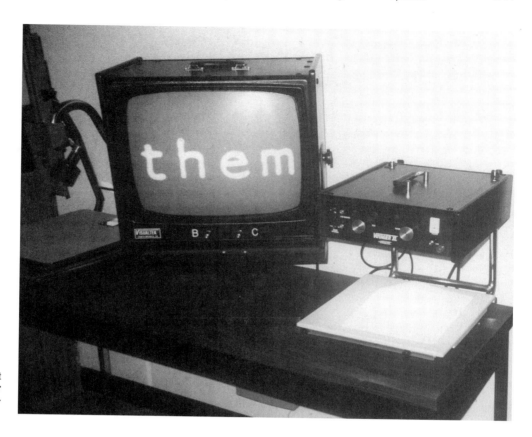

FIGURE 11-2. **A closed-circuit television with a large monitor that is placed alongside the camera unit.**

print. This technique may also be an effective way to reduce glare reflecting from the monitor.

The overline and underline features may be controlled manually in the horizontal and vertical orientation when available. It appears on the screen as a straight line. It may be useful as a line marker for reading and for aligning math problems, as well as other applications (Figure 11-3). One disadvantage with windows and line features is their flicker, which is due to the manner in which the window and line are electronically created. Placing a dark line marker directly on the reading material (i.e., typoscope) can serve the same purpose without creating the annoying flicker.

Older CCTV systems that are adapted for use with a typewriter have accessories to create the reversal or mirror image needed for viewing the typed material on the paper when in the typewriter. This feature was more common before electronic access to computer technology.

A dual-camera system provides the simultaneous viewing of two different sources for reading or writing tasks. A single screen is electronically split into two sections to allow two separate cameras to project their outputs at the same time on the same adaptable monitor. For example, one camera can be focused onto a geometry textbook while another camera is focused on the paper where the geometry problems are being drawn and calculated. Not all monitors are split-screen capable.

All CCTVs enable the patient to select regular polarity (black letters on a white background) or reverse polarity (white on black) for reading. In addition to the polarity change, some black-and-white CCTV systems have

a "photo mode," which when selected, reverts the camera to a preset contrast and brightness mode that is ideal for viewing photos (in black and white). One option available on some systems allows the patient to select one of a number of preset color combinations (e.g., yellow on blue). Another

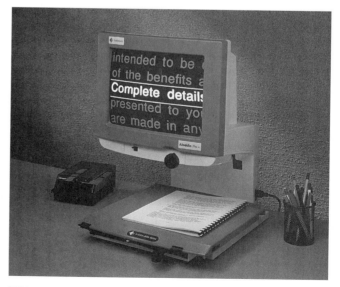

FIGURE 11-3. **The overline and underline features help isolate a line of print, making it easier to read and maintain one's place. (Courtesy of Telesensory, Mountain View, CA.)**

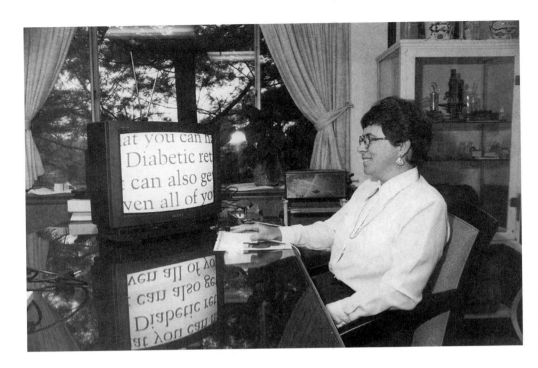

FIGURE 11-4. **A portable black-and-white camera can easily be connected directly to any television and used as a closed-circuit television system.**

option allows material placed on the reading table to be viewed in full color. Full-color systems reproduce all of the colors in the original pictures and offer the patient access to photographs, maps, color-coded graphs, and materials not as easily recognized with black-and-white systems.

Portable Closed-Circuit Televisions

Portable, monochrome (black-and-white) and color cameras are available that may be connected directly to any television set (Figure 11-4). These systems are ideal for the low vision patient who travels often or who may need a portable system for work- or school-related tasks. In many cases, the camera can be powered by a rechargeable battery. With most systems, the camera is small and easily held in a patient's hand, which makes scanning and reading easy. Magnification is variable and can be changed by raising or lowering the camera from the reading material. Additional magnification can also be achieved by using a larger television screen. As the screen size is enlarged, so too is the magnification of the print projected onto the screen. For example, when the print size on a 19-in. screen is projected onto a 27-in. screen, 1.42× magnification is obtained (27/19 = 1.42).

These small camera systems can be adjusted for contrast, which enables enhancement of photographs and newspaper print. They also have the ability to change the image from a positive image to a negative image (*reverse polarity*), which allows the print to be viewed by the patient as black print on a white background or white print on a black background. A large percentage of patients with low vision appear to prefer white print on a black background.

Some manufacturers of portable CCTVs have recently introduced head-mounted systems that take portability

one step further (Figure 11-5). The headset is connected directly to the camera and a battery pack. The headset can be worn over a patient's spectacle lenses. The image from the camera is projected onto the head-mounted display system and can produce magnification up to approximately 25×. The manufacturer of Magni-Cam (Innoventions, Inc., Littleton, CO) reports that the magnified image of their system is comparable to a patient viewing a 20-in. television screen from a distance of 3 ft.

One of the major advantages of these systems is that they allow patients total portability. For example, patients can now read prices and labels when shopping, students

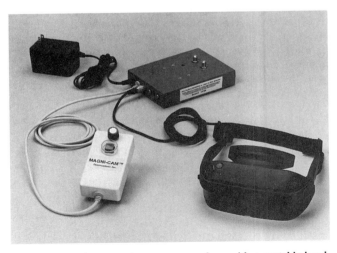

FIGURE 11-5. **The monochrome camera along with a portable head-mounted system allows total portability when used with a battery unit to supply the power. (Courtesy of Innoventions, Inc., Littleton, CO.)**

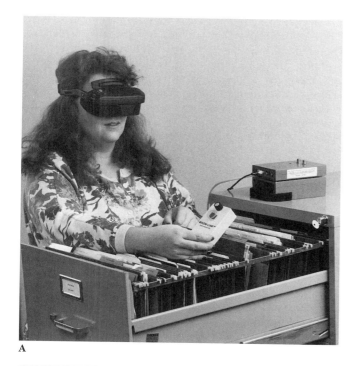

A

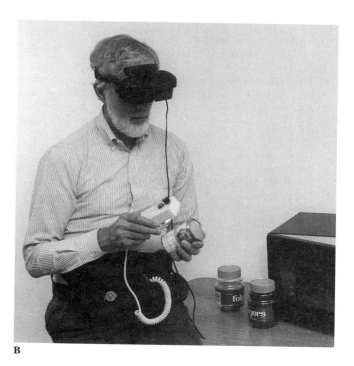

B

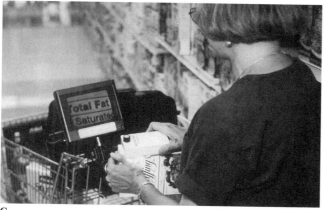

C

FIGURE 11-6.   **A. A patient using the portable head-mounted system for job-related tasks. B. A patient using the portable head-mounted system for home use. The system has excellent depth of focus, which allows the print to be in constant focus when reading the print on a can of food. C. A patient using the portable camera with a small television while grocery shopping. (Courtesy of Innoventions, Inc., Littleton, CO.)**

can read their books or notes in class, and individuals at work have the ability to read files, mail, and other business-related material without being confined to a monitor (Figure 11-6). The major disadvantage of the portable head-mounted system is that it cannot be used when walking. The headset can be positioned above the patient's eyes, however, so that he or she can walk and then be repositioned back over the eyes when reading again (e.g., when grocery shopping).

INITIAL STEPS IN THE USE OF A CLOSED-CIRCUIT TELEVISION

It is notably easier to adapt to reading with a CCTV than to reading with an optical device. Therefore, it is suggested that appropriate optical devices be first introduced for initial instruction, practice, and adaptation. If

the first introduction to optical devices is to an easier reading system, such as a CCTV, it may be more difficult for the patient to adjust to the limitations and recognize the merit of other magnification instruments. When it is appropriate to introduce CCTV systems to a patient, the following outlines the basic steps used in the evaluation process.

1. The unit should be plugged into an electrical outlet and the power turned on.
2. The patient's preferred viewing distance should be determined. If the patient is unable to accommodate for the viewing distance, an appropriate near correction should be used to ensure maximum clarity.
3. The reading material should be placed on the X-Y table. One technique is to move the X-Y table outward toward the patient and to the right. The material is then placed in the upper left corner of the table.

From that position, things can be easily adjusted and aligned under the camera. A piece of Plexiglas placed over a magazine or book may keep it smooth and flat on the X-Y table.

4. The image is focused on the screen. When focused at the greatest level of magnification, the image will remain focused when magnification is reduced.
5. The focused image is reduced to the magnification level preferred by the patient. It is suggested that the patient use the least amount of magnification visually comfortable for the type of print being read, as that approach will enhance the field of view.
6. The preferred polarity or color combination, if available, of the background and foreground should be selected by the patient.
7. The patient should practice manipulation of the X-Y table for localization, horizontal tracking, and scanning back to the margin.
8. Correct body posture and monitor positioning (many screens can be tilted) should be encouraged. Patient fatigue, which may be indicated by the patient moving closer to the monitor and by changes in the original print size, quality, or contrast, should be noted. When fatigue occurs, the patient should be encouraged to rest or reschedule for another visit if the initial session was not sufficient or if other options need to be explored.

APPLIED USE OF CLOSED-CIRCUIT TELEVISION SYSTEMS

CCTV systems are used for educational, vocational, recreational, and personal pursuits. They serve multiple purposes for an array of activities that include reading, writing, typing, specific daily living skills, leisure time activities, and computer technology access.

Materials of assorted print sizes and varying contrast should be selectively incorporated in the evaluation and instructional sessions. Materials specific to patient goals and needs are to be introduced at appropriate levels of difficulty in the sequence. A suggested reading task sequence for instruction and practice is as follows: single-sheet, typed print sentences; single-sheet, typed print short story; magazine print; book print; newsprint; dictionary; computer printout; photographs; maps; and labels and instructions on cans and boxes. Reading handwritten notes is a challenging task that may be laborious and sometimes impossible to achieve. The complication usually lies with the illegibility of handwriting that resembles hieroglyphics more than decipherable familiar language. Patients in distress may appreciate reassurance that reading the handwriting of others may indeed be futile due to penmanship rather than visual capacity.

Adaptation is essential for working on two planes when using the CCTV for handwriting tasks. Locking the reading platform in place is often useful and should be the first step that the patient completes. The patient should be instructed not to look down at his or her hand, paper, and

pen while writing but to look at the CCTV monitor to view the position of the pen, paper, and written information. The angle of the writing paper as well as that of the writing hand and pen will need some exploration and practice to achieve the best writing position. A suggested hand-writing task sequence for instruction and practice is as follows: lined paper, letters, envelopes, bank checks, forms, math problems.

Some patients find that the extensive use of CCTV equipment causes headaches, eye tearing, and fatigue. It is important that patients be advised to take periodic breaks to prevent unwanted effects.

Patients having constricted visual fields, decreased visual acuity, and decreased contrast sensitivity secondary to advanced glaucoma, retinitis pigmentosa, or ischemic optic neuropathy present a challenge to the low vision practitioner. In some cases, the only option is a CCTV. This system benefits these patients due to the ability to adjust contrast, brightness, and magnification. Magnification should be kept to a minimum to more effectively use the patient's remaining field. Also, the potentially increased working distance with a CCTV may enable the patient with advanced retinitis pigmentosa or glaucoma to see more words or letters at one time.

MAGNIFICATION AND EQUIVALENT POWER OF A CLOSED-CIRCUIT TELEVISION

There are several approaches to determining how much magnification a patient is achieving with a CCTV. A precise method requires specific measurements entered into a calculated formula. The measurements that must be taken are the print size of the enlarged image on the CCTV monitor, the actual print size, and the working distance (spectacle plane to CCTV screen). The traditional approach is to determine the total magnification provided by the CCTV system. The formula for calculating the total magnification is as follows:

$$M = (X)(Y)$$

where X = print size on the monitor divided by actual print size, and Y = reference distance (25 cm or 40 cm) divided by the working distance in centimeters.

It is important to note that the total magnification will vary depending on the reference distance used.

Example 1
What is the total magnification that a patient requires when he or she reads 3-cm print on the monitor screen when viewed from a distance of 20 cm? The actual size of the print is 3 mm.

Answer:
Print size = 0.3 cm
Print size on the monitor = 3 cm
Working distance = 20 cm
When 25 cm is the reference distance:

$$\left(\frac{3}{0.3}\right)\left(\frac{25}{20}\right) = (10)(1.25) = 12.5\times$$

When 40 cm is the reference distance:

$$\left(\frac{3}{0.3}\right)\left(\frac{40}{20}\right) = (10)(2) = 20\times$$

As seen in the preceding example, magnification can be somewhat confusing because different magnifications will result from the same data (when different reference distances are used). When the reference distance is not specified it becomes difficult, if not impossible, to determine the precise magnification. Therefore, the best approach is to determine the equivalent power provided by the system. Use of equivalent dioptric power will enable the practitioner to obtain the dioptric equivalent of the projection magnification–relative distance magnification interaction. The calculated dioptric equivalent can then be used in the comparison and selection of other systems of equivalent power, such as microscopes, handheld and stand magnifiers, and telemicroscopes, during the evaluation sequence. The formula for determining equivalent dioptric power (D_{eq}) is as follows:

$$D_{eq} = (X)(Z)$$

where X = print size on the monitor divided by actual print size, and Z = dioptric equivalent of the working distance or the reciprocal of the working distance (100/working distance [in cm]).

Example 2

What is the equivalent power needed for a patient who reads 3-cm print on the monitor screen when viewed from a distance of 20 cm? The actual size of the print is 3 mm.

Answer:

Print size = 0.3 cm

Print size on the monitor = 3 cm

Working distance = 20 cm; therefore, the reciprocal is 100/20 = 5.00 D

$$D_{eq} = (X)(Z)$$
$$= \left(\frac{3}{0.3}\right)(5) = (10\times)(+5.00\ D) = +50.00\ D$$

Another approach to obtaining a quick projection magnification estimate does not factor in the working distance. To obtain this measurement, a piece of graph paper is placed under the camera of the CCTV after the appropriate size print had been established on the screen for the patient's needs. Another piece of the same size graph paper is then held up to the monitor and the number of regular size graph squares that fit into the length of one or two magnified graph squares on the screen can be counted. By dividing the resultant smaller number into the larger number, the projection magnification can grossly be determined. It must be remembered that this estimation does not account for the relative distance magnification.

ASSESSMENT AND SELECTION CONSIDERATIONS

Patients to be evaluated with CCTV technology have varying circumstances.

1. For the visually impaired patient who has never used a CCTV system, the practitioner should provide a demonstration or an orientation to the equipment and then evaluate the individual's potential to use this magnification option.

2. For the visually impaired patient who does have a CCTV system and is experiencing problems, the practitioner should review the patient's understanding and use of the system and address problem-solving strategies.

3. For the visually impaired patient who has or had a CCTV system and would like an "update" of new products and equipment features, the practitioner should provide demonstrations of such available equipment and give product resource literature to the interested consumer.

For practitioners who do not have CCTV systems available to them, most manufacturers have local salespeople who will demonstrate their equipment in the doctor's office or at a patient's home.

Practitioners may also elect to use a CCTV as a diagnostic tool to determine the appropriate equivalent power necessary to achieve a reading goal. This approach is helpful when traditional visual acuity testing procedures provide inconsistent or variable findings or when the patient is inconsistent in responding to standard magnifying devices. The CCTV provides the advantages of variable magnification, contrast and brightness control, and enhanced field of view, which frequently result in more consistent and repeatable findings. The CCTV may also be used to differentiate reading deficits from visual deficits. The patient who continues to have difficulty when all other variables are controlled on a CCTV system may manifest behaviors suggestive of visual memory deficits, cognitive lapses, or low literacy skills.

A CCTV may be the preferred visual option when copious amounts of reading are to be accomplished. Nonvisual options may include braille, recorded, or CD-ROM versions of novels, manuals, textbooks, and magazines when available.

The selection of a CCTV system should be a methodical process during which the patient should be given sufficient time to fully evaluate all appropriate systems. During the selection process, the patient should be encouraged to voice any current needs that he or she may have as well as explore possible future needs that may arise in the educational or vocational setting. Considerations to be taken into account by the low vision patient before the final selection of a system are the following:

1. The patient should be encouraged to contact the representatives of various manufacturers to arrange for personal demonstrations of equipment in the environment that the CCTV system will be used, if possible.

2. The patient's goals and personal performance with a CCTV should be reviewed so that it can be determined if a specific system enables the intended user to fulfill those necessary tasks.

3. The patient should decide which features are important to him or her: two-color text option (e.g., yellow let-

ters on blue); full-color option; monitor size; overlining, underlining, or windowing features; computer compatibility; in-line or handheld camera systems; and availability of automated viewing table, among other features.

4. The patient should investigate the availability of further instruction for the use of new equipment through the manufacturer or the practitioner's office.

5. The patient should explore the arrangement of the equipment (the system's camera, monitor, X-Y table, and light source) on the ease of reading the types of materials that need to be read.

6. The patient should inquire about the availability of a typewriter attachment, computer compatibility, or accessories for a dual-camera hookup if there is future need for such.

7. The patient should explore the physical place available and whether the preferred system will fit in that space.

8. The patient should compare the companies and models for repair service and the manufacturer's warranty or guarantee. Is a loaner CCTV supplied while the patient's system is being repaired?

9. The patient should examine and compare equipment portability, if needed now or in the future.

10. The patient should explore the cost of the system and whether payment can be made in installments.

ADVANTAGES AND DISADVANTAGES OF CLOSED-CIRCUIT TELEVISION SYSTEMS

A CCTV system has a number of advantages and disadvantages. The practitioner should provide this information to patients so that they can determine if this type of system is appropriate for their needs.

Advantages

The following is a list of advantages of the CCTV system.

1. Adjustable projection magnification levels (range from 4× to 45× on smaller screens and from 5× to 65× with some larger-screen systems).
2. Reading distance is more variable than most other low vision devices.
3. Polarity change is available.
4. An illumination system is designed with most units.
5. Brightness and contrast intensity controls are available.
6. An adjustable field of view is possible by manipulating the magnification or screen size.
7. Binocularity is possible with large amounts of magnification.
8. Standard-size print may be instantly accessible.
9. A patient's reading endurance and efficiency may be increased.
10. A CCTV may be the only option for print access for some severely impaired low vision patients.
11. Photographs may be easily viewed.

Disadvantages

The CCTV system, however, also has some disadvantages. The following are possible disadvantages of the CCTV system.

1. Physical size may hinder portability and maneuverability.
2. Training and practice time is needed to become a proficient user.
3. Limited availability of maintenance services for components.
4. Initial cost may be higher than most low vision devices, yet CCTV distributors may require full payment on delivery of equipment to the patient.
5. The use of high magnification reduces the field of view; patients may become dependent on overmagnification when less magnification may be appropriate for a particular task.
6. Local and regional distributors and company representatives have varied business styles. Some representatives may be high-pressure salespersons, which may reflect negatively on the practitioner's low vision practice.

HEAD-MOUNTED SYSTEMS FOR DISTANCE AND NEAR

New high-technology head-mounted systems have been developed for patients with low vision. Using computer technology and miniature cameras, these systems improve a patient's vision via magnification and enhancement of the visual images.

Low Vision Enhancement System

The LVES (pronounced *Elvis*) was the first of its kind developed for low vision patients. The LVES was initially developed by a team of doctors and researchers at Johns Hopkins School of Medicine (Baltimore, MD) along with the National Aeronautics and Space Administration and the Veterans Administration. This electronic vision system weighs 2.5 lb and is worn as a head-mounted system similar in appearance to a virtual reality headset (Figure 11-7). The system has two fixed, high-definition monochrome video cameras that provide a three-dimensional unmagnified wide-angle view. The approximate field is 50 degrees in the horizontal direction and 38 degrees in the vertical. The headset also contains one automatic-focus camera in the center that has the ability to focus in or out, along with the ability to produce magnification at distance from 1.7× to 7.5×. The manufacturer has likened the equivalent view of this system to watching television on a 60-in. black-and-white screen from a distance of 4 ft. At near, the camera can produce up to 10.5× magnification, and when a special reading cap is added, the system will provide magnification up to 25×.

The headset is connected to a portable control box by a 40-in. cable. The control box houses the battery, which lasts approximately 90 minutes, along with the magnification, contrast, and brightness controls. The control box also contains the image polarity control, which allows the image to be displayed as white on black or black on white. The control box and battery weigh 2.6 lb and can be worn on a belt pack or hung from the shoulder on a shoulder strap. LVES also has the capability of being plugged into an outlet and operated using electrical current.

When the system is used for watching television or seeing print on a computer screen, it can be connected directly into the television or computer and thereby bypass the LVES unit's cameras. This setup enables the enlarged image to be displayed directly on the video screen in front of the patient's eyes. The LVES also has a video-out port that allows the patient to be connected to a television so that the practitioner can see what the patient is seeing through the LVES. This feature is especially useful when the patient is initially being taught how to localize and scan through the system.

The LVES is recommended for patients with visual acuity ranging from 20/100 to 20/800. For patients requiring a refractive correction, prescription lenses can be incorporated directly into the headset.

Advantages

This type of system has several advantages.

1. The system is a revolutionary new idea.
2. The device can provide magnification, contrast, and brightness enhancement.
3. The device can provide a wide range of magnifications.
4. The system can be used for distance, intermediate, and near.
5. The device has an automatic focus ability.
6. The system can be connected directly to a television or computer system through the use of a cable.
7. The system is completely portable with the use of a battery.
8. The system has the ability to change polarity for increased contrast at near.

Disadvantages

The LVES system also has some disadvantages.

1. The headset is heavy with extended wear.
2. The headset is cumbersome.
3. The headset can cause claustrophobia.
4. The control box and battery pack are heavy and cumbersome.
5. The battery has the capacity to last only a maximum of 90 minutes.
6. The system requires extensive instruction.
7. The system can be intimidating to some patients.
8. The system provides only black-and-white images.
9. The system is very expensive.
10. The system is not widely available.
11. The practitioner is required to have an extensive inservice to learn how to use the system.

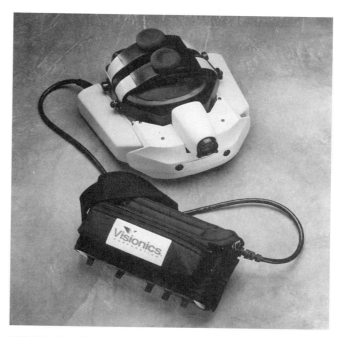

FIGURE 11-7. **The Low Vision Enhancement System is a first-of-its-kind, head-mounted electronic magnification system. It provides a monochrome image and has automatic focus capabilities at distance, intermediate, and near. (Courtesy of Visionics Corporation, Vadnais Heights, MN.)**

V-max

The V-max is the next generation of a head-mounted assistance device that addresses distance, intermediate, and near vision (Figure 11-8). It is an automatic-focus system with a range of magnification, at distance, from 0.8× to 20×. This system also has the capability of having five customized, preset magnification levels (set by the practitioner) for the patient's specific needs, allowing the patient to change quickly from one level of magnification to another. The manufacturer has likened the equivalent view of this system to watching television on an 80-in. color screen from a distance of 10 ft.

One high-resolution color camera is set at the center of the head-mounted unit with the weight of the system ergonomically designed so that it rests over the patient's center of gravity, minimizing neck and back strain. The headset weighs 23 oz.

The camera has a built-in vision stabilization system that compensates for small head movements and head tremors, thereby providing a more steady image. The camera and display system use state-of-the-art digital technology to provide enlarged, color-enhanced images. The field of view of this system is 47 degrees in the horizontal and 36 degrees in the vertical. The V-max also features edge-enhancement technology, whereby the edges of the image are given an increased contrast level that results in easier overall image recognition.

The V-max requires no special fitting procedures. It can be easily evaluated by placing it on the patient's head,

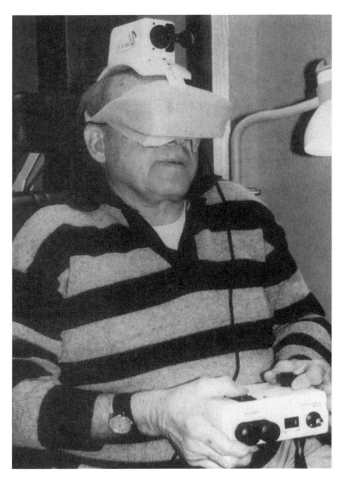

FIGURE 11-8. **The V-max provides a color image with automatic focus capabilities. It can be worn directly over a patient's spectacles. (Courtesy of Enhanced Vision Systems, Costa Mesa, CA.)**

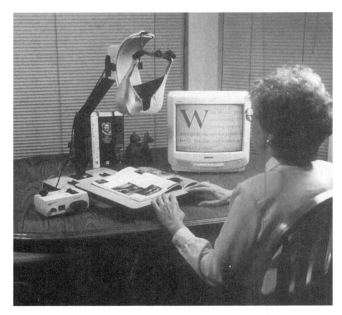

FIGURE 11-9. **The V-max is converted into a reading system by placing the headset on a docking stand (with an X-Y table) and attaching the system to a television monitor. (Courtesy of Enhanced Vision Systems, Costa Mesa, CA.)**

fitting over the patient's prescription spectacles. Therefore, any patient can be evaluated with this system, regardless of prescription.

The head-mounted unit is connected to the control box by a 5-ft cable. The control box houses the battery (which lasts approximately 90–120 minutes) along with the magnification, polarity, edge enhancement, and on-off controls. The control box also contains a video-in port, for direct connection to a television set, and a video-out port, which provides the connection to a television for the conversion into a CCTV as well as a connection that permits the practitioner to view what the patient is looking at. The control box (and battery) is worn on a belt pack that weighs 27 oz. The system can also be plugged directly into an electrical outlet.

V-max is actually two systems in one. The system can be converted to a very advanced color CCTV by simply sliding the headset into the docking stand attached to an X-Y table (Figure 11-9). At all levels of magnification, the system will automatically adjust by means of the automatic focus. Objects can be enlarged up to 60 times their original size, which also depends on the size of the television screen. The camera requires no additional external light

source, and it has the ability to reverse polarity. When in the positive mode, the patient can view the images on the screen in color; when in the negative mode, the images on the screen can be displayed as white on black or black on white. Like all low vision systems, the V-max has a number of advantages and disadvantages.

Advantages
The advantages of the V-max system are the following:

1. The system can be used for distance, intermediate, and near.
2. The device can provide a wide range of magnifications.
3. The system can provide edge enhancement to increase contrast of objects.
4. The system has an automatic focus capability.
5. The camera has a vision stabilization system.
6. The camera has color capabilities.
7. The camera automatically adjusts for brightness.
8. The system is ergonomically designed to minimize neck and back strain.
9. The system is completely portable with the use of a battery.
10. The system can be customized to provide preset levels of magnification.
11. The system has the ability to change polarity for increased contrast at near.
12. The headset can be worn over a patient's spectacles.
13. The headset is designed to allow peripheral vision, therefore minimizing claustrophobia.
14. The system can be connected directly to a television or computer system.
15. The system is easy to fit and operate.

Disadvantages
The V-max has several disadvantages.

1. The headset is cumbersome.
2. The control box and battery pack are heavy and cumbersome.
3. The battery has the capacity to last only a maximum of 90–120 minutes.
4. The system may be intimidating to some patients.
5. The system is expensive.
6. The system is not widely available.

CONCLUSION

A tremendous amount of progress has occurred in a very short time in the area of electronic magnification. It is anticipated that much more progress will occur as researchers and manufacturers attempt to build the ultimate low vision system. There is no doubt that the most potential for the advancement in low vision devices lies within the area of electronic magnification systems.

SELF-ASSESSMENT QUESTIONS

1. The total magnification of a CCTV incorporates the following magnifications:
   (a) relative size magnification
   (b) projection magnification
   (c) relative distance magnification
   (d) a and b
   (e) b and c

2. When a patient with absolute presbyopia is viewing the monitor of a CCTV, an appropriate near correction should be used to ensure maximum clarity.
   True or False

3. When the CCTV is initially focused at the lowest level of magnification, the image will remain focused when the magnification level is changed.
   True or False

4. Which type of patient with low vision would possibly be successful in using a CCTV for reading bills?
   (a) a patient with constricted peripheral fields (10-degree central field remaining)
   (b) a patient with decreased visual acuity (20/600 acuity)
   (c) a patient with decreased contrast sensitivity
   (d) b and c would probably be successful
   (e) a, b, and c would probably be successful

5. What is the equivalent power of the system when a patient is reading 30-mm print on a CCTV monitor from 15 cm away? The original size of the print is 5 mm.
   (a) +10.00 D
   (b) +22.50 D
   (c) +40.00 D
   (d) +60.00 D
   (e) +90.00 D

6. What equivalent power microscope would you predict is needed for an 80-year-old emmetropic patient who is wearing +3.00 D reading lenses to read 4-mm print projected onto a CCTV screen on which the print is 5 cm (assume that all factors, such as brightness, contrast, and so forth, are the same when comparing the CCTV to the microscope)?
   (a) +26.66 D
   (b) +37.50 D
   (c) +42.75 D
   (d) +60.00 D
   (e) +82.00 D

7. Both the LVES and the V-max can be used by patients with advanced retinitis pigmentosa to help in their mobility.
   True or False

Appendix A

MANUFACTURERS AND SUPPLIERS OF ELECTRONIC MAGNIFICATION SYSTEMS

Note. This information does not denote a complete list of manufacturers and suppliers in the United States.

Acrontech, Inc.
Williamsville Executive Center
5500 Main St.
Williamsville, NY 14221
(716) 854-3814
800-245-2020

American Printing House for the Blind, Inc.
1839 Frankfort Ave.
P.O. Box 6085
Louisville, KY 40206
(502) 895-2405
800-223-1839

C Tech
2 N. William St.
Pearl River, NY 10965
(914) 735-7907
800-228-7798

Enhanced Vision Systems (maker of V-max)
2915 Redhill Ave., Suite B201
Costa Mesa, CA 92626
(714) 957-0155
800-440-9476

Gracefully Yours, Inc.
12527 Ulmerton Rd.
Largo, FL 34644
(813) 593-1010
800-331-2211

Innoventions, Inc.
5921 S. Middlefield Rd., Suite 102
Littleton, CO 80123
(303) 797-6554
800-854-6554

Okaya Electric America, Inc.
503 Wall St.
Valparaiso, IN 46383
800-325-4488

Optelec
P.O. Box 729
Westford, MA 01886
(508) 392-0707
800-828-1056

Reinecker Reha-Technik
c/o 4× Products, Inc.
P.O. Box 555
Millwood, NY 10546
(914) 762-3555

SeeWell Reading Enhancers
P.O. Box 5962
San Clemente, CA 92674
(714) 366-3188
800-660-0804

TeleSensory
P.O. Box 7455
Mountain View, CA 94039-7455
(415) 960-0960
800-227-8418

Visionics Corporation (Maker of the Low Vision Enhancement System [LVES]. As of this writing, LVES is no longer being manufactured.)
380 Oak Grove Parkway
Vadnais Heights, MN 55127
(612) 483-3408
800-507-4448

CHAPTER TWELVE

Rehabilitation of Peripheral Field Defects

Richard L. Brilliant and
Leonard H. Ginsburg

The treatment and management of patients with peripheral field defects is multifaceted, with the ultimate goals of the practitioner being an increase in the patient's comfort and visual functioning. To reach these goals, five major areas must be addressed:

1. Maximized visual acuity.
2. Reduction of the effects of glare and photophobia both indoors and outdoors.
3. Use of magnification.
4. Field enhancement techniques.
5. Referrals for additional rehabilitation services.

ATTAINING MAXIMUM VISUAL ACUITY

The importance of performing a thorough refraction and obtaining the maximum visual acuity cannot be overemphasized. If there is any acuity loss, it must be due to the pathology and not to a poor refraction. Although the concepts of the examination and refraction procedures are routine, there are some aspects and areas that are unique and therefore different from those of the fully sighted patient. A thorough discussion of refraction procedures is provided in Chapter 3.

Visual Acuity

The visual acuity must be measured on charts with many increments of acuity and using variable illumination. During the visual acuity examination, particular attention should be paid to the size of the optotype (letter or number) and the distance the acuity is initially shown so as not to introduce an optotype that is too large for the patient's constricted field (Figure 12-1). This situation may occur because a patient's remaining central visual field is cone-shaped (it gets proportionally larger the further away from the eye), and therefore, if the peripheral field is reduced, the patient may have a problem seeing a larger target at near.

There will generally be a preference for bright or midrange illumination on the acuity chart, depending on the extent of the peripheral field loss, other ocular disorders (e.g., cataracts), and certainly on individual preference.

Refraction

A trial frame should be used for all subjective refractive procedures to allow the patient the opportunity for habitual scanning or, if necessary, eccentric viewing. It is important to measure the monocular pupillary distance for each eye and to set the trial frame at the appropriate angle. Many patients with restricted visual fields will be sensitive to errors in centering of the lens cells, especially those with significant refractive error.

Before beginning the subjective refraction, information from the objective refractive findings, such as static or radical retinoscopy and keratometry, is always helpful. When standard subjective techniques are not possible, the just noticeable difference technique along with bracketing is recommended.

Binocularity

It is important to evaluate the fusional ability for all conditions, especially in those patients demonstrating large differences in acuity (>2 lines) between the two eyes. A Maddox rod is a good disassociating lens and can be used to determine vertical and lateral imbalances. The binocular evaluation can also be done on a toposcope or any other type of stereoscope with small, medium, and large targets. In addition to the psychological advantage of using both eyes, binocularity can also provide better visual acuity, greater depth of focus, and a larger field of view.

GLARE AND PHOTOPHOBIA CONTROL

The evaluation of glare and photophobia control is just as important as a refraction for the remediation of the effects of peripheral field defects. Glare and photophobic sensitivities are common problems with field restrictions

 700 foot optotype seen at 10 feet

patient's remaining
field at 10 feet

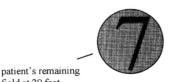 700 foot optotype seen at 20 feet

patient's remaining
field at 20 feet

FIGURE 12-1. **A patient with an extremely reduced peripheral field would have difficulty identifying the number 7 at 10 ft in this example.**

because of reduced contrast sensitivity, slower responses to light and dark adaptation, and secondary media defects (e.g., cataracts). Another factor with conditions such as retinitis pigmentosa and glaucoma, is that as the disorder worsens, the retinal pigment epithelium tends to absorb less light and, therefore, glare and photophobia are increased due to light scatter. Glare affects the middle and low spatial frequency levels of a patient's contrast sensitivity and therefore has an impact on contrast and mobility but may show no effect on visual acuity (which is related more to high spatial frequency).

The theory of glare control seems vague and obscure. To understand glare fully, one must have an understanding of flare and scatter. Flare and scatter are caused by media or retinal involvement. The effect is similar to seeing through atmospheric dust or fog. Rosenberg's[1] study of relative scatter as a function of wavelength indicated that the shorter wavelengths cause the most scatter and the longer wavelengths cause relatively little scatter in the human eye. Additional significance can be drawn from the Bezold-Brücke phenomenon and Abney's effect,[2] which indicate that a wavelength of 578 nm is unaffected by brightness and a wavelength of 570 nm is unaffected by saturation. Perhaps it is the constancy of these wavelengths that accounts for the success of some patients with the Kalichrome (Bausch and Lomb, Rochester, NY [may be ordered through local laboratories]), Corning Photochromatic Filter (Corning Medical Optics, Elmira, NY), and NoIR (NoIR Medical Technologies, South Lyon, MI) amber lenses that have peaks in these ranges (yellow and amber). Yellow or amber lenses absorb blue light (shorter wavelength) that is responsible for light scatter or glare.

The evaluation of a glare- or illumination-control lens should be subjective and task specific. There is no reason to believe that one lens tint can be applied to all patients. In addition, varying types of outdoor illumination must be considered when prescribing any absorptive lens for outdoor glare or photophobia. In many parts of the country, two or more weather conditions contributing to glare can occur over the span of a single day. The evaluation for outdoor glare should take place under actual conditions by taking the patient outdoors and judging his or her response to various tinted lenses. It may be necessary to evaluate patients under several weather conditions to fully understand glare comfort needs. Problems of ambient light can be resolved using NoIR and Solarshield (Dioptrics, Irvine, CA) lenses or using side shields that can be attached to most frames. Slip-in, wraparound, absorptive lenses can alleviate the ambient light and may also be used in combination with spectacle tinted lenses for greater light absorption. The patient may require more than one pair of absorptive lenses to help alleviate the effects of varied lighting conditions.

Photochromatic lenses must be considered carefully. Although these lenses may be helpful for their absorptive quality, they require some time to complete their fading process. For many ocular disorders involving a reduced amount of rod function, this length of time may be a major inconvenience and possibly even dangerous in some circumstances. A gradient tinted lens may be considered so that the patient can adjust the amount of absorption by changing his or her eye position when looking through the lenses (see Chapter 13 for a full description of sun lenses and filters).

Although a sun visor is not an absorptive lens, it should be considered for some patients because of its effectiveness in controlling the ambient glare. The sun visor or peaked cap can be used alone or in combination with absorptive lenses.

Glare testing indoors should also be task specific. For example, general room glare should be tested separately for each individual task, such as reading, watching television, or using a computer or closed-circuit television (CCTV). The practitioner should not assume that the tint preference will remain the same for all indoor tasks.

To evaluate the tint needs for a CCTV, it is necessary to first determine the polarity preference (i.e., black letters on a white background or white letters on a black background). Tinted lenses can then be evaluated for further comfort. A tint for a CCTV or computer screen can be provided in one of three ways:

1. The appropriate spectacle correction can be combined with the preferred tint.
2. A colored acetate filter can be placed over the entire screen.
3. A color CCTV or computer monitor can be prescribed that would allow for different color combinations (e.g., yellow print on a blue background, red print on a green background).

Glare from printed material can be controlled using a typoscope or a lamp with which the angle of the light source and the bulb distance to the reading material can be changed. The value of the typoscope can be increased by attaching a yellow acetate filter to the window opening, thereby further reducing glare as well as increasing the contrast of the print.

ILLUMINATION

Illumination needs for patients with visual field constrictions must strike a balance between the demands of their photopic vision and the use of their remaining scotopic vision. Illumination sources must also satisfy many needs and goals, such as reading, hobbies, activities of daily living, and mobility.

Illumination sources should have specific requirements:

1. The amount of illumination must be variable by rheostat or height adjustment of the light source. The use of a goose-neck or spring-balanced, flexible-arm lamp is recommended for reading and other near tasks.
2. Desk lamps should include a shade that covers the bulb deeply enough to shield the patient from glare and wide enough to prevent overheating. On-off switches should be accessible and convenient.
3. The wattage of the desk lamp should not be more than 75–100 W of incandescent illumination. Typi-

cally, incandescent lamps are preferred, although some patients may favor fluorescent lighting.

4. For mobility purposes, the light sources should be as bright and wide beamed as the design of the unit will allow. These units should be portable and rechargeable.

The low vision practitioner should think in terms of a variety of lamps to illuminate different areas for near tasks. Desk lamps are necessary for reading and writing, but attention should also be given to the other major areas of the home, such as the kitchen (where lights under cabinets and bright lights above the stove may be quite helpful) and dining areas as well as hallways and the bedroom. Penlights are excellent as portable sources of illumination and can be used for spot reading (often serving the secondary function as a pointer to maintain continuity in reading) as well as finding the keyhole in the door at night.

For reading, the appropriate lighting along with a thorough understanding of the field loss will help in the prescribing strategies. A patient exhibiting a right hemianopic field loss may experience problems in finding the end of a sentence because he or she is reading into a blind area. When the scotoma is to the left side, as seen in a patient with a left hemianopic field loss, he or she may experience problems in finding the beginning word of a new sentence. The use of a typoscope, ruler, or even a finger may provide refined tracking and thereby allow the patient improved functioning. It may also be recommended that the patient orient the reading material to a position that eliminates reading into a scotoma by having the material angled at a 45-degree angle or even a 90-degree angle. This position may appear awkward in the beginning, but with practice and persistence, patients can become accustomed to reading in this manner.

Illumination sources for mobility are one of the major contributions a low vision practitioner can make toward the rehabilitation of the patient with a constricted field. There are two approaches to consider in this regard.

The first is the enhancement of scotopic vision through a device that creates a brighter image. The best known of these devices is the ITT Nightscope (Night Vision Aid Distributors, Randallstown, MD). (See Chapter 13 for information on this device. Figure 13-15 shows a Nightspy, an Israeli night-vision device.) In spite of the impressive view through a night-vision device, there are some objections to this device:

1. The device is only helpful when the patient holds it in front of the eye; for extremely constricted fields, the patient must hold the device in front of the eye constantly while walking at night or in dim light.

2. Although the device is relatively lightweight, holding it steady in front of an eye for any length of time is fatiguing.

3. The field of view through the system is relatively limited. Therefore, this limits the patient's scanning ability through the system. Fields of view vary from 10 degrees to as wide as 40 degrees, depending on the system design.

4. Not all night-vision devices are created equal. There is both a wide range of prices and performance in the units now on the market. The sharpness of the image will vary with the quality of both the optics and the electronics.

5. A top-quality system will maintain the same levels of brightness and sharpness across the entire viewing field, whereas older and less expensive units may show a marked drop in brightness and image sharpness around the edge of the system.

6. When a night-vision device reaches the end of its useable life, it does not simply quit working, it just gradually goes dimmer. This effect may result in some patients fearing that their vision has further decreased.

7. Turning a night-vision device on in full daylight can cause permanent damage in a very short time if not equipped with a brightness protection circuit.

8. The Generation II technology night-vision device is available from a limited number of U.S. manufacturers and is fairly expensive. (Generation III models are the most sophisticated and are reserved for U.S. government use only.)

The second method of illumination addresses the problem more directly. A bright flashlight or a Wide-Angle Mobility Light (WAML) (Innovation Rehabilitation Technology, Inc., Mountain View, CA) may be recommended for night travel. The WAML is a wide-beam light source that illuminates an area approximately 10 ft (30 degrees horizontally and 20 degrees vertically) in front of the patient (see Figure 13-14). It has a halogen bulb that provides an intensity of 1,400 candlepower. This unit satisfies the needs of many patients because it is portable, rechargeable, bright, and wide beamed. The major disadvantages of this system are its weight and size. Although shoulder straps are provided, the patient should be evaluated for its portability because the device weighs 5 lb. Another disadvantage with the WAML is its tendency to burn out relatively quickly (it is in fact a diver's lamp designed for underwater use and is constantly water cooled when used for this purpose).

Comparative studies between the WAML and the ITT Nightscope indicate a preference for the WAML when used for general mobility purposes.[3–5]

A halogen flashlight or camcorder light can be used as portable illumination sources as well. Although these units are lighter and more comfortable to hold, the intensity of the beam is not as strong as the WAML, but they may serve the purpose well for some patients. Flashlights are now available with adjustable beams (e.g., the Mag-Lite [MAG Instrument, Ontario, CA] series of flashlights). These flashlights vary in size from pocket size, using one AAA battery, to units using up to six D batteries. Naturally, the light intensity increases with the number of batteries, providing an intensity up to 20,500 candlepower.

MAGNIFICATION

Retinal magnification must be used with care and discretion in cases of peripheral field constriction. The amount of magnification should be restricted to the minimum amount that satisfies the patient's immediate needs.

In the earlier stages of peripheral field loss, a patient's central vision is generally not impaired (other then a possible refractive error). When reading, therefore, nothing more then a low-powered reading lens may be required. In cases of glaucoma or retinitis pigmentosa, as the condition progresses, resulting in increased constriction of the peripheral fields along with reduced central vision, a low-powered reading lens may no longer be sufficient. If the patient now requires a high-powered reading lens (microscope) to read, he or she is then forced to hold the reading material at a much closer distance. Because the patient's remaining field is more constricted at a close distance (field is cone shaped), the patient may be able to see only a few letters at a time, making reading tedious and frustrating. Other factors, such as maintaining the appropriate lighting and decreased depth of focus with more powerful reading lenses, also adds to the frustration. Therefore, other low vision devices should be demonstrated that would allow the patient to move the reading material further away from his or her eye.

The use of handheld and stand magnifiers should be investigated if reading lenses are not accepted by the patient. When using magnifiers, the patient must be instructed to adjust the overhead illumination or angle the magnifier to avoid reflections from the front surface of the magnifier. These reflections may hamper the patient from using the magnifier. Handheld and stand magnifiers with attached illumination are often the preferred alternative.

The use of electronic or projection-type magnification, such as a CCTV, for writing, reading, and other tasks is a major consideration for patients with peripheral field constrictions. The CCTV has the advantage of providing more magnification, which can be tolerated by the patient with peripheral field loss because of the greater viewing distance. The choice of polarity and ability to control the brightness and contrast, as well as scroll the reading material across the patient's field of view (while the patient maintains a straight-ahead fixation), are important factors in the successful use of these systems. In some cases, a patient may require a minimum amount of magnification; however, his or her need for illumination and contrast enhancement may be so great that only a CCTV will allow the patient to read comfortably (see Chapter 11 for more details on a CCTV).

Magnification to improve distance vision through the use of a telescope is more restricted and may be considered inappropriate treatment for severe constrictions of peripheral field loss by some low vision practitioners. It is important, however, that each patient be given the opportunity to evaluate low-powered telescopes to address his or her needs and to determine the merits of such a device. It is not uncommon for patients with remaining fields as small as 5 degrees to use handheld telescopes to increase the quality of their distance vision.

Another source of distance magnification can be seen in the use of a Fresnel-type television magnifier. This magnifier is placed in front of the television set and provides 2× magnification. Patients may reject this system, however, due to the loss of contrast and brightness that is inherent in this type of magnifier. Another recommendation is to have the patient view a larger-screen television, thereby obtaining a slight increase in magnification while maintaining a good quality image. For example, if a patient switches from a 20-in. screen to a 27-in. screen, he or she will be obtaining 1.35× magnification (27/20 = 1.35).

For patients who may benefit from a slight increase in magnification, spectacle magnification may be considered. By manipulating various parameters of a spectacle lens, the amount of magnification can be increased to a very small degree. This increase may, however, be sufficient to allow an increase in the quality of the patient's vision. Spectacle magnification (M_{spec}) is given by the following formula:

$$M_{spec} = \left[\frac{1}{1 - D_1(t/n)}\right]\left(\frac{1}{1 - hD_2}\right)$$

where D_1 = the front surface power of the lens, t = the thickness of the lens, n = the index of refraction of the lens, h = the distance from the back surface of the lens to the entrance pupil of the eye (vertex distance + 3 mm [front surface of the cornea to entrance pupil]), and D_2 = the back vertex power of the lens.

The first section of this equation is called the *shape factor*, because it relates to the form or shape of the lens. The second section is called the *power factor*. A summary of the results that can be obtained through the spectacle magnification formula is as follows:

1. Increased magnification can be attained by using a steeper base curve.
2. Increased magnification can be attained by using a thicker lens.
3. Increased magnification can be attained by increasing the vertex distance.
4. Increased magnification can be attained by using lens material with a lower index of refraction.

VISUAL FIELDS TESTING

Accurate visual fields must be plotted to understand the nature of the visual impairment and to follow the course of the pathology. In general, when peripheral field loss exists, it can be classified into two groups:

1. Constricted, circular loss usually associated with some form of tapetoretinal degeneration or glaucoma. In cases of hysterical blindness or malingering, a patient will also demonstrate peripherally constricted circular fields or "tunnel vision." These patients, however, will demonstrate the same size constriction at different testing distances. This field is unlike that of a patient with retinitis pigmentosa, for example, who will show a geometrically expanded field with increased test distances (cone shaped).

2. Sector loss usually associated with retinal detachments or neurologic disorders (e.g., stroke, head trauma,

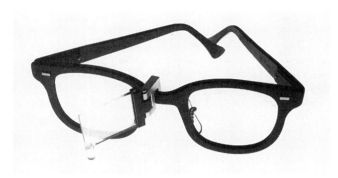

FIGURE 12-2. **This semireflective plano mirror placed on the nasal aspect of the spectacle frame would aid a patient with a right temporal field loss. Because the mirror is semireflective, the patient can also view through the mirror, thereby eliminating a potential nasal scotoma created by a full reflective mirror.**

tumors). These fields are generally represented as quadrantanopsias or hemianopsias.

Regardless of the cause of the visual field loss, a determination should be made as to whether static or kinetic testing should be performed. In static perimetry, the size and location of the target are constant, whereas the brightness of the target is increased until the patient reports seeing it. With kinetic perimetry, a target is placed in the periphery (nonseeing area) and moved toward the fixation target (seeing area) until the patient reports seeing it. The target is moved along a set meridian with the procedure repeated along other major meridians using the same target. By joining the points in the various meridians where the patient reported first seeing the target, an isopter is formed. The isopter is nothing more than an outline of the patient's peripheral sensitivity to a given size target.

A number of studies have compared static perimetry testing to kinetic perimetry testing.[6, 7] The results indicate that both forms of testing are sensitive and accurate in evaluating field defects.

Confrontation fields provide a rapid and fairly accurate kinetic test. Confrontation fields are best performed when instruments of perimetry are not available or when certain circumstances warrant the test—for example, with patients who are bedridden or those who do not respond to conventional instrument testing (see Chapters 16 and 17). A confrontation field is best suited for estimating the size of a central scotoma or peripheral field loss as well as hemianopic or altitudinal field losses. It cannot, however, provide information on subtle changes that may occur over time in patients with glaucoma or retinitis pigmentosa.

Goldmann's bowl perimetry uses both static and kinetic testing and has throughout the years proved reliable in demonstrating the subtle changes required for evaluating retinitis pigmentosa and glaucoma patients. Automated fields using static testing, however, such as in the Humphrey field analyzer, appear to have supplanted Goldmann's bowl perimetry testing. In any case, either of

the two forms of testing (kinetic or static) as well as a number of field instrumentation may be used to obtain accurate and reliable information of peripheral field defects.

When performing peripheral field testing (as in any type of field testing), it is important to realize that accuracy and reliability are dependent on many factors, for example,

1. *Refractive error.* Uncorrected refractive errors can cause a blur of the target with decreased retinal sensitivity. If high prescriptions are involved, the habitual frame, trial frame, or trial lenses may hamper accurate results.
2. *Patient elements.* Fatigue, experience in field testing, degree of understanding the instructions, and motivation are all important factors.
3. *Patient anatomic structures.* Some forms of cataracts or corneal dystrophies, ptosis, pinhole pupils, and prominent orbital structures may have some effect on field results.
4. *Targets.* Size of the target, illumination levels of the target, length of time, or speed in which targets are presented are all factors that must be standardized or may result in different findings at any given time.

Some patients with peripheral field loss show improved mobility and near-point skills (e.g., reading, locating objects easier) with greater illumination. One explanation may be that the patient has a relative scotoma and will function better with increased illumination. Thus, valuable information concerning a patient's functioning may be obtained if he or she is occasionally evaluated with large targets or very bright illumination levels (maximum sensitivity) when field testing. Educating the patient as to the effects of the interplay of fields, lighting, contrast, and glare on everyday functioning is crucial. With this awareness, the patient may be able to analyze his or her own work and home environments and modify them as needed.

FIELD ENHANCEMENT

The earliest reference to field enhancement is seen in a paper by Bell,[8] who, in 1919, described the placement of a mirror on the nasal area of a spectacle for a patient with a bitemporal hemianopsia. This plano mirror reflected the image of an object on the nonseeing side (temporal area) to a more nasal area of the same eye, where the patient had functional retina (Figure 12-2). The mirror system, however, has a number of disadvantages that are discussed in Chapter 17.

Considering the awkwardness of the mirror system and the confusion caused by the dual imaging (from a semireflective mirror) and the reversal of an image, a prism system appears to be the more accepted system for peripheral field enhancement. The benefit of a prism is similar to that of a mirror. It causes a displacement of an object in the patient's blind area to an area on the retina where there is useful vision. A major advantage of a prism over that of a mirror, however, is that the prism is placed on the area of the eye that is nonseeing and therefore does not cause an additional blind spot or dual image. The displacement of the image is toward the apex of the prism, with the angle of deviation in degrees equal to approximately half the dioptric power of the prism (1 prism diopter = 0.57 degrees). For example, a 30.00 D prism will deviate an image approximately 15 degrees (actually 17.10 degrees) toward the apex of the prism. When a prism is used for a patient with a hemianopic temporal field loss, the prism is placed on the temporal portion of the carrier lens with the base of the prism toward the temporal area and the apex of the prism toward the nasal area. When the patient glances into this prism, he or she does not have to look as far toward the blind side because the image has been displaced nasally onto viable retinal tissue. The patient is able to reduce his or her eye movement, thereby reducing the amount of required versions.

Fresnel Prisms

Fresnel press-on prisms have become the most commonly used prisms for field enhancement. A Fresnel prism is a 1-mm plastic (polyvinyl chloride) material that can be applied to the back surface of a spectacle lens by nothing more than surface tension. This allows for easy application of the prism to a carrier lens along with the ability to reposition the prism as many times as is necessary (Figure 12-3). Other advantages of a Fresnel prism are the following:

1. Minimal weight
2. Minimal thickness
3. Minimal cost
4. Wide range of available powers (from 0.5 prism diopter to 30 prism diopters)

Fresnel prisms do, however, have some disadvantages. These disadvantages are as follows:

1. They can cause a decrease in visual acuity.
2. They can cause a decrease in contrast sensitivity at all spatial frequencies and especially at the high spatial frequencies.
3. The prisms will discolor over time.
4. The prisms may lose the surface tension over a period and fall off.
5. The prisms demonstrate greater distortion and chromatic aberration than an equal-powered ground-in prism.

When using a Fresnel prism, it is important that the patient understand that the purpose of the prism is not to sharpen the image but rather to enhance the awareness of peripheral objects. The amount of prism and the initial placement of the prism are subject to some controversy and professional opinion. The most commonly prescribed prism is found in one of three powers: 15 prism diopters, 20 prism diopters, or 30 prism diopters. The decision as to proper power depends on the patient's

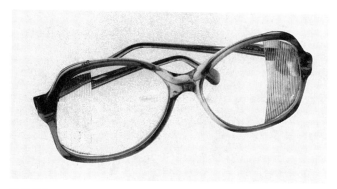

FIGURE 12-3. **A Fresnel prism placed base out in each spectacle lens for a patient with a bitemporal hemianopic field loss.**

goals, amount of peripheral field loss, and adaptation to the displaced image. Successful use of the prism system also mandates an extensive instructional program. A technique for placement of the Fresnel prism is found in Appendix A; the specific parameters of instruction are discussed in Appendix B.

As Fresnel prisms were evaluated, prescribed, and reported on in the literature, it became evident that not all peripheral field defects responded equally. The successful cases were with those patients having a hemianopic field loss, and the most success was with bitemporal hemianopic field loss. In these cases, prisms placed base out at the temporal aspect of the carrier lenses were well received. To address the concentrically reduced fields of retinitis pigmentosa and glaucoma, it seemed reasonable to surround the remaining field with prism. The degree of success with this concept ranged from small to none. Some practitioners have verbally reported success with these systems, but none of the reports has become part of the literature. Even in cases in which the prism was placed only in the temporal area (to help avoid objects and people to the side of the patient), success for those with concentrically reduced fields has been limited. It has become apparent that not all peripheral field defects are sensitive to the same methods of field enhancement. Patients with a hemianopic field loss do not have the same needs as those with a reduced field due to retinitis pigmentosa, and therefore, should not be categorized as one homogeneous group. The differing results may be due to the sudden field loss associated with strokes and brain injury versus the more gradual field loss associated with retinitis pigmentosa or glaucoma. Patients having a gradual field loss may learn to be more efficient with their scanning ability and therefore have less need for prisms or mirrors.

Scanning is often emphasized for all visually impaired patients exhibiting a peripheral field loss. A study of scanning patterns for patients with retinitis pigmentosa reveals interesting results.[9] When patients with absolute 5-degree fields were presented with a target that subtended an angle greater than their visual fields, they reported being able to see the entire target by using fine-scanning techniques. The nature of the scanning had several characteristics:

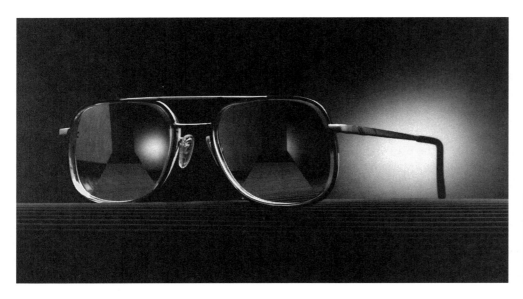

FIGURE 12-4. **The Inwave Field-Expanding Channel Lens is composed of two 12 prism diopter lateral prisms and an inferior 8 prism diopter lens. The size of the channel is dependent on the patient's remaining central field. (Courtesy of Inwave Optics, Inc., Janesville, WI.)**

1. The extent of the scanning covered a very small range as opposed to the larger scanning range of nystagmus, for example.
2. The extent of this fine scanning was not observed during a routine examination.
3. The fine scanning was effortless and appeared to be an involuntary response. The scanning occurred in the horizontal, vertical, and oblique positions of the target.

Field-Expanding Channel Lens

Inwave Optics, Inc. (Janesville, WI) has designed a lens system that is composed of two 12 prism diopter lateral prisms and one 8 prism diopter inferior prism with the apex of each prism toward a central nonprismatic channel (Figure 12-4). A distance prescription (available to ± 8.00 sphere and ± 7.00 cylinder) can be incorporated into the front surface of the lens along with a bifocal, if needed. This lens system is designed for various degrees of peripheral field loss by having the patient use a specific-sized channel that is dependent on the size of the peripheral field that is remaining (Table 12-1). It is recommended that the lens channel be aligned with the peripheral edges of the functional retina so that as the fields decrease in

size so, too, does the width of the channel. The inferior prism is placed at a similar height to that of the bifocal segment.

The Field-Expanding Channel Lens was designed for improved mobility with the patient viewing objects through the channel while having the advantage of temporal, nasal, and inferior awareness. This lens is recommended for glaucoma and retinitis pigmentosa (tapetoretinal degeneration) patients. For patients who have fields less than 6 degrees, it is recommended that the temporal channel edge of the lens (of a 6-mm channel lens, see Table 12-1) be positioned so that it aligns with the edge of the patient's temporal functional retina.

Inwave also makes a Hemispheric Field Loss Lens, which is specifically designed for patients with hemianopic field losses. This lens is discussed in Chapter 17.

Reverse Telescopes

In addition, there must be some differentiation between field enhancement for *mobility* and field enhancement for *sighting*. The word *mobility* refers to a dynamic situation in which the patient must travel efficiently and safely from one place to another. A patient demonstrating a reduced peripheral field loss may improve his or her mobility by using scanning, prisms, or mirrors. The concept of *sighting* indicates observations being made while the patient is stationary. The use of a reverse telescope when sitting or standing but not when walking is an example of this difference. A patient may use a reverse telescope to spot the number of people in a room, to locate his or her children on a busy playground, to scan an environment for potential obstacles, to find objects on a desk, or even to locate a doorway in a building. A reverse telescope is nothing more than a Galilean or Keplerian telescope in which the patient views through the objective lens (as opposed to looking through the ocular lens, or eyepiece), thereby causing minification. This minification is approximately

TABLE 12-1
Channel Width of Inwave Field-Expanding Channel Lens*

Field Loss	Recommended Size of Channel (mm)
Beyond 20 degrees	14
To 20 degrees	12
To 15 degrees	10
To 10 degrees	8
To 6 degrees	6

*Available from Inwave Optics, Inc., Janesville, WI.

equal to the power of the telescope. For example, looking through the objective lens of a 2× telescope will increase the patient's field by approximately 2 times, but will also decrease visual acuity (through minification) by approximately 2 times. In general, the patient with reduced peripheral fields has not experienced success with a reverse telescope for mobility because of the peripheral distortion found in these systems. Another problem is that depth perception, so critical during mobility tasks, is greatly impaired by minification. Problems in correctly judging the position of stairs, curbs, and irregularities on the walking surface render the system impractical for continuous viewing while in motion. Finally, these systems prevent the patient from scanning. For example, a patient with a 5-degree central field may be able to scan 5 degrees to either side of his or her field and thereby achieve a functional field of 15 degrees. When a 2× reverse telescope is placed in front of this patient, his or her field is confined to the 10 degrees that this particular telescope provides this patient, and therefore, the patient has a smaller field through the reverse telescope than he or she would have with his or her remaining field and scanning combined.

A reverse telescope can be prescribed as a handheld device, or it can be mounted in a spectacle and worn as a full-diameter or bioptic system (Figure 12-5).

Amorphic or New Horizon Lens

In an attempt to minimize visual acuity degradation, a meridional minification system called the Amorphic or New Horizon Lens (Designs for Vision, Inc., Ronkonkoma, NY) was designed by Dr. William Feinbloom. By properly spacing positive and negative cylindrical lenses, minification is limited only to the horizontal meridian. This results in the creation of a retinal image unchanged in the vertical meridian and compressed in the horizontal meridian by a factor of the minifying power of the lens (Figure 12-6). Full-field Amorphic lens systems are available in powers of −1.2×, −1.4×, −1.6×, −1.8×, and −2.0×. The use of the minus sign indicates minification by the manufacturer and not an inverted image. As a matter of fact, the Amorphic lens is a reverse Galilean system. These lenses were mounted in a spectacle and were originally intended for full-time viewing by the patient with reduced fields and poor mobility (Figure 12-7). Most patients reported dizziness, depth of field confusion, distortion, and disorientation, however, when using the lenses for a period. The full-field Amorphic lens was later redesigned into a bioptic form to allow patients to alternate between the cylindrical minifier and the carrier lens while in motion (see Figure 1-4). (As of this writing, the Amorphic lens is no longer manufactured.)

Image Minifier

Ocutech, Inc. (Chapel Hill, NC) has designed the Image Minifier, which is a reverse Galilean telescope that pro-

duces a one-third image size reduction without producing the excessive barrel distortion commonly seen in most reverse telescopes (Figure 12-8). The Image Minifier is focusable and lightweight and can be used as a handheld, clip-on, or spectacle-mounted system (Figure 12-9).

Concave Lenses

Another sighting device worth mentioning is a handheld minifier (concave lens). When a concave lens is held at a specific distance from the eye, a minified image is created, and the patient must provide some accommodation (or use an add) to see the image clearly. This system is therefore nothing more than a reverse Galilean telescope. The ratio of the dioptric power of the concave lens (D) to the amount of accommodation or add (A) will determine the amount of minification (M_{in}).

Example
A patient holds a −10.00 D lens at a given distance from his +2.00 D bifocal and views a clear minified image. What is the total amount of minification obtained?
   Answer:

$$M_{in} = \frac{D}{A}$$
$$= \frac{-10.00}{2.00}$$
$$= -5 \times \text{ (minification)}$$

The Field Viewer by Ocutech is a 45-mm-diameter, biconcave, coated glass lens mounted in a plastic ring (see Figure 12-9). This lens, which can be worn around the neck using a neck strap, is available in three minifications (2.50×, 3.25×, and 4.50×) and should be held approximately 16 in. from the eye.

Convex Mirrors

When placed on a desk or kitchen work area, convex mirrors allow patients with field constrictions to be aware of people approaching them from the side or behind and also reduces the shock of the unexpected tap on the shoulder (especially for patients with Usher's syndrome). These same convex mirrors can be placed in hallways or rooms to provide information about open closet doors, people coming through halls or doorways, or any other obstacles that may create a hindrance.

REFERRAL FOR ADDITIONAL PROFESSIONAL SERVICES

Low vision rehabilitation for patients with peripheral field constrictions cannot be considered complete without the involvement of other professionals. The most commonly used professional services are listed in the following sections, but by no means is this list complete. The low vision

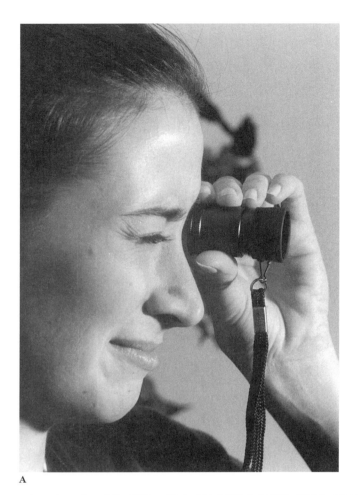

A

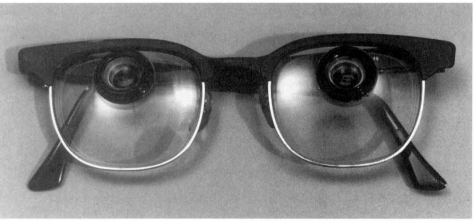

B

FIGURE 12-5. **A. A patient using a reverse handheld telescope (patient is looking through the objective lens) to obtain an increased field through minification. B. A spectacle-mounted bioptic reverse telescope.**

practitioner must analyze all aspects of the patient's problems and frustrations and make the appropriate referrals.

State Agency for the Blind or Visually Impaired

A state agency for the blind and visually impaired is found in every state in the United States with variations of its name from state to state. This agency can be the starting point for many patients in terms of receiving professional services, such as counseling, mobility instruction, rehabilitation teaching, and an adaptive technology evaluation. This state agency can also provide assistance to the patient seeking a job placement or the patient who may have to change careers due to vision loss (see Chapter 19 for more information).

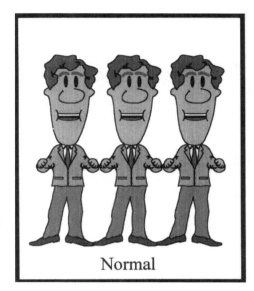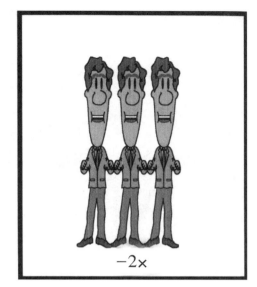

FIGURE 12-6. **The Amorphic lens (Designs for Vision, Inc., Ronkonkoma, NY) in this figure is producing 2× minification in the horizontal direction with no change in the vertical direction. There is, therefore, no change in the visual angle in the vertical meridian.**

Counseling

Patients with reduced peripheral field often retain good central vision for a long time. Many of them have psychological difficulty dealing with their situation. Too often, the frustration of accepting impairment is complicated by family and friends who doubt that the condition exists because of the relatively good central vision or because "their eyes look normal." Statements regarding depression and threats of suicide are not uncommon. The practitioner must be sensitive to this frustration and arrange for counseling before these feelings reach uncontrollable levels. A referral to a psychiatrist, psychologist, or social worker may be indicated when a patient is unable to cope with these frustrations (see Chapter 2 for more information).

Genetic counseling is extremely important in cases in which there are genetically transmitted problems. The decision to have children is a very personal one. Patients with retinitis pigmentosa and their mates, for example,

should be fully informed about the chances of passing this disorder to their offspring.

Mobility

The use of the long cane, guide dog, or other mobility aids can only complement what may be done visually. Professionals known as *orientation and mobility therapists* are trained to provide mobility services. The name of this specialty describes its main function. *Orientation* refers to a familiarization with and adaptation to a position or point in the environment, whereas *mobility* refers to the safe travel from one point to another. Patients with visual impairments that affect their ability to get around should be educated about these services. Many patients with reduced peripheral fields believe that the long cane is only for those who are totally blind. They are often surprised to learn that they are indeed appropriate candidates for a cane. Many patients indicate that they travel with much greater confidence and freedom

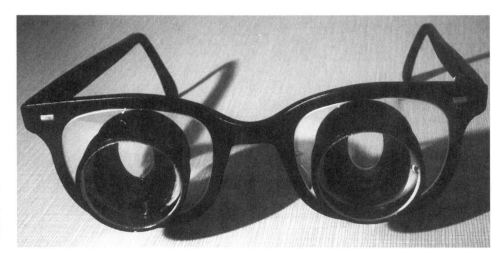

FIGURE 12-7. **The original Amorphic lens (Designs for Vision, Inc., Ronkonkoma, NY) was designed as a full-diameter system through which a patient with reduced peripheral fields would view on a full-time basis.**

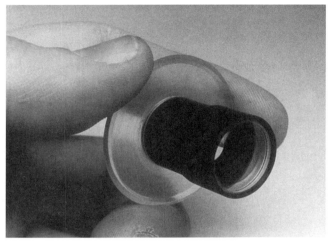

A

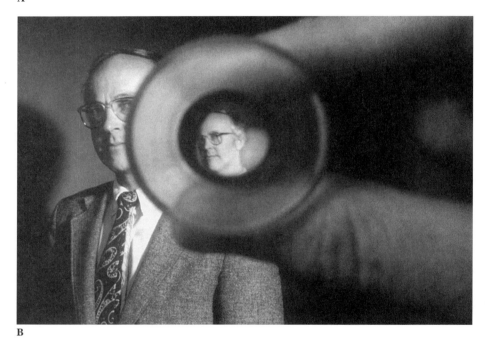

B

FIGURE 12-8. **A. The Image Minifier is a reverse Galilean telescope. B. The Image Minifier produces a flat field with a minimum of barrel distortion. (Courtesy of Ocutech, Inc., Chapel Hill, NC.)**

after receiving mobility and cane instruction. If they have learned to use a long cane, their vision may be "freed" for scanning the environment and thus improve on their orientation in the environment. In many cases, before using the cane, all the patient's visual energy was spent in attending to the area directly in front to avoid walking into obstacles.

It is equally important that all patients and their family members and friends be well skilled in sighted guide techniques (see Chapter 3 for more information).

Audiometry

Due to the possibility of Usher's syndrome, retinitis pigmentosa patients should have audiometry tests to identify any

hearing loss. Karp and Santore[10] indicated that deafness in Usher's syndrome is not always severe. Moderate hearing impairments are significantly represented. The early detection of any hearing loss for these patients is essential to their rehabilitation and must not be overlooked.

Rehabilitation Teacher

Braille instruction may be necessary to assist patients with severe field constrictions. It should be considered for patients whose impairment prevents them from reading print as well as for those who might request an alternative to reading print as a precautionary measure for the future. Talking books, typing, and high-technology equipment

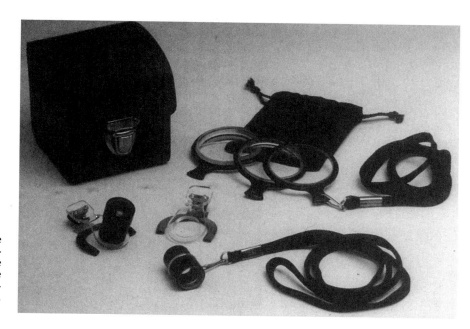

FIGURE 12-9. **The Image Minifier can be prescribed as a handheld, clip-on, or spectacle-mounted system (lower portion of figure). The upper portion of the figure demonstrates the Field Viewer. These lenses are biconcave, handheld lenses that are used as spotting minifiers. (Courtesy of Ocutech, Inc., Chapel Hill, NC.)**

should also be considered. Many of these alternative methods to reading print can be instrumental in continuing a patient's education as well as obtaining or maintaining gainful employment.

The lack of peripheral fields may make common tasks difficult. Alternative techniques may need to be explored for activities of daily living, such as household chores, grooming, cooking, and shopping. Concerns relating to accessibility of items in cupboards or refrigerators and arranging the kitchen and bathroom areas for greatest safety must also be considered. All of the preceding services can best be provided through rehabilitation teachers.

Consumer and Support Groups

Consumer groups (e.g., American Council for the Blind, National Federation of the Blind, and the Council of Citizens with Low Vision International) can be valuable sources of information, support, and social activity. These groups provide publications, may have local affiliates with regularly scheduled meetings, and offer yearly national conferences as well.

Support groups can be invaluable as well. They provide a forum in which the patient can share his or her concerns with those who understand those concerns through firsthand experience. Many patients find support and consumer groups invaluable, simply because through these groups they learn that they are not alone in facing vision loss.

Patients with vision loss due to retinitis pigmentosa should be referred to the Foundation Fighting Blindness for information about retinitis pigmentosa, national con-

ferences, and local affiliates. This organization was founded in 1971 to find a cure for retinitis pigmentosa and was previously called the Retinitis Pigmentosa Foundation Fighting Blindness. This organization now raises substantial moneys every year to fund research into retinitis pigmentosa and other hereditary retinal degenerations, such as macular degeneration.

ASSISTIVE TECHNOLOGY EVALUATION

Patients who require computer access for educational, vocational, or leisure activities but whose vision loss creates difficulty reading a standard computer monitor with a low vision device should be referred for an assistive technology evaluation. In this evaluation, they can explore various alternative modes of computer access, such as electronic display magnification, vocalization input and output systems, or braille systems. They may ultimately benefit from one of these alternatives or from several in combination (see Chapter 14 for information on computer assistive technology). The state agency for the blind and visually impaired is an excellent referral source for a patient seeking assistive technology services.

DRIVING

It is vital that the low vision practitioner address the issue of driving with patients who have reduced peripheral fields. Many patients do not report functional difficulties until their fields are quite constricted, often less than 20 degrees. The patient should understand that driving is as much a visual field task as it is a visual acuity task. It may never have occurred to the patient to ask or comment about driving. Thus, it is incumbent on the practitioner to initiate such a discussion. This topic is a very emotional one, as most patients are not fully aware of other transportation options, nor are they willing to give up their independence. Giving up driving is one of the hardest steps to accept for many patients who are still attempting to deal with their adjustment to vision loss. The practitioner who addresses the issue of driving with sensitivity and empathy, yet firmly and clearly explains why the patient must stop driving, does the patient (and society) an important service.

CONCLUSION

Greater understanding of the pathologies causing field constrictions and how they interfere in the normal functioning of low vision patients is necessary to allow more specific treatment and improved rehabilitation. The variations in glare and photophobia, the use of meridional minification as opposed to overall minification, and the understanding of prism deviation and its application to field enhancement must be further investigated. Only after a better understanding of when and why these systems work can the practitioner be better prepared to help patients with any form of peripheral field loss.

Acknowledgment
The authors would like to acknowledge the assistance of Dr. Norman J. Weiss in the writing of this chapter. Dr. Weiss was extremely generous in providing much of the original material for this chapter. It is greatly appreciated.

SELF-ASSESSMENT QUESTIONS

1. When glare affects the *middle* and *low* spatial frequency levels of a patient's contrast sensitivity, you would most likely expect this patient to experience problems with which of the following?
   (a) visual acuity
   (b) mobility
   (c) color vision
   (d) a and c

2. Which of the following recommendations should be made when evaluating a patient with end-stage glaucoma who has complaints of glare and photophobia?
   (a) The patient should be prescribed a photochromatic lens so that one lens can be used in different lighting situations.
   (b) A yellow or amber lens may be required in certain environments because it will eliminate the annoying effects of blue light.

   (c) A number of tinted lenses may have to be prescribed depending on the different environments or lighting situations a patient may be in at any particular time of the day.
   (d) a and b
   (e) b and c

3. When a patient with advanced retinitis pigmentosa attempts to read with a microscopic lens, he complains that he is able to see only two or three letters at a time. What other lens or device may be recommended that would allow him to read at least the same size print but see more letters at a time?
   (a) a CCTV
   (b) a handheld magnifier
   (c) a stand magnifier
   (d) all of the above
   (e) None of the above because the patient's field is too small to allow any increase in the number of letters seen at one time.

4. When a prism is recommended for a patient with a bitemporal hemianopsia, the base of the prism should be placed toward which aspect of the spectacle lens?
   (a) nasal
   (b) temporal
   (c) inferior
   (d) superior
   (e) central

5. Which statement is *incorrect* in regard to a Fresnel prism?
   (a) It may cause a decrease in a patient's contrast sensitivity.
   (b) It may discolor over time.
   (c) It is free of distortion and aberrations.
   (d) It may cause a decrease in a patient's visual acuity.
   (e) It is attached to a spectacle lens by surface tension only.

6. If a patient has difficulty locating objects on a desk, which of the following low vision device(s) may be recommended?
   (a) a Fresnel prism
   (b) a reverse telescope
   (c) an Amorphic lens
   (d) a ground-in prism
   (e) b and c

7. How much minification is obtained when a patient views through a −12.00 D lens held 40 cm from the eye?
   (a) 3.0×
   (b) 3.3×
   (c) 4.2×
   (d) 4.8×
   (e) 5.6×

REFERENCES

1. Rosenberg R. Light, Glare and Contrast Sensitivity in Low Vision Care. In E Faye (ed), Clinical Low Vision (2nd ed). Boston: Little, Brown, 1984;197–212.
2. Benson WE. An Introduction to Color Vision. In T Duane (ed). Clinical Ophthalmology (Vol 3). New York: Harper & Row, 1981;1–19.
3. Morisette DL, Goodrich GL. A study of the effectiveness of the night vision aid for legally blind people with night blindness. J Vis Impair Blindness 1978;72:67–70.
4. Morisette DL. The Wide Angle Mobility Light: an aid for night blindness. J Vis Impair Blindness 1983;77:393–395.
5. Morisette DL, Goodrich GL, Marmour MF. A study of the effec-
tiveness of the Wide Angle Mobility Light. J Vis Impair Blindness 1985;79:109–111.
6. Katz J, Sommer A. Reliability indexes of automated perimetric tests. Arch Ophthalmol 1988;106:1252.
7. Werner EB, Petrig B, Krupin T, Bishop KI. Variability of automated visual fields in clinically stable glaucoma patients. Invest Ophthalmol 1988;30:1083.
8. Bell E. A mirror for patients with hemianopia. JAMA 1919;140:1024.
9. Weiss NJ. The low vision management of retinitis pigmentosa. J Am Optom Assoc 1991;62:42–52.
10. Karp A, Santore F. Retinitis pigmentosa and progressive hearing loss. J Speech Hearing Disord 1983;48:308–314.

Appendix A

PLACEMENT OF THE FRESNEL PRISM

Patient

Before determining the position of the Fresnel prism, the patient is seated in an ophthalmic chair with his or her head comfortably placed in the primary position, supported by the headrest. He or she is wearing the best spectacle distance correction (plano lenses if no prescription needed) with one eye occluded. The patient's fixation is on a small distance object on an uncluttered wall. The patient is instructed to maintain constant fixation on this central object. He or she is further instructed to report when he or she begins to see a straight edge (see numbers 1 and 2 in the next section) impinging on his or her vision. It is important that the patient maintain constant head position during this procedure.

Procedure

The following steps should be used when placing a Fresnel prism on the temporal portion of a spectacle (carrier) lens. The steps that follow are for a patient with a bitemporal hemianopic field loss. The same principles can be used for any other peripheral field loss; however, the position of the prism would have to be changed depending on what area of the field has to be enhanced. Patients with bitemporal field loss tend to show the greatest success with Fresnel prisms. It is important to remember that the prism does not cover the entire carrier lens but is placed on only part of the lens.

1. An opaque self-sticking material, such as an adhesive note pad is used, and the edge of the paper is gradually moved from the patient's blind area (temporal periphery) toward the seeing area (central nasal).
2. The movement of the paper is stopped when the patient reports seeing the leading edge of the paper. This point is marked on the spectacle lens with a fine-tip felt marker.
3. Steps 1 and 2 are repeated several times for reliability.
4. The edge of the paper is placed 1–2 mm temporal to the mark that was initially placed on the spectacle lens.
5. If the correction is to be binocular, steps 1–4 are repeated for the fellow eye. (The patient must be reminded to maintain the same straight-ahead position.)
6. As the patient looks straight ahead, he or she should not notice the edge of the paper. If the patient notices the paper (when looking straight ahead), it should be moved 1 mm more in the temporal direction or until the leading edge of the paper is no longer visible to the patient.
7. The patient is instructed to walk around with the paper still attached to the lenses. The patient should not notice the edge of the paper with his or her normal eye movements (if noticed, move the paper 1–2 mm more temporal). He or she is then instructed to make a small saccadic movement to the right or left to view the edge of the paper.
8. Once this final position is determined, a straight vertical line is placed on the front of the spectacle lens (with a fine-tip felt marker) indicating the edge where the apex of the prism will be placed.
9. The prism should be cut so that the apex of the prism lines up perfectly with the straight line placed on the lens, whereas the remainder of the prism is cut to the same shape as the spectacle lens, with the base of the prism at the temporal edge of the spectacle lens.
10. The spectacle lenses are cleaned, removing all residue. Rubbing alcohol is spread on the inside surface of the spectacle lens. The prism is placed in the appropriate position (on the ocular lens surface). Gentle force is applied to the whole prism, eliminating all air bubbles. The Fresnel prism should set in approximately 20–30 minutes.
11. The orientation of the prisms should be reconfirmed to check that they are in the proper direction (in this case, base out) and that no edge of the prism is overlapping the frame.
12. The patient is now ready for instruction (see Appendix B).

Cleaning the Prism

The spectacles and prisms can become dirty over time. It is important to instruct the patient in how to maintain the cleanness of the system without removing the prism.

1. The patient should be instructed not to remove the prism.
2. The spectacles (and prisms) can be rinsed under a gentle stream of warm water, with a small amount of liquid soap (dishwashing soap) if needed. A soft toothbrush can be used to clean the grooves in the prism.
3. The spectacles and prisms can be blotted dry with a soft, lint-free cloth and allowed to thoroughly dry before wearing them.

Appendix B

INSTRUCTIONAL PROGRAM IN THE USE OF THE FRESNEL PRISM

Four basic instructional steps should be accomplished before a patient who is using a prism for enhanced peripheral awareness is to be discharged. The following information pertains to the instruction of a patient with a bitemporal hemianopic field loss. Again, similar steps could be performed for a patient demonstrating any other field loss in which a prism is used to increase peripheral awareness. The patient may require several practice sessions of 1 hour or more, with home practice in between, before mastering prism use.

I. Patient stable; object stable
   A. The patient is seated with the instructor facing the patient.
   B. Figure-ground confusion should be minimized when presenting objects. The object should have good contrast with the background.
   C. The patient is told to look through the Fresnel prism and is made aware of the loss of clarity and brightness through this lens system.
   D. As the patient continues to look through the prism, the instructor holds his or her finger or a pencil in the temporal periphery of the patient. The patient is asked to point directly at the object. It is expected that the patient will initially point more nasally than the actual position of the object. While the patient maintains his or her hand in this initial position, he or she is instructed to look through the carrier lens (outside of the prism) to determine the amount of displacement that is achieved when looking through the prism.
   E. The same activity is repeated; however, this time the patient is asked to compensate for the displacement and to point where he or she thinks the object is truly located.
   F. Step E is continued with the object placed at various positions within the patient's periphery. The patient is able to proceed to step II when he or she achieves 100% accuracy in judging the prism displacement.
II. Patient stable; object moving
   A. The patient is seated with the instructor facing the patient.

   B. The patient is again instructed to look through the prism.
   C. The instructor moves his or her finger or a pencil in the peripheral temporal area of the patient. As the finger or pencil is being moved at a constant speed, the patient is instructed to grab the object when the instructor says "now."
   D. Steps A–C are repeated until the patient attains 100% success in accurately grabbing the object.
III. Patient moving; object stable
   A. The perfect environment for this step is a long hallway with many doorways opening into the hallway (or a large room with obstacles placed along the side). Lighting should be even and fairly bright.
   B. The patient is instructed to walk slowly down the hallway, looking straight ahead through the carrier lens. As the patient walks down the hallway, he or she is told to keep his or her head straight ahead but to make swift saccadic movements into and out of the prism (similar to using a side view mirror on a car when driving).
   C. The patient is to repeat the preceding steps until he or she is proficient in identifying the doorway (or obstacles) in a more efficient (head and eye movements) and quicker manner than if he or she was not using the prisms.
IV. Patient moving; object(s) moving
   A. The patient is placed in a complex "normal" or "crowded" environment such as a busy sidewalk, store, or shopping mall.
   B. The patient must successfully maneuver through this crowded environment, while using the prisms, with no bumping into people or objects.
   C. The patient can be dispensed the prisms when he or she has successfully satisfied both him- or herself and the instructor in using the prisms. (To prove the effectiveness of the prisms, it is recommended that the Fresnel prism be removed or reversed to determine if there is a noticeable decrease in the patient's performance.)

Before the patient is finally dispensed the Fresnel prism, the option of replacing it with a cemented spheroprism should be discussed.

CHAPTER THIRTEEN

Nonoptical and Accessory Devices

Douglas R. Williams

Nonoptical devices play an important role in the successful use of many low vision optical devices. Often, when optical devices present limitations to the patient, nonoptical devices may facilitate their use. Frequently, nonoptical devices are used alone, long before optical low vision devices are prescribed.

Many of these nonoptical devices were not specifically developed for the visually impaired. In many cases, they were developed from commonly used items that were modified or adapted after an individual lost some degree of functional vision. Nonoptical devices, by their name, do not rely solely on lenses for their effects and usefulness but rather use relative size, illumination, position, contrast, color, or other sensory input for their effects.

TYPES OF NONOPTICAL LOW VISION DEVICES

Nonoptical devices can be grouped by how they produce their effects. Although there are a host of products, many of the commonly used and recommended devices can be placed into the following categories:

1. Relative size and larger assistive devices
2. Glare, contrast, and lighting control devices
3. Posture and comfort maintenance devices
4. Handwriting and written communication nonoptical devices
5. Medical management nonoptical devices
6. Orientation and mobility management techniques and devices
7. Sensory substitution devices

Relative Size and Larger Assistive Devices

The largest category of nonoptical devices may be referred to as *relative size devices*. The use of relative size involves the concept of using a larger size object. If an object is made larger, it will be easier to see. The amount of magnification obtained depends on a comparison of the new larger object compared with the "standard-size" object. This type of magnification is termed *relative size magnification* and is

a measure of the ratio of the angular size of the enlarged object to that of the original object (Figure 13-1). No lenses are used in making the object larger. There is also no change in working distance. The angular size of the objects can be compared directly; however, this is sometimes difficult to do if the standard is not readily available for comparison.

Large Print
By far, the largest category under relative size devices is large print. Most large print is measured in point type. Large type generally is 14-point type or larger but rarely exceeds 24-point type. Ellerbrock[1] has suggested using 10 point as the standard for normal-sized type, and thus an estimate of how much magnification is achieved can be easily determined by dividing 10 into the size of the larger type.

The concept of large print involves not only the size of the print but also the spatial layout of the print. The margins, gutters, spacing, and type style are some of the characteristics that demand special attention in large-print publications. Caution must be exercised in reproducing a book by simple photo-offset enlargement. Eakin and McFarland[2] cautioned that, "without concern for standardizing type size, any publisher is free to label his product a 'large print book' as long as the type has been reproduced in any size greater than the original."

Various criteria have been established for the desirable features in large-print publications. The National Association of Visually Handicapped[3] recommends the following:

1. A maximum sheet size of 8½ in.×11 in.
2. An off-white, opaque, vellum paper
3. Gutter margins at least ⅞ in., with outside margins smaller, but not less than ½ in.
4. Type size not smaller than 16 point, preferably 18 point
5. Adequate leading (white space between lines of print)
6. Adequate density (no gray ink)
7. No broken letters

In addition to the preceding features of large print, legibility is improved when attention is given to contrast.

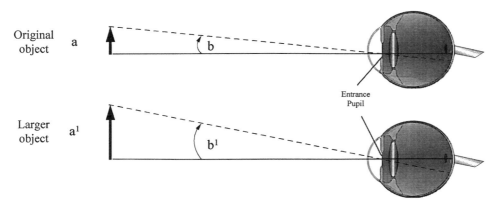

Original object   a

Larger object   a¹

Entrance Pupil

FIGURE 13-1. **Relative size magnification can be calculated using the following formula:**

$$M_{rs} = \text{Tan } b'/\text{Tan } b$$
$$\text{or}$$
$$a'/a$$

where a = the size of the original object, a' = the linear size of the larger object, angle b = the angular subtense of the original object, and angle b' = the angular subtense of the larger object.

High contrast is recommended for maximum legibility. For many low vision patients who have conditions that cause a loss of contrast sensitivity, light print on a dark background may be more readable than the customary dark print on a white background.

ADVANTAGES OF LARGE PRINT.   The advantage of using large print lies in its easy acceptance by the low vision patient. Large print is sometimes used along with a low-power optical device to provide the proper combined magnification. This combination allows the patient to develop the proper fixation and scanning techniques that are easier to learn with lower-power optical devices. Once these skills have been developed, a higher-power optical device may be prescribed, providing the patient greater access to more common standard-size reading material. Although evidence shows that some children with low vision can read standard-size print if held closer, custom and tradition dictate that large print is easier to see and is easier on the eyes.

Another advantage of large print is its acceptance by patients who show poor or reduced contrast sensitivity. The large print allows the low vision patient to read the print because of the change in spacing between letters and words, spatial frequency, and contrast due to the large letters.

DISADVANTAGES OF LARGE PRINT.   One major disadvantage of large print is that of limited magnification. It is common for large-print books not to exceed 18 point, which produces only 1.8× magnification. With this amount of magnification, only a small segment of the low vision population can rely solely on large print alone as a solution to its reading problems. Fonda[4] has emphasized that large-print books have too often been used when regular size type could have been easily read by the same person by holding the book closer, perhaps with the assistance of lenses. A patient with 20/200 reduced Snellen at 16 in. could read 10-point print at 4.85 in., 12-point print at 5.84 in., 14-point type at 6.8 in., 18-point at 8.76 in., and 24-point type at 11.67 in.

Another disadvantage is in the availability of large-print material that is of interest and importance to the patient. Although there are many books published in large print, immediate access is not always possible. Barraga[5] indicated that large-print educational books are seldom available to a child once he or she advances to higher grade levels. A further disadvantage is that large print takes additional space to print, making it thicker and heavier than standard-size print. The number of pages required to print a book in large print is approximately equal to the standard print format times the square of the magnification represented by the large print; thus, financial considerations become important factors.

There are many sources of large-print material. Magazines, newspapers, reference books, and music scores as well as fiction and nonfiction titles are available from a variety of publishers and distributors. Magazines in large print include *Reader's Digest*, *Good News*, and *Young and Alive*. For children, large-print magazines include *Flash* and *In Focus*. Newspapers include the *New York Times Large Type Weekly* and the *World at Large*. Dictionaries, thesauri, atlases, cookbooks, encyclopedias, and Bibles are all available in large-print format.

One important source for both information and supply of large print is the National Library Service for the Blind and Physically Handicapped (NLS). The NLS has several reference circulars that list extensive sources for various large-print and other special media material. In addition to the NLS, the American Printing House for the Blind (APH; Louisville, KY) offers an extensive variety of large-print publications. One of the largest commercial large-print book publishers is G.K. Hall & Co., which has been consolidated with another large-print book publisher, Thorndike Press. These companies regularly publish selections from the best-sellers lists in large print and also offer fiction and nonfiction selections, biographies, classics, adventure and suspense, mystery, romance, westerns, self-help, and inspirational writings. G.K. Hall has also introduced two additions to its large-print offerings: the Perennial Bestseller series featuring long-standing best sellers in a mixture of classic and contemporary options and the Inspirational/Religious Series featuring books on all faiths.

Music selections can be found in the *NLS Reference Circular, Large-Print Scores and Books Catalog*. This circular lists several sources of large-print music and is divided into two general sections, one for scores and the other for books. The scores are further divided into six categories: brass, keyboard, percussion, strings, voice, and woodwinds.

Large print can be produced by computer. With the advent of computer technology, many visually impaired individuals have need for large-print computer access. Various fonts, in both sans serif and serif type styles, can be selected in sizes ranging from 4 point to 40 point. A font is a set of characters in one size and one typeface. Type styles can be varied and enhanced with bold face to provide enhanced contrast. Although these printer options produce good output in a hard copy, the patient with low vision also needs access to computer input as well as data appearing on the monitor screen. Software programs have been written specifically to enlarge the display of the information appearing on the monitor. Large-print access tools for computers are available for both Macintosh and IBM-compatible systems. Berkeley Systems, Inc. (Berkeley, CA) manufactures a large-print access software program for Macintosh computers called InLARGE 2.0. This software will magnify characters from 2 to 16 times. Magnification can be entered in several ways through the keyboard or the Apple control panel. InLARGE 2.0 will work on all current models of Macintosh running System 6.07 or higher. Ai Squared (Manchester Center, VT) produces VisAbility, a software program that turns a personal computer and a scanner into a magnification and reading system. The VisAbility's display mode allows the user to see a magnified window and the regular image simultaneously. Reading material can be magnified up to 32×. Printing can be done in regular size or magnified sizes up to 8×. Zoomtext Plus, also manufactured by Ai Squared, allows for the magnification of DOS-based graphics from a 2× to an 8× level in 1× increments and 2× increments from 10× to 16×. Other large-print access systems available include Artic and Business Focus (Artic Technologies International, Inc., Troy, MI), LPDOS (Optelec, Westford, MA), and BIGED (Turbo Power Software, Colorado Springs, CO). It should be noted that large-print software must be compatible with the type of computer one is operating (e.g., Macintosh, IBM, or clone).

Large-print typewriters offer the ability to produce large print when there is no computer access. For patients who are intimidated by computer technology, acceptance of a large-print typewriter may be a practical alternative. The size of typewriter print is often designated by the term *pitch*. Pitch is a measure of the number of typewriter characters per horizontal inch. The smaller the pitch, the larger the type size. Vertical dimension is not given by pitch, and thus point and pitch must be used together to determine print size. Many typewriter manufacturers use the designation *Bulletin* to describe a large-type type style. Bulletin typestyles vary from 10 pitch to 6 pitch with 3–5½ lines per vertical inch. The type styles may be sans serif or serif depending on the manufacturer. Generally, typewriter type styles are available from the manufacturer. Enlarged alphanumeric stick-on keys are available for the computer and typewriter keyboard. These stick-ons (Zoom Caps, Meeting the Challenge, Colorado Springs, CO) increase the size of the keys to 38-point size and fit IBM-compatible keyboards.

Other Relative Size Devices

There are a number of other relative size devices. One commonly used system is the large-size telephone dial. With the use of touch-tone telephones, the need to see the small buttons on the phone can be a formidable task for the visually impaired. The use of the large touch-tone telephone overlay makes dialing much easier. Large-print rotary telephone dials are also available. It should be noted that there still may be a problem reading the letters on the large-print telephone overlay. This problem could be considerable if a telephone number is given in letters rather than in numerals. Voice-activated automatic dial telephones may solve this problem.

Banking is another task that may present problems to the visually impaired patient. Writing a check can be made easier with large-print checks. Deluxe Check Printers (St. Paul, MN) makes the Guideline style of check that uses a business-size check with large print and raised bold lines, producing a tactile cue. Some banking institutions also make available services for large-print statements through customer service departments.

Crossword puzzles provide pleasure for many low vision patients. Large-print editions are available from many sources and can be found weekly in the *New York Times Large Type Weekly* and the *World at Large* newspapers. Both the *New York Times* and Charles Preston produce large-type crossword puzzles as separate publications as well. In addition to crossword puzzles, games that have been prepared in large-type editions are useful for patients' recreational interests. Scrabble (Milton Bradley Company, Springfield, MA), chess, checkers, backgammon, and bingo as well as many types of playing cards are available in large-print format.

A number of adapted devices are available to assist patients with sewing activities. These sewing aids use relative size magnification. It is often assumed that sewing requires a good degree of vision. This leisure activity, however, can often be accomplished by the visually impaired with a few aids. Self-threading sewing machine needles and automatic needle threaders make this often-curtailed activity possible for many patients. Sticking sewing needles into a piece of cork is a method that can simplify manipulation. Handling pins can be made easier with the use of large-head or large-bead pins. Sewing seams can be aided with the use of magnetic tape cut in a strip and applied under the seam, providing both increased contrast as well as a tactile cue for keeping the seam straight.

Relative size magnification is used in watches with large faces, in wall clocks and timers, and on light-emitting diode (LED) electronic displays for calculators. The task of telling time can be a problem with a small wristwatch or a clock that is situated in a room in which the lighting is inadequate. Both analog instruments and digital displays are available in a variety of formats. Large-face, high-contrast, digital "flip" format, LED format, and liquid crystal display (LCD) are available. Caution should be used with the LCD display, however, as the dark numbers on a gray background rarely provide enough contrast for individuals with reduced vision. It is suggested that the low vision practitioner have several catalogs of these products available for patients to borrow or keep so that they can order devices for their individual needs.

Glare, Contrast, and Light Control

Low vision encompasses many types of ocular pathology. Each condition has properties that may impact the functional vision loss for the patient. Loss of contrast sensitivity is often encountered after laser photocoagulation and in patients with cataracts. Glare may be encountered by patients with posterior subcapsular cataracts. Scattering is often encountered by patients with anterior cortical cataracts. Glare and photophobia are seen in albinism, achromatopsia, retinal cone dystrophies, optic atrophy, aphakia, glaucoma, and retinitis pigmentosa. In most cases, glare causes a greater reduction in contrast than in visual acuity.

When an object cannot be resolved, the size of the object may be increased to the point at which resolution can be made, which in turn changes its spatial frequency. Enlargement lowers spatial frequency. An increase in contrast may be accomplished by decreasing the spatial frequency as well. Low vision rehabilitation uses various devices that often involve a change in spatial frequency, a change to alter the contrast sensitivity, or a combination of both (see Figure 4-1).

Glare can be classified as discomfort glare or disability glare. *Discomfort glare* is light that, because of its intensity, misdirection, or exposure time causes discomfort or fatigue. *Disability glare* is glare that interferes with vision by blinding, veiling, or dazzling, and results in reduced visual performance. Both types of glare may exist simultaneously.

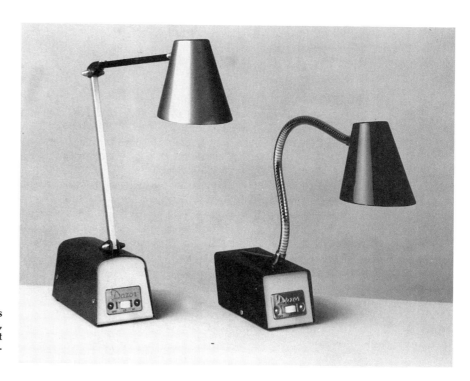

FIGURE 13-2. **Dazor Hi-intensity models 3612 and 3615 provide for adjustable, intense, incandescent light in a compact and lightweight unit. (Courtesy of Dazor Manufacturing Corporation, St. Louis, MO.)**

Glare management begins with a comprehensive history directed at the identification of particular glare sources and individual solutions that the patient may have already attempted. A major source of indoor glare comes from light entering through a window. Proper window treatment must never be overlooked when discussing possible solutions to indoor glare with a patient. Indoor lighting is another major source of glare. In general, the greater the wattage of the light source, the greater the glare. Positioning the light source away from the line of sight will also help reduce glare. A light source that may not be disturbing for an exposure of a few minutes may become disturbing when used for an extended period. Counseling the patient in the proper position and wattage of the light source is critical and may require a lighting engineer to provide the appropriate information.

Illumination
Many low vision patients require more light when indoors. Due to the effects of aging, it has been found that the older population requires twice the amount of illumination than that required by a younger population. This difference is significant in that a large majority of low vision patients are older adults.

As the eye ages, physiologic changes occur that involve a loss of media transparency. Nuclear sclerosis produces a yellowing of the lens and a loss of short wavelengths reaching the retina. These short-wavelength luminosity losses can be exaggerated by inappropriate lighting. Incandescent lamps, having more energy output in the long wavelengths than does daylight, and loss in the short wavelengths, tend to enhance reds, oranges, and yellows and subdue blues and greens. The "white" fluorescent lamps (with the exception

of the generic Warm Light and Deluxe Cool White), tend to accentuate the blues, greens, and yellows and have a graying effect on reds.

Fluorescent lighting is used a great deal in commercial and business applications because it is energy-efficient and cost-effective. Fluorescent lighting is normally considered harsh, however, because its output is in the blue portion of the spectrum. Patients often complain that fluorescent lighting is disturbing, causing discomfort glare. The use of diffusers and indirect fluorescent lighting tends to minimize these problems. Because incandescent light is more directional and has its main spectral output in the longer wavelengths, it generally provides more contrast. Another light bulb, the neodymium bulb, emits 30% less UV and blue and 20–28% less infrared light than does the incandescent bulb. This bulb has shown a significantly improved performance over the standard incandescent bulb for short-term near tasks.[6] The neodymium bulb is marketed as Chromalux (Lumiram Electric Corp., Mamaroneck, NY) in the United States. In use, the perception is that white appears whiter and black appears blacker because of the decreased yellow and blue spectral output.

Halogen light has also been introduced, and many patients believe that the use of halogen light is appropriate because it is new, high-intensity, and available in small, portable lamps that they find practical and functional. In reality, halogen light may present some concern because of cost and the high UV output with the potential for erythemal effects. High-intensity incandescent portable lamps may present a more practical solution to the need for flexible placement of lighting in a cost-effective manner (Figure 13-2).

From a functional point of view, the position of the light source is a greater factor than the actual wattage of the bulb, demonstrated by use of the *inverse square law of illumination*. *Illuminance* is the amount of light falling on an object or surface. The unit of illuminance is measured in *lux*, when the distance of the light source to the surface is measured in meters; or *foot-candles*, when the distance of the light source to the surface is measured in feet. One lux is equal to 0.0929 foot-candles, whereas 1 foot-candle is approximately equal to 1 watt (W). The concept of the inverse square law of illumination can be shown to the patient by moving a light closer to his or her reading material, thereby providing more illumination. The inverse square law is demonstrated in the following formula:

$$\text{Illuminance} = \frac{\text{Candle power of source}}{\left(\text{Source to surface distance}\right)^2}$$

This law can be useful in calculating the illumination from individual point sources on surfaces perpendicular to the source. It should be understood that halving the distance between the source and the illuminated surface will quadruple the illuminance.

Example 1
How much illumination is obtained when a 100-W bulb is held 4 ft perpendicular to a newspaper?

$$\text{Illuminance} = \frac{100}{\left(4\right)^2} = 6.25 \text{ W}$$

Example 2
How much illumination is obtained when a 100-W bulb is now placed 2 ft perpendicular to the newspaper?

$$\text{Illuminance} = \frac{100}{\left(2\right)^2} = 25 \text{ W}$$

When the light source is not perpendicular to the surface or reading material, the *cosine law* must be used. The cosine law states that the illuminance varies with the cosine of the angle between the source and the perpendicular to the surface. The inverse square law and the cosine law can be combined into one formula:

$$\text{Illuminance} = \frac{\text{Cosine angle a (candle power of source)}}{\left(\text{Source to surface distance}\right)^2}$$

Example 3
How much illumination is obtained when a 100-W bulb is held 2 ft from a newspaper at an angle of 45 degrees?

$$\cos 45 \text{ degrees} = 0.7$$
$$\text{Illuminance} = \frac{\left(0.7\right)\left(100\right)}{\left(2\right)^2} = 17.5 \text{ W}$$

In most cases, the light source should be directed over the shoulder of the better seeing eye and held close to the reading material to get maximum illumination. The bulb should have an air-cooled shield surrounding it to protect the patient from the heat of the bulb and to eliminate any possible glare.

Filters
Filters have been used in an attempt to enhance visual performance. Filters will attenuate excessive light to comfortable levels and reduce both discomfort and disability glare. In addition, filters can selectively transmit the wavelengths that the compromised eye may be more sensitive to and absorb those wavelengths that may be potentially harmful. Filters can alter color perception, enhance contrast by reduction of glare and scattering, and act as a refractive medium to correct refractive errors. Filters have a variety of properties. The material, color, transmission or density, photochromaticity, polarization, and coatings can impart unique properties to the filter depending on its desired application.

Color alone is not a determinant of the function of the filter but will tend to direct its application. Although the dyes and additives in the material determine the absorptive properties, the final color of a filter depends on the wavelengths transmitted after white light passes through the filter. The use of filters in low vision rehabilitation has little research to confirm improvement in visual function. The practitioner is left with the theoretical and hypothetical models as well as the research on similar animal models to draw conclusions for an ideal filter. Anecdotal reports and testimonials of the preference of various filters tend to offer some credence to the value of filters; however, much remains to be understood about how the functional vision of a patient with a particular ocular disorder is remediated by a specific filter.

Some of the spectacle lens filters used for glare reduction and contrast enhancement as well as protection for the eye are the result of extensive research on animal models. Among researchers who study retinal degenerations, there seems to be some optimism in the studies of several animal models that show genetically linked degenerative disease. Adrian and Schmidt[7] experimented with filters and proposed criteria for a filter that would hypothetically protect and minimize the damage thought to occur by excessive light levels in patients with retinitis pigmentosa. This research, along with other hypothetical and animal model research,[8–10] led the way to some of the initial filters developed for particular ocular degenerative diseases. Filters were designed with specific criteria. Desirable features included low light level transmission, spectral transmissions to protect the rod visual receptors more than the cone visual receptors, minimal color distortion, absorption of both infrared and UV rays, and a material capable of being fabricated into a prescription if needed. The Adrian filter was produced in Aalen, West Germany by the Carl Zeiss Company and consisted of an absorptive layer between two surfaces of glass, the outer surfaces of which contained antireflection coatings. Due to the limited accessibility of the Adrian lens, other filters were investigated for similarity, and with time, various filters have been identified as having many desirable features

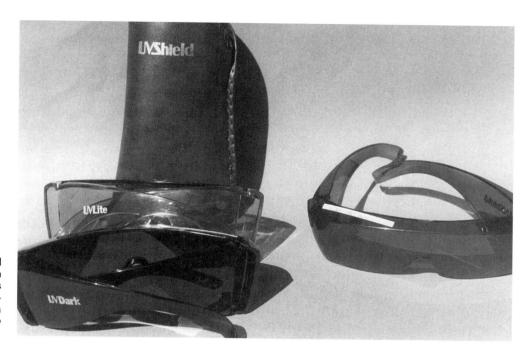

FIGURE 13-3.   The NoIR UVShield (NoIR Medical Technologies, South Lyon, MI) is a fit-over filter. It is available in many colors and transmissions. This plastic goggle has a top shield along with side shields to filter extraneous light.

incorporating some of the original hypothetical design properties of the Adrian lens.

NoIR MEDICAL TECHNOLOGIES.   NoIR Medical Technologies (South Lyon, MI) manufactures a wide variety of plastic filters that are commonly prescribed for low vision patients experiencing problems with photophobia and glare.

Originally, the NoIR filters were described as chemical sunglasses designed to absorb the near UV (200–400 nm) and the near infrared (800–1,400 nm) regions of the spectrum. NoIR Medical Technologies currently manufactures an extensive line of plastic filters of several transmissions in both goggle and frame styles (Figure 13-3). The NoIR UVShield styles offer a variety of transmissions with complete UV blockage while the NoIR filter styles offer complete UV as well as significant infrared reduction. It has been shown that the NoIR Model 107 has similar properties to the original Adrian lens.[11] Retrospective studies of the NoIR filters[12, 13] showed patient preference in descending order for Models 101, 102, and 107. Diabetics preferred Models 101 and 102. Patients with nonexudative macular degeneration, retinitis pigmentosa, and glaucoma showed a preference toward Model 101. Darker NoIR filters (Model 108 with 1% total light transmission and Model 109 with total light transmission 2%) were not preferred when acuity dropped below 20/400. Table 13-1 lists the models and specifications for the currently available filters from NoIR Medical Technologies.

CORNING PHOTOCHROMATIC (GLARE CONTROL) FILTERS.   The development of Corning Photochromatic Filters (CPF, Corning Medical Optics, Elmira, NY) grew out of attempts to design a filter to aid in the protection of eyes with progressive retinal degenerations. In 1981, Corning introduced the CPF 550-S lens specifically designed for retinitis

pigmentosa patients. The spectral cutoff of this glass photochromatic filter is 550 nm and hence the name of the filter. CPF stands for Corning Photochromatic Filter, and the number designates the spectral cutoff wavelength below which virtually all light is absorbed and above which substantial transmission occurs. This filter was designed to reduce the scotopic transmittance and allow a much higher level of photopic transmittance, resulting in the highest photopic to scotopic transmittance ratio possible. Adrian[7] had proposed that this ratio, known as the *cone/rod* or *R ratio*, should be as high as possible yet still be compatible with useful vision.

The CPF 550 filter is manufactured from a borosilicate glass (Corning Photogray Extra), which is ground and surfaced in the patient's prescription. After initial surfacing, the lens is treated in a 2-day firing involving a high-temperature hydrogen gas diffusion process. This process alters the absorption of the lens by creating a thin (less than 0.2 mm thick) color layer having tiny metallic silver particles that produce the coloration. The color is then removed from the nonocular surface because leaving it on would prevent the actinic sensitivity and thus prevent the lens from being photochromic. By varying the time and temperature, each product in the Corning CPF filter line produces its own unique transmission and filtering characteristics. Corning followed the CPF 550 lens with the introduction of the CPF 511 and CPF 527 lenses in 1983. These two filters have met with considerable acceptance.

The Design Series coating was added as a feature to the CPF 511 and CPF 527 lenses 3 years after their initial introduction. The Design Series coating consists of a multiple layer of special flash mirror coating combined with an antireflection coating. According to Corning, the addition of the special coating makes the filters more stylish while

TABLE 13-1
NoIR Medical Technologies Key to Filters by Transmission[a]

Color of Filter	Total Light Transmission (%)	Models of Frame Styles and Series Available[b]
Clear	90	210, 410, S10, U10, L10, N10, 10L
Light yellow	65	258, 458, S58, U58, L58, N58, 58L
Light red	59	298, 498, S98, U98, L98, N98, 98L
Light grey	58	220, 420, S20, U20, L20, N20, 20L
Light grey	58	228, 428, S28, U28, L28, N28, 28L
Yellow	54	250, 450, S50, U50, L50, N50, 50L
Light amber	53	248, 448, S48, U48, L48, N48, 48L
Light orange	52	268, 468, S68, U68, L68, N68, 68L
Light grey-green	50	238, 438, S38, U38, L38, N38, 38L
Orange	49	260, 460, S60, U60, L60, N60, 60L
Red-orange	47	275, 475, S75, U75, L75, N75, 75L
Red	45	290, 490, S90, U90, L90, N90, 90L
Pink	44	270, 470, S70, U70, L70, N70, 70L
Light amber	40	111, 211, 311, 411, 711, 911, 11L
Light grey-green	40	112, 212, 312, 412, 712, 912, 12L
Light green	40	131, 231, 331, 431, 731, 931, 31L
Light yellow	40	151, 251, 351, 451, 751, 951, 51L
Light orange	40	161, 261, 361, 461, 761, 961, 61L
Light plum	40	288, 488, S88, U88, L88, N88, 88L
Light red	40	191, 291, 391, 491, 791, 991, 91L
Medium grey	32	221, 421, S21, U21, L21, N21, 21L
Medium plum	20	281, 481, S81, U81, L81, N81, 81L
Medium grey-green	18	102, 202, 302, 402, 702, 902, 02L
Amber	16	240, 440, S40, U40, L40, N40, 40L
Medium green	14	135, 235, 335, 435, 735, 935, 35L
Medium yellow	14	155, 255, 355, 455, 755, 955, 55L
Medium orange	14	165, 265, 365, 465, 765, 965, 65L
Medium red	14	195, 295, 395, 495, 795, 995, 95L
Dark grey	13	222, 422, S22, U22, L22, N22, 22L
Medium amber	10	101, 201, 301, 401, 701, 901, 01L
Grey grey-green	10	232, 432, S32, U32, L32, N32, 32L
Grey-green	7	230, 430, S30, U30, L30, N30, 30L
Dark grey	4	223, 423, S23, U23, L23, N23, 23L
Dark grey-green	4	233, 433, S33, U33, L33, N33, 33L
Dark green	4	139, 239, 339, 439, 739, 939, 39L
Dark amber	4	243, 443, S43, U43, L43, N43, 43L
Dark yellow	4	253, 453, S53, U53, L53, N53, 53L
Dark yellow	4	159, 259, 359, 459, 759, 959, 59L
Dark orange	4	263, 463, S63, U63, L63, N63, 63L
Dark orange	4	169, 269, 369, 469, 769, 969, 69L
Dark plum	4	280, 480, S80, U80, L80, N80, 80L
Dark red	4	293, 493, S93, U93, L93, N93, 93L
Dark red	4	199, 299, 399, 499, 799, 999, 99L
Dark amber	2	107, 207, 307, 407, 707, 907, 07L
Dark grey-green	1	108, 208, 308, 408, 708, 908, 08L

[a]Available from NoIR Medical Technologies, South Lyon, MI. The NoIR filter has transmission protection in both the UV and infared, whereas the UVShield has protection primarily for the UV range and short wavelength blue.
[b]Key to filters: 400 series: fashion frames. NoIR Fit-Overs: 100 series (small); 700 series (medium); 900 series (large); 200 series (wrap-around); 300 series (with side shields/skull temple). UVShield Fit Overs: L series (large); U series (medium); S series (small); N series (side shield with skull temple).

not altering the spectral cutoff points from the original CPF 511 and CPF 527 filters. The overall transmittance, however, is slightly reduced.

Further research resulted in the CPF 450 and the CPF 550XD (extra dark) filters in 1989. These filters extended the CPF family of filters to seven. They also extended the range of filtering applications to patients who needed a lighter lens with only moderate blue filtering with the CPF

450 and to those patients with extreme photophobia and extraordinary light sensitivity with the CPF 550XD. The CPF 450 filter tends to have application in patients experiencing glare from fluorescent lighting and is helpful in reading. The CPF 550XD has shown considerable application in aniridia and achromatopsia.

The latest addition to the Corning series of lenses is the Glare Cutter lens. The Glare Cutter is designed as an outdoor lens only. The lens has improved cosmetic appearance in that the lens appears less red and more of a pleasant copper-red-tan color. In the light state, the lens is somewhat lighter than the CPF 550 lens (ranging from 19% transmittance for a 2.0-mm thickness to 21% transmittance for the thinner 1.5-mm thickness). Outdoors, the scotopic transmittance value is similar to the CPF 527 filter.

The Glare Cutter has been designed with more transmittance in the 390–410 nm range than the other CPF filters. Transmittance in this range is above 10%. Because of this higher transmittance, there is minimum color distortion compared to most other CPF filters. The Glare Cutter blocks 100% of UVB and greater than 99% of UVA.

All the lenses in the original CPF series were termed *CPF*. Corning changed the name of the product line to Corning Glare Control lenses in April 1987. The terms "CPF" and "Glare Control" are now becoming synonymous. All of the filters in the CPF series have the features of short wavelength (blue and UV) filtering with complete filtering of UVB (290–315 nm) and not less than 97% of UVA. They also have the unique property of being photochromatic, thus allowing for darkening in bright conditions and clearing in lighter indoor conditions. Additional advantages include the capability of incorporating a prescription into the lenses if needed and the durability of a glass lens. Disadvantages include weight (glass being heavier than plastic), additional cost, and additional time for processing. Table 13-2 lists the filtering characteristics of the CPF filters.

YOUNGER PROTECTIVE LENS SERIES. The Younger Protective Lens Series (PLS) (Younger Optics, Torrance, CA) also grew out of the search for a filter that would be protective by filtering UV and short-wavelength blue light. Rayleigh's law states that scattering is inversely proportional to the fourth power of the wavelength such that the shorter blue wavelengths are scattered more than the longer red wavelengths. Younger PLS filters work by blocking the shorter wavelengths, thus reducing scattering encountered within the ocular media. Studies by Zigman[14] showed that UV radiation and blue light have been linked to cornea, lens, and retinal damage and are believed to be major causes of yellow-brown nuclear cataracts.

Younger Optics introduced the PLS series and manufactured specialized lenses that were designated as the PLS 530, PLS 540, and PLS 550. The filters were made of CR-39 and were made with protective additives to filter the short wavelengths of light. The three filters provided the practitioner with a choice of filtering levels to meet the needs of the patient. The lowest level of filtering was achieved with the PLS 530; it was recommended for patients with developing cataracts, corneal dystrophies, and mild light sensitivities. Additional protection and fil-

TABLE 13-2
Corning Glare Control Filter Characteristics

Filter Characteristics	CPF 450	CPF 511-S	CPF 511-Dn	CPF 527-S	CPF 527-Dn	CPF 550-S	CPF 550-XD	Glare Cutter
Transmittance lightened (%)	73	47	34	34	26	20	8	19.0
Transmittance darkened (%)	18	12	10	9	8	5	3	6.0
UV filtering (%)								
UVB (290–315 NM)*	100	100	100	100	100	100	100	100.0
UVA (315–380 NM)*	97	99	99	98	99	99	99	97.6

*Percentages shown are minimum. Actual values are typically higher.
SOURCE: Reprinted with permission from Corning, Inc., Corning Medical Optics, Elmira, NY.

tering were achieved with the PLS 540, which had a brown color and was formerly called the *PLS 530-B* lens. The fullest range of filtering action for the short-wavelength blue light is given by the PLS 550 lens. The PLS 550 was recommended for patients having retinitis pigmentosa, glaucoma, extreme photophobia, or aniridia.

Due to low demand and escalating costs, Younger Optics has now phased out the PLS series of selective filters and has discontinued manufacturing them. As an alternative to these filters, Brain Power, Inc. (Miami, FL), a manufacturer of ophthalmic dyes, has developed dyes for plastic lenses that simulate the characteristics of both the Corning CPF filters and the Younger PLS.

OTHER FILTER CHARACTERISTICS. The need for protection from UV radiation is well documented.[15–17] Evidence supports filtering out all UVA (315–380 nm) and UVB (290–315 nm) and up to 400 nm in the visible spectrum. The risks from exposure to UV radiation may be expected to increase in the future due to damage of the earth's ozone layer.

Figure 13-4[18] shows the UV transmission of commonly used ophthalmic materials. It should be clear that Crown glass is not a good choice for eliminating UV light unless a UV inhibitor is incorporated into the melt or applied separately as a vacuum-coated addition. Likewise, CR-39 without an inhibitor begins transmittance at approximately 350 nm, and polycarbonate, in its raw polymer state, transmits UV readily. When inhibitors are added to CR-39 and polycarbonate, both lens materials provide excellent protection. UV coating should be recommended for patients who have aphakia, retinitis pigmentosa, or macular degeneration. (See Chapter 8 for more information on UV coating.)

Antireflection Coatings
When light passes through a lens, the majority of the light is transmitted, but some of the light is reflected. Depending on the index of refraction of the lens material, approximately 3.87–5.32% of the light is lost at each surface. To reduce this light loss, the use of antireflection coatings can be applied to the lens surface in either glass or plastic materials. As the index of the lens increases, the amount of light loss through the lens will also increase. In addition to the index of the material, the lens form often contributes to reflections. Many prescriptions for low vision patients often

require very steep or very flat curvatures or doublet lenses in various lens designs. These lenses produce reflections that distract from the visual performance of the lens. Antireflection coatings help to reduce the amount of lens reflections. Antireflection coatings are available in single- and multiple-layer coatings. Single-layer coatings applied to one-fourth-wavelength thickness will be effective for a narrow band wavelength of light. Two-layer coatings increase the effectiveness of the antireflection by widening the band of wavelengths canceled out and allowing greater light transmission. Current technology has produced multiple-layer antireflection coatings that further increase the transmission over a broad range of the visual spectrum. The higher the index of the lens material, the greater will be the need for antireflection coatings. Ideally, the coating mater-

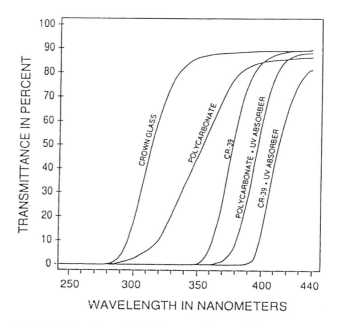

FIGURE 13-4. **Clear ophthalmic crown glass provides minimal UVA and UVB protection, whereas clear polycarbonate transmits less than 10% of UV radiation. CR-39 lenses provide full protection against UVB and partial protection against UVA. Polycarbonate and CR-39 lenses incorporating UV absorbers provide full UVA and UVB protection. (Printed with permission of Dr. Donald G. Pitts.)**

ial should have an index of refraction equal to the square root of the material on which it is to be applied. Commonly used coating materials include metallic chlorides and fluorides, metals such as lithium and sodium, and alkaline earth metals such as magnesium (see Chapter 8).

Polarization
Polarization may be included with a filter to improve the glare reduction. Polarization reduces the glare from reflected surfaces. Light reflected from shiny, highly polished, or smooth surfaces becomes plane polarized. Examples include light reflected off a wet street, snow, or water. When viewed through a polarizing filter, this reflected light is canceled out because of the orientation of the Polaroid filter, which is acting as an analyzer. One problem with the Polaroid filter is the change in light intensity that is transmitted through the filter as the user changes head positions. The polarizing filters that are commonly used today are made from what is referred to as an "H-sheet" Polaroid. This H-sheet is made from a clear sheet of polyvinyl alcohol that has been heated and stretched in one direction. During the stretching, the sheet's long hydrocarbon molecules become aligned. The sheet is then dyed in an ink solution containing iodine that impregnates the plastic and attaches itself to the straight long-chained molecules. The absorption axis of the Polaroid is aligned with the iodine chains, while the transmission axis is perpendicular to the iodine chains. Thus, when the alignment of the chains is vertical, the transmission axis is horizontal. There are a variety of lens forms incorporating polarized filters. Examples are seen in single vision, bifocal, trifocal, and progressive styles in glass laminate and molded plastic forms (see Chapter 8).

Mirror Coatings
Placing a mirror coating on a lens will reduce the transmittance and act as a filter. Mirror coatings can be full or partial. A flash mirror coating is a partial mirror coating and thus has only minor reflective properties. Flash mirror coatings can be placed on colored filters to improve their appearance. Mirror coatings can be placed on the ocular side of photochromatic filters without interfering with the properties of the filter. Mirror coatings enhance the performance of the absorption by also adding the property of reflection.

Accessory Forms of Light Control
Attempts at changing illumination to improve contrast often bring about increased glare. A delicate balance exists between these two factors. Glare is occasionally created while attempting to increase the illumination on reading material with a portable lamp. Glare from the paper counteracts the effect of the additional contrast provided by the illumination. With the use of a typoscope, some of this problem may be eliminated (see Figure 3-17). The typoscope is a small rectangular card that has a horizontal slot to allow for the viewing of two to three lines of printed text. The card can be made from a nonreflective material, such as black paper or poster board. Prentice[19] described the original typoscope as a device that "excludes

all light reflected from the surface of the paper that except which actually affords the necessary contrast between it and the type within the slot." Yellow acetate filters can be attached to the window of the typoscope to further increase contrast.

PINHOLES AND STENOPAIC SLITS. The pinhole has been suggested as a low vision device. It makes use of the principle of paraxial rays to reduce the size of the blur circle on the retina. Peripheral distortion and reflection, primarily from ocular media involvement, find the largest application for the pinhole. Pinholes can vary widely in size. When used in contact lenses, they may act as artificial apertures and improve vision (see Chapter 8 for more information on artificial apertures in contact lenses). Rosenbloom[20] suggested pupil sizes in contacts ranging from 1.0 mm to 6.0 mm. If placed in spectacles, experimentation is the best guideline for the size. According to Abney,[21] the size of the pinhole diameter can be calculated by the following formula:

$$y = k\sqrt{x}$$

where x and y represent the distance from the pinhole to the retinal plane and the diameter of the pinhole in millimeters respectively, and k denotes a constant of 0.1275. For an 11-mm vertex distance (plus distance from cornea to retina of approximately 24.75 mm), the diameter of the pinhole is found to be 0.76 mm. Fonda[22] suggested a diameter from experimentation of 1 mm. Depending on the ocular condition, multiple pinhole spectacles may give better results than the single pinhole (Figure 13-5). The distance between holes should be equal to or greater than the size of the patient's pupil under normal illumination. If the distance between the holes is less than the pupil diameter, diplopia may result. When vision impairment is due to macular pathology, pinholes may not work well because of the lowered retinal illuminance. The best effects of multiple pinholes are seen under high illumination with medial opacities, corneal involvements, or possibly cataracts.

The stenopaic slit may be of some use in controlling illumination. These horizontally positioned slits were used centuries ago as a form of sunglass. Today their use is limited. Cohen and Waiss[23] described a horizontally louvered black sun lens for glare reduction.

Posture and Comfort Maintenance

Prescribing an optical device for the low vision patient often does not succeed when the patient is uncomfortable due to the postural demands imposed by the prescriptive device. When high-powered optical systems are prescribed to make use of relative distance magnification, the reading material must be maintained at a close and fixed working distance. For the elderly, infirm, arthritic, multiple sclerotic, or patient with a tremor, a correct postural position must be maintained to help prevent premature fatigue.

Posture involves a process of constant adjustment and readjustment and the use of low vision devices has a direct

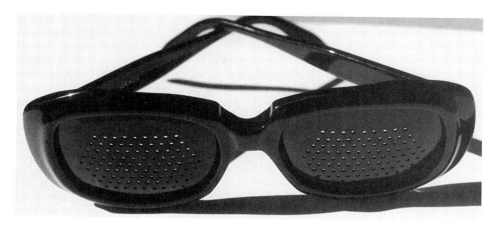

FIGURE 13-5. **Multiple pinhole glasses may be helpful to patients with reduced vision secondary to anterior segment involvement.**

bearing on an individual's posture. Hoover[24] related that posture "has direct relation to the comfort, the mechanical efficiency, and the physiologic functioning of the individual." Harmon[25] suggested that the ideal posture when attempting a near activity while seated is to hold the material at a distance equal to the length of the individual's elbow to middle knuckle (Harmon distance) and to have the material tilted approximately 70 degrees off the vertical. Tinker[26] suggested the ideal angle is approximately 45 degrees down from the vertical. Although the Harmon distance cannot be used when dealing with high-powered optical systems, the positioning of material at a proper angle will improve legibility and reduce fatigue. Reading racks, book stands, lap desks, and copy holders make the maintenance of these postures easier.

Reading racks and book stands can aid in the placement of books and other material at unusually close working distances to achieve relative distance magnification. If the material or book is not too heavy, ordinary racks and stands may suffice. If, however, the material is heavy, and the patient is unable to sustain the weight and thus unable to maintain the correct positioning, a stand or rack capable of holding a heavier book may be indicated. The rack should allow for tilting of the material to positions 45–70 degrees from the vertical.

The Able Table (Weir Enterprises, Santa Cruz, CA; Figure 13-6) is completely adjustable and multipurpose. It may be used as a work easel or table, book stand, or music rack. The Lap Desk (Sharon's Lap Desk, Woody, CA; Figure 13-7) is particularly helpful because it allows the print

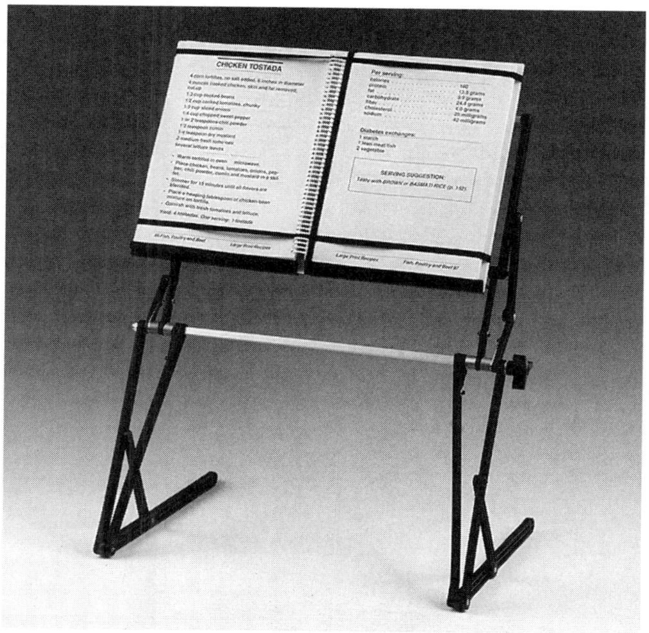

FIGURE 13-6. **The Able Table (Weir Enterprises, Santa Cruz, CA) is an extremely adjustable table that adjusts up or down, side to side, and can also tilt to various angles. It can hold material up to 30 lb.** (Courtesy of The Lighthouse, Inc., Long Island City, NY.)

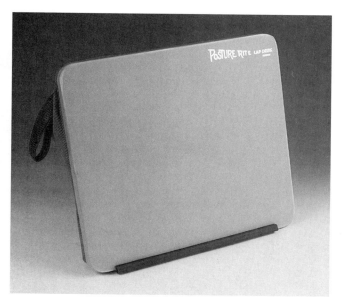

FIGURE 13-7. **The Lap Desk (Sharon's Lap Desk, Woody, CA) has a beanbag-type base with a hard table top for writing and reading purposes.** (Courtesy of The Lighthouse, Inc., Long Island City, NY.)

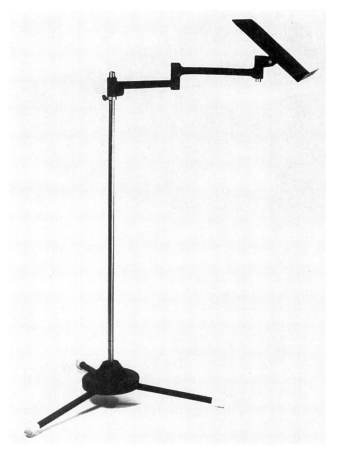

FIGURE 13-8.   **The Shafer reading stand is an adjustable stand capable of holding heavy books. (Courtesy of American Printing House for the Blind, Louisville, KY.)**

to be positioned in situations in which there is no flat surface, such as reading in bed or where no table is available. The device rests on the lap with a bean bag pillow arrangement that is attached to a flat, inclined surface. The Shafer reading stand (APH; Figure 13-8) is extremely useful. The metal tray is adjustable in both tilt and height and the weighted base offers a stable stand capable of holding heavy books.

When handheld telescopic devices are prescribed and prolonged viewing may be indicated, the use of a ring stand may be indicated. A special wide hand grip may also help in handling and positioning the monocular. With telescopes above 4× magnification, holding the telescope steady may be facilitated by the use of a stand. Chest pods and variations of ring stands can be fashioned to hold monoculars. A special headband may be fashioned with a clamp to hold a monocular (Figure 13-9).

Handwriting and Written Communication Nonoptical Devices

Although a large part of communication is verbal, written communication still is prevalent and is a concern for many visually impaired patients. Being able to sign one's name or write a letter or a simple grocery list can be a formidable task. Special products are available to make writing tasks easier.

Large-print typewriters often make written communication easier for patients who may have a hand tremor or arthritis and who cannot hold a pen or pencil or keep their place on the paper. The use of Bulletin type or a low-pitch type style make for easier reading. A heavily inked ribbon will provide for additional contrast.

Handwriting and signature guides can assist in the proper placement of the handwritten signature. These guides can be custom made and cut with a sharp knife to

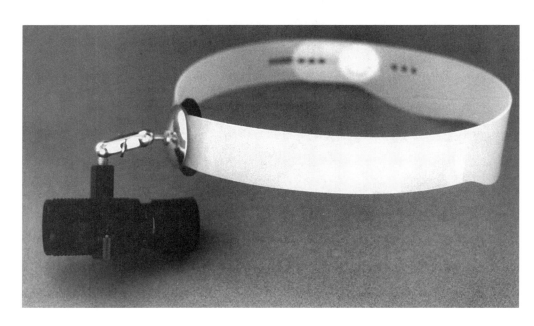

FIGURE 13-9. **A telescope attached to a headband mounting with a pivot joint provides for complete adjustability of position.**

allow for an opening that aligns the signature in proper placement. Depending on the written task, these guides are termed *signature guides, envelope addressing guides,* or *letter writing guides.* They can also provide steadiness for the patient whose manual dexterity may be limited (Figure 13-10).

Signature guides usually consist of either rigid metal bars separated by approximately one-half in., or a cut-out template that allows about the same size opening. One problem with guides when used for writing, however, is that letters that extend upward or downward are constrained by the window or opening. The use of a guide, such as Easy Writer (Richcreek Enterprises, Astoria, OR), offers a partial solution to this problem by using string that does not restrict upward or downward handwriting as much as a rigid restraint on a signature or letter writing guide. The Marks Script Guide (Sewell Metal Processing Corp., Woodside, NY) also has flexible wires allowing less interference.

Use of bold, felt-tip pens provides additional contrast. Black ink generally provides the best contrast; however, some patients may prefer to use blue or other colors. The 20/20 pen with an extra-wide tip produces good contrast. A visit to the local stationary store often provides enough variety to select a pen offering better contrast. These pens can be used on large-print checks and with the various guides for further assistance. Patients with poor grip due to paralysis, paresis, or arthritis may find wide-barrel pens, larger-bodied pens, or pens stuck into a rubber ball useful in providing enough bulk to allow for good manipulation.

The type of paper used by a patient with low vision for writing should be considered as well. The lines on the paper should provide the necessary contrast and spacing. Generally, the best contrast is provided by white, nonglossy paper that is thick enough to prevent ink from bleeding through the paper. Colored paper is not recommended. Keeping one's place can often be facilitated by merely folding the paper to provide creases. Additional help can be obtained from lined paper, and the heavier the lines on the paper, the better the contrast. APH provides many types of special paper for the low vision patient.

Medical Management Nonoptical Devices

Many activities of daily living involve the management of medical necessities. Daily tasks may involve identifying medications, measuring dosages, taking blood pressure, checking one's weight, self-monitoring blood sugar levels, examining the body for signs of illness or change, and taking temperatures. Studies have identified reading medicine labels as a significant problem for the visually impaired. The most common solution to this problem is reliance on others to perform the task.[27] Activities involving medical management are affected by lack of central acuity and possible changes in color vision. It is not uncommon for the visually impaired to have other systemic conditions in addition to their visual disorder(s). It is also common for many visual etiologies to produce situations requiring medical management. Other sensory

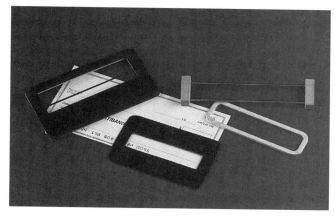

FIGURE 13-10. **A number of reading and writing guides are available to the patient with reduced vision. (Courtesy of The Lighthouse, Inc., Long Island City, NY.)**

input cues, such as hearing and tactile sensitivity, may commonly be affected in such conditions as Usher's syndrome (retinitis pigmentosa with deafness) and diabetes exhibiting peripheral neuropathy.

A large portion of the nonoptical devices for medical management are designed for the visually impaired with diabetes. For the insulin-dependent diabetic, medical management involves daily monitoring of blood glucose and injection of insulin. Urine monitoring for glucose may also be part of the medical maintenance tasks required of the diabetic. Other aspects of medical management in the control of diabetes encompass foot care and observation of skin lesions.

Monitoring blood glucose allows for an immediate determination of the need for insulin and enables the diabetic to alter the dosages to maintain strict control. Monitoring blood glucose involves obtaining a drop of blood, placing the drop of blood onto a test strip, and reading the test strip visually, by comparing the color to a color chart, or by inserting the test strip into a glucometer that provides a numeric output. These tasks present many vision problems. Obtaining the blood sample can be a problem for some patients. The use of lancet aids may solve this problem. Currently used lancet devices include Autolancet (Palco Labs, Santa Cruz, CA), Autolance (Becton Dickinson, Franklin Lakes, NJ), and Autolet (Owen Mumford, Marietta, GA). Glucometers can read test strips and indicate if the amount of blood on the strip is enough to provide a reading. The glucometer may have a large display screen or an auditory output, or both. Glucometers with large displays (Figure 13-11) include the Accu-Chek, Advantage, and Accu-Chek Instant (Boehringer Mannheim Corp., Indianapolis, IN), the Lifescan One Touch, Profile, Sure Step, or First Take (Lifescan, A Johnson & Johnson Company, Milpitas, CA), and the Precision Q.I.D. (Medisense, Inc., Bedford, MA). If auditory output is required, the Accu-Chek Easy or Lifescan One Touch Profile can be used.

The actual administration of insulin involves many visual tasks for diabetic patients. These tasks may include the following:

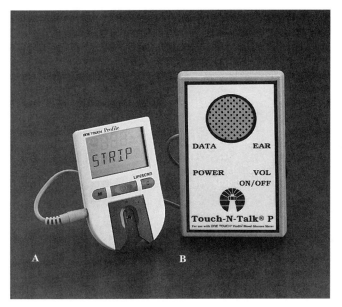

FIGURE 13-11.   **A. The Lifescan One Touch Profile Blood Glucose Monitoring System (Lifescan, A Johnson & Johnson Company, Milpitas, CA) has a large display for reading the blood glucose level. B. The system also has the capacity for the addition of a Touch-n-Talk Voice Synthesizer. (Courtesy of The Lighthouse, Inc., Long Island City, NY.)**

1. Selecting the proper insulin if a mixed dosage is used
2. Determining the amount of insulin remaining in the vial
3. Reading the syringe markings to determine the number of units to be given
4. Placing the needle into the center of the vial cap
5. Drawing up the insulin to the proper level and avoiding air bubbles
6. Injecting the insulin subcutaneously

Each of the preceding tasks can present special problems for the visually impaired diabetic patient. One of the purposes of using nonoptical devices for the medical management of diabetes is independence. Placing a rubber band on a vial to help identify one type of insulin is a possible solution to identification. Nordisk (Novo Nordisk Pharmaceuticals, Inc., Princeton, NJ) insulin vials have markings on the metal rim of the vial to assist individuals with reduced vision in identification of insulin type.

When the visual impairment is not too severe, the use of lights and a contrasting background color can assist in reading the syringe scale. Syringe magnifiers, while not strictly a nonoptical device, can be used for identification of syringe markings. For patients who cannot see the markings even with a magnifier, the Meditec Insulgages (Meditec, Inc., Denver, CO) are available (Figure 13-12). Insulgages are hard plastic gauges that fit over the head of the syringe plunger and are sized according to the number of units to be drawn into the syringe. The markings on the plastic Insulgage can be in braille, large print, or raised numbers. Individual insulin gauges that fit onto the syringe can be made. The gauge is fashioned so that its length is calibrated for the spacing distance between the

head of the syringe plunger and the base of the syringe barrel for a specific insulin dose to be drawn. Gauges should be specific for the type of syringe being used. Homemade gauges may be fashioned from paper clips, Popsicle sticks, straws, or wooden tongue depressors.

When a single dose is required, the use of a device that has a preset dosage may be useful. Inject Aid (Maxi-Aids, Farmingdale, NY) is available and is useful for a diabetic with unsteady hands. The device is preset to one dose and holds the vial in position, allowing for proper needle placement into the vial cap. When multiple doses or mixed doses are required, the Count-a-dose (Jordon Medical Enterprises, South Pasadena, CA) or Load-Matic (Palco Labs) devices can be used. The Count-a-dose and Load-Matic use disposable syringes and have geared calibrations that allow clicks to be felt and heard. The Load-Matic, with two calibrated wheels, a thumb setting for 10-unit increments, and a click wheel for 1-unit increments, is especially useful for drawing large dosages.

Prefilled syringes require that the patient place a glass cartridge into the penlike device, place the needle on the pen, and rid the system of air bubbles. The Autopen (Owen Mumford) has visual, tactile, and auditory sensory clues and comes in two models. One measures 2–32 units in 2-unit increments and the other measures 1–16 units, in 1-unit increments. Another prefilled syringe glass cartridge pen includes NovolinPen (Novo Nordisk), in which the dose is dialed and is injected when a button is pressed. The settings can range from 2 units to 36 units and are accompanied by a clicking sound when the measurement is made. A disadvantage of the NovolinPen is that the clicking may become less pronounced with use and should not be solely relied on for the confirmation of the drawn dosage. Novolin Penfill cartridges are available for 70/30, regular, and neutral protamine Hagedorn insulins. Other manufacturers are currently planning to market prefilled syringes with dialing systems.

Urine monitoring for diabetic patients is not as prevalent as blood glucose monitoring. When incorporated into the medical management, however, the readings are routinely performed before insulin injection or at the time of peak insulin action. Urine monitoring can consist of monitoring for glucose or ketones. Ketone testing is still considered an important part of self-monitoring to evaluate unexplained hyperglycemia irrespective of blood glucose monitoring.

Urine testing involves either mixing urine with water and a reagent and matching the color of the final solution to that on a color chart or dipping a specially treated test strip into the urine and comparing the color of the moistened strip to a color chart. Vision loss can often make this color comparison difficult, and the problem is compounded when the hues are close for the various readings. Using a plain white background and good illumination can make this color comparison task easier.

Another medical management task is that of monitoring blood pressure. A sphygmomanometer normally involves listening for sounds and reading a calibrated gauge. For many patients who may have hearing difficulties, this is an impossible task. The Cardio Vox (The Lighthouse, Inc.,

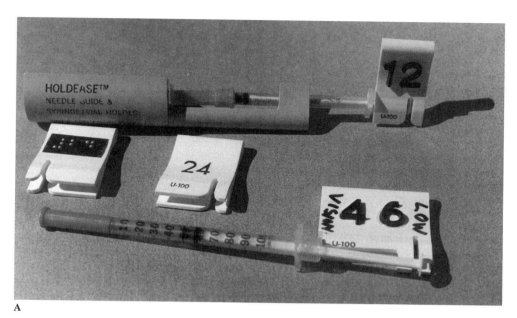

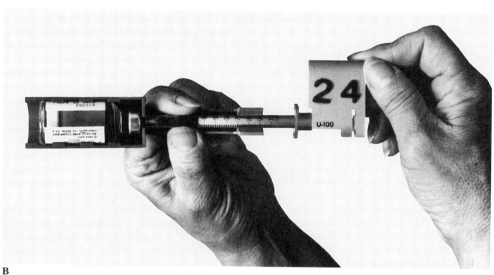

FIGURE 13-12. **The Meditec Insulgage (A) and Holdease (B) (Meditec, Inc., Denver, CO) are available to the patient who is unable to see the markings on a syringe.**

A

B

Long Island City, NY) is one of several specially designed sphygmomanometers with sensors placed in the inflatable cuff that detect both the systolic and diastolic pressures and announce the output (Figure 13-13). Large output displays or large LED displays feature jumbo readouts for the visually impaired.

Large readout thermometers and talking thermometers make taking temperature measurements easier. Pill organizers and large labels make the identification of medications more manageable. Relative size items, such as large-face watches, can be used for timing, and special scales can be used for measuring food or weight control that have large display outputs or voice output.

Although some medical products may be used by the visually impaired diabetic, the U.S. Food and Drug Administration requires a separate approval for a product to be marketed specifically for the visually impaired. For this

reason, some manufacturers have discontinued, withdrawn, or no longer promote some of the products in their line as products for the visually impaired even though some patients may still find the product useful.

Orientation and Mobility Management Techniques and Devices

Mobility and orientation are two vital functions that an individual needs for survival. Mobility deals with the process of moving within the environment, whereas orientation involves knowing how to move purposely within that environment. Although visual acuity is important for both functions, it is probably safe to say that the integrity of the visual field plays a more significant role than does visual acuity in the determination of the visual need for

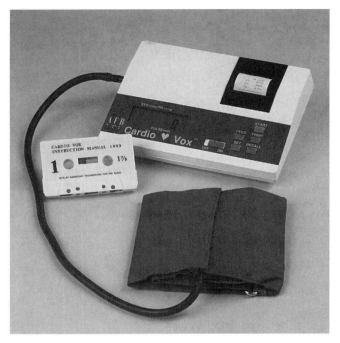

FIGURE 13-13. **The Cardio Vox large display sphygmomanometer not only has a large print-out display but is also equipped with auditory output. (Courtesy of The Lighthouse, Inc., Long Island City, NY.)**

orientation and mobility assistance. A visual field of approximately 20–50 degrees is required for good mobility with safe orientation.[28] Movement within the environment, when adequate visual cues are not present, may require the assistance of other people, canes, a dog guide, or electronic travel aids.

Sighted Guide Technique

Dependence on others for mobility involves the use of the sighted guide technique.[29] With this technique, a sighted individual can assist a person with a visual impairment using nonverbal cues for safe and efficient travel (see Figures 3-1 through 3-3). The sighted guide technique allows the guide and patient to navigate narrow passageways, stairways, and doorways, and to accommodate different seating situations (see the section Sighted Guide in Chapter 3).

Canes

Canes can also provide assistance for mobility. Through the early work of Dr. Richard Hoover in the 1940s at the Valley Forge Army Hospital, the foundations of mobility techniques using the long cane were formed. The long cane differed from the previously used support cane in that it was longer, had no support function, and was specifically designed to sense the environment. The long cane has the advantages of being highly maneuverable, reliable, and requires virtually no maintenance except for the occasional replacement of a tip. Folding and collapsible canes allow easy storage or carrying when not in use. Disadvantages of the long cane are its ineffectiveness in providing

adequate protection to the upper portions of the body (no warning of possible hazards until contact is made) and the range of information received by the user is limited by the length of the cane.

Common folding canes have from four to eight sections and either single or multiple cords to provide the necessary tension to hold the cane securely together. With more sections, the cane will be more compact but less rigid. Cane lengths will vary, but the usual length is measured from 1½ in. above the breastbone of the user to the ground at the side of the foot when it is in a forward position.

Dog Guides

Throughout history, humans have enjoyed a special and close relationship with dogs, not only as a companion but also as a helper. Dorothy Harrison Eustis is considered to be the mother of the dog guide movement in America.[30] She established Seeing Eye, Inc., in Morristown, New Jersey, in 1929. After the establishment of this school, other dog guide schools were established in the United States and Europe. A total program for the dog guide involves not only the skills that are taught between the user and dog guide, but also involves the breeding and training of the dogs, as well as matching the dog with a person. Typical breeds used for dog guides are the German Shepherd, Golden Retriever, and Labrador Retriever. Although some schools use both male and female dogs, most are females who demonstrate even temperaments and have short coats to allow for easy grooming.

Electronic Travel Aids

Electronic mobility devices or travel aids (ETAs) grew out of the need to provide more information to the visually impaired individual than was provided by the long cane or dog guide. Ideally, ETAs provide information that allows determination of size, range, and direction of an object or hazard. Although the history of the development of ETAs shows remarkable ingenuity, communication between researchers, developers, and funding organizations as well as users and mobility specialists has been sparse, and only a few devices have managed to survive. Even today, the use of ETAs is limited by cost, the need for extensive training, and the small number of trained professionals with enough experience to provide the instruction for these devices. In addition, ETAs can often provide the user with too much sensory information, which may complicate the problem. A few of these devices, despite these problems, do merit mention.

The Pathsounder was an electronic travel aid that was used to complement the long cane. It consisted of an ultrasonic device that was chest mounted and that emitted waves to aid in the dectection of obstacles. The device, invented by Lindsay Russell and no longer being manufactured, detected reflected waves when an object was within approximately 6 ft of the user and provided sound changes to provide a warning in the form of an auditory, vibratory, or combination of both outputs. Today, the Wheelchair Pathfinder (Nurion Industries, Paoli, PA) uses these principles but is permanently mounted on a wheelchair, scooter, or walker to provide these sensory clues. Another, similar device, the Polaron (Nurion Industries) detects objects within 4, 8, or 16 ft and is specifically designed as a navigation aid to be worn around the neck of the partially sighted, blind, deaf-blind, and visually impaired wheelchair user.

Similar to the Pathsounder is the Sonic Pathfinder (Pulse Data International Limited, Christchurch, New Zealand). This device is also a secondary mobility aid that evolved out of the work of the Blind Mobility Research Unit at Nottingham University in England.[31] It consists of a head-mounted pulse-echo sonar system controlled by a microprocessor. The device does not give information about surface texture of objects, but does provide auditory feedback from five transducers that is fed to the right, left, or both ears depending on object location. It also has an "artificial intelligence" built into its electrical system, which, by way of digitized information, is analyzed by decision-making algorithms to display only relevant information to the user. It is purported to avoid informational overload, which was a common problem with many earlier electronic travel aids. Currently, the Sonic Pathfinder is distributed in the United States by Mobility Services, Inc., Atlanta, Georgia; Baum Electronic Gmbh., Schloss Langenzell, Wiesenbach, Germany in Europe; and Perceptual Alternatives in Victoria, Australia.

The Laser Cane (Nurion Industries) is another form of electronic device that combines auditory feedback with the use of a long cane to provide additional sensory information that cannot be provided by a long cane alone. Three small lasers that emit pulses from 40 to 80 times per second provide what are referred to as an *upper channel, forward channel,* and *downward channel.* The upper channel provides information in an upper zone to warn of overhead obstacles. The forward channel gives information in the travel path and immediate periphery. Information about drop-offs is provided by the downward channel. Output is in the form of auditory pitched tones according to the channel and is coupled with a tactile vibratory output. Limitations of the Laser Cane include difficulty of use in heavy rain or snow and difficulty in receiving reflections from some smooth and highly polished surfaces. In addition, training time is lengthy.

Another device that may have some use as a mobility aid is the Mowat Sensor (Pulse Data International Limited). The Mowat Sensor was developed by G.C. Mowat in 1970. The device consists of a handheld transmitter that sends out a high-frequency ultrasonic cone 15 degrees wide and 30 degrees high, roughly approximating the shape and form of a person.[32] The reflected beam is detected and causes the Mowat Sensor to vibrate. A switch allows a change in the range of the device and an earphone attachment is available for an optional auditory output. The Mowat Sensor is designed to be used in conjunction with the conventional long cane or dog guide to help in the detection of hazards, public transportation signs, doorways, or other landmarks.

Mobility for the individual who has poor acuity or a limited field becomes increasingly difficult in dim illumination. In patients with poor dark adaptation, rod-cone

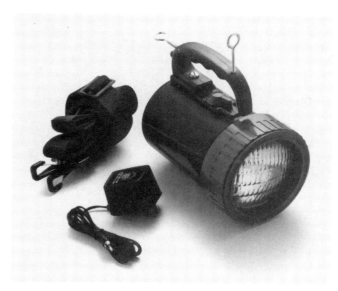

FIGURE 13-14. **The Wide-Angle Mobility Light (Innovation Rehabilitation Technology, Inc., Mountain View, CA) provides a wide beam of illumination that may aid in mobility under dim illumination. (Courtesy of The Lighthouse, Inc., Long Island City, NY.)**

dystrophies, retinitis pigmentosa, or advanced glaucoma, successful mobility often depends on providing adequate illumination. The *WAML*, which is an acronym for *Wide-Angle Mobility Light* (Innovation Rehabilitation Technology, Inc., Mountain View, CA) (Figure 13-14), provides a source of portable illumination. Directed downward and worn as a waist-level, wide-beam flashlight, the WAML can be a valuable mobility aid in dim environments. The unit weighs approximately 5 lb and is available with a rechargeable battery, allowing for portable operation. The field dimensions are 20×30 degrees.

Providing additional illumination is one solution to the problem of poor night vision, while another solution is increasing the level of sensitivity to lowered illumination through the use of an ITT Nightscope (Night Vision Aid Distributors, Randallstown, MD) light amplification device. Night-vision devices (NVDs) (Figure 13-15) for mobility in dimly lit environments grew out of the developments of military and surveillance in the United States and the former Soviet Union. These new systems use a Generation III technology in which a thin microchannel plate (MCP) is used to aim or direct the electron flow within the intensifier for added brightness. Russian Generation III NVDs incorporate a fiber-optic bundle between the MCP and phosphor screen, whereas the U.S. version typically uses a gallium arsenide (GaAs/AlGaAs) coating on the photo cathode, which has a higher photosensitivity, rather than the multi-alkali coating used in Generation I and Generation II models. The U.S. Generation III models typically show a black-and-white image and are more costly than the Generation III scopes of Russian technology, which show a greenish image. Studies show that the best candidates for the NVD devices are patients demonstrating visual acuities of better than 20/200 and visual fields of at least 20

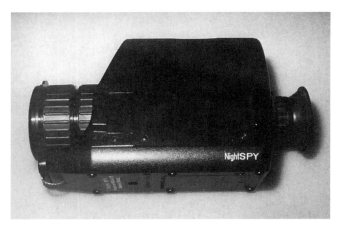

FIGURE 13-15.   **NightSPY (Nogalite, Tel Aviv, Israel) is a night-vision device that may aid mobility under dimly lit environments.**

degrees.[33] In one study comparing the WAML to the NVD, the NVD did not significantly improve the subjects' mobility at night, and the majority preferred the WAML.[33] Despite this data, the value of the NVD should not be discounted for all individuals who are night blind.

Sensory-Substitution Devices

When working with the low vision population, it is not uncommon to occasionally encounter a patient who has such poor vision that no low vision optical device is helpful. In these cases, other sensory inputs may be used to assist these patients. Hearing, touch, taste, and smell can all be used for sensory substitution. The two largest categories of sensory-substitution devices are those that use hearing and touch.

Auditory Substitution
Of the sensory-substitution devices for vision, the largest number of devices fall into the category of auditory substitution, which includes products with voice output, or nonverbal output devices in the form of tones, beeps, bells, or other auditory forms. Compared to other forms of sensory-substitution devices, the sense of audition in the form of synthesized speech ranks high as a form of sensory input, favored over tactile input and nonverbal input. Auditory-substitution devices consist of talking books, voice output products, nonverbal auditory output products, and reader and descriptive services.

TALKING BOOKS.   Talking books are the largest category of auditory-substitution devices. Talking books consist of audio recordings on cassettes, discs (records), and tape (reel-to-reel). Today, most of the selections are distributed through cassettes. With the advent of computers and synthetic sound, the world of computers and CD-ROMs can also provide auditory substitution.

Sources for talking books are many, but perhaps the largest collection is available free of charge through the NLS. Free distribution includes a cassette or record player

and free postage to and from NLS or its subregional libraries. Through this network of regional and subregional libraries, distribution is accomplished for what is referred to as material in *special media*, which could be talking books, large-print publications, or braille. Under the current regulations, optometrists and ophthalmologists can certify the need for these materials if the patient has difficulty reading conventional material. The individual does not have to be legally blind to qualify for these services. Selections can be made from catalogs listing numerous recordings on a variety of current topics. Reference circulars are available from NLS and include religious material and current magazines. In addition to NLS, commercial distribution of special media is available through some publishers such as Thorndike Press/G.K. Hall, which has a wide selection of the most popular bestsellers in fiction and nonfiction.

Four methods are available for the blind to "read" printed material: braille, tape and disc recordings, direct translation reading devices (optical scanners), and the sighted reader. Of these methods, reading by way of cassettes is the fastest and approaches 150–175 words per minute. Even this method, however, has some problems: It takes a blind person longer to read by tape than it does for a sighted counterpart to read print. There is no active participation, as listening is passive, and the blind reader has no control over the rate at which the material is being presented. Reading rates for a sighted reader approach 200–400 words per minute. A faster reading rate for the blind reader would therefore save time and eliminate inattention. Because of this difference in reading rates, the ability to speed up the tapes would be desirable. The major problem with speeding up the recording is a loss of tonal quality and increased pitch, resulting in a distortion of the speech. A speech compressor allows for an adjustable playback speed for faster or slower listening over a range of approximately one-half times normal to 2½ times normal while restoring the pitch. Speech compressors are available for open reel-to-reel, cassettes, and discs (records).

Another problem with auditory recordings is the lack of spatial layout. If a particular passage must be located, the user is forced to search back and forth on the tape until the material is located. One solution to this is voice indexing or tone indexing. Chandler[34] was the first to introduce voice indexing as an assistive technique for accessing recorded material for the visually impaired. With voice or tone indexing, auditory cues or other information is placed on the tape. Recording for the Blind and Dyslexic, Inc. (Princeton, NJ) uses very-low-pitched beeps to indicate page and chapter headings. Other systems use two tracks, spaced a few seconds apart. Indicators are spoken at every 10-second interval on the fast track. Thus with this system, the user can find material very quickly.

Voice indexing or *V-Dex*, a term coined by Chandler,[34] is another system that uses recordings performed at a fast speed on the track parallel to the track used for text material. Still other methods use the same track played at two different speeds. The indexing is done at the fast speed and the information is recorded at the slower speed. This method has proved to be effective for works such as dictionaries. Voice indexing should be more widely used to allow the full potential of auditory substitution to be appreciated.

TALKING PRODUCTS. With the invention of synthesized speech, voice output for many common products used around the home has become commonplace. Clocks, watches, calculators, scales, computers, and telephones are just a few of the common devices that are available with speech output. Often, many of the voice-output products will also have a large display incorporating relative size magnification along with voice output. This combination makes for an extremely useful product.

Speech synthesis technology has had its greatest impact for the visually impaired in the area of computer technology. With speech technology, the entire field of computer-assisted occupational, vocational, educational, and recreational opportunities are now a reality. Products include speech synthesizers, speech adapters, terminals with voice output, and microcomputers with voice output.

Speech synthesizers are devices that will take the ASCII codes generated by the host computer and convert them into speech. The separate speech synthesizer or voice-output device must be connected to a host microcomputer or terminal to receive the information to convert into speech. Most of the devices are said to be in a "real-time" mode because the device speaks as the text is typed and transmitted. Most of the speech synthesizers also have a small buffer capacity that momentarily stores data as it is vocalized. Review functions largely depend on the computer system to which the synthesizer is connected. Most speech synthesizers can distinguish upper and lower case letters and can vocalize text as words or letter by letter.

Speech adapters that are peripheral devices to a host computer provide real-time speech output much like speech synthesizers but have a larger buffer capacity and built-in software to allow additional functions to be performed. Cursor location, punctuation, announcement of upper and lower case, and choice of speech rate are some of these additional functions, which enable the visually impaired user to scan the material on the computer screen.

Talking terminals have hardware and software that allow both input and output to a host computer. They have all the functions that speech synthesizers and speech adapters have in addition to having the ability to edit text before it is sent to a host computer. Talking terminals have large buffers that allow for up to five screens of data to be randomly vocalized.

With the advent of optical character recognition (OCR), "reading machines" were developed. One of the first was the Kurzweil Reading Machine (KRM) developed by Kurzweil Computer Products (a Xerox company). The KRM is no longer available, but its development led to the reading machines of today. An optical scanner was used to convert printed characters on a page into speech output. Other reading machines that are currently available include the Reading Edge (Telesensory, a Xerox Strategic Partner, Sunnyvale, CA), Expert Reader (Telesensory),

and An Open Book (Arkenstone, Sunnyvale, CA). The OsCaR system (Telesensory) is an OCR system that can scan printed material into text that can be used in off-the-shelf word processing, desktop publishing, database, or spreadsheet programs. Coupled with a computer speech output program, OsCaR can turn a personal computer into a reading machine. The Versatile Image Processor (VIP) (JBliss Imaging Systems, Los Altos, CA) combines the latest in software to provide both image enhancement and enhanced auditory output of computerized information. The input can be from computer created files, scanned text material, or material received from electronic mail or the Internet.

READER SERVICES. Personal readers can be used by the visually impaired; however, the disadvantages are obvious. Lack of privacy, the loss of independence, and availability of on-hand readers are major drawbacks. Other reader services include radio reading services and audio reading services for theatrical, television, and video performances. The Radio Information Service makes printed material available to the blind and other visually impaired by using the broadcast facilities of an existing radio station or the subcarrier of an FM station. A special receiver is necessary because the current U.S. Federal Communications Commission regulations prohibit reading copyrighted material over the radio. Radio receivers are also available that can receive the audio portion of television stations and thereby allow blind individuals to access television broadcasts without the cost of purchasing a television.

Audio Descriptive Services is available in a few locations. This service uses a weak-powered radio transmission to provide an audio descriptive commentary for theatrical productions. The user wears earphones and a special receiver to hear the descriptive service.

Descriptive Video Service (DVS) is a newer service that provides a carefully programmed commentary describing the action, sets, locations, facial characteristics, mannerisms, and costumes. It is programmed and planned so as not to interfere with the main dialogue of the performance. Currently, DVS is broadcast free of charge to more than 80 public television stations nationally. To receive DVS, the user must have either a video receiver or recorder, television, or special receiver with the second audio program feature.

Tactile Substitution

The second largest sensory input that is used when the visual sensory input is not functional is the sense of touch. The most common form of providing this sensory input is through braille. Other forms of tactile substitution include basic touch, Moon, the Fishburne alphabet, and paperless braille (refreshable braille).

Stereognosis or tactile form recognition is not an acute sense in humans, and does not provide a chief sensory input. When the visual system is nonfunctional, however, basic touch can provide supplemental information to the other senses. The texture of surfaces, hardness or softness of objects, or temperature of an object perceived through the fingertips are some examples of the information that can be gained through somesthesis and kinesthesis.

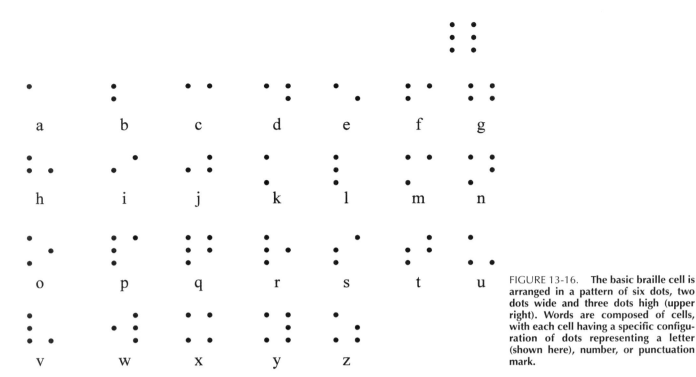

FIGURE 13-16.   **The basic braille cell is arranged in a pattern of six dots, two dots wide and three dots high (upper right). Words are composed of cells, with each cell having a specific configuration of dots representing a letter (shown here), number, or punctuation mark.**

BRAILLE.   Braille is the best example of tactile substitution. Developed in 1834 by Louis Braille, the system of reading and printing consists of raised dots that are tactually identified.[35] The pattern of dots represents letters or symbols of a language that has been almost universally accepted by blind individuals. The braille cell is arranged in a pattern of six dots, two dots wide and three dots high. When originally developed, braille consisted of only characters of the alphabet, numbers, and punctuation marks. Material was transcribed letter by letter (Figure 13-16). This was and still is known as *grade I braille*. Grade II braille consists of combinations of 63 possible dot orientations and combinations, many of which have more than one meaning. By using contractions and more combinations, material produced in grade II braille uses only approximately 60% of the space that grade I would require, saving space and production time and allowing for an increased reading speed. Most braille is produced in grade II. Grade III is a higher contracted form of braille, containing more than 500 contracted forms and used for note taking and by blind stenographers.

Reading braille requires good tactile sensation. For this reason, when there is a peripheral neuropathy from diabetes or other conditions giving rise to tactile aphasia, learning to read braille is not recommended. Another consideration in using braille is a slower reading speed. Average reading speeds are approximately 90–100 words per minute. Due to the slow speeds compared to sight reading (200–400 wpm) and voice recording (175–200 wpm), blind individuals rarely rely on braille alone but use readers and other sensory input along with braille.

Additional problems with braille consist of difficulty in transcribing certain materials, distribution, and storage problems. Transcription requires a highly trained braillist who is familiar with the rules governing translation. Many of the individual orders for braille books involve manual translation. Some of these problems, however, are being overcome with braille printers and braille translation software, such as Duxbury (Duxbury Systems, Inc., Littleton, MA), which allows a user to produce grade II braille from printed copy. The lack of ability to provide spatial layout with braille or present graphic representation has been a special problem. Some of these spatial layout problems are addressed with special embossers, which are capable of producing graphical output, such as Versa Point Duo Braille Embosser, available through Telesensory.

Braille reading selections are available from a variety of sources. Two of the main sources of braille publications are the NLS and the APH. Other sources include several religious advocacy and support groups, which provide charitable services for the visually impaired.

MOON.   Moon, another system of embossed printing, was invented by William Moon in 1847, and uses large, simplified Roman letters.[36, 37] The Moon alphabet is made up of nine characters (portions of Roman letters) that are used in different positions. The lines are read and set so that the first line is read from left to right and the second line is read from right to left. The pattern repeats itself; however, the letters are not reversed.

The main advantages of Moon over braille are that it is easy to learn and does not require a good tactile sense. One disadvantage is that the letters are relatively large and bold, making Moon books large and bulky. Another disadvantage of Moon is that it cannot be written by hand.

Production of Moon involves setting print by hand, moistening paper before the printing and then embossing and drying the paper in a mechanical gas-heated drier. With the almost total acceptance of braille, Moon is rarely seen and its distribution is very limited. The number of Moon readers is very limited as well. The small number of Moon readers (approximately 2,000 British readers and possibly 500 outside of England) continue to perpetuate this system. For those unwilling or unable to read braille, the Moon system has proved to be effective. It is easier to read than braille and is easier for individuals with impaired touch. Currently, the Royal National Institute for the Blind in England is the primary producer of Moon.

OTHER TACTILE SUBSTITUTION.   The Fishburne alphabet is similar to braille in that it uses specific patterns or embossed dots and lines to represent the various letters of the alphabet. Fishburne characters are approximately twice the size of their braille counterparts. The Fishburne alphabet can be self-taught by means of programmed cassettes. This method is useful for individuals who do not read braille. The Fishburne alphabet has found its greatest use in labeling; however, the space required for its letter size is the major drawback to its expanded use.

The preceding tactile methods use impressions on paper that are then read by touch. Although this provides a "hard-copy" print for study and review, the major drawback is one of space and storage. Braille, which is produced via a mechanical display without actual impressions on paper, is termed *paperless braille* or *refreshable braille*. Mechanical displays consist of an array of electronically controlled "pins" arranged in specific patterns. These patterns can be a braille cell in a six- or eight-dot configuration or in a multipin tactile array. The display allows for a one-to-one duplication of the input from either a camera-sensor device or direct translation into grade II braille from computer input. When these displays are positioned as a series of braille cells (from 20 to 81 in a row), the user can read braille output. By controlling the position of the pin in the individual cell, the positions are recorded on magnetic tape and thus can be stored easily, overcoming the storage problem of conventional braille. This method of braille display is common with many applications, including computer interfacing, and is often combined with speech synthesis for both input and output, allowing a blind user to "see" and hear what is being both input and output.

SELF-ASSESSMENT QUESTIONS

1. The largest category of nonoptical devices is probably which of the following?
   (a) relative distance devices
   (b) writing devices
   (c) relative size devices
   (d) lighting and illumination control
   (e) mobility devices

2. Illumination controls used for distance vision include all of the following *except*
   (a) side shields
   (b) typoscopes
   (c) multiple pinhole spectacles
   (d) tints and coatings
   (e) visors or hats

3. The greatest advantage of large-type materials is that they
   (a) have better contrast and therefore greater visibility
   (b) are available in relatively large amounts of magnification
   (c) are less cumbersome than most means of magnification
   (d) are relatively inexpensive and available in a wide range of formats
   (e) permit more habitual and therefore comfortable reading

4. The most common form of sensory substitution for low vision patients involves the use of
   (a) audition
   (b) tactile sensation
   (c) olfaction
   (d) taste
   (e) sight

5. Which of the following nonoptical device groupings is *incorrect?*
   (a) large-print book, *New York Times Large Print Weekly*, jumbo playing cards
   (b) Corning Photochromatic Filter, typoscope, UVShield, rheostat on lights
   (c) guide dog, Nightscope, Laser Cane
   (d) Expert Reader, talking books, WAML
   (e) braille, Moon, paperless braille

6. Patients with visual fields of less than __ degrees may not demonstrate improved mobility with night-vision devices.
   (a) 20
   (b) 30
   (c) 40
   (d) 50
   (e) 140

7. A visual field of approximately _____ is the minimum required for good mobility with safe orientation.
   (a) 10–20 degrees
   (b) 20–50 degrees
   (c) 90–140 degrees
   (d) 140–180 degrees
   (e) no peripheral constrictions

8. Of the following filters, which one has the properties of being photochromatic and having the ability to incorporate a patient's refractive correction?
   (a) NoIR 107
   (b) CPF 550
   (c) UVShield
   (d) neutral density gray
   (e) flash mirror on Polaroid

9. Mobility under dim illumination conditions is best assisted with the
   (a) Mowat Sensor
   (b) Dog guide
   (c) WAML
   (d) Mobility cane
   (e) Sonic Pathfinder

10. Moving a light source that is perpendicular to a surface from 4 to 2 ft away will
    (a) double the illumination
    (b) triple the illumination
    (c) quadruple the illumination
    (d) halve the illumination
    (e) more than double but less than triple the illumination

11. Monitoring blood glucose levels in diabetics can be done with
    (a) U-100 syringe
    (b) Autopen
    (c) One Touch Profile
    (d) Insulgage
    (e) Count-a-dose

12. Reading speeds for sighted readers will be between _____ words per minute, whereas listening rates or "reading rates" by blind persons using cassettes without speech compression average _____ words per minute.
    (a) 150–175 and 300–500
    (b) 200–400 and 150–175
    (c) 200–400 and 80–100
    (d) 100–300 and 300–500
    (e) 80–300 and 500–1000

REFERENCES

1. Ellerbrock VJ. Partial Vision and Optical Aids. In MJ Hirsch, RE Wick (eds), Vision of the Aging Patient: An Optometric Symposium. Philadelphia: Chilton, 1960;174–201.
2. Eaken WM, McFarland TL. Type, Printing and the Partially Seeing Child. Pittsburgh: Stanwix House, 1960.
3. National Association for the Visually Handicapped. Uniform Standards and Equipment Recommended for the Preparation of Large Type Materials. San Francisco: National Association for the Visually Handicapped, 1963.
4. Fonda G. Management of the Patient with Subnormal Vision. St. Louis: Mosby, 1965;6–10.
5. Barraga N. Large type books versus regular size type and visual aids. International Council for Education of the Visually Handicapped Educator 1974;2:6–7.
6. Cohen JM, Rosenthal BP. An evaluation of an incandescent neodymium light source on near point performance of a low vision population. J Vis Rehabil 1988;2:5–21.
7. Adrian W, Schmidt I. Photic damage in retinitis pigmentosa and a suggestion for a protective device. J Am Optom Assoc 1975;46: 380–386.
8. Berson EL. Light deprivation for early retinitis pigmentosa: a hypothesis. Arch Ophthalmol 1971;85:521–529.
9. Noell WK, Walker VS, Kang BS, et al. Retinal damage by light in rats. Invest Ophthalmol 1966;5:450–473.
10. Gorn RA, Kuwabara T. Retinal damage by visible light: a physiologic study. Arch Ophthalmol 1967;77:115–118.
11. Everson RW, Schmidt I. Protective spectacles for retinitis pigmentosa. J Am Optom Assoc 1976;47:738–744.
12. Maino JH, McMahon TT. NoIRs and low vision. J Am Optom Assoc 1986;57:532–535.
13. Hoeft WW, Hughes MK. A comparative study of low vision patients: their ocular disease and preference for one specific series of light transmission filters. Am J Optom Physiol Optics 1981;58:841–845.
14. Zigman S. Vision enhancement using a short wavelength light absorbing filter. Optom Vis Sci 1990;67:100–104.
15. Pitts DG. A comparative study of the effects of ultraviolet radiation on the eye. Am J Optom Arch Am Acad Optom 1970;47: 535–546.
16. Pitts DG, Cameron LL, Jose JG, et al. Optical Radiation and Cataracts. In M Waxler, VE Hitchins (eds), Optical Radiation and Visual Health. Boca Raton, FL: CRC Press, 1986;5–41.
17. Pitts DG, Cullen AP, Hacker PD. Ocular effects of ultraviolet radiation from 295 to 365 nm. Invest Ophthalmol Vis Sci 1977;16: 932–939.
18. Pitts DG, Kleinstein RN. Environmental Vision: Interactions of the Eye, Vision and the Environment. Boston: Butterworth–Heinemann, 1993;274.
19. Prentice CF. The Typoscope (1897). Republished in Ophthalmic Lenses, Dioptric Formulae for Combined Cylindrical Lenses, the Prism-Dioptry and Other Papers by Charles Prentice (2nd ed). Philadelphia: The Keystone Publishing Company, 1907.
20. Rosenbloom AA. The controlled-pupil contact lens in low vision problems. J Am Optom Assoc 1969;40:836–840.
21. Southall JP. Mirrors, Prisms, and Lenses. New York: Macmillan, 1918;5.
22. Fonda GE. Management of Low Vision. New York: Thieme–Stratton, 1981;6, 164.
23. Cohen JM, Waiss B. An evaluation of horizontally louvered black sunwear for glare reduction in a glare sensitive low vision population. J Vis Rehabil 1991;5:61–68.
24. Hoover RE. Orientation and Travel Techniques for the Blind. New York: American Association of Workers for the Blind, 1947:27.
25. Harmon DB. The Co-ordinated Classroom. Grand Rapids, MI: American Seating Company, 1949.
26. Tinker MA. Effect of sloped text upon the readability of print. Am J Optom Arch Am Acad Optom 1956;33:189–195.
27. Genensky SM, Berry SH, Bikson TH, et al. Visual Environmental Adaptation Problems of the Partially Sighted (CPS 101-HEW). Santa Monica, CA: Santa Monica Hospital. Center for the Partially Sighted, 1979.
28. Faye EE. Clinical Low Vision. Boston: Little, Brown, 1976:243.
29. Hill E, Ponder P. Orientation and Mobility Techniques. New York: American Foundation for the Blind, 1976:12–26.
30. Eustis DH. The seeing eye. Saturday Evening Post, 5 November 1927.
31. Heyes T. Perceptual Alternatives [personal communication]. 1994.
32. Morrissette DL, Goodrich GL, Hennessey JJ. A follow-up study of the Mowat sensor's applications, frequency of use, and maintenance reliability. J Vis Impair Blind 1981;75:244–247.
33. Morrissette DL, Goodrich GL. The night vision aid for legally blind people with night blindness: an evaluation. J Vis Impair Blind 1983;77:67–70.
34. Chandler JG. Voice indexing of tape recordings. J Vis Impair Blind 1979;73:191–192.
35. Goldish LH. Braille in the United States: Its Production, Distribution, and Use. New York: American Foundation for the Blind, 1967.
36. Gill JM. New moon. Br J Vis Impair 1985;3:85–86.
37. Yeadon A. Moon—A contemporary appraisal. J Vis Impair Blind 1979;73:341–343.

CHAPTER FOURTEEN

Computer Assistive Technology for the Low Vision Patient

Glenda V. Such and
Stephen G. Whittaker

In the past, individuals with severe visual impairment were severely restricted in what they could read and write. They needed to wait for a scheduled radio broadcast or the arrival of an audiotape or brailled materials. The closed-circuit television (CCTV) and advances in optical systems have enabled patients with residual vision to access normal print, but with higher magnification, some patients experience difficulty searching, scanning, and writing with these devices.

At this time, for many with low vision, assistive computer systems have the potential to remove many of these restrictions. With specialized assistive equipment, some patients with low vision can use the home computer to convert digitized text into a format that compensates for any degree of visual impairment, enlarging text on a screen or converting it to speech. With a computer, the patient can locate specific information using search or find functions and type his or her messages and correspondence. Once the information is found, the patient can "read" by listening to synthetic speech at rates of 200–300 words per minute, which is about as quickly as someone with normal vision reads continuous text visually.[1] Financial transactions and banking can be conducted with computers. Most important, nearly all written information at some point exists in digital form. Newspapers and magazines are available on the World Wide Web or on commercial on-line information services. Even material available only in print form can be converted to a digital file that can be read by a computer. Thus, the personal computer has become an important assistive device that allows for accessing and processing information, and therefore, a world of limited vision may no longer be a restrictive environment.

TYPES OF COMPUTER ASSISTIVE DEVICES

For individuals with low vision, four basic types of adaptations may enable them to read a computer screen:

1. Optical magnification
2. Electronic display magnification (through the use of software)
3. Vocalization or synthetic speech systems (that translate text into speech)
4. Braille display systems (that convert text into braille and vice versa)

Patients with mild to moderate vision loss may use optical magnification systems (e.g., magnifiers, telemicroscopes) in conjunction with either a standard or larger computer screen or may find electronic display magnification preferable. For patients with severe vision loss, vocalization systems that convert text displayed on the screen to an audible output may be more effective and prolong usage without fatigue. Although many of these systems are expressionless and often robotic sounding, some of the more expensive computer speech synthesizers produce speech that is as intelligible as natural speech.

Optical Magnification

In many cases, a patient's problem with reading print on a computer monitor can be solved by simply using an optical device. Reading lenses (microscopes) may be helpful for patients who are willing to view the monitor from a close distance, sometimes as close as 5 cm from the screen. The relative distance magnification obtained at this 5-cm working distance (+20.00 D lens) is 5× when compared to a "normal" 25-cm working distance (25/5 = 5). Patients using this reading lens, however, may soon experience fatigue from positioning themselves so close to the monitor screen. To reduce some of the effects of poor body posture, the use of special monitor stands positions the monitor close to the patient so that he or she can sit straight when reading the print. An antireflective coating and possibly a tint on the lenses may eliminate glare and possibly help in reducing fatigue as well (see the section on tinted and photochromatic lenses in Chapter 8).

When patients are resistant to the use of a microscope, handheld magnifiers may be considered to view the computer monitor. It is best to recommend a handheld magnifier with as large a lens diameter as possible, and, most important, one with a minimum amount of peripheral distortion. A handheld magnifier may be of most benefit to a patient who is able to read print on the monitor screen but has problems in identifying the icons, which are smaller in size.

Another optical device that may be considered is a Fresnel-type lens that is positioned in front of the monitor a given distance from the screen (Figure 14-1). This plus lens system is capable of increasing the character size on the screen approximately 2×. The lens may also provide the benefit of glare reduction by way of a tint or coating.

In addition to the optical devices mentioned in the preceding paragraphs, a telemicroscope may be a possible option in allowing patients with low vision to identify print on a computer monitor. The telemicroscope has the added advantages of providing more magnification and allowing a greater working distance than any of the preceding devices. As the magnification is increased, however, the field of view decreases. Therefore, to make the telemicroscope a viable device, a compromise must be reached between the maximum magnification of the system and the maximum field of view needed for the patient to function comfortably.

Electronic Display Magnification

Many operating systems provide electronic display magnification by increasing the character font size. Newer operating systems for the IBM compatible and Macintosh systems offer features that enlarge the print as well as the graphics. Special electronic magnification software packages, such as Zoom Text Xtra (Ai Squared, Manchester Center, VT) (for IBM and IBM-compatible systems) magnify text and graphics in off-the-shelf word processing, spreadsheet, and database programs from 2× to 16× in size. This special software also allows for mouse tracking, color changes, and split and full-screen magnification. InLARGE (Berkeley System, Inc., Berkeley, CA) is a screen magnification system for the Macintosh. This program has similar features to Zoom Text Xtra and also provides magnification from 2× to 16×.

Electronic display magnification, through the use of software, has many advantages over the use of optical devices. It can

1. Provide greater magnification
2. Provide contrast enhancement
3. Provide luminance control
4. Provide reverse contrast
5. Modify font types and letter spacing
6. Change the color combinations of the characters as well as the background
7. Permit a greater working distance
8. Automatically scroll text into the patient's field of view (review mode)

When using software to provide electronic display magnification, only a small portion of the magnified printed material can be displayed on the screen at any given time. Obviously, as the magnification increases there is a proportional reduction in the amount of printed material seen on the screen.

When considering the various electronic display magnification programs, there are several factors to consider. These factors are (1) the sizes of print available (most provide 2–16× magnification), (2) the display colors and appearance, (3) the method to review and track text, and (4) font characteristics and presentation modes. An explanation of these features follows.

Presentation Modes
The magnified portion of the screen can be displayed in several ways.

1. *Full.* The print on the screen is magnified and fills the entire screen much like a CCTV magnifies a page of text. To help the patient orient him- or herself on the screen, the magnification can be toggled on and off. When off, a normal display is sometimes presented with the area outlined that will be magnified.

2. *Split.* The normal unmagnified display is presented on one-half of the screen and an enlarged portion on the other half of the monitor screen. These "halves" can be vertically or horizontally presented on user demand.

3. *Quadrant.* This feature uses only one-fourth of the screen to show magnified print while the remaining area of the screen displays normal unmagnified print.

Display Colors and Font Characteristics
The colors that are available on the screen are influenced by the monitor capabilities and the software program. At present, some of the features offered are the following:

1. *Foreground.* The color of the characters on the screen may be changed to one or more of a variety of predetermined selections.

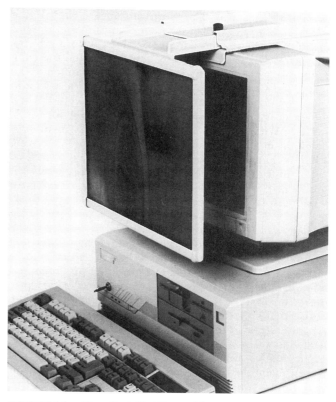

FIGURE 14-1.   **The adjustable EZ magnifier provides magnification levels from 1.2× to 2.4×. The lens assembly consists of a convex lens sandwiched between a Clarifier lens in front and optical glass in back. This arrangement provides protection and easy cleaning with ordinary glass cleaners. It is attached to the monitor with an adjustable slide bracket using Velcro and a bungee cord for additional support. The lens assembly simply lifts off for cleaning. (Courtesy of Less Gauss, Inc., Rhineback, NY.)**

2. *Background.* The field on which the characters are displayed may be changed to one or more predetermined color selections.

3. *Spacing.* The spacing between characters and lines may be increased in some programs to reduce letter crowding effects.

4. *Font.* The type style of displayed print on the screen may be changed to a number of selections (both size and style). Fonts vary in "smoothness"; some become "pixelated" with high magnification.

5. *Color rendition.* Electronic display magnifiers vary in the number of colors (e.g., 16 colors, 256 colors) they can display.

Reviewing Text
Once information has been entered into a computer system, it is necessary to review the text or graphics on the screen. As mentioned under Presentation Modes, screen magnification programs actually involve two screens, the normal unmagnified display and the magnified display. The unmagnified print display is similar to a "printed page," whereas the magnified display will enlarge only a

portion of the printed page on the screen, similar to a CCTV. As with the CCTV, the patient must master the orientation of the magnified material without losing his or her place. For example, the patient can switch the computer display back and forth from the unmagnified to the magnified view. When in a magnified view, the program will move the display into the magnified region just as one moves a page into the narrow field of a magnifier or CCTV camera. With some magnifiers, the patient can move a magnification window over the display much like moving a handheld magnifier over a stationary printed page. The latter strategy allows the patient to orient more easily but the field of the magnifier is narrower than if the entire screen displays the magnified text.

Review versus Programming Cursors

A *cursor* is a flashing line or arrow that indicates where text is to be entered, or the section of the screen that is to be displayed. With many screen magnification programs and all screen readers for speech, there are two cursors: a program cursor and a review cursor. The *program cursor* is the cursor that indicates where information is being entered. An example of a program cursor is the blinking bar or vertical line in a word processing program that indicates where text is going to be inserted. In addition, some screen magnifiers have a *review cursor*. The review cursor indicates what portion of the normal screen is being magnified by the screen magnifier. For example, an individual might be typing a word positioned in the lower left of the screen. The program cursor, therefore, would be sitting in the lower left of the screen indicated by a blinking line or highlight. If the patient wanted to read something in the upper right corner of the screen, the review cursor would be moved (usually by moving the mouse) to the upper right corner of the screen and read under magnification (without moving the program cursor). Thus, the review cursor allows the patient to review text and easily return to the spot where he or she had stopped typing.

Automatic Review Mode

Some screen magnification programs allow the patient to use an automatic review mode. If the patient wishes to read an entire screen under magnification, the computer can be programmed into an *automatic (or scrolling) review mode*. The text on each line will be automatically scrolled from right to left across the screen, similar to news marquees. This is a very convenient feature for patients reading a screen under very high magnification (seeing a few letters at a time) as it keeps track of the reader's place in the text. Important features that differentiate the various software programs are how smoothly the text moves and how easily a patient can control the scrolling speed—for example, slowing it down when the reading is difficult and speeding it up to skim the material.

The features that are most important when selecting a screen magnification system are the following:

1. *Magnification.* As previously mentioned in Electronic Display Magnification, most programs range from 2× to 16× magnification.

2. *Contrast.* White or yellow letters on a black or dark background provide better contrast for many low vision patients who have reduced overall contrast sensitivity. In some cases, it will allow these patients to read faster and more comfortably.

3. *Fonts.* Smooth letters or fonts, such as Times Roman or Arial, are easier to read in many cases. With higher magnification, fonts often become pixilated and more difficult to read.

4. *Smooth motion.* When text is scrolled on the screen by moving the mouse or when in automatic review mode, it should be smooth. This depends, in part, on the processor speed and the amount of video random-access memory and general random-access memory in the computer.

5. *Font spacing.* Increased letter spacing enables some patients to read with more ease when crowding is decreased. Many patients with metamorphopsia or central field loss appear to read more easily with this modification.

Vocalization or Synthetic Speech Systems

Speech systems should not be considered as a last resort or only for those with severe vision loss. Speech systems may be considered for patients with moderate vision loss because some patients can "read" as quickly and comfortably with a speech system as a normally sighted computer user can read visually, whereas other patients prefer visual reading to listening even if it means they are slower in the overall task. Choice of speech is very much a matter of individual preference.

For speech systems, it is, of course, important to screen for significant hearing loss. If, in a quiet room, a patient who cannot see the practitioner's face (to read lips) cannot fully hear normal conversational volume at 20 in., then this patient may have a moderate hearing loss and an audiologic evaluation should be recommended. It is, however, important not to automatically rule out using a synthetic speech system if a patient has a significant hearing loss. Individuals with impaired hearing should not be expected to have greater difficulty with synthesized speech than with natural speech.[2] Learning to understand computer speech is much like learning to understand a speaker with a foreign accent. Comprehension improves greatly with practice.

There are two components to all computer speech systems: a speech synthesizer and a screen reader. The speech synthesizer translates digital text to speech, much like a printer translates digital text to print. A speech synthesizer requires a piece of hardware that plugs into the computer and a speaker that plugs into the speech synthesizer. A screen reader is a software program that enables the patient to select which portion of the text, displayed on a screen, will be read by the speech synthesizer. An example of using a speech synthesizer and screen reader can be seen with a patient who wishes to enter a certain command into his or her word processing program. As the patient types the command, the screen reader relays each letter typed to the synthesizer, which in turn speaks each letter as it is typed. The patient also has the option of typing the entire word, sentence, or paragraph and then striking a key combination to instruct the synthesizer to read the entered command aloud. Satisfied that the correct command has been typed, the patient strikes the enter key to instruct the word processing program to execute the command. The screen reader can be instructed to read the entire text, some portion of the text, or just the first sentence of the printed material on the monitor screen. The patient is also able to speed up the reading rate or change the voice from male to female using commands to the screen reader. In addition, the patient has the ability to ask the screen reader to pause and spell a word that is not recognized or to have it phonetically pronounced.

Speech Synthesizers

Like a printer or the speakers in a stereo system, the speech synthesizer is an output device. Synthesizers differ considerably in the types of voices, voice pitch, and reading speeds produced, as well as how natural the speech sounds.

Even though speech synthesizers have improved over the years in discerning one word from another, they still do not take context into consideration in deciding how to pronounce a word. For example, when encountering the word *lead*, even the most sophisticated synthesizer might confuse the two potential meanings and pronunciations of this word. With practice, however, the patient, in many cases, can quickly adapt to these mispronunciations, and as mentioned in the preceding section, he or she does have the ability to have the computer spell out the word.

In most cases, the cost of the synthesizer usually correlates with how human the voice sounds. Although no synthesizer has the ability to sound absolutely human in all inflections, the most expensive systems produce speech that is as recognizable as natural speech. One of the most sophisticated synthesizers is used by the telephone company. Newer speech synthesizers, which use multimedia sound cards, correlate well with how the human voice sounds and are becoming relatively inexpensive.

Screen Readers

As with electronic display magnification software, screen reading programs with synthetic speech systems involve two pointers or cursors: a *program cursor* that indicates where text will be typed and a *review cursor*, which indicates where on the screen text will be read. For example, when an individual is typing in a word processing program, the text is inserted at the program cursor. The individual using a screen reader can, with a keystroke, direct the review cursor to the top of the screen (which contains the page number) to have the page number read aloud or direct the review cursor to the beginning of the paragraph to read what was just typed.

Similar to the electronic display magnification systems, vocalization systems have an *automatic review mode* and a *manual review mode*. In automatic review mode, the review cursor can automatically scroll through the text and read at a rate specified by the individual. Screen readers can read line by line (stopping at the end of each line), sentence by sentence, and paragraph by paragraph. In the manual mode, the patient can move the review cursor one word or even one letter at a time.

Problems with Vocalization Systems

The primary problems associated with vocalization systems are their inability to access graphics and a patient's difficulty in navigating an application (orientation on the monitor). Although speech systems are now available that read text displayed in Microsoft Windows or the Macintosh Operating System, the patient may have difficulty finding a particular program to fill a special need. The individual with some functional vision may benefit from combining optical magnification or electronic magnification with vocalization systems using the optical or electronic display magnification to navigate the screen and the speech systems to read longer passages.

Voice Input

The newest of the vocalization devices available to the visually impaired patient is the voice input system. This system allows the patient to speak a command, select an option, or dictate text. The system itself is comprised of a microphone (mounted, clipped, or handheld); software that interprets the tones and translates them to symbols, letters, or commands; and the application software that performs the desired operations for which the input was intended. Voice input systems are rapidly improving in their capabilities. When considering such a system, the patient should pay particular attention to the speed of the system and its reliability, especially as it relates to any extraneous noise that may be in the room when the system is being used.

Braille Display Systems

The choice to use braille is not as uncommon as one might believe. For some patients, braille may not be a primary mode for reading; however, these same patients may choose braille for correspondence because it empowers them with information processing ability that is both quick and accurate. Braille is a language in which a given letter or combination of letters is represented by a specific configuration of dots. For example, the letter *a* is represented by a single dot in the first position of the braille cell. Similarly, the letter combination *st* is represented by another unique configuration of dots. Thus, braille is a kind of shorthand system (see Chapter 13).

Braille can be typed into a computer by use of a braille keyboard. This special keyboard uses only six keys, and each key corresponds to one dot of the braille cell. Thus, by pressing some combination of keys, any letter or letter combination (known as a *contraction*) can be created. Braille involves many contractions, and therefore a word such as *rust*, which contains *st* (a contraction) can be typed into the computer by using only three braille cells.

Braille systems have the capability of translating standard word processing material directly into braille format. In addition, for individuals who are not familiar with braille, written print can be typed into a computer and is automatically converted to braille and read by a visually impaired patient on a braille output device or is embossed (printed) onto braille paper. Braille printers require software that translates the printed signal to the appropriate braille character. A braille output device is a braille display system with "refreshable" braille cells. With a refreshable braille device, a series of braille characters is electromechanically "popped up" along a rubberized rectangular strip. As the visually impaired patient moves his or her finger over the display, the cells of the display are electromechanically "flattened." Once the individual has read the information, the next set of braille cells automatically pop up as the braille output device continues to translate the printed material on the computer.

In the past, one of the major disadvantages of a braille display system was its inability to produce graphics. Software is now available to create tactile graphics by either drawing them or scanning them directly from a book. Once the graphic is stored on the hard drive or disk, it can easily be printed on paper into a tactile representation.

MONITORS

The quality of the monitor can greatly affect the clarity of text. One measure of monitor quality is the dot pitch, or the aperture-grill pitch. *Dot pitch* refers to the distance, measured in millimeters, between pixels. *Pixels* are the number of dots that make up the monitor's image. The more pixels on the screen, the higher the resolution and the more detailed the screen image will be. The smaller the dot pitch, the closer the pixels and the sharper the image. If the dot pitch is too wide, the image will look blocky. A dot pitch size of 0.28 mm is acceptable; a size of 0.26 mm is better. Another factor that determines the quality of the monitor is the vertical display refresh rate, which measures in hertz how quickly screens are painted on the monitor. A refresh rate of 72 Hz is acceptable; a rate of 75 Hz is better. Most individuals are bothered by annoying screen flicker when the refresh rates are at 60 Hz or lower.

Patients with certain visual impairments are sensitive to glare on the monitor, and antiglare treatment of the monitor can help alleviate some of these problems. Some patients may find that the antiglare treatments reduce the brightness of the displays, however. For those monitors without any antiglare treatments, separate filters can be used. Glare and monitor illumination can also be controlled by the brightness, contrast, and color adjustments found on the monitor. The patient's needs can sometimes be met simply by judiciously adjusting these settings.

The display size of the monitor screen can be used as an effective magnifier of print. The most important benefit of using a larger monitor is that the low vision patient can attain greater magnification. For example, when a patient switches from a 14-in. monitor to a 21-in. monitor, he or she is able to achieve an increase in magnification of 1.5× (21/14 = 1.5). Monitors typically are available in 14-in., 15-in., 17-in., 20-in., or 21-in. sizes (diagonally measured) with actual display sizes of approximately 12.7 in., 13.8 in., 15.7 in., 18 in., and 20 in., respectively. As the screen size increases, however, the resolution should be maintained or increased as well. The resolution of the monitor is defined by the number of pixels on the screen. As presented, higher amounts of pixels (more densely spaced pixels) will produce greater resolution and better legibility. Low-density resolution monitors tend to present poor quality characters with background bleeding.

TECHNICAL ASSESSMENT

Evaluating a patient for an assistive computer system may be considered a three-step process: (1) a low vision assessment, (2) a computer specialist's assessment, and (3) instruction. During the low vision assessment, the practitioner, in conjunction with the patient, initially determines if there is a need for an assistive computer system. If a need is established, the low vision practitioner should help to determine the need for optical magnification, electronic display magnification, a speech system, or possibly some combination thereof. If an optical device is involved, the practitioner should determine the appropriate amount of magnification along with the type of device and working distance.

In the computer assessment, the computer specialist should demonstrate and help to configure the complete computer system by recommending specific components that are compatible with one another as well as being compatible with the patient's needs. The recommended computer components should also be based on the low vision practitioner's recommendations and any optical devices that the patient expects to use with the computer system.

The final process in this triad technical assessment program is instruction. The patient should be provided with adequate instruction in the assistive components (e.g., electronic display magnification, telemicroscope) that are required for efficient use of the computer system as well as instruction in the software application program (e.g., word processing program). This service can be provided by various professionals such as rehabilitation teachers, vision rehabilitation therapists, or computer specialists.

Low Vision Assessment

The first step in a low vision assessment is to determine if a patient needs a computer to accomplish his or her goals. In many cases, patients may not have expressed a need for a computer system because they might have thought that they could not use one because of their poor vision, or they might not have been aware that they could benefit from such a system. For example, a patient who wishes to read the newspaper may not know that newspapers can be accessed through the computer via on-line information services. Someone who wishes to write letters can do so more easily on a computer than a typewriter or by hand. Many may not consider computers because of the cost. The patient may not be aware that a school system or employer may be required to supply computers as necessary "reasonable accommodations" under the Americans with Disabilities Act. Practitioners should be knowledgeable of the local, state, and federal services that may benefit low vision patients and should provide this information to the patient when appropriate. (See Chapter 19 for information on local, state, and federal services.)

Recommending the Appropriate System

Once the practitioner has established the need for an assistive computer system, the next step is to determine if an optical device, electronic display magnification program, or vocalization system is required. The purpose of this assessment is to collect information for the patient so that he or she can make an informed decision. Simply demonstrating systems is inadequate for most patients because considerable training is required before they achieve their potential with most computer assistive devices. The low vision assessment, therefore, should enable the practitioner to predict performance potential and provide the patient a feel for what it is like to use such a system. Such predictions of performance could be based on both the patient's performance and measures of visual functioning, such as visual acuity, contrast sensitivity, oculomotor control, and visual fields.

The practitioner can quickly ascertain the probable acceptance of an optical or electronic display magnification system based on a direct performance assessment. Using reading cards (e.g., MNRead or Sloan cards [The Lighthouse, Inc., Long Island City, NY]), the patient is asked to read passages of decreasing size print using his or her customary near spectacles. If fluent reading (smooth, accurate reading at approximately 150 words per minute) is attained with any size print, even as large as 8 M (meter system), then it is very likely that either an optical or screen magnification system would be acceptable. These reading cards can also be used by the practitioner to estimate the required magnification for fluent reading on a computer screen. The amount of magnification is determined by dividing the patient's best reading acuity (recorded in M or point) by 1.6 M or 12 point (the approximate size of computer print on a monitor). For example, if a patient is able to fluently read 6.4 M continuous print then he or she would require 4× magnification to read standard-size computer print on the monitor. The practitioner should also evaluate the patient's contrast sensitivity to determine the need for special illumination, contrast, and glare control. With the preceding information, the practitioner can then demonstrate the appropriate magnifying system to the patient.

A comprehensive review of the basic research literature on vision and reading yields a tentative set of visual requirements for fluent reading.[1] This research was not based on clinical results; however, the following recommendations, in combination with patient performance, should provide the practitioner with a good starting point. The recommendations are based on the assumption that the patient's reading demands mandate fluent reading. Fluent visual reading is possible if the following conditions are met:

1. An optical magnification device or a video display (electronic display magnification) magnifies continuous text print at least two times larger than letter acuity threshold.
2. Video display print contrast is 10 times better than letter contrast threshold.
3. The patient has a central scotoma that is smaller than 8 degrees in diameter.
4. The patient is able to see more than six characters (or letters) at one time on the monitor screen.

Optical and electronic display magnification systems differ in the magnification and contrast enhancement they provide. Given the visual requirements in the preceding list, there is a range of visual acuity, contrast sensitivity, and visual fields in which the patient can fluently read with either an optical or an electronic magnification system. If both assistive systems meet the visual requirements for fluent reading, then there should not be a significant difference in reading rates. When visual acuities and contrast sensitivities are too poor to allow fluent reading with an optical device, electronic display magnification may provide the necessary requirements. With more severe loss in visual acuity and contrast sensitivity, not even the text enhancement characteristics of electronic display magnification are adequate and, therefore, only reading with synthesized speech or braille will be fluent.

With postexudative maculopathy, higher reading rates usually are observed more often with electronic display magnification systems than with optical magnification devices.[2] Patients with advanced maculopathy can read enlarged text with either optical or electronic display magnification, but even with electronic magnification, the reading rate is normally no faster than 100 words per minute and rarely faster than 80 words per minute.[2] Thus, for many patients with low vision, optical and electronic magnification systems can restore the ability to read, but reading may be slow and uncomfortable and well below fluent levels. On the basis of this research, recommendations may be derived to help guide the low vision practitioner toward evaluating and recommending assistive systems for patients (Table 14-1).

Contrast Recommendations
When assessing a patient with low vision for a computer system, contrast and glare problems may be an important factor. Patients with media problems usually perform slightly better with white or yellow letters on a dark background. Those with significantly reduced overall letter contrast sensitivity (worse than 5–10%) would require monitors to be set up with maximum contrast and illumination.

TABLE 14-1
Guide for Evaluating and Recommending Assistive Systems for Patients with Low Vision

Consider optical devices if all of the following conditions are met:
1. Visual acuity is better than 20/200.*
2. Letter contrast threshold is better than 8.5% (see section on contrast sensitivity testing in Chapter 4).
3. Central scotoma is smaller than 8 degrees in diameter.

Consider electronic display magnification systems if one of the following conditions is met:
1. Visual acuity is worse than 20/150.*
2. Letter contrast threshold is worse than 8.5%.
3. Central scotoma is greater than 8 degrees in diameter.

Consider vocalization or braille systems if one of the following conditions is met:
1. Visual acuity is worse than 20/500.*
2. Letter contrast threshold is worse than 10.0%.
3. Central scotoma is greater than 10 degrees in diameter.
4. A field of view with electronic magnification of less than six characters.

*Best visual acuities through conventional lenses.

If reduced contrast sensitivity is due to media problems or cataracts, the patient will be susceptible to glare. Room lighting in combination with the computer screen luminance may create a glare problem. To control room illumination, windows should have appropriate window treatments to prevent too much light from entering the room. Overhead lighting, if possible, should be controlled by a rheostat or have deflectors attached. Lights should neither be in the patient's field of view nor should they be seen as a reflection on a darkened monitor screen. If glare from room illumination is unavoidable, a visor or hood around the monitor or a glare reducing screen that covers the entire monitor screen may be a viable solution. Another possible solution is to change the brightness and contrast of the monitor to enhance the letters on the screen. A final solution may require the computer being moved to an area of the room that has reduced room illumination and glare.

Final Selection Process
Once the visual assessment is complete, it is important that the patient have sufficient time to thoroughly evaluate all of the advantages and disadvantages of the appropriate systems. To evaluate the performance with an optical magnification device, the practitioner should be able to easily adjust monitor distance and height. A monitor stand on an arm is highly recommended and can be purchased from an office furniture supply house. The patient should be seated comfortably, the reading material on the screen should have the appropriate size font, and all glare should be minimized or eliminated. The recommended optical magnification device should be placed on the patient and the required working distance maintained. A reading rate should be taken and the patient should be asked to comment on his or her experience with the device in question. This same procedure should be repeated with all of the optical devices that the practitioner plans on evaluating.

To evaluate an electronic display magnification program the practitioner would require the necessary software. Samples of software can generally be obtained from the manufacturers or local distributors at no charge. Once the software is installed, the patient is seated comfortably at the recommended distance from the monitor (which is sometimes dictated by a patient's reading spectacles). The patient should first be shown different print contrasts on the monitor until a preferred contrast is chosen. He or she is next shown the different magnified font sizes and encouraged to work with the smallest print size that can comfortably be seen. The patient is shown how to control the scrolling speed, pause, and back up when necessary. A reading rate can be easily determined by having the patient read while the text on the monitor is in an automatic review mode. In addition to information on the patient's reading rate, the patient is asked to comment on his or her experience with this system. If the performance is not acceptable, the same procedure should be repeated with different font sizes. To demonstrate reading with a vocalization system, cassette tapes having various forms of synthetic speech can be obtained from a distributor of assistive computer technology or one of the authors of this chapter.

Only after a patient has experienced the various options can the practitioner and patient make a final decision concerning which system is best suited for a patient's visual goals. In some cases, it may be recommended that the patient also be evaluated at an assistive technology center that specializes in evaluating and teaching individuals who are visually impaired to use a computer.

DEVELOPING NECESSARY REFERRALS

Few low vision practices have the resources to provide comprehensive adaptive computer solutions. Practitioners can refer patients to an assistive technology center that has access to equipment and computer specialists who can provide this service. The ideal center will provide all of the following services:

1. Speech and braille systems for those with severe vision loss
2. Electronic display magnification systems
3. Instruction in all assistive technology

The selection of an assistive computer system requires the input of a computer specialist because effective computer-based adaptive technology cannot be purchased "off the shelf." Rather, systems must be tailored to the needs and capabilities of each patient. In addition, specially trained instructors who are familiar with assistive computer technology are needed to instruct patients to use the technology, because it is complicated and requires time to learn to use. Assuming the individual has touch-typing skills and no computer experience, the following in-class instruction time can be expected:

1. 5–50 hours to learn an assistive speech system

2. 3–15 hours to learn a display enhancement system (electronic display magnification)
3. 15 hours to learn how to negotiate the user interface of an online information service

Finding a local assistive technology center often requires some research. The state rehabilitation agency is a good place to start. It will usually have a list of such technology centers, and the state agency may also provide a source of funding for the low vision patient.

Referral for a computer evaluation requires clear and effective communication between the low vision practitioner and the computer specialist. A letter of referral therefore is the critical communication link that helps to determine an overall successful outcome. This letter should clearly provide the patient's goals, explain the patient's visual problems in lay terms and, most important, provide information on necessary optical equipment (e.g., reading lenses with a tint and antireflective coating) that may be required in conjunction with the computer equipment. By suggesting the general type of assistive devices that meets the patient's visual needs (electronic display magnification, vocalization or braille systems), the letter of referral can save the patient and computer specialist several frustrating hours of trial and error with unworkable systems.

A summary of important information that should be included in the referral letter is as follows:

I. Specific tasks the patient wishes to perform
II. Whether electronic display magnification or nonvisual (vocalization or braille) systems (or any combination) are suggested for further exploration with the computer specialist
III. If an optical system has been recommended (to be used in combination with electronic display magnification or vocalization systems) the following should be indicated:
   A. Type of device(s)
   B. Monocular or binocular system (if monocular, which eye)
   C. Working distance
   D. Minimum print size that the patient can see on the screen (inches or centimeters) and the optimum print size for reading
   E. Contrast and lighting requirements
   F. Color preference of characters and background on monitor screen (if it has been assessed by the practitioner)
   G. Need for a reading stand, monitor stand, or other special equipment
   H. The patient's fluency with visual reading. For example, "The reading rate with a 5× reading lens on the right eye was smooth and accurate" or "The reading rate with a 5× reading lens on the right eye was halting and slow with numerous errors." It will also be helpful to mention the actual reading rates with the various devices, if available.
IV. Any central scotoma or field restriction should be described in lay terms. For example, "Mrs. Jones has a blind spot in her central vision approximately the size of a fist at arm's length. Visual targets may disappear if she looks directly at them." Note that the "rule of thumb" is that a thumb nail (2 cm) at arm's length (50 cm) is approximately 2 degrees, while a fist is approximately 5×10 degrees.
V. Other observations about visual function, such as color preference, photophobia, or glare problems, should also be included in the letter.

CONCLUSION

Many practitioners are not aware of the general types of assistive technology that exist for their low vision patients (see Appendix A). Also, in many cases, the patients themselves are unaware that they can benefit from such systems. Although computers are usually associated with those who are employed, such systems should not be ruled out for visually impaired students and adults. On-line information services should become popular among the visually impaired population because shopping; banking; managing retirement portfolios; corresponding and acquiring news, weather, and sports information can be performed easily within the confines of their home. Two factors, however, may discourage use of computers by low vision patients. For individuals with no prior computer experience, assistive systems may appear very complicated and intimidating. Assistive computer systems may also require proficient touch-typing skills. Newer systems, however, are becoming easier to use and some do not even require touch-typing skills.

Because computers will be playing a more integral part in the life of most individuals in the future and because so many low vision patients can benefit from using computer systems, it is imperative that low vision practitioners be aware of the newest assistive technology available. It is equally important that practitioners work closely with other specialists (e.g., computer specialists, rehabilitation teachers) who work with this technology to provide the appropriate recommendations to the patients.

SELF-ASSESSMENT QUESTIONS

1. Which optical device(s) will possibly help a low vision patient read the print on a computer screen?
   (a) a reading spectacle (microscope)
   (b) telemicroscope
   (c) handheld magnifier
   (d) all of the above

2. Which statement(s) is correct when a low vision patient uses electronic display magnification?
   (a) with increased magnification there is a corresponding reduction in the amount of material displayed on the screen at any given time
   (b) there is only a minimum amount of magnification (4×) that may be obtained
   (c) font types cannot be modified
   (d) letter spacing cannot be modified
   (e) a and d

3. A review cursor, in an electronic display magnification program, will indicate what portion of the printed material on the screen is being magnified.
True or False

4. A screen reader is similar to electronic display magnification in that they both have a program cursor and a review cursor.
True or False

5. The following components make up a computer vocalization system:
   (a) screen reader
   (b) speech synthesizer
   (c) scanner
   (d) all of the above
   (e) a and b

6. Braille software systems have the capability of translating written word processing material directly into braille format.
True or False

7. Which of the following is *not* true when using a vocalization system?
   (a) a patient may experience orientation problems on the monitor screen
   (b) all word processing programs are capable of speech output
   (c) the speech may be difficult to understand
   (d) speech systems are not able to access graphics

8. When recommending a monitor for a patient, it is best to recommend the highest dot pitch available because this will provide a sharper image on the screen.
True or False

9. The higher the vertical refresh rate of a computer monitor, the poorer the quality of the image, and the more likely a patient is to notice the annoying screen flicker.
True or False

10. If a low vision patient has a visual acuity of 20/100 through his spectacle lenses, which computer adaptation system should be initially evaluated?
    (a) optical devices
    (b) electronic display magnification system
    (c) vocalization system
    (d) braille display system

REFERENCES

1. Whittaker SG, Lovie-Kitchin J. Visual requirements for reading. Optom Vis Sci 1993;70:54–65.
2. Stelmack J, Reda D, Ahlers S, et al. Reading performance of geriatric patients post exudative maculopathy. J Am Optom Assoc 1991;62:53–57.

Appendix A

RESOURCES TO CONTACT FOR INFORMATION ABOUT AVAILABLE ASSISTIVE TECHNOLOGY COMPUTER SYSTEMS

Note. Most manufacturers and distributors have Web pages. Current Web addresses can be located by entering the name of each agency with the key terms, such as *disability*, and *blindness*, into a Web browser.

AbliTech
Assistive Technology Department
4040 Market St.
Philadelphia, PA 19104
(215) 243-2033

Accextion Information
P.O. Box 700
Bloomington, IL 61702
(309) 378-2961

American Foundation for the Blind
15 W. 16th St.
New York, NY 10011
800-232-5463

Closing the Gap
P.O. Box 68
Henderson, MN 56044
(612) 248-3294

Disability Rights Education and Defense Fund
222 Sixth St.
Berkeley, CA 94710
(415) 644-2555

Human Resources Center
10 Willets Rd.
Albertson, NY 11507
(516) 747-5400

Less Gauss, Inc. (maker of EZ computer magnifier)
187 E. Market St., Suite 160
Rhineback, NY 12572
(914)876-5432

The Trace Center
RM S-151 Waisman Center
1500 Highland Ave.
Madison, WI 53705-2280
(608) 262-6966

CHAPTER FIFTEEN

Driving with Low Vision

Richard L. Brilliant,
Sarah Deborah Appel,
and Bill G. Chapman

Giant strides have been made in the field of low vision rehabilitation. Optical and electronic magnification systems that are routinely prescribed enable the low vision individual to function more effectively and independently at home, school, and work. There is one area, however, that continues to frustrate the visually impaired population. Modern society demands freedom of mobility, and the individual who cannot drive often encounters limitations in vocational and avocational options. At the same time that financial and social independence appear to be realistic goals, visually impaired individuals are denied a vital key to that independence—licensure to drive.

Psychological studies of visually impaired young adults have found that transportation problems were strongly linked with conflicts between dependence and the emergence of independence.[1] Such conflicts are often destructive, impacting negatively on the emerging self-concept of these young adults. Adults who lose driving privileges as a result of acquired vision loss may experience a lowering of self-esteem and a declining level of social status, which often has a major negative impact on the individual's relationship with friends and family members as well as employment-related interactions and issues.[2]

LICENSURE REQUIREMENTS

Driver's licenses are issued to a wide range of physically challenged individuals.[3] Visually impaired individuals, however, are frequently denied licensure due to their inability to satisfy the high visual acuity standards established by regulatory agencies nationwide. This denial of licensure is in spite of studies comparing the driving records of various groups of handicapped drivers that consistently report a favorable ranking of visually impaired drivers.[3] A comparison of accident ratios per hundred drivers conducted by the Texas Medical Advisory Board revealed ratios of 8.50% for drivers with neurologic impairments, 5.63% for drivers with cardiovascular impairments, and 4.86% for drivers with visual impairments.[3]

Although visual acuity standards for an unrestricted license vary, most states require best-corrected visual acuities of 20/40 or better through conventional prescriptions. The recommendation for the minimal standard of 20/40 was made in a report developed by the American Medical Association's Section on Ophthalmology in 1925.[4] More recent reports in the ophthalmic and optometric literature suggest that a 20/20–20/40 level of visual acuity is not as important for safe driving as state laws appear to indicate. Fonda[5] and Weiss[6] maintained that the 20/40 requirement is arbitrary and is not based on actual visual acuity demands while driving. The often heard argument justifying the 20/40 requirement is that all highway signs are calibrated for 20/40 visual acuity. This, however, is not the case. Highway signs vary greatly not only in letter size, but also in contrast, letter style, and spacing between letters. Traffic symbols are more uniform in their size, shape, and color. A visually impaired individual who is familiar with these characteristics can identify the symbols without reading the sign. Fonda[5] maintains that a person with 20/200 daytime visual acuity traveling at 40 mph can recognize a stop sign in sufficient time to react safely.

Traditional visual acuity is a static test. Research by Burg[7] has shown that accident rates have a 10 times higher correlation with dynamic acuity than static acuity (dynamic acuity is measured when the patient is stationary and the targets are moving). When driving, the individual is in relative motion with objects in the visual field. Therefore, one might argue that a dynamic acuity test would be a far better predictor of visual performance while driving. Dynamic acuity, however, is not measured on either normally sighted or low vision drivers.

A survey by the authors of motor vehicle agencies nationwide confirmed that there is no uniformity of vision standards for licensure (Table 15-1). When vision is present in both eyes, visual acuities for unrestricted driving privileges range from 20/40 to 20/70. In cases in which the driver is monocular, visual acuity requirements range from 20/25 to 20/70. A majority of states require the same visual acuity level for drivers with spectacles and those driving without correction. It is interesting, however, that a small number of states differentiate between corrected and uncorrected drivers by specifying that acuity can be worse when corrected. In Texas, for example, it appears that a monocular person may drive with 20/50 acuity with a correction, but must have 20/25 acuity to drive without a correction.

There is a lack of standardization for the issuance of restricted licensure as well (not included in Table 15-1). Fonda[5] listed 17 states that provide restricted licenses to individuals with visual acuities of 20/70 or worse. Seven states provide restricted licenses to individuals with 20/100 acuities. Two states, Missouri and Washington, issue restricted licenses to individuals with visual acuities that are poorer than 20/100.

Feinbloom[8] stated that it is possible for a trained individual to drive safely with visual acuities as low as 20/200. He conducted a study in which 12 normally sighted, experienced drivers were fogged to 20/200 with +3.00 D lenses. Over a 1-week test period, these subjects drove from 1 to 4 hours per day under varied traffic and weather conditions and encountered no driving-related difficulties. They drove at the speed limit in both highway and city environments. Pedestrians, animals, bicyclists, and traffic lights were all reported to be visible. The only problem encountered was the inability to read signs. An important consideration is the difference that exists between a visual system that is fogged by +3.00 D lenses and the visual system of a low vision patient in which in-focus images are only blocked centrally by a hypoplastic or atrophied macula. Peripheral image quality for these low vision individuals is equal in clarity to that of an emmetropic healthy eye, whereas the fogged individual experiences peripheral blur.

Many practitioners have heard of patients with acuities ranging from 20/60 to 20/200 admitting that they are presently driving and experiencing no difficulties seeing other cars and pedestrians or reacting to potential prob-

TABLE 15-1
Vision Standards for Unrestricted Licensure and Use of Telescopic Bioptic Lenses in the United States

State	Visual Acuity (does not include restricted license)				Visual Field			Comments
	Both Eyes without Glasses	Both Eyes with Glasses	One Blind Eye without Glasses	One Blind Eye with Glasses	Left Eye (degrees)	Right Eye (degrees)	Both Eyes (degrees)	
Alabama	20/70	20/70	20/60	20/60	NS	NS	NS	Telescopes not recognized. Individually evaluated by Medical Advisory Board (ABCD[1]).
Alaska	20/40	20/40	20/40	20/40	NS	NS	NS	Allows telescope lenses: 20/40 through telescope; 60–90% field (ABCD[1]).
Arizona	20/40	20/40	20/40	20/40	NS	NS	NS	Does not permit use of telescopes.
Arkansas	20/40	20/50	20/30	20/40	NS	NS	110	NS—Individually evaluated by Medical Advisory Board (ABCD[1]).
California	20/40	20/40	20/40	20/40	NS	NS	NS	Allows bioptic telescopes: 20/40 through telescope; 75-degree lateral field in each eye (ABCD[1]).
Colorado	20/40	20/40	20/40	20/40	NS	NS	NS	Allows bioptic telescopes: 20/40 through telescope; 20/100 through carrier (ABCD[2]).
Connecticut	20/40	20/40	20/30	20/30	NS	NS	NS	Does not permit use of telescopes (ABCD[2]).
Delaware	20/40	20/40	20/40	20/40	NS	NS	NS	Allows bioptic telescopes: 20/40 through telescope (ABCD[1]).
District of Columbia	20/40	20/40	20/40	20/40	NS	NS	130	NS—Individually evaluated by Medical Advisory Board (ABCD[1]).
Florida	20/70	20/70	20/40	20/40	NS	NS	140	Does not permit use of telescopes.
Georgia	20/60	20/60	20/60	20/60	140	140	140	NS—Individually evaluated by Medical Advisory Board (ABCD[1]).
Hawaii	20/40	20/40	20/40	20/40	70	70	140	NS—Individually evaluated by Medical Advisory Board (ABCD[1]).
Idaho	20/40	20/40	20/40	20/40	NS	NS	NS	NS—Individually evaluated by Medical Advisory Board (ABCD[1]).
Illinois	20/40	20/40	20/40	20/40	70	70	140	Allows bioptic telescopes: 20/40 through telescope; 20/100 through carrier (up to 3x telescope only); 140-degree binocular field; 105-degree monocular field (ABCD[1]).
Indiana	20/40	20/50	20/30	20/50	NS	NS	NS	Does not permit use of telescopes (ABCD[1]).
Iowa	20/70	20/70	20/70	20/70	NS	NS	NS	Does not permit use of telescopes (ABCD[1]).
Kansas	20/45	20/45	20/30	20/30	NS	NS	NS	Does not permit use of telescopes (ABCD[1]).
Kentucky	20/45	20/45	20/33	20/33	NS	NS	NS	Does not permit use of telescopes (ABCD[1]).
Louisiana	20/40	20/40	20/40	20/40	NS	NS	NS	"Telescopic lenses are treated same as other corrective lenses"*—20/40 with telescope (ABCD[2]).
Maine	20/40	20/40	20/40	20/40	NS	NS	130	No longer allows the use of a telescope.
Maryland	20/40	20/40	20/40	20/40	140	140	140	Allows bioptic telescopes: 20/100 through carrier lens; 20/70 through telescope. 150-degree binocular field; 100-degree monocular field (ABCD[1]).
Massachusetts	20/40	20/40	20/40	20/40	90	90	120	Allows bioptic telescopes: 20/40 through telescopic lens (ABCD[1]).
Michigan	20/40	20/40	20/40	20/40	NS	NS	110	Allows bioptic telescopes: 20/40 through telescopic lens (ABCD[1]).
Minnesota	20/40	20/40	20/40	20/40	NS	NS	NS	Does not permit use of telescopes (ABCD[2]).
Mississippi	20/40	20/40	20/30	20/30	60	60	120	Does not permit use of telescopes.
Missouri	20/40	20/40	20/40	20/40	NS	NS	NS	Allows bioptic telescopes: 20/160 through carrier lens; 20/40 through telescope (ABCD[1]).
Montana	20/40	20/40	20/40	20/40	NS	NS	NS	Allows bioptic telescopes: 20/160 through carrier lens; 20/40 through telescope (ABCD[1]).
Nebraska	20/40	20/40	20/40	20/40	70 degrees temporal	70 degrees temporal	140	Does not permit use of telescopes (ABCD[1]).
Nevada	20/40	20/40	20/30	20/30	NS	NS	NS	Allows bioptic telescopes: 20/120 through carrier lens; 20/40 through telescope; 130-degree field of view (ABCD[1]).
New Hampshire	20/40	20/40	20/30	20/30	NS	NS	NS	NS—Individually evaluated by Medical Advisory Board (ABCD[1]).
New Jersey	20/50	20/50	20/50	20/50	NS	NS	NS	Allows bioptic telescopes: 20/50 through telescope.
New Mexico	20/40	20/40	20/40	20/40	NS	NS	140	Does not permit use of telescopes (ABCD[1]).
New York	20/40	20/40	20/40	20/40	NS	NS	NS	Allows bioptic telescopes: 20/100 through carrier; 20/40 through telescope (ABCD[1]).

Continued

TABLE 15-1
Continued

State	Visual Acuity (does not include restricted license)				Visual Field			Comments
	Both Eyes without Glasses	Both Eyes with Glasses	One Blind Eye without Glasses	One Blind Eye with Glasses	Left Eye (degrees)	Right Eye (degrees)	Both Eyes (degrees)	
North Carolina	20/40	20/50	20/30	20/40	NS	NS	70	NS (ABCD[2]).
North Dakota	20/40	20/40	20/30	20/40	NS	NS	NS	Allows bioptic telescopes: 20/40 through telescope; 20/130 through carrier. Full peripheral fields (ABCD[1]).
Ohio	20/40	20/40	20/30	20/30	70	70	NS	Does not permit use of telescopes (ABCD[1]).
Oklahoma	20/40	20/60	20/30	20/50	NS	NS	NS	Does not permit use of telescopes.
Oregon	20/40	20/40	20/40	20/40	NS	NS	110	Does not permit use of telescopes (ABCD[1]).
Pennsylvania	20/40	20/60	20/40	20/60	NS	NS	NS	Does not permit use of telescopes.
Rhode Island	20/40	20/40	20/40	20/40	115	115	115	NS.
South Carolina	20/40	20/40	20/40	20/40	NS	NS	NS	NS—Individually evaluated by Medical Advisory Board.
South Dakota	20/40	20/40	20/40	20/40	NS	NS	NS	NS—Individually evaluated by Medical Advisory Board (ABCD[1]).
Tennessee	20/70	20/70	20/40	20/40	NS	NS	NS	Allows bioptic telescopes: 20/200 in carrier lens (must be binocular); 20/60 through telescope (up to 4x telescope); 150-degree field.
Texas	20/40	20/50	20/25	20/50	NS	NS	NS	Allows bioptic telescopes (ABCD[1]).
Utah	20/40	20/40	20/30	20/30	NS	NS	NS	Does not permit use of telescopes (ABCD[2]).
Vermont	20/40	20/40	20/40	20/40	60	60	120	Allows bioptic telescopes: 20/100 through carrier lens; 20/40 through telescopes (ABCD[1]).
Virginia	20/40	20/40	20/40	20/40	100	100	100	Allows bioptic telescopes: 20/200 through carrier lens; 20/70 through telescope; 70-degree field (ABCD[1]).
Washington	20/40	20/40	20/40	20/40	NS	NS	140	Does not permit use of telescopes.
West Virginia	20/40	20/40	20/40	20/40	NS	NS	NS	NS—Individually evaluated by Medical Advisory Board (ABCD[1]).
Wisconsin	20/40	20/40	20/30	20/30	70	70	140	Does not permit use of telescopes.
Wyoming	20/40	20/40	20/40	20/40	NS	NS	NS	NS—Individually evaluated by Medical Advisory Board (ABCD[1]).

*Quote from motor vehicle agent at the Louisiana motor vehicle agency.

NS = not specified; (ABCD[1]) = American Bioptics Certified Drivers Association reports the use of bioptics for driving is officially sanctioned by state; (ABCD[2]) = American Bioptics Certified Drivers Association reports the use of bioptics for driving is unofficially sanctioned by state.

lem situations quickly enough to avoid accidents. These responses are in line with Kelleher's observation that a 4-ft child at 1,200 ft subtends a visual angle greater than 20/200. As in Feinbloom's study, the main difficulty that these individuals encounter consistently is their inability to read road signs and see street lights.

There are no laws in any state prohibiting driving during weather conditions resulting in poor visibility such as heavy rain and fog. The normally sighted driver often functions under these conditions with a more significant impairment than that of many low vision individuals who are denied licensure to drive during "normal" weather conditions. By electing not to prohibit driving under these conditions, the motor vehicle agencies recognize that proper defensive driving strategies minimize the risk of accidents even under conditions of extremely poor visibility.

In addition to the wide range of visual acuity requirements, there is an even wider disparity in visual field requirements. From Table 15-1, it is interesting to note that 58% of motor vehicle agencies do not specify visual field requirements for driving. Of the remaining states, 40% require binocular fields ranging from 110 to 140 degrees and one state requires a binocular field of only 70 degrees. This lack of emphasis on testing of the peripheral field area is disturbing in light of the fact that one of the most important functions of peripheral vision when driving is motion detection. In fact, objects that are three to 10 times smaller than those resolved by the fovea can be detected in the periphery through motion. Retaining an intact peripheral field is essential for safe driving.[9]

A selection process is certainly necessary to eliminate those who are incapable of visually adapting to the stringent demands placed on drivers. Most agencies, however, fail to take into account important information about the nature of the visual impairment in their determination of what constitutes an acceptable candidate for licensure. Low vision individuals with stable ocular conditions unaccompanied by any peripheral field limitations may be good candidates for driving. Ocular disorders, such as albinism, rod and blue cone monochromatism, aniridia, and congenital nystagmus, tend to be nonprogressive and generally have no accompanying visual field defects. Individuals with vision loss related to macular degeneration may also be good candidates, depending on the extent of their central scotoma and the stability of the condition, as well as the efficiency of their eccentric viewing skills.

Table 15-1 indicates that a number of motor vehicle agencies allow for the licensure of visually impaired drivers. Twelve states permit unrestricted driving with visual acuities ranging from 20/45 to 20/70. Sixteen states presently permit driving with bioptic telescopes and eight states will permit testing on a per-case basis. Other surveys indicate higher numbers. (For example, the American Bioptic Certified Drivers Association [ABCD] provides an information sheet that indicates that 28 states officially sanction the use of bioptic telescopes for driving and seven states unofficially permit the use of telescopes for driving. See Appendix 19B for the address and phone number of ABCD and to obtain updated information.)

TELESCOPIC DEVICES AND DRIVING

Telescopic devices have been an integral part of the low vision armament of optical devices. They are routinely prescribed to improve the distance visual efficiency of individuals with low vision. Full-diameter telescopic devices, through which the individual looks full time, exhibit too many disadvantages to allow their use during driving. Problems, including apparent nearness, magnification, increased apparent motion, and restrictions of field, make it impossible to use a full-diameter system for full-time use while driving.

The bioptic telescopic spectacle was first developed by Dr. William Feinbloom to enable the low vision individual to use telescopes for full-time use. The bioptic is essentially a dual optical system in which a telescope is mounted superiorly in a standard prescriptive carrier lens. Objects are readily localized in the unmagnified field (carrier lens) below the telescope. By slight movement of the eyes and head the individual can change fixation and locate the magnified image of the desired object within the telescopic portion of the system (Figure 15-1). The low vision driver spends a majority of the time viewing the environment through the nonmagnified carrier lens. The telescope is only used when it becomes necessary to read signs or achieve enhanced resolution of a distant visual target.

The early telescopic bioptics consisted of afocal Galilean systems of 2.2×, 3.0×, and 4.0× magnification (see Figure 9-B4). Although the magnification of these devices resulted in increased visual discrimination for the low vision driver, the field of view was compromised due to the optical characteristics of the Galilean telescope. A majority of critics that discuss the negative impact of the restricted field of view of bioptic telescopes on driving only refer to the early Galilean telescopic devices.[3, 10–12] In the mid 1970s, Feinbloom developed a Keplerian "camera lens" system that exhibited several significant advantages over the Galilean bioptics. These telescopic units (see Figure 15-1) are focusable, available in magnifications ranging from 2.0× to 10.0×, and have a larger field of view and smaller ring scotoma than Galilean devices of equivalent magnifications.

The use of bioptics for driving was not implemented until 1969.[13] At that time, Korb[14] selected 32 out of 67 low vision individuals who failed to meet visual acuity requirements set by the Department of Motor Vehicles of Massachusetts. These individuals received extensive training in the use of the bioptic device and 26 ultimately obtained driver's licenses. Korb reported that the 26 individuals, driving with bioptics, compiled a record of 32 man-years of automobile operation without any incidents.

A great deal of controversy has surrounded the issue of driving with bioptic telescopic devices since the initial licensure of visually impaired drivers. Advocates and critics of driving with bioptic telescopes present their cases with equal fervor, which is not surprising in light of the impact that this issue has on freedom of mobility for the visually impaired individual and the perceived threat to the public welfare.

Those who oppose the use of bioptic telescopic systems for driving have cited several criticisms that they believe

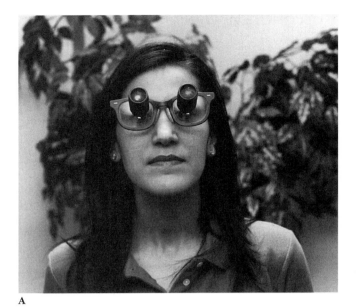
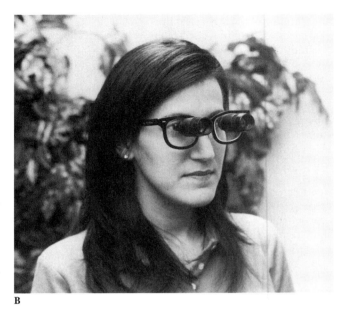

A   B

FIGURE 15-1.   A. The low vision driver spends a majority of the time (approximately 90%) looking through the carrier lens when driving. B. When the low vision driver wishes to read a street sign or see a traffic light from a great distance, he or she looks through the telescope for a short period (similar to the time taken to view through the rearview mirror of the car). The telescope is also very helpful to the driver when viewing distant traffic patterns or traffic flow. This patient is using a Keplerian camera lens bioptic telescope.

render the system dangerous and impractical for driving tasks.[10–12] Critics often point to the restrictions in field of view and ring scotomas that are created while viewing through a telescope. These ring scotomas are experienced while viewing through a binocularly mounted telescope. Advocates of driving with bioptics, however, maintain that when the bioptic telescopic device is used correctly, the ring scotoma is generally never experienced. If it is, however, it is only experienced for the brief period that is necessary to execute a spotting task.[8] They relate the effect of such scotomas to those that are created when a driver looks through a rearview mirror, a frequent monitoring action vital for safe driving.

Another criticism is the "Jack-in-the-box effect." This effect is created when the driver is spotting through the telescope and an automobile passes from the field of the carrier into the field of the telescope. The perceived effect is that of a car suddenly appearing and moving at great speed into the driver's central field. Critics maintain that errors in judgment are possible because magnified images appear to be closer and these objects appear to move faster.[10] Proponents think that proper monitoring of rear view and side view mirrors alert the driver to an approaching automobile, thereby greatly reducing the startling effect of its sudden appearance.[8, 14] They further argue that the visually impaired driver can adapt to any magnification-induced perceptual difficulties, such as objects appearing to be closer with increased apparent motion, in the same way that drivers adapt to the reversal and minification of mirror systems routinely used while driving.

Several other factors should also be considered when evaluating the safety of driving with bioptic telescopic devices. Visual acuities that are measured with a telescope in clinical practice may not realistically represent actual acuity while driving. Image instability induced by vibrations while driving may significantly reduce acuity below static measurements.[15] Clinical observations demonstrate that this effect increases in significance as the magnification of the telescope is increased. Another consideration is the amount of time needed to shift fixation from the carrier lens to the telescope. Clinical observations as well as preliminary clinical trials demonstrate that significant variability exists in such changes in fixation, depending on the design and magnification of the bioptic telescopic system. In addition, subject-related factors, such as reaction time, overall physical and cognitive condition, and size and configuration of central scotomas, may result in an increase in the time needed for changing fixation.

Advocates of the use of bioptic telescopic devices for driving agree that proper adaptation to the bioptic telescopic device is essential to its appropriate use while driving. An instructional sequence concentrating on proper scanning and localization through the bioptic telescope as well as rapid changes in fixation between the carrier lens and telescopic device is essential. Additionally, a driver's training program that teaches visually impaired drivers to drive while using a telescope would also significantly improve the prognosis for safe driving practices.[8, 16] Such programs are presently available in West Virginia and New York. (See Appendix A for an outline of a driver training program.)

It is recognized that the issue of licensure of visually impaired individuals is both complex and controversial. A number of areas should be further explored, however, before any final conclusions can be drawn. Studies involving the effect of contrast sensitivity, dynamic acuity, and visual fields on safe driving could provide essential information. Ironically, the usefulness and importance of proper usage of peripheral fields of view, which are useful in approximately 90% of the total driving time, are underestimated and often not included in the visual screening as part of the driver's license application process. Other factors specifically related to visually impaired drivers, such as efficiency of blur interpretation; the effects of central scotoma size, density, configuration; efficiency of eccentric viewing skills; and photostress-related issues, also should be evaluated. Additionally, research evaluating the necessary reaction time for safe driving and the effect of various levels of visual impairments on reaction time would assist motor vehicle agencies in establishing more realistic visual criteria for licensure.

This information is necessary to adequately evaluate driving with telescopic devices. Telescope-related factors, such as vibration induced image instability, duration of carrier to telescope fixation changes, and the effects of telescope-induced ring scotomas and Jack-in-the-box phenomena, should be evaluated. Research should also include evaluation of the effectiveness of presently available bioptic telescopic devices for driving, with recommendations for modification of these systems. The results of these studies would be invaluable in designing and administering an individualized evaluation and instructional program geared toward the special needs of the visually impaired driver.

CONCEPTS AND TECHNIQUES IN BIOPTIC DRIVING

Most low vision patients receive little or no instruction on how to use their bioptic telescopes for driving. This lack of instruction results in drivers who may lack confidence in their abilities, therefore imposing restrictions on where or when they will drive.

The most important concept that must be emphasized is that the patient is not viewing through the telescopic portion of the spectacles at all times. As a matter of fact, the telescope is used only 10% of the time by the driver; the rest of the time he or she is looking through the carrier lens. The main use of the telescope, in addition to seeing street lights and road signs, is aiding the partially sighted driver to survey conditions at a distance. There are two techniques that help accomplish this task through the telescope: scanning and spotting.

Scanning

Scanning through a telescope is probably the most difficult technique that the visually impaired driver must master. This technique allows the driver to inspect the traffic conditions at a distance (approximately 100 yd or more) that could not be seen without the telescope. In other words, the purpose of the scanning movement is to identify situations or hazards that the driver should be aware of while driving. Although the scanning technique allows the driver to ascertain whether there is an object or hazard in the distance, spotting helps to identify that object.

Spotting

It is vitally important for the partially sighted driver to thoroughly master spotting. Learning to "hit" a given target immediately without any searching takes practice, but this skill must be acquired if one is to drive safely. To spot an object, the driver initially localizes the object (while looking through the carrier lens), then drops his or her head straight down while moving his or her eyes up to align the telescope on the object. Once the object is identified through the telescope, the driver raises his or her head to move the telescope out of the way and to continue viewing through the carrier lens. This entire spotting movement should be executed within one-half of a second. Every sign, when first identified by the scanning technique, is an "unknown," because it is too far away to be read. A few seconds later, however, the sign is spotted and read because the visually impaired driver will have a visual acuity through his or her telescope equivalent to that of a "fully sighted" driver.

The difficulty of driving on a given street relates to three variables: "object vision," "visual clutter," and speed.

Object Vision
When driving, objects do not always have to be identified to drive safely. For example, if a visually impaired driver sees an object roll onto the street, it does not matter whether it is a baseball, tennis ball, or football, the driver should be prepared for a child to follow that ball onto the street. In other words, to drive safely the driver must have "object vision" (not "detail vision"). An exception to "object vision" is when the driver must read street or highway signs.

Visual Clutter
Visual clutter occurs when unimportant objects interfere with those objects that must be identified to drive safely. For example, as one drives down a street, telephone poles or trees may interfere with the process of identifying important objects such as street signs and street lights.

Speed
To control both "object vision" and "visual clutter," the driver should reduce the speed at which he or she is traveling. It is not necessary to slow one's speed so much that the driver becomes a hazard to other traffic, but reducing speed by 5–10 mph below the speed limit will provide the necessary speed to master "visual clutter" and "object vision."

With all of these variables in mind, it becomes obvious that it is far easier to drive familiar streets than it is to drive in unknown areas.

Before providing an instructional program for the visually impaired driver, one final situation should be addressed. The average user of the bioptic telescope cannot read the speedometer. In most cases, the needle of the speedometer can be seen, but the number indicating the actual speed cannot be read. (If the needle cannot be seen, a speedometer repair shop can sometimes fit the system with a wider needle. Another solution may be painting the needle in a color that creates more contrast, thus making it easier to see.) There are a few solutions to this problem:

1. The patient can memorize the position of the numbers on the dial by initially viewing it with a magnifier. For example, the needle pointing to the 9 o'clock position may indicate a speed of approximately 30 mph, and the 12 o'clock position would indicate 60 mph.

2. The patient can paint a line or mark on the protective covering of the speedometer indicating various speeds. One line, at the appropriate position, would indicate 30 mph, whereas another line further up on the dial might indicate 45 mph.

3. During highway driving in some cars, the cruise control can be preset to a desired speed.

4. On some cars, the speedometer has electronic digits that may be easier to read than the standard system. For those visually impaired drivers who are unable to see the standard speedometer, it may be in their best interest to purchase a car with an electronic digit speedometer.

5. A reading cap, set for the appropriate distance, can be slipped over the front of the telescope. This may be hazardous as the telescope is not available for distant viewing at that time; however, the reading cap does provide the advantage of being used to read other gauges on the dashboard as well. With the advent of the Ocutech Autofocus (Ocutech, Inc., Chapel Hill, NC) telescope (see Chapter 9, Appendix B), the problem of seeing near or intermediate objects, such as the odometer or radio dial, as well as distance objects may be eliminated.

SELF-ASSESSMENT QUESTIONS

1. The minimal standard acuity of 20/40 to drive with an unrestricted license is based on the fact that all highway signs are calibrated for 20/40 acuity.
   True or False

2. Having an intact peripheral field is essential for driving.
   True or False

3. Which low vision patient would most likely experience the *most difficulty* in driving with city traffic?
   (a) a patient with congenital nystagmus
   (b) a patient with ocular albinism
   (c) a patient with advanced glaucoma
   (d) a patient with blue cone monochromatism
   (e) a and d

4. Which optical device is recommended for low vision patients who are permitted to drive in some states?
   (a) a full-diameter telescope
   (b) a handheld telescope
   (c) a bifocal telescope
   (d) a bioptic telescope
   (e) a and d

5. When using a low vision device for driving, the majority of the time (approximately 90%), the patient is viewing through the spectacle (carrier) lens.
   True or False

6. When a low vision patient uses a low vision device for driving, he or she must perfect the following technique(s):
   (a) scanning
   (b) stratifying
   (c) spotting
   (d) all of the above are correct
   (e) a and c

7. When a low vision patient who is driving looks into a rearview mirror to see cars far behind him or her, he or she should be using the telescopic portion in conjunction with the mirror.
   True or False

REFERENCES

1. Mehr EB, Fried AN. Low Vision Care. Chicago: Professional Press, 1975.
2. Mehr HM, Mehr EB, Ault C. Psychological aspects of low vision rehabilitation. Am J Optom Physiol Opt 1970;47:605–612.
3. Lippmann O, Corn AL, Lewis MC. Bioptic telescopic spectacles and driving performance: a study in Texas. J Vis Impair Blindness 1988;82:182–187.
4. Keeney AH. The visually impaired driver. Am J Ophthalmol 1976;82:799–801.
5. Fonda G. Legal blindness can be compatible with safe driving. Ophthalmology 1989;96:1457–1459.
6. Weiss N. The visually impaired driver in New York state. J Vis Impair Blindness 1979;73:228–232.
7. Burg A. Vision and driving, a report on research. Hum Factors 1971;13:79–87.
8. Feinbloom W. Driving with bioptic telescopic spectacles. Am J Optom Physiol Opt 1977;54:35–41.
9. Kelleher DK. Driving with low vision. J Vis Impair Blindness 1979;73:345–350.
10. Johnson CA, Keltner JL. Incidence of visual field loss in 20,000 eyes and its relationship to driving performance. Arch Ophthalmol 1983;101:371–375.
11. Fonda G. Bioptic telescopic spectacles for driving a motor vehicle. Arch Ophthalmol 1974;92:348–349.
12. Keeney AH, Weiss S, Silva D. Functional problems of telescopic spectacles in the driving task. Trans Am Ophthalmol Soc 1974; 72:132–138.
13. Keller JT, Eskridge JB. Telescopic lenses and driving. Am J Optom Physiol Opt 1976;53:746–749.
14. Korb DR. Preparing the visually handicapped person for motor vehicle operation. Am J Optom Physiol Opt 1970;47:619–628.
15. Kelleher DK. Driving with Low Vision from a Patient's Perspective. Read at the Annual Meeting of the American Academy of Optometry, December 14, 1975.
16. Keeney AH. Driving at high risk! The Sightsaving Review 1979; 48:167–174.

Appendix A

DRIVER TRAINING PROGRAM

I. Target practice
   A. From a stationary position, learn to spot stationary targets:
      1. The driver should locate the target through the carrier lens, then drop his or her head while moving eyes upward to spot through the telescope. Once the target is identified, the driver moves his or her head back to the original position (maintaining fixation through the carrier lens).
      2. The driver works for accuracy first, then speed.
      3. This spotting speed should be accomplished within one-half of a second on a consistent basis.
   B. From a stationary position, spot and track moving targets:
      1. The driver should spot a moving target through the telescope and follow (track) it as it moves through the environment.
      2. It should be observed that the closer the target, the faster the driver must move his or her head to get the target within the field of the telescope.
II. In-car training (as a passenger)
   A. From a moving car, the patient should spot stationary targets.
   B. From a moving car, the patient should spot and track moving targets.
III. In-car training (as a driver)
   A. First driving experience should be on a four-lane, controlled-access highway (having no cross traffic or stoplights) because this is the easiest on which to drive in terms of "object vision" and "visual clutter":
      1. The driver should know in advance where to exit.
      2. The driver must learn to identify, but not necessarily read, every sign that is passed.
      3. The driver must learn to make scanning movements with the telescope to view traffic conditions approximately 1 mi. ahead. This scanning movement should occur three to six times per minute.
      4. The driver should begin to use the mirror to keep track of traffic to the side and behind. When spotting objects far behind, he or she should use the telescope in conjunction with the mirror. For objects close behind, the carrier and the mirror should suffice.
   B. Driving the residential street (25–30 mph zone)
      1. This type of street has a lot of visual clutter; however, the speed is slow enough to allow time to see and identify everything.
      2. The driver must use good scanning movements, sweeping to both sides of the street.

      3. The driver must be alert because he or she is most likely going to encounter pedestrians, pets, and children playing.
   C. Driving the major traffic artery (45–65 mph zone)
      1. The speed is faster with less visual clutter.
      2. The driver should *initially* use a familiar road, knowing where to exit and avoiding rush hour.
      3. The driver should never let the speed drop to a point more then 10 mph below the posted speed limit (with free-moving traffic).
   D. Driving the residential street (30–45 mph zone)
      1. Speed once again drops as visual clutter increases.
      2. The particular street and time of day should be carefully determined so as not to encounter school buses picking up or dropping off children.
   E. Driving downtown rush-hour traffic (bumper-to-bumper traffic: ≤30 mph)
      1. There is a psychological barrier that must be overcome at this stage, and that is the belief that heavy traffic makes driving more difficult.
      2. The route should initially be familiar and pre-planned.
      3. The driver should initially stay in the right lane at all times.
      4. If the driver is first in line at a light, he should point the telescope at the proper light, wait for the light to change, then check through the carrier lens for pedestrians and cars possibly crossing his or her space (cars making a turn or cars attempting to beat the light) before continuing on.
      5. The driver should never move close enough to the car in front that he or she loses sight of its rear tires (tailgating).
   F. Driving the commercial street or business district (30–45 mph zone)
      1. These streets are generally the most difficult to drive because there is a lot of visual clutter with many things to identify (e.g., street lights, pedestrians, cars pulling in and out of parking spots)
      2. The driver should carefully pick the street and time of day, initially avoiding rush hour and streets with heavy traffic.
   G. Driving on a variety of streets and highways
      1. Up until this point, only one type of roadway had been driven on at one time. There is a mental set associated with each driving condition. This step requires a mental shift as well as a shift in using the telescope.
      2. Initially, potential trouble spots should be anticipated beforehand and avoided.
   H. Driving the four-lane highway:
      1. This highway has cross traffic and traffic lights.
      2. Scanning is one of the most important techniques used on this type of roadway.

I. Driving the two-lane highway
   1. This highway typically has narrow shoulders and follows the contour of the land.
   2. When passing another car, the driver should judge the distance of the car in front through the carrier lens and use the telescope to spot up ahead to determine if it is clear to pass.
   3. When passing, the driver should continue to view through the carrier lenses. Every second or two, however, he or she should spot through the telescope to check oncoming traffic.

J. Driving the city freeway (many states that permit low vision patients to drive have a restriction on city driving)
   1. This roadway usually has very little visual clutter; however, there are a lot of things to identify.
   2. This type of roadway also has a psychological barrier associated with it that must be overcome: the fear of drivers going from lane to lane jockeying for position.
   3. Tailgating is also common, and defensive driving is a must.

CHAPTER SIXTEEN

Low Vision Special Populations I: The Multiply Impaired Patient

Elise B. Ciner,
Sarah Deborah Appel,
and Marcy Graboyes

In 1977, there were 29,403 school-age individuals registered with the American Printing House for the Blind. In less than a decade (1977–1984), that number increased approximately 50% to 44,313.[1] This trend, which continues today, is due at least in part to the enormous medical advances made in prenatal care, enabling the survival of very young or very sick premature infants. The literature abounds with reports of pediatric syndromes that have associated ocular abnormalities. Intrauterine infections, such as rubella, syphilis, and cytomegalovirus, are frequently associated with significant levels of visual impairment. Syndromes, such as Down, Hallermann-Streiff, and Laurence-Moon-Biedl, and Crouzon's disease present with a host of ocular disorders. Although infants with these syndromes survive, they often exhibit lifelong handicapping conditions, such as hearing loss, cerebral palsy, and learning disabilities along with frequent severe visual impairment. This trend of increasing numbers of multiply handicapped infants and young individuals is not likely to reverse in the near future.

Evaluating the visual functioning of severely disabled individuals and partially sighted infants has long been a source of frustration for many eye care practitioners. A reflection of this difficulty is seen in the number of multiply handicapped patients who are labeled *untestable* or *blind* by eye care practitioners, although parents, teachers, and caregivers report that these patients appear to have some residual vision. This difference of opinion has led to three undesirable outcomes:

1. Rehabilitation professionals and special educators who distrust the information contained in reports from eye care practitioners and who then overlook even the valuable, valid information contained in them.
2. Parents, educators, and rehabilitation personnel who are confused by the conflict in their informal assessment of the individual's vision and the formal assessment of the eye care practitioner, and who therefore often develop inconsistent rehabilitation and educational programs.
3. Parents, teachers, and other rehabilitation professionals who accept the judgment of the eye care specialists and ignore the potential of the individual's residual vision.

All three of these outcomes result in decreased learning potential and quality of life for the special needs individual.

Serious visual impairment is often a significant component of multiply handicapping conditions affecting individuals. A problem professionals still face today is how to reliably and validly test visual ability in these individuals. These special needs individuals may not be responsive to standard testing procedures for a variety of reasons.[2] Stress-related behaviors, orthopedic and neuromuscular disorders, mental retardation, and preverbal levels of development often greatly interfere with communication and cooperation levels.

As parents, educators, and rehabilitation professionals have become aware of the importance of vision in the development of any individual, the demand for comprehensive functional vision evaluations has substantially increased. The goal of a functional vision evaluation is to treat each individual holistically, taking into consideration a wide variety of factors extending beyond visual functioning. The interdisciplinary approach, however, may not always be feasible, especially for the private practitioner. It is therefore important for eye care specialists to formulate their own examination procedures and provide a framework from which comprehensive services can be delivered in conjunction with available community resources.

INFORMATION GATHERING

To ensure a holistic approach in the evaluation of the special needs individual, information should be compiled from a variety of sources. The assessment process should ideally begin before the actual office visit. An information packet may be sent to the individual or agency requesting the evaluation. The purpose of this packet is severalfold:

1. It provides the family with a better understanding of services and their application to the patient.
2. It attempts to stimulate thought on the part of the family or significant others as well as other professionals working with the patient (e.g., eye care practitioner, teacher, rehabilitation specialist, occupational therapist) regarding the use or potential of vision in different environments.
3. It provides the evaluator(s) with valuable information that assists in screening potential candidates and meeting any special needs throughout the evaluation sequence.

Three forms may be included in an information packet:

1. *Background data.* The background data form is designed to discern how an individual is functioning visually from the perspective of the primary caregiver (e.g., parent, other relative, day care worker). Questions regarding understanding of diagnosis, reaction to light and other sensory stimuli, and level of expressive and receptive communication serve as a guide in the initial determination of how the individual may be using vision. The form also provides the primary caregiver with an opportunity to list questions or concerns regarding the use of vision, previous diagnosis, and expectations from the evaluation.

2. *Eye care data.* Eye care information should ideally be provided by previous or current eye care providers. Baseline data, such as diagnosis, visual acuities, refraction, and fields, are requested. Frequently, the information provided is limited due to the special needs individual's inability to respond to conventional testing.

3. *Educator's checklist.* The last piece of information is collected for individuals who are currently in an educational or workshop setting. It is to be completed by the individual's teacher, rehabilitation specialist (i.e. physical, occupational, or speech therapist) or other professionals involved in the individual's care. Questions include commenting on unusual visual postures, illumination prob-

lems, use of previously prescribed lenses or aides, and the type of setting(s) in which the individual is involved. Any other sources of information should be explored, and all professionals should be encouraged to express questions, concerns, and frustrations regarding the individual's use of vision and how this might affect the achievement of learning or working potential.

Patient History and Observation

The history is designed to collect pertinent information regarding visual and medical history as well as observed levels of visual and other sensory functioning. Information is also obtained on current education or vocational status and daily living skills. The history should include goal setting so that the evaluation addresses the specific needs and concerns of the patient. In addition to the patient and family, any accompanying professionals should be strongly encouraged to participate in this phase as well as throughout the entire evaluation, thus becoming an integral part of the interdisciplinary team.

General Medical History

Background information concerning the patient's systemic and ocular history is collected. Conditions, such as Down syndrome, hydrocephalus, cerebral palsy, and rubella, are frequently encountered in the special needs population.[3] These and other conditions are often associated with marked ocular as well as systemic abnormalities.[4] It is therefore essential to be fully cognizant of potential systemic and visual implications before initiating any evaluative diagnostic procedures. The practitioner should also be aware, however, that individuals labeled with diagnoses, such as Leber's congenital amaurosis and cortical blindness, may have been erroneously labeled as such due to a lack of any clear-cut ocular signs indicating the pathology. Only with confirmation by the appropriate electrodiagnostic tests (electroretinogram and visual-evoked response [VER]) does the level of confidence rise in these two diagnoses.

For individuals who have a history of seizure activity, a neurologic report as well as information from accompanying caregivers should indicate the type, frequency, duration, severity, last onset, and level of control of seizure activity. It is not unusual to encounter individuals who have mistakenly been reported to be seizure-free because of a change in the type of seizure activity exhibited. Their new, milder seizure activity is interpreted by their caregivers to be fluctuations in visual attention. Throughout the evaluation sequence, the practitioner should be alert to such focal seizure activity in which an active, responsive individual will lose fixation and momentarily become passive and inattentive. If this is noted in an individual with a past history of seizure activity, a neurologic consultation should be considered.

Medical Alerts
Although various conditions may already have been noted in the evaluation record, it is useful to separately highlight those conditions that may be categorized as medical alerts. The presence of diabetes, swallowing difficulties, allergies, and eating of inedibles must be emphasized in preparation for activities that may include food and small objects that are used as visually motivating targets. The presence of cardiopulmonary abnormalities, seizure disorders, and shunts should be kept in mind during testing procedures requiring vestibular stimulation, strenuous physical activity, and the administration of ocular drugs.

The practitioner should also be aware of the higher prevalence of infectious disease in institutional settings. It is therefore important to be alert for conditions, such as hepatitis B or human immunodeficiency virus carriers, and take proper precautions when evaluating all patients.

Medications
As a result of the high percentage of seizure activity, psychoses, and other psychomotor abnormalities found in this population, a careful systemic and ocular medication history should be obtained. Antipsychotics, such as chlorpromazine (Thorazine) and thioridazine hydrochloride (Mellaril), are often administered on a long-term basis at institutions for the mentally retarded. Short-term usage of these drugs creates few lasting side effects. Long-term usage and high short-term dosage, however, create a dramatic increase in the incidence of ocular side effects (>3-year usage, 30%; >10 years, nearly 100%), which may include marked retinopathy and optic nerve disease. Phenobarbital, a drug often used as an anticonvulsant, may, with chronic use, precipitate nystagmus, paresis of the extraocular muscles, and ptosis.[5] The practitioner should also be aware of potentially harmful interactions between tricyclic antidepressants and phenylephrine, a combination that may precipitate adverse cardiovascular effects.[5]

Modifications of Examination
Accompanying physical disabilities often necessitate modifications in the evaluation procedure for the special needs individual. Conditions, such as cerebral palsy and spinal cord injury, may interfere significantly with gross and fine motor activities. Severe hearing loss, commonly associated with a variety of syndromes, including rubella, will necessitate a modification of both communication techniques and sensory stimulation throughout the evaluation. Greater emphasis may be placed on tactual, gustatory, and olfactory stimulation. One should also be aware of emotional and cognitive disorders that may interfere with an individual's response to testing. Individuals that manifest behavioral disorders, mental retardation, or developmental delays necessitate modifications both in the level of testing and its duration.

Behavioral Observations

After the collection of pertinent background information, four areas must still be explored to ensure a more positive initial contact with the special needs individual:

1. Manifest behaviors
2. Optimal position(s) for attentiveness

3. Appropriate reinforcement(s)
4. Reported visual behaviors

It is important to record the following information as reported by parents, teachers, or direct care providers.

Manifest Behaviors
Manifest behaviors, such as assaultive behavior or aggression, self-abuse, tactual defensiveness, hyperactivity, and fearfulness, are factors the doctor should be aware of before the onset of the evaluation. Without this information, the practitioner who uses a firm-touch approach during initial contact with an individual who is tactually defensive to this touch may lose any positive rapport before the testing procedure begins.

Throughout the evaluation sequence, the practitioner should record any visual behaviors manifested by the individual being evaluated. A consistent eccentric viewing posture may indicate the presence of a central scotoma. Head turns or tilts should alert the observer to the possibility of severe visual field deficits, photophobia, compensation for extraocular muscle abnormalities, or the presence of a null point in an individual with nystagmus. The practitioner also should not ignore systemic conditions that may create such turns or tilts. Severe arthritis, cerebral palsy, and spinal cord injuries commonly cause skeletal malformations. Consistent squinting may indicate the presence of refractive error or severe photophobia. Although each observed visual behavior may not be specific to only one causative factor, by comparing all observed behaviors to test results, a more concise picture should develop concerning an individual's visual system.

Optimal Position(s) for Attentiveness
To evaluate the greatest potential of visual functioning, the practitioner should ascertain the best position in which the special needs individual is most attentive or responsive. These may include the following positions: fetal, propped, prone, supine, lying on one side, sitting, standing, or crouched. Consultation with an occupational or physical therapist may yield additional helpful information.

Appropriate Reinforcement(s)
Positive reinforcement is vital in ensuring optimal responses. The practitioner should determine the most appropriate reinforcement for maximizing an individual's response to instructions or the presentation of stimuli. Possible reinforcement may include auditory (e.g., music, ringing), tactual (e.g., light or firm touch), vestibular (e.g., rocking, spinning), olfactory, gustatory, visual (e.g., lights, colors), verbal praise, favorite object, or a token system.

Reported Visual Behaviors
The first indication of the presence of visual functioning may be apparent during the collection of reported visual behaviors or during the practitioner's initial observations of the special needs individual. It is useful to explore the presence of visual behaviors, for example, squinting, light gazing, eye-poking, finger flicking, head turning or tilting, and closing of one eye. In addition, questions should be raised regarding the individual's mobility and movement patterns. Items such as ease and speed of motion, shuffling of feet, walking with head down, and avoiding or bumping into objects should be determined. Further visual behaviors to be observed or inquired about may include postural responses to stimuli such as neck or facial straining, exploration of the environment by the individual (e.g., tactual, visual, auditory, olfactory), eye preference while visually exploring the environment, maximum distance at which the individual exhibits visual recognition, and response to different lighting conditions. Inquiries should also be made about the best time of day for attentiveness. It is not uncommon for the special needs individual to exhibit optimal visual functioning during meal time. The individual's caregivers may have noted whether the patient opens his or her mouth as the utensil approaches and whether he or she uses vision to locate food on the table or uses a totally tactual approach to eating.

Psychosocial Information

The practitioner should attempt to elicit feelings and concerns regarding the individual's problems as well as expectations from the evaluation. Efforts are also made to identify other needs of the individual or family that may not be met through the evaluation sequence. Appropriate community resources can be identified and referrals to other services can be made at this time. The practitioner may also observe the following during the intake process: interaction between the patient, family, or accompanying professional; posture and presence of the patient; and the patient's ability to communicate verbally and nonverbally.

The importance of this initial background information cannot be overemphasized. It ensures more time-efficient and goal-directed examination procedures. It also enables the practitioner to draw from untold hours of observation that are impossible to achieve in an evaluation sequence. By combining this background information with the following clinical information, a truly comprehensive picture will evolve as to the visual functioning of the special needs individual.

EXAMINATION PROCEDURES

The actual examination of the special needs individual involves many aspects of visual functioning. The different areas assessed as well as the optimal tools to complete the evaluation are often dependent on the individual's cognitive and visual skills. The various visual functions that should be considered in the assessment of the special needs individual include visual acuity, refractive error, ocular alignment and binocularity, ocular motilities, accommodation, visual fields, contrast sensitivity, color vision, photosensitivity, and ocular health.

Visual Acuity

In discussing the various techniques used for visual acuity measurement, one should keep in mind that one test alone is often insufficient to determine visual acuity levels. Combining the results of several tests and recording observations of the individual's visual behavior during testing will yield far more valuable results. In addition, it is important to understand the differences between recognition (e.g., Snellen optotypes), resolution (e.g., grating acuity) and detection (e.g., candy bead) visual acuities. Each of these types of visual acuities requires different levels of cortical functioning and therefore may result in different acuity measurements for a given individual. This distinction is important when providing certification for visual impairment and in the implementation of educational programs.

Recognition Acuities

All too often, the standard Snellen visual acuity test is not applicable to this population. For those individuals who have some language skills, various options for assessing a recognition type of acuity are available. Generally, recognition visual acuities would be attempted with any individual whose cognitive skills were at least at the 3-year level. Matching activities may elicit useful results if the individual is not verbal or is unable to communicate by signing. Best results are usually obtained when testing is first performed under binocular conditions. This technique minimizes trauma, especially for individuals who are tactually defensive and fearful of being patched. A disadvantage of this approach is that the individual often has a limited attention span, and the practitioner may be unable to obtain both binocular and monocular acuities in one test session. In cases in which amblyopia or other unilateral vision loss is suspected, it may be necessary to have the individual build up tolerance to wearing a patch so that monocular acuities can be taken at a subsequent visit. Results are also enhanced when near acuity testing is per-

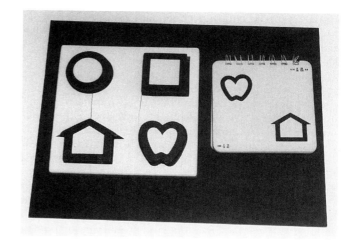

FIGURE 16-1.   **LEA Symbols visual acuity test (right) (Precision Vision, Villa Park, IL) with puzzle (left).**

formed first, as visual attention is easier to achieve when the visual stimulus is within arm's reach.

Two standardized and easy to administer recognition visual acuity tests are the LEA symbols (Precision Vision, Villa Park, IL) (Figure 16-1), with matching puzzle and the Broken Wheel Cards (Vision Training Products, Inc., Mishawaka, IN) (Figure 16-2). Both of these tests are calibrated for a 10-ft working distance. Other advantages include cost and portability. The matching puzzle, which is available with the LEA symbols, does require some motor skills but has the added advantage of engaging the individual directly in the task, allowing for sustained attention and enhanced motor involvement by the individual, which may result in more accurate findings.

Resolution Acuities

The technique that is considered to be most clinically useful in the determination of visual acuity in nonverbal indi-

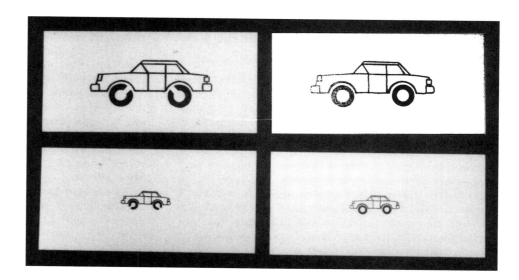

FIGURE 16-2.   **Broken Wheel Visual Acuity Cards (Vision Training Products, Inc., Mishawaka, IN).**

viduals is forced choice preferential looking. This test can provide the practitioner with valuable objective information concerning the special needs population. Research has shown that infants, when simultaneously presented with a patterned stimulus and a homogeneous one, will preferentially view the patterned stimulus.[6] The technique involves the presentation of two stimuli, one an unpatterned field and the other a black-and-white grating. Both fields are of equal size and average luminance. If the patient cannot resolve the grating, both fields will appear to be unpatterned and discrimination between the two will be impossible. The patient's viewing posture is observed through a peephole in the screen and a judgment as to the position of the grating is made by the doctor (who is unaware of the location of the stripes) based on the patient's first fixation, number and length of fixations, and overall viewing posture (Figure 16-3A). The width of the stripes is diminished with subsequent trials. Testing continues until the individual no longer fixates on the patterned background with any consistency. A visual acuity level is thus determined from the highest spatial frequency to which the patient consistently responded. The advantages of this test are its portability, ease of administration, and high success rate in obtaining repeatable, measurable acuities in the special needs population. Forced choice preferential looking is especially beneficial in individuals with cortical visual impairment,[7] delayed visual maturation,[8] and developmental disabilities.[9, 10] Again, the practitioner should be aware of several limitations of resolution acuities:

1. Grating acuities do not always correlate with recognition acuities and may overestimate the acuity obtainable with a Snellen optotype.
2. Grating acuities, such as preferential looking, are typically performed at a near working distance as compared to recognition acuities, which can be performed at either distance or near. Grating acuities may therefore miss decreased visual acuity due to myopia or moderate astigmatism.
3. Acuities obtained with preferential looking have been found to be insensitive to the detection of strabismic amblyopia and acuity loss due to macular abnormalities. They are, however, sensitive in detecting vision loss due to optic nerve or cortical involvement.[11]

Preferential looking is typically performed using cards, such as the Teller acuity cards, in a stage. This set-up allows for direct eye contact and interactions between the doctor and the patient being tested. The stage decreases the presence of distracting visual stimuli in the room and helps maintain the patient's attention on the task. Puppets, noisy toys, food reinforcement, or bubbles have frequently been used when performing preferential looking to enhance and maintain attention to the task (Figure 16-3B). In addition, there are several modifications of the preferential looking procedure that are specifically designed for special needs populations. These include the following:

1. Presentation of the cards outside of the stage allows the test to be administered to individuals who may not be able to achieve optimal positioning in front of the stage. This would include individuals who are in special adaptive chairs or those who are most alert when in a fully supine or prone position.
2. Vertical presentation of the cards often allows for easier observation of eye movements and is especially useful for individuals with nystagmus or those with strabismus who are being tested binocularly (where it may be difficult to differentiate which way the eyes are looking) (Figure 16-4).
3. For individuals who are unresponsive to the preceding testing, the doctor can present the patient with the blank side of the card and observe the individual's behavioral response. The striped side of the card is then presented to the patient, and the doctor then looks for a change in the individual's behavior when he or she sees the stripes.

Detection Acuities

Individuals who cannot respond to a two-dimensional symbol or grating may perform better with three-dimensional acuity targets. A test, such as the STYCAR Graded Ball Test (Nfer-Nelson Publishing Co., Windsor-Berks, England), is targeted for these individuals. This test uses white Styrofoam spheres of various diameters that are rolled perpendicular to the patient's line of sight. As they are individually rolled along a black cloth strip, the practitioner varies the speed, distance, and side of roll. A record is made of the smallest sphere that the patient follows at a set distance and an acuity level is calculated. Two factors should be considered in determining the accuracy of this test:

1. The STYCAR Graded Ball Test is a dynamic and not a static acuity test. Acuity level determination may therefore not correlate well to standard Snellen acuity.
2. A white ball set against a black background becomes easier to identify with increasing blur such as that created by refractive errors. A more neutral background, such as gray, may yield more reliable results.[12]

For individuals needing additional reinforcement to localize three-dimensional objects, edibles, such as chocolate-coated candies, candy beads, or raisins, are often highly effective motivators. The practitioner presents both hands to the patient, making sure that rings and watches have been removed. Only one hand contains the candy. If the patient cannot verbally or through gestures indicate which hand contains the candy, the practitioner may determine if there is visual recognition by observing fixation patterns. It is helpful to let the patient eat one candy before testing commences to ensure proper motivation. Although this gross acuity technique may not arrive at the threshold of visual acuity (a 1-mm bead located at 33 cm only requires a minimum separable acuity of approximately 20/200), it provides both parents and teachers with information about the size and contrast of solid objects (e.g., blocks, pegs, balls, bolts) that an individual should be able to see at a normal working distance. This knowledge is helpful in sorting and other eye-hand coordination activities.

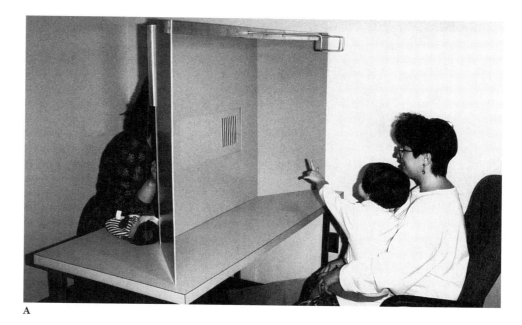

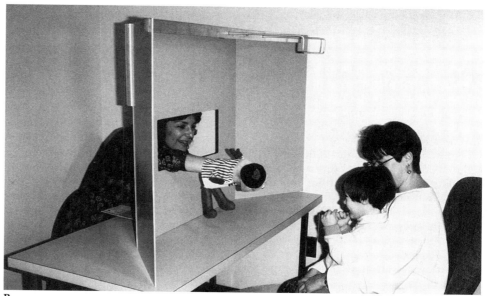

FIGURE 16-3. **Teller acuity cards for forced choice preferential looking. A. Presentation of cards using stage. B. Presentation of puppet in stage to attract child's attention.**

Electrodiagnostic Testing of Visual Acuity

When electrodiagnostic facilities are available to the practitioner, the VER technique is an excellent method for determining visual acuity levels. Stimuli, such as gratings, flashed checkerboards, and alternating checkerboards, are presented to the patient, and the occipital cortical responses are monitored and averaged by a computer. Analysis of the computer-averaged waveforms and amplitudes yields acuity level estimates. In assessing the significance of VER acuities, several points should be considered:

1. The VER response is in large part a measure of macular functioning. With patterned stimuli, information from the retinal periphery is not significantly reflected in the results.

2. This technique, although monitoring primary reception areas, cannot monitor higher cognitive functions. In working with the special needs population, the practitioner should always keep in mind the acute difference that often exists between visual acuity data and overall visual functioning.

3. The VER may provide limited useful information in individuals with cortical visual impairment.[7]

4. As with all tests mentioned, cooperation of the subject is essential for valid results. In all testing, the special needs individual may need to be slowly habituated to the procedure before the test is administered.

5. In cases of hypsarrhythmia, in which random high voltage slow waves and spikes arise from multiple foci and affect all cortical areas, VER results may not be reliable.

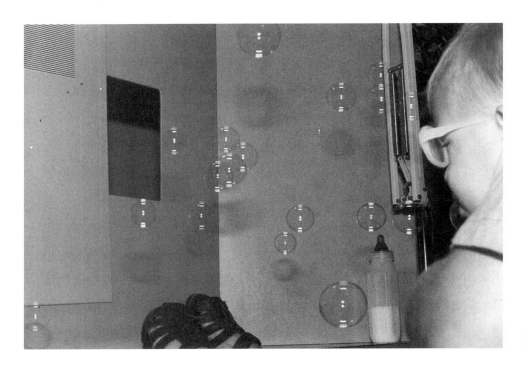

FIGURE 16-4. **Vertical presentation of Teller acuity cards with bubbles to maintain attention.**

Signs that will alert the doctor to this condition are continuous muscle spasms or quivering spells (myoclonus). This disorder is commonly associated with patients who have mental retardation.

Involuntary Visual Responses
The optokinetic nystagmus (OKN) drum has been used as an auxiliary test of visual functioning. Theoretically, if an individual can visually discriminate the series of bars moving across his or her visual field as the drum is rotated, an involuntary OKN is elicited and may be observed by the doctor. A rough visual acuity estimate may be made based on the stripe width and the distance at which the nystagmus is elicited.

Controversy surrounds this procedure for several reasons:

1. This is a dynamic and not a static visual acuity test.
2. Results may be more representative of peripheral acuity than central acuity.
3. Resolution may not be the function that is tested, but rather a subcortical response of the superior colliculus.

There are also some practical drawbacks involving the lack of visual attention beyond a limited fixation distance. This technique should still be considered when a quick screening method is needed to determine the presence of a gross visual response to stimuli. In addition, evaluation of OKN can be invaluable in determining the etiology of nystagmus, which is frequently present in special needs individuals. When nystagmus is congenital and benign, there is an inverted OKN response, meaning that the fast phase of the nystagmus is in the same direction as the rotating stripes. In a normal OKN response, which may be seen in pathologically or neurologically based nystagmus, the fast phase is in the opposite direction of the rotating stripes.

Light and Form Perception
If an individual shows no visual response to any objects or patterns, the practitioner should explore responsiveness to light stimuli. A helpful screening technique for form perception uses an open hand that is thrust in front of an individual's face. A consistent response, such as a blink reflex, closing of the eyes, or an avoidance behavior, is viewed as a positive sign of visual discrimination. Care should be taken to have the fingers spread apart to avoid the introduction of air currents that can elicit the same responding behaviors.

Although pupillary responses should be noted, they should not be used as the sole determinants of visual responsiveness. The presence of pupillary contraction to light and near objects will generally indicate a visual response. Relatively normal pupillary responses to light, however, have been noted in cases of no light perception due to suprageniculate lesions. Conversely, the absence of pupillary responses does not indicate the absence of a visual response. Drug-induced mydriasis or miosis, synechiae, or neurologic pupillary abnormalities, for example, can all adversely affect the pupillary responses in a visual patient.

One final test of visual responsiveness involves the use of a light stimulus to elicit a fixation reflex. Often, the individual will show facial or postural changes or an enhanced level of alertness when the lighting is altered. A useful tool for eliciting responses to light is a flicker bulb ("ball of fire") (Figure 16-5). Children who do not respond to other types of illuminated or nonilluminated visual stimuli may demonstrate a response to a colorful flickering light. Although several colors are commercially available, a red light is often most effective in eliciting a response. In addition, caution must be exercised when turning the light on and off to avoid an accompanying auditory stimulus. Monitoring the distance of the bulb to the individual's face or hands to avoid a tactile stimulus from the heat of the bulb must also be considered. Finally, it is often useful in individuals who show little response to other types of visual stimuli to watch for behavioral changes as room lights are turned on or off. A blink reflex to any type of light should also be noted. Positive responses will generally indicate visual responsiveness. Although a positive response should indicate that vision is grossly intact, one should remember that studies have shown responses to light and OKN in individuals without a functioning visual cortex. Consideration should therefore be given in these cases to educating parents and caregivers regarding level of functioning and prognosis.

It may be noted from this discussion of involuntary visual responses that no test viewed in isolation can yield indisputable results. Only by combining results from several tests and comparing them to behavioral observations obtained throughout the entire evaluation sequence can the practitioner arrive at an accurate assessment of visual functioning.

Refractive Error

Conditions often seen in special needs individuals, such as albinism, Down syndrome, retinopathy of prematurity, and rubella, are frequently associated with marked refractive error (see Chapter 3, Table 3-3). In addition, patients younger than 5 years commonly have significant refractive errors and often show large fluctuations.[13] For individuals older than 5 years, refractive error continues to change gradually during the school years.[14] A careful refraction and appropriate correction is important in ensuring the attainment of an optimal retinal image and maximum sensory input.

Although conventional refraction can often be completed with certain special needs individuals, modifications to the standard distance retinoscopy technique are advisable. These include the following:

1. Performing a trial lens or lens rack refraction instead of using the phoropter. Individuals who are tactually defensive may feel threatened with the phoropter close to their face. In addition, it is important for the doctor to maintain good facial and eye contact with the patient to obtain maximum cooperation.

2. If the individual is not tactually defensive and will tolerate spectacles, then accommodation can be better controlled by using "refracting glasses," which are colorful, comfortable frames that incorporate the doctor's "working distance" lens (e.g., +1.50 or +2.00 spheres OU). By using these glasses, the net refraction is whatever the doctor scopes in each meridian.

3. To maintain fixation and minimize accommodation, an appropriate distance target suitable for the individual is desirable. This target can include an interesting video-

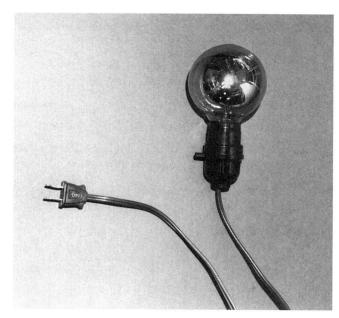

FIGURE 16-5. **Flicker bulb.**

tape, a talking toy, or the caretaker or parent standing across the room and speaking to the individual.

Due to the short attention span of a majority of special needs individuals, viewing angles and accommodative postures are in a continual state of change. Cycloplegic refraction is beneficial in individuals with whom steady fixation is particularly difficult. It should also be considered when a fluctuating reflex is present, when the individual presents with a significant degree of hyperopia, or when an eso deviation is present. Although cycloplegic refractions will reduce the accommodative variability, it may also produce psychotic reactions in some individuals. Care must therefore be taken in the concentration and type of cycloplegic agent used. In general, tropicamide, particularly in low doses, will rarely cause side effects, although it is not considered a very effective cycloplegic agent. A more effective drug is cyclopentolate. In general, although 0.5% or 1% is the maximum dosage to be considered for most special needs individuals, psychotic reactions can occur even at these low dosages.

A near retinoscopy technique (Mohindra) has been offered as an alternative to cycloplegic refraction. Retinoscopy is performed at a 50-cm working distance in a completely dark room free of extraneous light sources. Fixation is directed to the beam of the retinoscope. Sound effects, such as singing or other interesting noises, are often helpful when performing this technique. No fogging lenses or drops are required and −1.25 D is added to the spherical component of the neutrality lens value.[15] This technique is an attractive one for the special needs population in that the viewing angle is better controlled due to total elimination of visual distractions.

A new technique that is being used in screening refractive error in the special needs population is photorefrac-

TABLE 16-1
Summary of Guidelines for Prescribing in Special Needs Individuals

Refractive Error	Concern for Amblyopia	Effect on Binocularity	Interference with Learning	Consider Prescribing
Myopia	>5.00 D	Undercorrect esotropia Fully correct exotropia*	Depends on patient's age	>5.00 D
Hyperopia	>2.00 D	Undercorrect exotropia Fully correct esotropia*	>2.50 D	>2.00 D
Astigmatism	>1.25 D	Depends on other factors	Depends on visual acuity	>1.25 D >2 yrs
Anisometropia	>1.00 D	Monitor stereopsis	>1.00 D	>1.00 D and stable

*To maximize binocularity.

tion. The advantages of this technique are that it is quick, noninvasive, and nonthreatening to the individual. Photorefraction requires little expertise to administer, produces a permanent record of the individual's refractive status, and can detect as little as 0.50 D of ametropia. Photorefraction is also useful in detecting other visual abnormalities, including strabismus, anisocoria, and media opacities.[16]

Several techniques of photorefraction are available. Photorefraction uses a camera, special lens, and strobe to simultaneously evaluate the refractive status of both eyes. When a picture is taken, the strobe light enters the individual's eye, is refracted by the media, strikes the retina, becomes focused or forms a blur circle on the retina, reflects off the retina, and is refracted by the media on the way out of the eye.[16] This light is then captured on the film. Although the pupil of an emmetropic eye appears as a homogeneous red reflex on the developed film, any ametropia appears as a whitish crescent. The larger the crescent, the higher the magnitude of the ametropia. When the ametropia is greater than 6.00 D, the pupil is entirely filled with the white crescent. The crescents of myopia, hyperopia, and astigmatism are distinguished by their positioning in the pupil relative to where the strobe was placed on the camera. Photorefraction holds much promise for large screenings and in pediatrician's offices. There are still several drawbacks for routine diagnosis and prescribing, however. One is the cost and time necessary for processing the film in one technique (which may take several days).[16] Other computerized techniques[17] that provide more instantaneous results are still very costly and less portable for routine clinical care or widespread screening. Finally, although photorefraction can detect refractive errors >6.00 D, some techniques are unable to obtain an actual measurement necessary for prescribing in these high magnitude refractive errors. The availability of commercial portable Polaroid photorefraction units, such as the MTI (Lancaster, PA) photorefractor, offer photographs of the blur circles within minutes. Although these instruments overcome the time factor and provide promise for expanded use of this technique in the future,[18] their validity and reliability have yet to be fully established.

Consideration should be given to correcting significant refractive error in special needs individuals regardless of their entering visual acuity or level of cognitive functioning. The times when correction of refractive error may not be indicated are in cases of individuals who are not showing significant responses to light and those with little or no pattern perception who also have a field defect. In this latter group, the placement of a frame on the individual may actually hinder his or her ability to respond to vision stimulation activities, especially if this therapy is aimed at improving tracking and peripheral awareness.

If a significant refractive error is discovered, the practitioner should note any changes in visual behavior when the correction is placed on the individual. Immediate rejection of corrective lenses may not be due to an inaccurate refraction but rather to frame intolerance or perceptual difficulty in adapting to a significantly altered visual environment. A frame toleration program using positive reinforcements, such as food, music, or enjoyed play activities, may help a tactually defensive individual to adapt. The same reinforcement may be used to gradually introduce a significant correction. This tolerance may take weeks or months to accomplish, but the results in terms of enhancement of sensory input are often rewarding. A summary of guidelines for prescribing for special needs individuals is given in Table 16-1.

Ocular Alignment and Binocularity

When evaluating binocularity in special needs individuals, two aspects should be considered. The two aspects are motor findings, which evaluate how the eyes look, and sensory findings, which evaluate what the individual is seeing. The motor findings, or ocular alignment, may have a significant impact on cosmetic appearance and therefore be an important consideration for parents and others who are trying to establish eye contact and bonding with a special needs individual. The sensory findings are important when considering visual development, orientation and mobility concerns, and behavioral responses to the environment.

Motor Assessment of Ocular Alignment
Identifying the presence of a large-angle strabismus is often a simple matter. Hirschberg's test, using a penlight or a flicker bulb to measure angle lambda, quickly indi-

cates the presence of a gross alignment deficit. When one considers, however, that 1 mm of deviation equals 22 prism diopters, this test becomes less accurate for measurement of smaller-angle strabismus.

When it is possible to maintain accurate fixation on a distance or near target, the cover test is much more reliable in detecting and measuring any phoria or tropia that may be present. The success of attaining this measurement lies in the ability of the patient to maintain accurate fixation. Although an assortment of appropriate fixation targets is desirable, measurements should be taken while the patient is fixating on as detailed a target as possible to control accommodation. In the presence of a strabismus, measurements should be taken at distance and at near, if possible, as well as in nine positions of gaze, to determine comitancy. When recording the presence of a phoria or tropia, it is important to identify the following when possible:

1. Onset (age when deviation was first detected)
2. Magnitude (in prism diopters)
3. Type (eso-, exo-, hypo-, hyper-)
4. Comitant versus noncomitant (along with presence of an A or V pattern)
5. Frequency (constant versus intermittent along with percentage of time eye is turning)
6. Laterality (unilateral versus alternating)

With the presence of variable fixation, poor pattern perception, eccentric viewing, and no verbal feedback, however, even a combination of both tests may yield confusing results. Bruchner's test is an additional technique that can aid the practitioner in confirming the presence of a strabismus. By using a bright coaxial light source (halogen ophthalmoscope), both the position of corneal reflexes and brightness difference of the fundus reflexes are evaluated. In the presence of strabismus, the fixating eye has a darker reflex, whereas the nonfixating, strabismic eye has a brighter, whiter, and lighter reflex. (Anisocoria, lens, and media opacities can also be evaluated with Bruchner's test).[19] A summary of motor tests for binocularity is given in Table 16-2.

Sensory Assessment
Sensory assessment involves the determination of the following aspects of visual development:

1. Amblyopia
2. Suppression
3. Diplopia
4. Fusion
5. Stereopsis
6. Anomalous retinal correspondence
7. Normal retinal correspondence

Amblyopia can initially be detected by performing visual acuity monocularly. An alternative technique that can be used to assess amblyopia when a constant strabismus is present is the observation of fixation patterns when a verti-

TABLE 16-2
Evaluation of Motor Binocularity in Special Needs Individuals

Test	Purpose
Bruchner's test	Compares color and brightness of red reflex between eyes
Hirshberg's test	Evaluates placement of corneal reflex
Krimsky's test	Measures placement of corneal reflex with prism
Four Base Out test	Detects presence of central suppression or microstrabismus
Vergence response	Use of prisms to evaluate negative and positive fusional vergence ranges
Convergence near point	Evaluates individual's ability to converge to a near target

cal 10–prism-diopter lens is placed over an eye. Abnormal patterns indicating amblyopia are identified when a nondominant eye will not hold or will only briefly hold fixation (1–3 seconds) after the other eye is unoccluded. Equal visual preference will show up as a spontaneous alternate fixation or steady fixation for at least 5 seconds by the nondominant eye once the dominant eye is unoccluded.

Tests that require subjective feedback (e.g., Worth's four-dot test, Stereo Fly test [Stereo Optical Co., Chicago, IL]) are often difficult to administer due to the cognitive level and limitations of receptive and expressive language skills of many of these individuals. The three-figure flashlight test is conceptually the same as Worth's four-dot test, except that three pictures appear on the flashlight instead of dots. While wearing anaglyphic (red-green) glasses, the individual must identify a girl (red), an elephant (green), and a ball (white). The presence of more or less than three figures usually indicates diplopia or suppression, respectively. The three-bear test is another simple test whereby the individual is shown several small (1-in.) bears (available at craft stores) while wearing anaglyphic glasses. The individual is asked to either name the colors of the bears or sort them by color. The individual is initially asked to sort the bears without glasses to demonstrate understanding of the task. Inability to subsequently sort the bears with the glasses indicates suppression (Figure 16-6).

Random dot stereograms are more useful in detecting small-angle strabismus and suppression. These include the Preschool Randot Stereo Test (Stereo Optical Co.), Lang Stereo Test I and II (Lang, Forch, Switzerland), the Viewer-Free Stereo Tests (US Optical, Mishawaka, IN), and TNO stereo test. The Stereo Smile Test (Stereo Optical Co.) is a preferential looking task that uses a smiley face target. This test has been shown to be useful in eliciting stereo responses in a clinical setting in infants, young children and special needs individuals[20] (Figure 16-7). As with any test using random dot stereopsis, resolution of the random dot pattern in individuals with significantly reduced visual acuity may be difficult despite the presence of good ocular alignment.

Other criteria, such as differences in acuity, refractive errors, visual fields, and head posture, may be useful in determination of eye dominance. Eye preference may be elicited by observations of an individual's behavior under

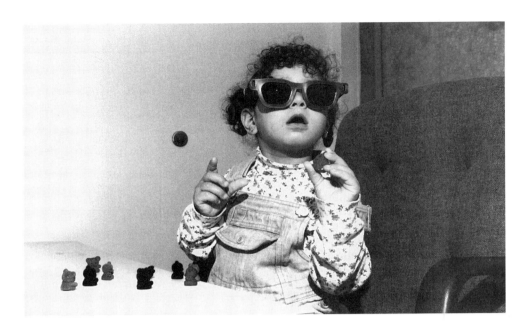

FIGURE 16-6.   **Three-bear test.**

monocular conditions. If more irritation or greater hesitation is displayed when one eye is patched versus the other, it may indicate eye preference or a difference in visual acuity between the two eyes. The practitioner should remember, however, that tactual defensiveness may also bring about similar behaviors. It is therefore very helpful to repeat this observation several times to habituate the individual to the procedure. A summary of significant tests for the evaluation of binocular sensory status is summarized in Table 16-3.

Ocular Motilities

Throughout the evaluation sequence, observations should be made of the individual's ocular tracking and saccadic skills. Targets, such as flicker bulbs, favorite toys or objects, preferred edibles, or a familiar face, will yield optimal results (Figure 16-8). A history of recent seizure activity should alert the evaluator to avoid extensive use of flickering stimuli. For each meridian, the practitioner should note whether there are any limitations in gaze, if movements are smooth or jerky and whether eye tracking, head tracking, or both are used. The presence and type of nystagmus should be noted, as well as if the nystagmus is present under monocular or binocular viewing. Midline problems, which are often encountered in the neurologically impaired individual, may show up as an alternating tropia or a startle reflex when the midline is crossed. If an individual exhibits acceptable tracking skills in the vertical meridian, but tends to head track after crossing midline in the horizontal meridian, a homonymous field loss should be considered as well as neurologic midline abnormalities. Saccadic tests will also provide the practitioner with valuable information, not only about ocular scanning, but also about possible field deficits. A technique that allows the doctor to examine both pursuits and saccadic skills as well as eye-hand coordination

and visual field integrity is one that uses a series of soap bubbles blown in front of an individual and observing the responding behaviors. Visual attention and overall cooperation is enhanced by incorporating such playtime activities into the examination procedure.

Accommodation

Accommodative skills are an important component to the special needs evaluation, especially for individuals who are learning or working with small, detailed targets at a near working distance. It has also been shown that accommodative skills are weaker in individuals with cerebral palsy and other types of disorders associated with special needs patients.[21] When the cognitive level is high enough (at least at a 3-year age level), the evaluation of accommodation is an important aspect of this evaluation.

Accommodation can be measured using several techniques. These include a simple push-up or pull-out amplitude. In the latter technique, a small, detailed, high-interest target is held very close to the patient's eye. The other eye is occluded. The doctor slowly moves the target away from the patient's eye until he or she is able to verbally identify the picture. It is important for the doctor to monitor changes in accommodation during this procedure by evaluating changes in pupil size. A change from a dilated to a constricted pupil will often indicate the point at which the patient begins accommodating, even if no verbal response to the target is elicited.

A second technique is to measure the lag of accommodation using the monocular estimation method (MEM) or near-point retinoscopy. For the special needs individual, a MEM card with high-interest pictures or simple letters is placed on the retinoscope. The retinoscope is held at arms' length from the patient and the patient is asked to describe the pictures on the card. In this manner, the doc-

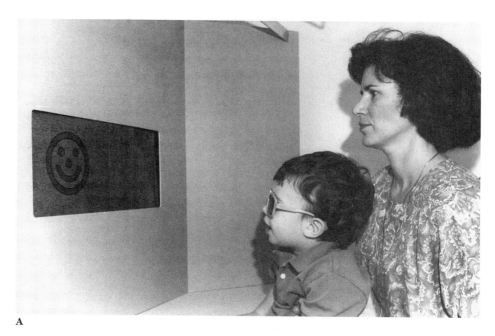

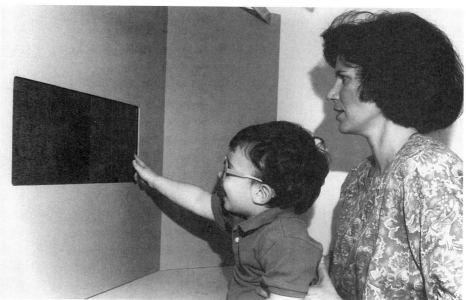

FIGURE 16-7. **Stereo Smile Test (Stereo Optical Co., Chicago, IL) training card (A) and test card (B).**

tor is able to evaluate where the plane of accommodation is relative to the MEM card. If the doctor measures with motion, the patient is under-accommodating. If the doctor measures against motion, the patient is over-accommodating. The normal lag of accommodation is approximately +0.25 to +0.75 D.

Visual Fields

The objective of visual field testing on the special needs individual is to uncover gross field deficits. Confrontation field tests are most appropriate for this population. Best

results are obtained when a practitioner and an assistant are involved in testing. The practitioner is seated in front of the patient and attempts to hold the patient's visual attention (e.g., flicker bulbs, toys, favorite food, familiar face) while observing visual responses to incoming stimuli. The assistant stands behind the patient and presents visually interesting objects in arcs delineating the principle quadrants. The patient is asked to name, point, or look at the object when it first appears in his or her visual field. If this is not possible due to the patient's developmental level, observations of consistent changes in fixation will indicate the point of visual awareness of the incoming stimuli (Figure 16-9). Standard precautions

TABLE 16-3
Evaluation and Interpretation of Sensory Binocularity in Special Needs Individuals

Test	Cognitive Ages	Task Required	Normal Retinal Correspondence	Suppression	Abnormal Retinal Correspondence	Diplopia
Worth's four-dot	≥5 yrs	Individual must count the number of dots	Four dots with no strabismus present during test	Two red dots or three green dots	Four dots with strabismus present during test	Five dots; exo = crossed, eso = uncrossed
Three-figure flashlight	2–5 yrs	Individuals must describe pictures they see	Three pictures with no strabismus present during test	Two pictures	Three pictures with strabismus present during testing	Four pictures; exo = crossed, eso = uncrossed
Three-bear	2–5 yrs	Individual must sort by color	Able to sort into red, green, and black groups	Sorts bears into only two groups	Sorts bears into three groups with strabismus present	May have difficulty accurately picking up bears
Stereo Fly (Stereo Optical Co., Chigaco, IL)	≥1 yr	Individual must reach out and pinch wings	Wings are pinched above page	Wings are pinched on the page	Wings may also be pinched above page	Wings are pinched on the page
Preschool Randot Stereo (Stereo Optical Co.)	1–3 yrs, depending on nature of test	Individual must point to or name stimulus	Individual correctly points to or identifies stimulus	Individual does not see stimulus (indicates no bifoveality present)	Individual does not see stimulus (indicates strabismus)	Individual does not see stimulus (strabismus, suppression, or poor visual acuity)
Stereo Smile (Stereo Optical Co.)	≥6 mos	Forced choice test—no language skills needed	Individual looks at smiley face target	Individual shows no preference for either side of card	Individual shows no preference for either side of card	Individual shows no preference for either side of card (strabismus, suppression, or poor visual acuity)

eso = esotropia; exo = exotropia.

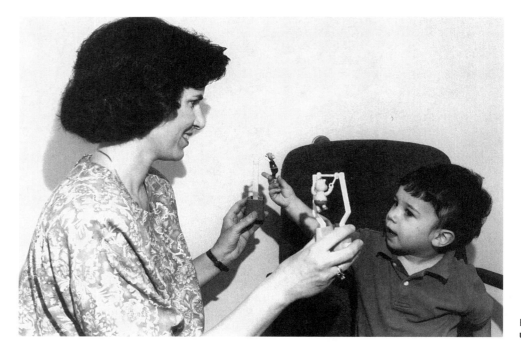

FIGURE 16-8. **Evaluating saccades using small swing toys for fixation.**

against the introduction of tactual and auditory cues should be taken.

An arc perimeter can also be used to more accurately measure the peripheral visual fields in special needs individuals. The double arc perimeter has been used with young children and is particularly useful as it provides both vertical and horizontal meridians for testing without changing the orientation of the instrument.

Repetition of tests is often necessary to ascertain the reliability of findings. As the testing should ideally be performed under both binocular and monocular conditions, it is helpful to have parents or caregivers simulate the pro-

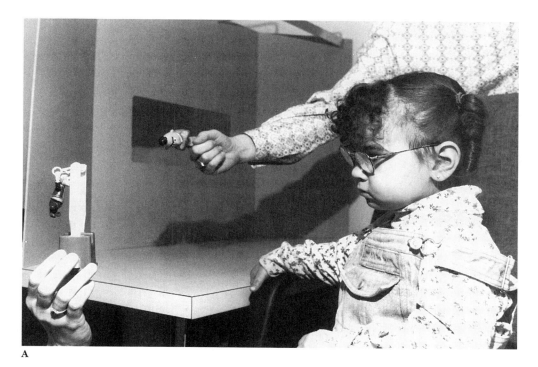

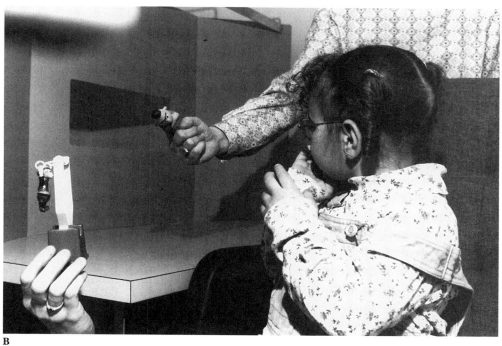

FIGURE 16-9. **Visual field testing with confrontation fields using small attractive toys. A. Child fixating straight ahead as target is brought in from periphery. B. Child detects peripheral target and turns head toward it.**

cedure in the individual's home environment. This will yield optimal results during repeat testing. Results should always be compared to observations noted throughout the entire evaluation sequence. Head and body turns as well as eccentric viewing postures are accurate indicators of possible field loss. Results should also be related to the systemic and neurologic history and ocular health finding. For example, congenital toxoplasmosis may be expected to create a large central scotoma, whereas hydrocephalus or brain trauma may create a homonymous hemianopic field loss.

Contrast Sensitivity

Special needs individuals often have difficulties in certain environments despite the presence of good visual acuity and unrestricted visual fields. Many are reported

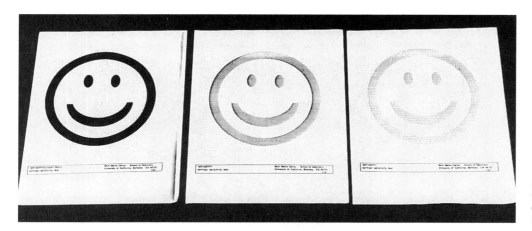

FIGURE 16-10. **Mr. Happy Contrast Sensitivity Test (University of California School of Optometry, Berkeley, CA).**

to have problems going up and down stairs, seeing objects in dim illumination, finding food on their plate, or stepping off a curb. Visual acuity measures spatial resolution under optimal, high-contrast viewing conditions, but many real-life situations present visual information in less than ideal or low-contrast viewing conditions. The evaluation of contrast sensitivity, therefore, can provide additional valuable information regarding an individual's functional vision capabilities. Knowledge of an individual's contrast sensitivity can be useful in providing answers to observed behaviors and should be considered when choosing educational materials. In addition, adaptations in the living or working environment, such as marking the beginning of stairs or curbs, for example, can often result in enhanced comfort and function as well as less stress for both special needs individuals and their caregivers. Although there are many commercially available methods to test contrast sensitivity, many are not suitable to the special needs individual. The following four have been found to be useful with this population, dependent on cognitive development.

Mr. Happy Contrast Sensitivity Chart
The Mr. Happy Contrast Sensitivity Test (University of California School of Optometry, Berkeley, CA) is a forced choice test that has several variations. Basically, the individual is shown two pictures, one with a homogeneous dot pattern, the other with a high-contrast happy face superimposed on the homogeneous dot pattern (Figure 16-10). Once a reliable response is established, the happy face card is exchanged for one with lower contrast. This procedure continues until the individual no longer shows a preference for the stimulus card. Training for this test and modifications to enhance responsiveness are similar to those used for the Teller acuity cards. This test can be used at any developmental age.[22]

Hiding Heidi
Hiding Heidi (Precision Vision, Villa Park, IL) is a variation of the Mr. Happy Contrast Sensitivity Test with a similar design and implementation (Figure 16-11).

LEA Symbols Contrast Sensitivity Chart
The LEA Symbols Contrast Sensitivity Chart consists of a large chart tested at a near working distance with the same optotypes used in the LEA visual acuity tests. The individual must identify or match the correct pictures at each contrast level until a threshold contrast sensitivity is reached. This test is primarily useful with patients whose cognitive level of functioning is at the 3-year level or better.

Preferential Looking Contrast Sensitivity Cards
These are cards modeled after the Teller acuity cards. The difference is that the contrast sensitivity cards present seven levels of contrast along with five levels of spatial frequency. A total of 42 cards are used, which allows the doctor to generate a contrast sensitivity curve for different spatial frequencies. Although these cards are not commercially available, they can easily be constructed using the Vis-Tech Contrast Sensitivity distance acuity chart (Dayton, OH) and gray cardboard. This test can be used at any developmental age.[23]

Color Vision

Due to often marked cognitive deficits, accurate color vision testing is often more challenging and may not always be successful with this population. Four different levels of color vision testing can be considered: color naming, color identification (pointing), color preference, and detection of color defects.

Color Naming
The ability to use language skills to name colors is directly related to an individual's development or cognitive abilities. Color naming is useful for individuals who can already point to colors and may be useful information for teachers and other members of the rehabilitation team when planning appropriate activities or programs for the special needs individuals.

When evaluating color naming, any type of consistent objects with varying colors can be used. These may include colored blocks, beads, balls, or bears. An assortment of colors in bright primary, pastel, and muddy colors is most use-

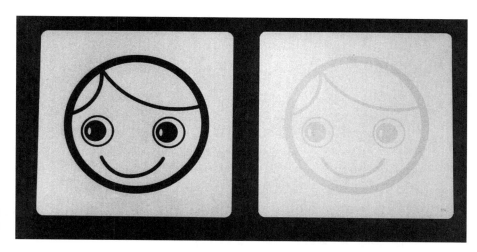

FIGURE 16-11. **Hiding Heidi Contrast Sensitivity Test (Precision Vision, Villa Park, IL).**

ful. It is important to provide good illumination for testing. The practitioner points to or isolates one of the objects and asks the individual to name the color. The practitioner should always begin with the primary colors and proceed to the pastel and muddy colors. This skill usually develops by the time the individual is at a cognitive age of 3–4 years old.

Color Identification

Color identification evaluates the individual's ability to point to various colors without the need for language skills. This information is important for both children and adults in helping the practitioner to identify appropriate educational materials and goals, as well as to determine appropriate self-help and work-related goals.

The same equipment and illumination that were used with color naming can be used for this evaluation. The patient is asked to point to each color, beginning with the primary colors and proceeding to pastel and muddy colors. This skill is dependent on appropriate receptive language skills and usually develops by age 3–4 years.

Color Preference

It is also valuable to determine if an individual responds better to certain colors and brightness because this can be helpful in identifying optimal targets to be used in vision stimulation activities. One way of accomplishing this type of assessment is to place different colored filters over a light source to determine if there is indeed a preference. Common attractive colors for special needs individuals are often bright red and yellow objects.

Detection of Color Vision Defects

Although color naming, color pointing, and color preference are all useful for educational and rehabilitative programs, it is important to remember that they are not considered acceptable indicators of true color vision deficits. There are several clinically useful tools for evaluating color vision defects in special needs individuals. These include the following:

1. *F2 Preferential Looking Plates.* The F2 Preferential Looking Plates (University of California School of Optom-

etry, Berkeley, CA) are a forced choice test of color vision that can be useful at any age or developmental level. No understanding of these tasks is required. They consist of pseudoisochromatic plates with a geometric shape visible to color normal individuals on one side (Figure 16-12). The doctor holds the plate in front of the individual and either asks him or her to point to the geometric shape or use preferential looking by observing his or her eye movements. These plates are designed to detect mild, moderate, or severe red-green defects and moderate to severe blue-yellow defects.[24]

2. *Portnoy Plates.* Portnoy Plates (University of California School of Optometry, Berkeley, CA) are also a forced choice test, but they require higher levels of receptive language, cognitive, and pointing skills than do the F2 plates. This test uses Munsell colors similar to those used in the D-15 test for adults. It differentiates mild from moderate and severe color defects as well as protan, deutan, and tritan anomalies. The plates consist of four colored circles (Figure 16-13). The individual must point to or identify which one of the four colored circles appears different. This test is suitable primarily for individuals with a cognitive age of at least 3 years.[25]

3. *Berson test.* The Berson test is identical in administration to the Portnoy Plates and is used if the individual is unable to pass the Portnoy Plates. It differentiates autosomal recessive complete rod monochromasy and sex-linked blue cone monochromasy.[25]

4. *Color Vision Testing Made Easy.* Color Vision Testing Made Easy (Vision Associates, Orlando, FL) consists of 10 pseudoisochromatic plates that present pictures instead of the traditional numbers used in adult color vision tests. The individual must identify or point to the picture. This test is useful in individuals with a cognitive age of at least 3 years and requires some degree of receptive and expressive language skills.

Photosensitivity

Photophobia has been found to be a side effect of several anticonvulsant medications. It is also associated with con-

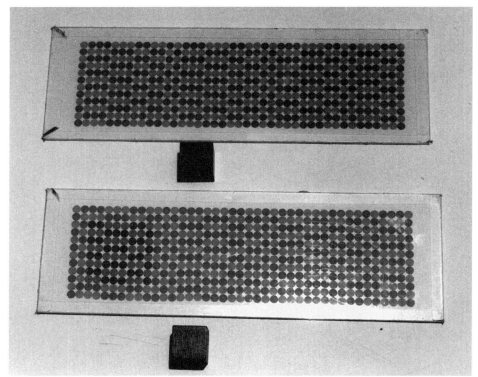

A

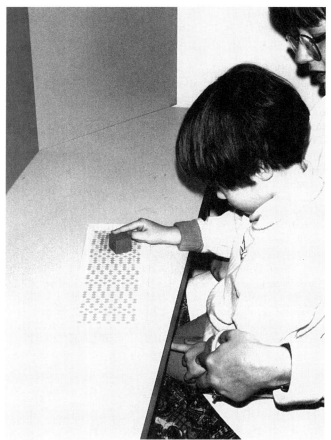

B

FIGURE 16-12. **F2 Color Plates (University of California School of Optometry, Berkeley, CA). A. Color plates with matching blocks. B. Child performing test.**

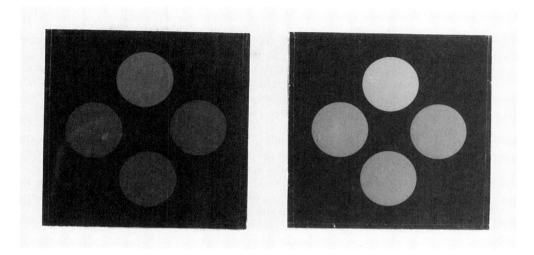

FIGURE 16-13.   **Portnoy Color Plates (University of California School of Optometry, Berkeley, CA).**

genital ocular disorders, such as rod monochromatism, congenital cataracts, albinism, and aniridia. Determination of photophobia may be arrived at through clinical observations. Any individual exhibiting a downward head tilt, squinting, increased irritability, or a degradation in visual behavior in brightly illuminated environments should receive a sun lens evaluation. During this assessment, nonverbal cues, such as relaxation of facial muscles, widening of palpebral apertures, and improvement in mobility, would indicate a positive response to sun lenses. NoIR filters (NoIR Medical Technologies, South Lyon, MI), the UVShield by NoIR, and Corning Photochromatic Filter (CPF) Lens series (Corning Medical Optics, Elmira, NY), as well as sun visors may be used in the evaluation under both artificial indoor and natural outdoor illumination conditions. Individuals with an ocular history of a tapetoretinal degeneration (e.g., Laurence-Moon-Biedl syndrome, Usher's syndrome, Leber's congenital amaurosis) should be observed under changing illumination conditions. If they exhibit light-dark adaptation problems, a sun lens evaluation may also be indicated (Figure 16-14).

Ocular Health

A comprehensive ocular health assessment should always be performed during the evaluation. Correct postural positioning and positive reinforcement are often critical, as this part of the evaluation tends to be traumatic for the special needs individual. Placing the individual in a caregiver's lap or special adaptive chair or enabling him or her to lie on a flat or tilted surface may facilitate the examination.

Anterior Segment Evaluation
The anterior segment can be evaluated initially by inspection, with assessment performed in a slit-lamp whenever possible. When a patient's physical abnormality or behavior prevents the use of a standard slit-lamp, alternative

tools include the use of a Burton lamp or, preferably, a portable, handheld slit-lamp. It is also important to evaluate ocular pressure in this patient population, as there is a high incidence of glaucoma from associated systemic and ocular conditions. Ocular pressures are ideally evaluated using a Goldmann tonometer that is either mounted on a slit-lamp or handheld. Other tools that are also useful include the portable, noncontact (air-puff) tonometer, Tono-Pen (Mentor, Inc., Norwell, MA), and Schiötz tonometer. Although each of these is fairly easy to administer, the Tono-Pen may require the least amount of physical contact or patient cooperation.

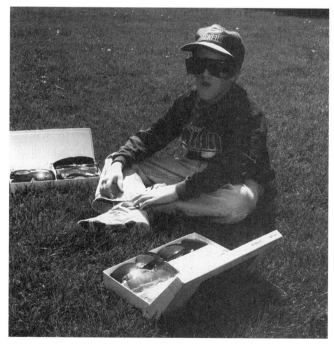

FIGURE 16-14.   **Sun lens evaluation.**

Posterior Segment Evaluation

Whenever possible, binocular indirect ophthalmoscopy should be attempted, especially in cases of high myopia, with individuals who exhibit chronic self-abusive behaviors that may result in posterior segment trauma, or with those who may have retinal involvement (i.e., retinopathy of prematurity, retinal detachment). When cooperation levels are poor, the practitioner may consider referral for evaluation under restraints or general anesthesia. A monocular indirect ophthalmoscope will often be better tolerated than a binocular indirect ophthalmoscope or standard direct ophthalmoscope due to the lower light intensity and increased distance between the patient and the practitioner.

The doctor should be sensitive to behaviors exhibited by the special needs individual that may indicate that his or her threshold level of tolerance has been surpassed. Input from accompanying parents or professionals will often help the doctor to accurately interpret such behaviors. Due to the comprehensive nature of this evaluation and the population that is being examined, it becomes evident that more than one evaluation session may be required. It is not unusual for the entire assessment to include one or two additional shorter sessions.

RECOMMENDATIONS

Once the visual information has been gathered and analyzed, it is important to develop an appropriate management plan, which is useful for medical, functional, and educational purposes. This management plan typically includes a series of recommendations that addresses each of the following areas.

Medical Recommendations

Medical recommendations closely mirror those made during any routine eye examination. It may include referral to tertiary care services such as retinal specialists, neurologists, or glaucoma specialists. Further evaluations may also be recommended such as electrodiagnostic testing. It is important for the caregiver to understand why a referral is being made and how soon the patient should be seen. It is often necessary to facilitate the scheduling of these appointments for the patient to expedite the appropriate care.

Functional Recommendations

Functional recommendations relate directly to the individual's developmental needs, how they are able to communicate with people, and how they will learn to interact visually with their environment. For example, it is not only important for caregivers or parents to know that an individual sees 20/80, but it is also important for them to understand how this level of visual acuity allows the patient to relate visually to his or her environment. It might be useful to have objects that subtend a visual angle equal to various visual acuities. The practitioner can then demonstrate to the caregiver what the patient is able to see by placing the equivalent sized object at different distances in the surrounding environment. Vision simulators depicting various acuity losses and field losses are also valuable tools in providing information to caregivers.

Beyond the actual description of an individual's functional level of vision, recommendations should be made regarding prognosis for improvement and guidelines for the development of appropriate vision stimulation programs. The following is a partial list of functional vision recommendations that might be made depending on the need:

- Appropriate refractive correction
- Appropriate sun shields
- Prescription of low vision devices
- Binocular vision therapy
- Accommodative therapy
- Patching therapy (e.g., to improve amblyopia or prevent diplopia)
- Eye tracking exercises (emphasizing size, color, and illumination of appropriate targets)
- Peripheral awareness therapy (emphasizing size, color, and illumination of targets)
- Contrast awareness
- Searching and scanning strategies
- Appropriate lighting
- Central or eccentric viewing strategies (depending on ocular diagnosis)
- Visual reach activities
- Appropriate games or toys, including size, color, shape, contrast, and developmental levels
- Office-based vision therapy
- Teacher of the visually impaired
- Orientation and mobility instruction

Educational Recommendations

Often, the doctor is asked to make appropriate recommendations regarding educational needs and placement. It is therefore important for the doctor to communicate the results of the evaluation with the school system using language that lay persons or educators can easily understand.[26] For example, rather than use the term *contrast sensitivity* it would be more helpful to describe the individual's ability to detect differences between light and dark areas. The following information from the visual evaluation is also useful for educational planning purposes:

- Level of lighting and sensitivity to glare
- Contrast of materials
- Positioning of the individual
- Size of material
- Placement of materials in optimal visual field

- Appropriate colors
- Brightness
- Need for clutter reduction
- Spacing of visual information
- Level of visual processing
- Orientation and mobility concerns

The doctor is often called on to make recommendations regarding the appropriate school or rehabilitation placement necessary for an individual. In these cases, it is not only important for the doctor to be part of the educational planning team but also to remember that vision is one component of the individual's overall profile. The doctor can therefore make recommendations for the type of program that would most benefit the patient based on the visual information; however, he or she should exercise caution in stating that a particular school or program is necessary.

Finally, it is important to provide information regarding when the patient is to return for further care. A yearly routine examination may be all that is indicated. For others, a specific follow-up time is recommended. For a number of patients, the appropriate follow-up appointment may be based on the achievement of specific visual milestones or changes that are noted by the vision teacher, therapist, or parent. It is, therefore, important for these individuals to feel comfortable calling the doctor and communicating any visual or developmental changes that have occurred.

CONCLUSION

Because vision plays a key role in the educational and rehabilitation of special needs individuals, the evaluation and management of the visual needs of this population can be a rewarding experience for the practitioner. It is important to remember that the practitioner is not only a provider of vision care but also a member of the rehabilitation team and should be actively involved in the coordination of visual services to this population.

When a special needs individual is brought in for an evaluation, the parent or teacher is often looking to the doctor to provide useful information that may go beyond the scope of a typical eye examination. It is obviously important to diagnose pathologic or neurologic conditions that might compromise ocular or systemic health. The value of this examination, however, can be enhanced tremendously by providing useful functional information that can enhance educational and rehabilitative efforts and improve the quality of life for special needs individuals.

SELF-ASSESSMENT QUESTIONS

1. When evaluating the visual skills of a special needs child, it is best to position the child so that he or she is sitting unsupported.
   True or False

2. The decision as to which visual acuity test is used with a special needs child should be based on the child's
   (a) chronological age
   (b) cognitive age
   (c) emotional status
   (d) environmental awareness
   (e) none of the above are correct

3. If a special needs child refuses to wear glasses that are prescribed, this may mean that
   (a) the prescription is too strong
   (b) the prescription is too weak
   (c) the child should not be wearing glasses
   (d) the child may need to learn to adapt to the frames on his or her face
   (e) a or d may be correct

4. A child who consistently turns his or her head toward one side usually has a visual field loss.
   True or False

5. The LEA symbols and the Broken Wheel test are appropriate for
   (a) children older than age 1 year
   (b) children older than age 3 years
   (c) children with a cognitive age >1 year
   (d) children with a cognitive age >3 years
   (e) children with a cognitive age >5 years

6. Which of the following is not true regarding the Teller acuity cards?
   (a) It is a near visual acuity test.
   (b) It can be insensitive to strabismic amblyopia.
   (c) It is equivalent to the LEA symbols.
   (d) It may not detect mild to moderate myopia.

7. Photosensitivity is commonly associated with which of the following disorders:
   (a) congenital cataracts
   (b) albinism
   (c) rod monochromatism
   (d) aniridia
   (e) all of the above

REFERENCES

1. Scholl GT. What Does it Mean to Be Blind? Definitions, Terminology, Prevalence. In Foundations of Education for Blind and Visually Handicapped Children and Youth, New York: American Foundation for the Blind, 1986;23–33.
2. Jose RT, Smith AJ, Shane KG. Evaluating and stimulating vision in the multiply impaired. J Vis Impair Blindness, 1980:74;2–8.
3. Zimmerman DR. Birth defects and visual impairment. J Vis Impair Blindness. 1977:71;2–12.
4. Scheiman M. Assessment and Management of the Exceptional Child. In AA Rosenbloom, MW Morgan (eds), Principles and Practice of Pediatric Optometry. Philadelphia: Lippincott, 1990; 388–419.
5. Fraunfelder FT. Drug-Induced Ocular Side Effects and Drug Interactions (2nd ed). Philadelphia: Lea & Febiger, 1982;97–101, 115–119, 225–257, 373–374.
6. Fantz RL. Pattern vision in young infants. Psychol Rec 1958:8; 43–47.
7. Birch EE, Bane MC. Forced-choice preferential looking acuity of

children with cortical visual impairment. Dev Med Child Neurol 1991:33;722–729.

8. Fielder AR, Russell-Eggitt R, Dodd KL, Mellor DH. Delayed visual maturation. Trans Ophthalmol Soc UK 1985:104; 653–661.

9. Mayer DL, Fulton AB, Sossen PL. Preferential looking acuity of pediatric patients with developmental disabilities. Behav Brain Res 1983:10;189–198.

10. Birch EE, Hale LA, Stager DR, et al. Operant acuity of toddlers and developmentally delayed children with low vision. J Pediatr Ophthalmol Strabismus 1987:24;64–69.

11. Mayer DL, Fulton AB, Hansen RM. Visual acuity of infants and children with retinal degenerations. Ophthalmic Pediatr Genet 1985:5;51–56.

12. Press LJ. STYCAR ball acuity in relation to contrast and blur. Am J Optom Physiol Opt 1982:59;128–134.

13. Ciner EB. Management of Refractive Error in Infants, Toddlers, and Preschool Children. In M Schieman (ed), Problems in Optometry. Philadelphia: Lippincott, 1990;394–419.

14. Baldwin WR. Refractive Status of Infants and Children. In AA Rosenbloom, MW Morgan (eds), Principles and Practice of Pediatric Optometry. Philadelphia: Lippincott, 1990;104–152.

15. Mohindra I. A noncycloplegic refraction technique for infants and young children. J Am Optom Assoc 1977:48;518–523.

16. Duckman R. Using Photorefraction to Evaluate Refractive Error, Ocular Alignment, and Accommodation in Infants, Toddlers and Multiply Handicapped Children. In M Scheiman (ed), Problems in Optometry—Pediatric Optometry. Philadelphia: Lippincott, 1990:333–353.

17. Braddick OJ, Atkinson J, Wattam-Bell, et al. Videorefractive screening of accommodative performance in infants. Invest Ophthalmol Vis Sci 1988:29S;60.

18. Freedman HL, Preston KL. Polaroid photoscreening for amblyogenic factors. Ophthalmol 1993:99;1785.

19. Tongue AC, Cibis GW. Bruckner test. Ophthalmology 1981:88;1041.

20. Ciner EB, Schanel-Klitsch E, Herzberg H. Stereoacuity development: 6 months to 5 years: a new tool for testing and screening. Optom Vis Sci 1996:73;43–48.

21. Duckman R. Accommodation in cerebral palsy: function and remediation. J Am Optom Assoc 1984:4;281.

22. Bailey I. Happy Face Contrast Sensitivity Test. Berkeley, CA: University of California College of Optometry Center for the Study of Visual Impairment School of Optometry.

23. Adams RJ, Mercer ME, Courage ML. A new technique to measure contrast sensitivity in human infants. Optom Vis Sci 1992:69; 440–446.

24. Pease PL, Allen J. A new test for screening color vision: concurrent validity and utility. Am J Optom Physiol Opt 1988:65;729–738.

25. Haegerstrom-Portnoy G. Color Vision. In AA Rosenbloom, MW Morgan (eds), Principles and Practice of Pediatric Optometry. Philadelphia: Lippincott, 1990;449–466.

26. Ciner EB, Macks B, Schanel-Klitsch E. A cooperative demonstration project for early intervention vision services. Occup Ther Pract 1991:3;42–56.

CHAPTER SEVENTEEN

Low Vision Special Populations II: The Stroke Patient

John S. Ray and
Michele A. Maahs

Approximately 5% of the United States population older than the age of 65 years is affected by stroke.[1] Considering this, one can reasonably project that the total number of individuals affected by stroke will continue to increase, given the aging "baby boom" generation. It has also been documented that there are frequently visual and visuoperceptual deficits that result from central nervous system damage.[2–4] A comprehensive visual and perceptual evaluation must, therefore, be included in the examination of any patient with history of stroke, enhancing the overall prognosis for successful rehabilitation of these patients.

The effectiveness of the ocular evaluation of the patient affected by stroke may be complicated by a number of concomitant deficits. Standard evaluation strategies often do not elicit accurate responses, as they do not factor in the effects of any concurrent deficits. Thus, modifications or adaptations of the standard ocular testing procedures are often needed. These adaptation strategies typically are not part of the standard ocular curriculum and are, therefore, not familiar to most eye care practitioners. An evaluation incorporating these modifications often yields valuable information about the individual's visual and perceptual status. This knowledge enables members of the rehabilitation team to structure appropriate treatment interventions for the individual exhibiting severe or multiple impairments secondary to neurologic loss.

Due to increased frustration, fatigue, decreased processing speed, communication deficits, or behavioral complications, complete evaluation of this patient population frequently requires extended sessions or multiple visits. If the low vision practitioner is part of the rehabilitation team, he or she must keep in mind that each discipline is performing ongoing evaluations with the patient as well. Information gathered from all evaluations should be available to all team members so that diagnosis and treatment may be refined. Sharing of information assures that all deficit areas are addressed and that the most appropriate intervention strategies are selected.

Familiarity with the deficits that may result from a stroke can assist the doctor in choosing the most appropriate evaluation strategies and enhance the information-gathering process. This chapter clarifies the types of concomitant deficits commonly found in stroke patients and presents a variety of evaluative and prescriptive techniques.

MOTOR DEFICITS ASSOCIATED WITH STROKE

A variety of physical deficits may result from nervous system (central or peripheral) damage. The motor deficits commonly resulting from stroke range from generalized weakness to total loss of function. The side of the body affected is typically contralateral to the central nervous system damage. The motor deficit may or may not be accompanied by abnormal muscle tone. Muscle tone may be flaccid (low tonus) or spastic (high tonus). Some of the atypical body positioning observed may be caused by muscle tone abnormalities and not necessarily result from visual or perceptual deficits.

The patient exhibiting flaccid, or low tone on the affected side of the body usually has one or both limbs on that side that appear lifeless. The limb or limbs may be noted to hang at the patient's side. If the practitioner attempts to move the extremity, he or she will feel that the extremity is very heavy and there is little or no resistance to the movement. If asked to move the extremity, the patient will most likely be unable, or the movement will be of poor quality. Posturally, the patient with flaccid tone tends to lean toward the affected side. If the patient is observed leaning to the opposite side, he or she is generally attempting to compensate for the low tone by increasing the tone on the unaffected side to hold his or her postural position and maintain balance.

The patient who exhibits spastic, or high, tone may also demonstrate the same type of postural leaning toward one side. The spasticity tends to pull the patient's body toward the affected side. The unaffected side may, in this instance, not be strong enough to counteract the effect of the spasticity. The pull, therefore, is toward the affected side. The individual with spastic tone typically holds his or her extremity close to the body in a flexed position. It is this tone that contributes to maintenance of the flexed position and not necessarily the volition of the patient.

Abnormal muscle tone and lack of movement on the affected side of the body may contribute to the fear a patient might exhibit when asked to move from his or her wheelchair into the examining chair. To ensure the best possible positioning for the examination, it is recommended that the practitioner not have the patient move into the examining chair. Instead, allow him or her to stay in the wheelchair, where the patient feels secure and where appropriate seating and positioning is maintained. An occupational or physical therapist may have provided the patient with a specialized seating arrangement that provides stability while optimizing function. Because the position of the wheelchair may reduce the usefulness of the established stationary equipment available in the doctor's examination room, modifications to the examination process are frequently necessary. To accommodate positioning issues, a variety of supplies and instrumentation is recommended, such as handheld charts, a portable biomicroscope, and a portable tonometer. Use of this equipment may be the only way to obtain accurate information.[5]

Another type of motor deficit that may result from stroke is apraxia. *Apraxia* is a motor planning deficit that more frequently results from left-sided central nervous system damage.[6] The patient with apraxia typically has difficulty automatically producing a movement in response to a verbal command or contextual cue. For example, when a patient is asked to demonstrate how to use a hammer, he or she is unable to respond. When the same patient is given a hammer, he or she automatically knows how to use it (given that the patient is familiar with the use of a hammer). There are multiple forms of apraxia, which are not discussed in this chapter. It is important for the practitioner to be familiar with general apraxia, however, as it could affect establishing useful communication. For example, in attempting to assess acuity from a patient with apraxia, the patient may be asked to point to the appropriate answer on a communication board. This patient may be unable to respond to the direction given, due to an inability to produce the movement that was requested. Demonstrating to the patient by pointing to the appropriate answer on the communication board may still not evoke a response. To gain a useful response, alternative testing measures must be determined. The doctor may consider using the Broken Wheel Cards (Vision Training Products, Inc., Mishawaka, IN) (see Figure 16-2). When holding the cards far enough apart, an eye movement toward the correct response can be the established communication. This alternative testing approach may assist in compensating for apraxia.

In most instances, the patient with apraxia poses the greatest challenge to the practitioner. With this patient, a keen sense of observation is the most effective strategy. It is also important to communicate with the rest of the team members, allowing observations to be gathered regarding the patient's functional ability, and therefore, enabling accurate judgments to be made regarding the patient's visual function.

COMMUNICATION DISORDERS AFTER STROKE

Aphasia, a communication deficit affecting the expressive or receptive components of language, is another concomitant loss associated with stroke. It is more commonly found with left-sided cerebral damage as opposed to right-sided damage. Aphasia can appear in a number of different forms. *Expressive aphasia* refers to difficulty with the expression component of speech. This deficit can vary from an occasional difficulty with word choice to total loss of speech. The patient with expressive aphasia finds it difficult or impossible to make his or her thoughts or needs known to others. A patient with expressive aphasia responds to a question with any of the following responses:

1. No verbal response
2. An inappropriate response, which the patient recognizes as wrong
3. An unintelligible flow of speech

In addition to speech, writing is usually also affected in expressive aphasia.

Receptive aphasia is the inability to understand verbal language presented by others. This deficit can also vary in severity from the occasional inability to comprehend to a total inability to understand spoken language. The patient with receptive aphasia finds it difficult or impossible to understand what others are trying to communicate. Understanding speech and written words is usually affected with this type of aphasia.

Finally, a combination of expressive and receptive aphasia can occur. This type of aphasia is termed *global aphasia*. The individual with global aphasia has seemingly equal difficulty in speaking, writing, understanding speech, and reading. Aphasia can complicate the evaluation process, creating difficulty in forming a means of communication between patient and practitioner. It is, therefore, important that the doctor be aware of this deficit to devise appropriate adaptations to the evaluation process.

SENSORY DEFICITS ASSOCIATED WITH STROKE

Of all the sensory deficits that can occur as a result of stroke, impairments of the tactile and visual systems appear to be the most common. Because both of these systems have a significant impact on motor performance, it is important to complete a thorough evaluation of each system. It is typically the responsibility of the physical or occupational therapist to evaluate the integration of the sensory systems. Results of these evaluations should be made available to all members.

Tactile loss may affect protective sensations, discriminatory sensations, proprioception, or kinesthesia. In the most severe form of tactile loss, there is hemianesthesia on the affected side, contralateral to the lesion.

Safety issues pose the greatest concern. For example, patients may unknowingly position themselves too close to a heat source and be burned, or they may not feel that their affected arm is hanging over the side of the wheelchair, thereby putting the extremity in jeopardy of injury. The loss of tactile sensation may lead to many potentially dangerous situations. The practitioner must, therefore, be prepared to intervene in the event of potential danger to the patient during the evaluation process.

The final sensory system frequently affected by neurologic loss is the visual system. Much has been written over the years about the visual deficits resulting from stroke and brain injury. Impairments that may occur are visual acuity loss, visual field loss, extraocular muscle (EOM) paralysis resulting in diplopia, and visual perceptual deficits such as unilateral inattention. The selection of effective evaluation modifications to aid in diagnosing these deficits for the stroke patient with aphasia or apraxia is quite challenging to the practitioner and well worth the effort. It is particularly rewarding to both the patient and practitioner when the patient had been previously labeled as "untestable."

Visual Acuity Evaluation

It is well understood that clarity of vision is crucial for daily functioning. Therefore, the visual acuity test should be one of the first evaluation measures completed. Most practitioners use a projector chart, as it is effective for the majority of patients. The stroke patient, however, responds differently than most patients evaluated. If aphasia is present, the patient will perform better if the practitioner is able to modify the visual acuity chart. Use of a number chart rather than one with letters provides a more successful tool. A letter chart is comprised of potentially 26 different letters or targets, whereas a number chart has the potential of only 10 different targets (Figure 17-1). The decreased number of targets is useful if a matching

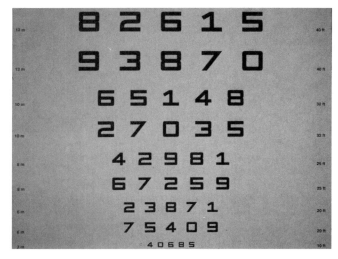

FIGURE 17-1.   **A number chart, in many cases, is easier for a patient who is neurologically impaired to identify. Because of the decreased number of targets, when compared to letters, it is also easier for patients to use when forced to use a matching technique.**

technique needs to be used to compensate for inaccurate verbal responses. Additionally, in many cases the aphasic patient has more success in verbalization of numbers than letters. When providing matching characters, it is recommended that the patient be provided with large, bold, black numbers written lengthwise on a standard 8½-in.×11-in. white paper. The practitioner should explain the matching procedure (several times if necessary), provide the patient with several trials, start at an acuity level well above the patient's threshold, and always provide verbal reinforcement for correctly following the directions and identifying the correct acuity optotype. The chart should be portable as well, so that it can be used at any distance and at any angle from the patient.

At times, especially when evaluating the severely aphasic patient, use of number or letter charts is still unsuccessful. Having access to the tumbling E, Landolt C, Lighthouse Picture chart (The Lighthouse, Inc., Long Island City, NY), or the Broken Wheel Cards can provide more opportunities to find some form of effective communication regarding patient responses. Having the patient point in the direction of the correct answer or separating targets so that an eye movement toward the correct response can be distinguished are other available options for testing.

Visual Field Evaluation

Visual field loss is another deficit that occurs after a neurologic insult. Because the majority of strokes occur behind the optic chiasm, most visual field losses tend to be homonymous in nature. Homonymous hemianopic field loss often involves a geniculocalcarine lesion. If the occipital lobe incurs damage, there is a higher incidence of macular sparing. With macular sparing, patients appear to

learn to compensate for the field loss at a much faster rate than if the macular fibers are damaged.

Visual fields are typically evaluated with the confrontation method, allowing the practitioner a quick procedure to determine if a loss exists. The most commonly used technique of confrontation is the finger count. With this technique, the patient is asked to maintain fixation on the doctor's nose and to use his or her peripheral vision to count the number of fingers on the doctor's hand as it is presented. Presentation of stimuli should occur in each quadrant, singly. Once each quadrant has been evaluated, double simultaneous presentation of stimuli is used, checking for the presence of the extinction phenomenon. This phenomenon is defined as an inability to perceive a stimulus in one area of the visual field when there is simultaneous stimulation elsewhere in the visual field. The condition is characteristic of unilateral inattention, in which the patient does not perceive one side of his or her environment, although there may not be a visual field deficit. With this test, the patient is asked to add the fingers being presented on both hands.

The confrontation test method of using finger counting is not usually effective for the aphasic patient, as the patient may be unable to verbalize the correct response. Use of a finger wiggle method may be more successful. Here the patient can communicate by pointing to or looking at the wiggling finger. This technique is most effective when double simultaneous presentation of hands is used, but only one hand at a time presents a wiggling finger. This method removes the peripheral cue of a moving target.

The flash method of presentation should be used in conjunction with the finger wiggle technique. This method uses a short presentation of a wiggling finger, followed by abrupt discontinuation of movement. The cue is thus removed before the patient's eye moves to fixate on the target, providing an adaptation for the patient who has difficulty maintaining fixation or who searches for the stimuli. This technique has also been effective in compensating for a communication disorder. The eye movement toward the position of the correct response can be used as a form of communication. It tells the doctor that the peripheral stimulus was noticed, because it produces a saccadic response that would not have occurred if there was a field deficit.

A second modification of the confrontation field is the dynamic confrontation field.[7] This method is performed by presenting a finger from one hand in one of the quadrants. The doctor asks the patient to touch the finger that is presented. In the case of unilateral inattention or hemianopsia, the patient often exhibits a combined head movement and saccade to successfully make contact with the doctor's finger on the affected side. When the target is presented on the unaffected side, the patient will generally exhibit a large amplitude saccade to make contact.

Penlight field testing is another useful technique for a severely impaired individual who is not capable of being assessed with the previously mentioned confrontation field tests. This technique requires two persons for effective administration. One person, serving as the fixation target and observer, stands or sits a few feet in front of the patient. The other person remains behind the patient with a penlight and is responsible for bringing the penlight from behind the patient into each quadrant: nasal, temporal, superior, and inferior. It is important to explain this test procedure to the patient before testing to enhance the accuracy of response. The person who is serving as the fixation target observes any responses that the patient may exhibit (e.g., head turn, eye turn, pointing). When a response is made by the patient, it is important to note which of the quadrants was tested and the actual position in which the target was first noted by the patient in each quadrant.

Another field test that may be helpful with this patient population is the functional field test. This test requires two individuals for accuracy. One individual serves as the fixation target and the other as the tester. The individual who serves as the fixation target positions him- or herself approximately 5 ft in front of the patient; the tester stands behind the patient. The tester slowly walks from behind the patient, along one side, until he or she is noticed. The tester then returns to the original position and repeats the procedure several times, walking to one side of the patient or the other. Variation in response time and position of the tester in relation to the patient provides the doctor with a gross indication of the patient's peripheral awareness. Before performing this test, all efforts should be made to explain the process that will occur so that test accuracy is enhanced. This particular test is also useful in demonstrating to the patient and others (e.g., therapists, family members) the presence of unilateral inattention or hemianopic field loss. It is helpful in teaching the patient awareness of these deficits as well. Furthermore, this test is the most effective to implement before evaluating and demonstrating the benefit of any form of prism to increase field awareness. The procedure, though simple, is certainly an integral part of the visual battery of testing for these patients.

Although most of the visual field tests discussed in this section reveal gross information, they may be the only way to obtain information. Many times, fatigue, frustration, lack of understanding or lack of impulsivity prohibit the patient with history of stroke from tolerating the extended procedure required for an automated field test. Having access to simple field tests and knowledge of the various modifications that have been successful provides the practitioner with valuable information within a reasonable time frame. This information, in turn, will positively affect the outcome of the rehabilitation process.

Extraocular Muscle Evaluation

EOM function can be difficult when attempting to assess this population as well. Observation is thus a very important component of the examination. Communication or motor planning deficits may not allow the stroke patient

to respond appropriately when using the conventional physiological H pattern to evaluate EOM function. Attempts at performing this pattern may be enhanced by having the patient hold the transilluminator along with the practitioner. Having the patient hold the transilluminator includes the patient in the examination process by adding tactile input to the procedure. This procedure is particularly helpful for patients with apraxia. If this procedure is unsuccessful, keen observation of the patient's eye movements throughout the evaluation process becomes necessary. If the practitioner is not satisfied with observational information, use of the doll's eye reflex (manually moving the patient's head side to side while he or she fixates on the doctor's face) may be the most successful resort. Head movement, while a person fixates on a target, elicits eye movements to compensate for the head's positional change. Therefore, a more automatic response is revealed, demonstrating the range of the eye's motility.

When an acquired strabismus exists (e.g., nerve palsy, gaze paresis, ophthalmoplegia), the practitioner may find neutralization of the eye turn using a prism bar and cover test procedure to be most effective. Use of the Maddox rod, in this instance, may be unsuccessful as it requires a verbal response. Observation of behavioral changes is usually the best indicator that fusion has been attained. The neutralization process may produce agitation if the practitioner provides "close" neutralization but not enough to produce fusion. For example, the existence of a severe eye turn may not produce complaints of diplopia because the disparity of the images is so significant that the patient is able to suppress or ignore the double imagery. Close neutralization only creates a more observable diplopia, which provokes agitation as the patient is no longer able to suppress the strabismic eye. Alternate patching may be the best intervention until further improvement is attained through neurologic resolution. Diplopia interferes with the patient's quality of life as well as creating nausea, postural imbalance, and eye-hand coordination deficits or mobility problems. The purpose of rehabilitation is to enhance independent functioning and increase the quality of life for a disabled individual, so all efforts to alleviate a distressing disorder, such as diplopia, will improve the prognosis for success.

Perceptual Deficits Associated with Stroke

It has been documented that there are significant visuoperceptual deficits that result from stroke.[2, 3, 8] The most widely researched and documented deficit is that of unilateral inattention, or neglect. In its purest form, *unilateral inattention* is defined as a condition in which an individual with normal sensory and motor systems fails to orient toward, respond to, or report stimuli on the side contralateral to the cerebral lesion. Unilateral spatial inattention occurs more often with right hemisphere damage. Inattention has been associated with lesions in both cortical and subcortical structures. Inattention is most com-

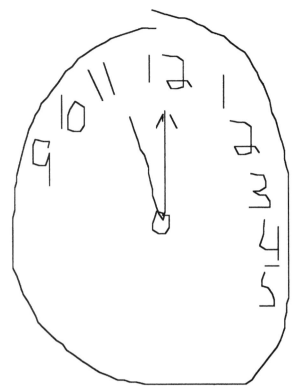

FIGURE 17-2.   **Drawing of a clock by a patient with inattention deficit.**

monly seen in inferior parietal lobe lesions and has also been observed in lesions of the dorsolateral frontal lobe, cingulate gyrus, thalamus, and putaminal hemorrhage.[8]

Unilateral inattention has been documented in persons demonstrating no accompanying visual field defect and limb sensory or motor loss. Unilateral inattention is not often seen alone, however, but is usually associated with accompanying sensory and motor defects such as homonymous hemianopsia or decreased tactile, proprioceptive and stereognostic perception, along with paresis or paralysis of the upper limb.[8] The effect of hemispatial inattention can be devastating. In fact, some researchers cite unilateral inattention as one of the main factors interfering with recovery and successful rehabilitation in stroke patients. In severe forms, the patient demonstrates complete hemispatial inattention to the extent that he may not dress or shave the affected half of the body. Questions addressed to the patient from the affected side may go unanswered. Navigation through an environment may be difficult as the patient collides with objects and is unable to orient him- or herself to new surroundings. In subtle forms, the patient demonstrates inattention only when faced with a complex task.[9]

EVALUATION PROCEDURES

The doctor's assessment should begin with simple observation of the patient. Patients with moderate to severe

inattention may demonstrate particular behavior patterns as they orient their body and activities toward the unaffected hemisphere.[9] The patient's posture when he or she enters the examining room and how he or she responds during the history interview should be noted. Observation of stance is very informative. If the patient's body weight is toward the unaffected side, or there is a lack of eye movement toward the affected side, the doctor should be alerted to the potential of an inattention deficit.

A commonly used screening procedure for inattention is the double simultaneous stimulation test (simultaneous finger count). A standard confrontation visual field is first conducted, using single stimuli presented in each quadrant of the visual field. If the response is abnormal, one cannot differentiate between a hemianopic visual field defect and a severe inattention disorder without further testing. In this case, the double stimulation test cannot be performed. If the responses are normal, the doctor then presents double simultaneous stimuli, one placed on each side of the vertical midline. Extinction occurs when the patient fails to perceive the stimulus in the field contralateral to the lesion, while correctly perceiving the stimulus in the ipsilateral field. It should be noted that this test sensitivity may be as low as 50%.[9] When results gained by confrontation leave a reasonable doubt in the practitioner's mind and the accuracy of the simultaneous stimulation finger count test is low, other tests should be considered to enhance the reliability of findings.

There are several test procedures that have been used and recommended by many authors, including the cancellation test, the line bisection test, and the drawing test.[8–14] These tests can be easily used in an office setting and require relatively little time and supplies. If the practitioner is interested in purchasing a standardized test, the Rivermead Behavioral Inattention Test (Western Psychological Services, Los Angeles, CA) is recommended. This test contains each of the preceding components, as well as a number of functional evaluation tasks such as reading a menu, identifying and sorting coins, and sorting cards.

Administration of the drawing test is initiated by placing a blank piece of paper and a pen in front of the patient and asking him or her to draw a clock, tree, house, or person. A patient without deficits should draw a relatively symmetric and accurate picture. A patient with inattention, however, will draw an asymmetric picture similar to those shown in Figures 17-2 and 17-3. Having more than one drawing sample per patient (e.g., house, tree, clock, and person) is recommended, as it gives the practitioner a larger sample on which to base the diagnosis.

The cancellation and line bisection tests are also recommended as components of the standard battery. Examples of these tests can be seen in Figures 17-4 through 17-7. The cancellation test is used to evaluate field awareness in patients with hemianopic field loss and hemispatial inattention. It further provides information on the patient's ability to compensate for the preceding problems by using eye and head movements. The Hart Chart (Vision Training Products, Inc., Mishawaka, IN), which may commonly be found in a practitioner's office, can be used as a cancellation test. This test is performed by having the practitioner identify one letter that appears on both the right and left side of the chart. The patient is then asked to "cross off" or "cancel" that particular letter throughout the chart. A ratio is produced in which the numerator represents the number of correct responses by the patient with the denominator being the total number of times that particular letter appears on the chart. The final score is represented by a percentage. At the same time, the practitioner observes whether a particular pattern of missed characters appears. This provides information as to whether the patient is aware of his or her field loss and whether he or she attempts to compensate for it.

The line bisection test is used to assess a patient's perception of visual space and midline awareness. A blank paper may be used for this test. The practitioner simply draws a number of lines on the paper at various locations and asks the patient to bisect each line at the midpoint. It is important for the placement of this paper to be directly at the patient's midline. The location of the patient's mark will help to indicate his or her perception of visual space. A patient having a hemianopic field loss or inattention deficit will skew the mark opposite to the affected side. For example, if the patient bisects the line more toward the right, it can be assumed that he or she has decreased perception of the left side. The degree at which the patient skews the line from the midpoint will indicate the extent of the defect. Observation of the patient when performing this test may also reveal an irregular scanning pattern or poor planning strategies that the patient is using for this near-task performance. These irregular patterns may also appear when the patient attempts to perform any distant task.

Dr. Henry Greene has presented two techniques that he found to be effective in the diagnosis of a unilateral inattention.[7,15] He demonstrated the use of both a phoria card, that had been increased in size to fit an 8½-in.×11-in. piece of paper, and a Hart Chart, as tools for evaluating near-point tasks. The phoria card was placed in the patient's midline, and the 0 point was emphasized with an X. He asked the patient to look at the X in the center, then to find the highest number located to the right of the X. When the right side was completed, he redirected the

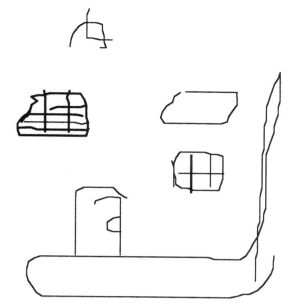

FIGURE 17-3. **Drawing of a house by a patient with inattention deficit.**

patient's attention to the X and then asked him or her to find the highest number to the left. When using this test, a patient with left unilateral inattention will accurately identify the highest number located on the right of the page but not on the left. Although this procedure is very simple, it gives the practitioner a good indication of the extent of a patient's peripheral constriction or visual awareness.

Use of the Hart Chart for testing peripheral constriction or unilateral inattention provides the practitioner with a percentage of a patient's constriction or inattention. The chart consists of 10 rows, having 10 letters in each row, thereby providing 100 targets (Figure 17-8). The Hart chart is placed in the patient's midline. The patient is asked to read the first letter on the left and the last letter on the right of each line until all of the first and last letters have been identified. Missing letters during the progression down the page provide the doctor with infor-

FIGURE 17-4. **An example of the E & R Cancellation Test from the Rivermead Behavioral Inattention Test (Western Psychological Services, Los Angeles, CA).**

AEIKNRUNPOERBDHRSCOXRPGEAEIKNRUNPB

BDHEUWSTRFHEAFRTOLRJEMOEBDHEUWSTJ

NOSRVXTPEBDHPTSIJFLRFENOONOSRVXTPEI

GLPTYTRIBEDMRGKEDLPQFERXGLPTYTRIBR

HMEBGRDEINRSVLERFGOSEHCBRHMEBGRDE

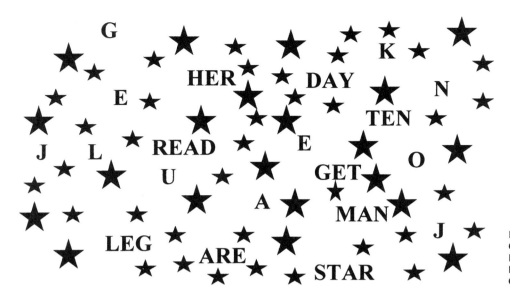

FIGURE 17-5.   **An example of the Star Cancellation Test from the Rivermead Behavioral Inattention Test (Western Psychological Services, Los Angeles, CA).**

mation of a field constriction or inattention. By counting all of the letters missed, the practitioner can determine a percent of deficit, or *drift,* as termed by Dr. Greene. If the patient misses 25 letters on the left side, that patient is said to have a 25% drift toward the right. A patient with unilateral inattention will typically start the task with good accuracy, because his or her attention has been directed to the left margin. Without further prompting from the doctor, the patient will begin to read letters that are closer to the midline of the page, rather than those located on the left. The doctor will notice a somewhat diagonal pattern forming during the test, and those letters to the left of the diagonal are counted as missed targets, thereby producing a percentage of right drift. Dr. Greene uses this procedure as a means of quantifying the field constriction or inattention and as a documented means of comparison between pre– and post–prism use determining whether prism is useful as a compensation tool.

Use of the functional field test has also been found to be effective in diagnosing unilateral inattention. This test demonstrates the functional impairment that is created by the inattention. It is important to perform both a static and a dynamic test procedure, as the severity of the inattention is frequently complicated by the complexity of the

task. The practitioner should begin with the technique discussed earlier in the section on field testing, as this is the static component of the test. When this part has been completed, the patient should be moved to an open area or hallway where he or she can ambulate or propel his or her wheelchair. As the patient moves within the test environment, the practitioner walks from behind (on either side) and notes when the patient responds to his or her presence. The patient with unilateral inattention will typically respond more rapidly to the doctor on the unaffected side than on the affected side. In most cases, there is a significant difference between sides in the distances the practitioner must walk before the patient notes his or her presence. For example, with some patients the response may be as great as 10–15 ft on the left as compared to 3–5 ft on the right.

LOW VISION TREATMENT STRATEGIES

When treating the visual problems resulting from stroke, it is best to use a combination of modalities from primary care, binocular vision, and low vision rehabilitation. Frequently, the most appropriate solution results from trial

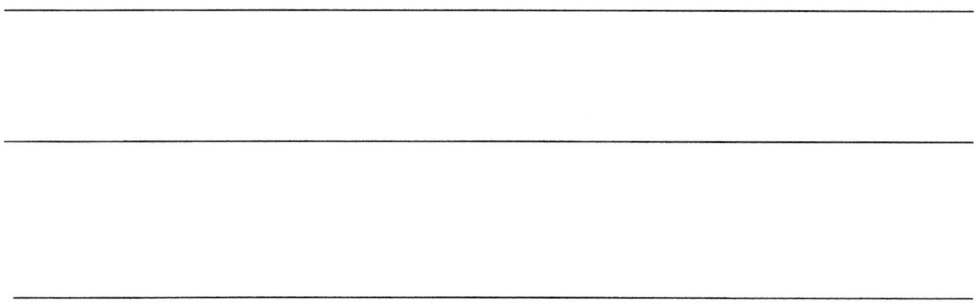

FIGURE 17-6.   **An example of the Line Bisection Test from the Rivermead Behavioral Inattention Test (Western Psychological Services, Los Angeles, CA).**

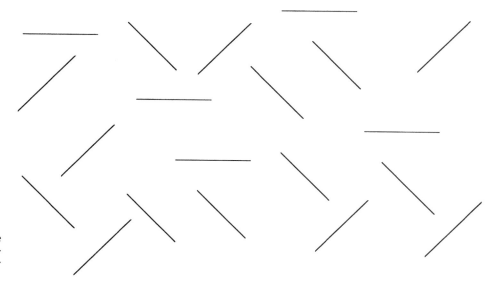

FIGURE 17-7. **An example of the Line Bisection Test from the Rivermead Behavioral Inattention Test (Western Psychological Services, Los Angeles, CA).**

and error, innovative and creative ideas, and experience. Management can incorporate optical as well as nonoptical devices, specific for the type of functional activity the patient wishes to perform. Some common visual concerns include reading and writing, eating, grooming, recognizing faces, viewing television, wheelchair propulsion, and ambulation. In many cases, low vision management strategies use separate treatments for each functional task. These same strategies can be incorporated into the visual management of the stroke population.

Provision for an extended evaluation and instructional period is imperative when working with patients exhibiting visual problems secondary to a stroke. This period allows time for the patient to become accustomed to a new approach. It also allows time for the team and family members to observe the patient's performance and to give feedback as to the effectiveness of the recommended treatment. Strategies for the treatment of decreased acuity, diplopia, homonymous hemianopsia, and unilateral inattention are presented in the sections that follow.

Decreased Acuity

Before establishing strategies for managing decreased acuity, the practitioner must first ascertain whether the decrease is refractive or pathologic. To make this determination, an accurate objective refraction must be performed. A subjective refraction may not always be possible with this population, due to decreased verbal communication or lack of patient understanding. Observation of behavioral changes may be the best indicator of subjective clarity, especially with the severely impaired patient. Time should be allotted for a trial period with the refractive prescription in place to allow for observation of the patient. During this period, it is the responsibility of the rehabilitation team and the family observers to report any noticeable changes in performance that may indicate a change in visual clarity. It may also be necessary to schedule

weekly follow-up visits to make changes in the lenses if appropriate, and reincorporate the changes into daily life tasks.

Once the refraction has been completed, it must be determined if the patient should wear single-vision or multifocal lenses. Personal goals, lifestyle, availability of assistance or supervision, and cognitive status are significant factors here. Previous spectacle wearing experience and adaptation, ocular motility functions, field loss or inattention, lens power, position of the activity, and layout of the workspace should be considered as well.

If a patient had been successful with either multifocal or single-vision lenses before the stroke and all other areas of concern are unchanged, the prevailing design should be retained. In contrast, if there are significant residual

	2	4	6	8	10
1	O F	N P	V D	T C	H E
	Y B	A K	O E	Z L	R X
3	E T	H W	F M	B K	A P
	B X	F R	T O	S M	V C
5	R A	D V	S X	P E	T O
	M P	O E	A N	C B	K F
7	C R	G D	B K	E P	M A
	F X	P S	M A	R D	L G
9	T M	U A	X S	O G	P B
	H O	S N	C T	K U	Z L

FIGURE 17-8. **The Hart Chart (Vision Training Products, Inc., Mishawaka, IN) can be used to test for peripheral construction or unilateral inattention.**

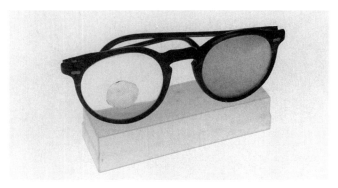

FIGURE 17-9.   **The right lens demonstrates a "spot" occluder that may eliminate a patient's diplopia when he or she is looking straight ahead (the left lens would have the patient's spectacle correction with no occlusion). In this same spectacles sample, the left lens is frosted, which is cosmetically more pleasing than a standard black patch when full occlusion is required.**

deficits, then another option may need to be chosen. Examples of situations in which single-vision lenses may be the lens of choice include limited extraocular range of motion, difficulty with infraduction, visual field loss, and the need for a high powered reading lens (above +4.00 D of add). When single-vision lenses are prescribed and the patient requires both distance and near correction, it is recommended that the patient choose two different spectacle frames to prevent using the wrong spectacle prescription.

Incorporating low vision systems to compensate for decreased acuity is also helpful. Simple changes, such as using a bold-line marker instead of a ball point pen to write, or increasing the lighting available by incorporating task lighting, may assist the patient in performing many tasks independently. Prescribing low-powered telescopes as well as microscopes and handheld and stand magnifiers is helpful in some cases.

Education plays an important role in many cases, paving the way to independence. When the patient understands the relevant concepts as they pertain to his or her specific needs, he or she can begin to formulate problem solving. With the severely involved patient, educating the family members is important, as it is they who will be responsible for assisting and setting up the environment for the patient.

Disconjugate Gaze and Diplopia

Disconjugate gaze with resultant diplopia can be a very disturbing complication from stroke. It has been found that gaze paresis occurs in 29% of right-sided stroke patients and 25% of left-sided stroke patients.[16] With this population, suppression rarely occurs, and therefore, this diplopic condition may cause significant effects on the patient's ability to participate in various tasks, including activities of daily living.

The residual diplopia can be horizontal, vertical, or oblique, and the course is often varied in duration, magnitude, and degree of resolution. Generally, 80% of prob-

lems associated with acquired muscle paresis resulting in disconjugate gaze have been found to resolve within 3–6 months.[17] Because this is typically the time period during which stroke patients receive rehabilitation, it is imperative that an ocular assessment be provided at the earliest possible time with the practitioner monitoring the patient for at least 1 full year.

Management of diplopia is most often a choice between occlusion and prism. The simplest to implement is occlusion. This technique, however, is not always acceptable to all patients as it may be uncomfortable, and is not cosmetically pleasing. Although the patient's peripheral field of view is decreased on the patched side, patching is the best option for those patients who cannot attain fusion with prism. It is also the most fitting management plan when there is still potential for neurologic improvement. Recommendation for ocular calisthenics should accompany the occlusion to assist in the prevention of contracture(s) of the EOMs.[18] Alternating the wearing schedule between eyes is also recommended.

In some cases of diplopia, along with the choice of patching, there is the choice of whether to completely or partially patch. Some patients may benefit from a small circular patch located on the spectacle lens, which occludes objects when the eye is in the primary gaze position. The patch can be constructed from an opaque piece of tape and applied to the ocular surface of the spectacle lens[19] (Figure 17-9). By applying this "spot" occluder, the practitioner may be able to eliminate the patient's diplopia when the patient is looking straight ahead and still allow the patient to maintain as much peripheral awareness as possible. In the case of noncomitant ocular misalignment, in which only specific positions of gaze produce diplopia, partial occlusion may be used. If the right superior oblique is paretic from a fourth nerve palsy and only inferior gaze produces diplopia, then only a patch in the lower portion of the right lens should be applied. The same would be true for a left lateral rectus paresis from a sixth nerve palsy. In this case, only left gaze would produce diplopia; therefore, a patch occluding the left portion of the lens should be applied. The edge of the patch in both cases should correspond to the position that initially produces diplopia. When the patient shifts gaze, no diplopia should result. If it does, then the patch should be moved closer to primary gaze to eliminate double vision.

Another option for the management of diplopia is the use of a prism. Both Fresnel prisms or ophthalmic ground-in prisms may be used. Each prism type has advantages and disadvantages. The advantages of Fresnel prisms as compared to ground-in prisms include their low cost, reduced weight, ability to be easily changed as the patient progresses, and the large variety of powers available. The major disadvantages are a reduction in contrast and a slight loss of acuity secondary to the inherent distortion. Fresnel prisms are generally more practical for the larger deviations of 8 prism diopters or more because of the reduced weight and thickness when compared to ground-in prisms.

When using prism to correct diplopia, the minimum amount necessary is advised. The practitioner should prescribe just enough power to produce fusion. This amount varies among patients but is typically between one-half to two-thirds of the total measured deviation.

For patients with noncomitancy, fusion may not be attainable in all positions of gaze. The primary goals are to produce single vision in primary gaze for distance, and inferior gaze at near.[18] These positions are considered priority because they correspond with most common functional tasks. This may require two separate prismatic prescriptions, because the power needed may be different for each position. Implementation can occur in either bifocal or single-vision form. Before prism is dispensed, however, it is necessary to investigate whether prism adaptation is present. This determination may be accomplished by having the patient wear the prism correction for approximately 1 hour, with continued cover testing every 15 minutes to rule out adaptation. If the deviation increases more than 3–5 prism diopters, adaptation is present, and prism should not be prescribed. In this situation, occlusion is then the management of choice.

The amount of prism may be prescribed in several ways. If the deviation is small (less than 8 prism diopters), then prism can be applied to or incorporated into one lens. The eye of choice is typically the one with less acuity.[20] With larger deviations, the prism can be evenly split between the two eyes. For horizontal deviations, the prism base should face the same direction when it is prescribed for both eyes. For example, if a patient has a deviation corrected with 6 prism diopters of base-out prism, then 3 prism diopters of base-out prism can be prescribed for the right eye along with 3 prism diopters of base-out prism for the left eye. For vertical deviations, the base must be inverted when split with the fellow eye. For example, if a patient has a deviation corrected with 4 prism diopters of base-down prism for the left eye, then 2 prism diopters of base-down prism in the left eye can be combined with 2 prism diopters of base-up prism in the right eye.

In the case of a horizontal diplopia caused by a sixth nerve palsy or a vertical deviation caused by a fourth nerve palsy, the Fresnel prism can be applied in the gaze position that elicits the diplopia, much like the partial occluder procedure. When diplopia occurs in most or all positions of gaze, as with a third nerve palsy, prism can be applied with one eye having the vertical component corrected while the fellow eye is corrected for the horizontal component. Moradiellos and Parrish also described a method for correcting oblique diplopia.[20] For their procedure, the patient wears a trial frame with the appropriate refractive correction while viewing through a Maddox rod placed in front of one eye. While fixating on a distant light source, such as the transilluminator, the patient rotates the axis of the Maddox rod until the red line travels through the middle of the light. The practitioner records this axis. Various powers of prism are then presented to the patient at this axis until the deviation is neutralized. Neutralization is reached when the patient sees the line centered on top of the light. The amount of prism and axis can then be prescribed.

Yoked prisms are another option for prismatic correction. Yoked prisms have been found to be helpful for patients who are unable to produce a desired eye movement due to paresis yet need awareness of information from that area of space. The prisms will shift the visual space away from the position of gaze with the greatest paresis. For example, in the case of a right lateral rectus paresis, the patient would be prescribed base-right prisms for each eye (base out OD, base in OS) to minimize the need to look toward the right.[18]

When prescribing prism, frequent follow-up visits are required. It is anticipated that many patients will demonstrate neurologic improvement, thereby requiring changes to the prescribed prismatic power. Only through follow-up services can the practitioner determine this need and provide the necessary change. A follow-up visit is recommended every 2–4 weeks.

Regardless of the choice of intervention, ocular exercises or calisthenics should be prescribed. In doing this, contracture can be avoided and improvement encouraged. It is recommended that these exercises be started monocularly, followed by binocular integration.

If disconjugate gaze does not resolve within 1 year, strabismus surgery can be considered. One can be reasonably certain that with lack of any improvement after 1 year, further neurologic recovery is unlikely. In educating the patient about options, he or she should also be informed that occlusion, lens frosting, and prismatic correction may be used indefinitely as potential options to surgical intervention.

Homonymous Hemianopsia and Unilateral Inattention

Homonymous hemianopsia and unilateral inattention are common visual field deficits resulting from cerebrovascular accident. Specifically, field loss has been found to be present after 36% of right-sided strokes and 25% of left-sided strokes. In contrast, unilateral inattention has been found in 82% of right-sided strokes and 65% of left-sided strokes.[16] Optical treatment for both of these conditions is similar and is aimed at providing peripheral awareness on the affected side.

Optical Displacement Systems

The systems that are commonly used with this patient population include Fresnel prisms, yoked ophthalmic prisms, the Visual Field Awareness System (REKINDLE, Stone Mountain, GA), the Inwave Field-Expanding Hemispheric Lens (Inwave Optics, Inc., Janesville, WI), and mirror systems. In all cases, these optical devices displace objects from the affected side, shifting them into view on the unaffected visual field. Due to the nature of the displacement, specific instruction in using any of the preceding systems must be provided, both verbally and in writing, before dispensing. See Appendix A for addresses and telephone numbers of manufacturers and suppliers of the preceding systems.

FRESNEL PRISMS. A description of Fresnel prisms and their advantages and disadvantages can be found in Chapter 12.

There are two schools of thought in the placement of a Fresnel prism to enhance field awareness. One technique positions the prism over the area of field loss, with the base of the prism positioned toward the field loss as described in Appendix A of Chapter 12. The other technique is to "crowd" the fit by making the Fresnel cover one-half of the pupil, so that any object in the affected peripheral area is constantly in view. In this situation, field awareness is enhanced without making any eye movement. This particular technique has been found to be helpful to individuals who have gaze paresis in addition to field loss or inattention. Again, the base should be directed toward the loss. Patient instructions on the adaptation of a prism can be found in Appendix B of Chapter 12.

Follow-up services should be provided in 2–3 weeks to determine how the patient is responding to the treatment and how successful he or she is in using the prism. If possible, input from a family member is often helpful in verifying the use of the prism.

Fresnel prisms may be successful for field enhancement for near tasks as well. The power of the Fresnel prism must be low (less than 15 prism diopters) to be effective in this case, however. For example, patients with a left temporal field loss often demonstrate difficulty finding the left margin of print. A Fresnel prism, held base left, can be positioned in front of the patient while reading. If this trial proves successful in assisting the patient to accurately return to the left margin, the prism may then be placed in the lower aspect of the spectacle for further evaluation.

YOKED PRISMS. Yoked prisms are a pair of identically powered prisms with the bases facing the same direction. They can be incorporated into a spectacle correction or are available in goggle form that can be worn over the patient's spectacles. Because these prisms are present across the entire field of view, there is no scanning necessary to gain peripheral awareness. They are particularly useful for patients with hemianopsia who have difficulty voluntarily scanning into the affected field for compensation. They have also been found to be beneficial for patients with unilateral inattention by giving the patient additional awareness of information on the affected side. Typically, only 4 prism diopters are needed in each eye, with the base of the prism facing the direction of the defect. For patients with hemianopsia, the objects not seen in the affected field are shifted toward the useable field. In cases of inattention, the prism realigns the patient's perceived midline of space to his or her actual anatomic midline. This realignment is called *midline shift syndrome*.

Yoked prism may be used for both distance and near tasks. Because there is little to no distortion and the displacement effect is throughout the entire lens, there is less time needed for specific instruction to successfully use this prism system.

VISUAL FIELD AWARENESS SYSTEM. The Visual Field Awareness System is a round, button prism that is cemented into a predesigned hole in the spectacle lens (Figure 17-10). As with other prism systems, the base is positioned toward the field loss. The prism lens, ranging from ⅞ in. to 1¼ in. in diameter, provides 18.5 prism diopters of power. This prism system has been shown to be beneficial for patients with hemianopsia and inattention.[21] Dr. Gottlieb has presented the use of this system for a young woman who wished to return to driving after experiencing a left temporal field loss.[22] Through placement trials, it was found that the best placement of the button prism was in the central left aspect of the spectacle lens. This position allowed the patient to momentarily view through the prism to gain peripheral information and to view in her side-view mirror.

This system was successful, and the patient was able to return to driving after specialized driver training. It should be noted that not all states allow driving with low vision optical devices. In this particular case, however, the state motor vehicle department accepted this situation after the individual demonstrated safe operation of the vehicle.

INWAVE FIELD-EXPANDING HEMISPHERIC LENS. The Inwave Field-Expanding Hemispheric Lens system consists of a hemi-field prism of 12 prism diopters. A patient's prescription can be ground onto the front surface of the Inwave lens. The base of the prism should be toward the field defect. It is positioned similar to the Fresnel prism, with the patient making a saccadic eye movement toward the prism when he or she wants to use it. The Inwave Field-Expanding Hemispheric Lens may be used on only one eye or may be prescribed binocularly (Figure 17-11).

When prescribing this lens system, any spectacle frame may be chosen. The lens material is CR 39 ophthalmic plastic, and, will therefore accept tints and coatings. A fitting set consists of 38-mm trial lenses that can be placed in a standard trial frame for patient evaluation.

MIRROR SYSTEM. A mirror, commonly attached to the nasal front surface of a spectacle frame (see Figure 12-2), may be used to shift objects on the blind side onto the functional, seeing retina of the same eye. This concept of image displacement is similar to that of using a prism, however, the mirror has some significant disadvantages.

1. When a mirror is placed on the nasal aspect of a frame, it produces a nasal scotoma. This problem can be reduced by designing the mirror with a semireflective or semisilvered backing, permitting the patient to view through the mirror while also maintaining a reflected image. The patient will therefore see two images, with the reflected image appearing brighter.
2. The mirror creates a reversed image, making it initially confusing to the patient.
3. The mirror system is more noticeable than the prism system and in many cases cosmetically not acceptable to the patient.
4. Fitting the mirror system and instructing the patient how to use it tends to be very tedious and time consuming.
5. Mirrors were initially made of glass, which added weight to the spectacles. There was also a greater chance of mirror breakage. Plastic mirrors are now used that reduce the weight and the breakage problem.

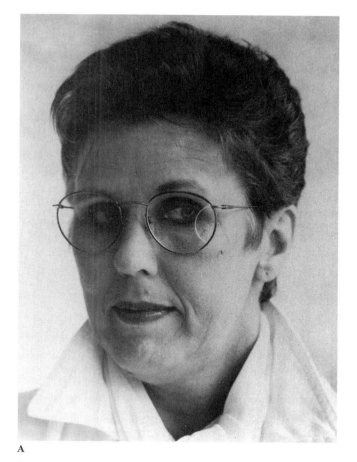
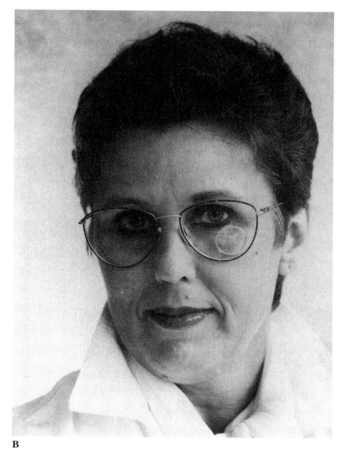

A   **B**

FIGURE 17-10. **A. An example of the Visual Field Awareness System used for a patient with field loss in the left temporal area. The prism is positioned base out. B. An example of a patient using the Visual Field Awareness System mounted base down in the inferior-temporal area of the spectacles for an inferior-temporal quadrant defect. (Courtesy of Dr. Daniel Gottlieb at REKINDLE, Stone Mountain, GA.)**

Because of the above mentioned disadvantages, the mirror system has not been widely used.

Nonoptical Systems and Scanning Strategies

In addition to optical intervention, there are several nonoptical systems that have been found to be helpful for patients with hemianopic field loss or unilateral inattention (see Chapters 12 and 13). A patient who experiences problems with finding the end of a line or the beginning of a new line may be helped by a typoscope or by incorporating borders. The border assists in finding the beginning or the end of a task through the use of brightly colored strips, which are placed along the edge of an activity in the affected field. By being aware of these borders, the patient is assured that he or she has scanned the full width of the activity. It is also helpful for some patients with bitemporal hemianopsias or inattention deficits to tilt the printed material toward the defect. By doing this, the field loss does not interfere with the patient finding the beginning or end of the sentence or paragraph.

It has been documented that some patients may demonstrate restricted scanning patterns secondary to a stroke.[23] To assist the patient in increasing his or her scanning skills, it is imperative that formal exercises be provided as "homework" assignments. Scanning should be practiced initially with simple tasks and in a limited environment. As the patient successfully demonstrates improved abilities, both the complexities of the activity and the environment should be increased. Incorporation of scanning strategies should be linked with functional activities such as reading, playing cards, and locating items in the store. Examples of scanning patterns include circular patterns to scan large spaces for orientation purposes, or left to right scanning as performed when reading.

SELF-ASSESSMENT QUESTIONS

1. Aphasia occurs in which of the following types:
   (a) expressive
   (b) receptive
   (c) global
   (d) all of the above
   (e) a and c

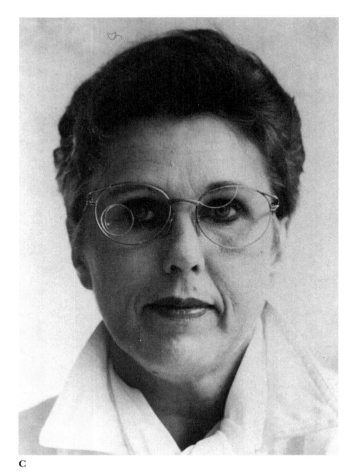

C

FIGURE 17-10. *Continued* **C. An example of a patient using the Visual Field Awareness System with the prism mounted base out in the right eye and base up in the left eye. (Courtesy of Dr. Daniel Gottlieb at REKINDLE, Stone Mountain, GA.)**

2. Acuity charts that have been most successful for use with the aphasic population are
   (a) letter charts
   (b) number charts
   (c) picture charts
   (d) b and c
   (e) none of the above

3. You are unsuccessful when testing a patient's EOMs using the conventional technique of having the patient follow the transilluminator. It appears that the patient is unable to understand the directions. You respond by
   (a) documenting that the patient is untestable
   (b) documenting that the patient is uncooperative
   (c) attempting the test again but this time have the patient hold the transilluminator while you guide the movement
   (d) testing the patient by using the doll's eye reflex
   (e) trying c first then resorting to d if unsuccessful

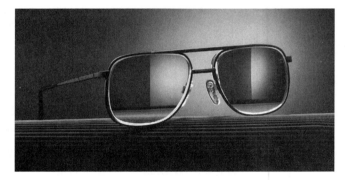

FIGURE 17-11. **The Inwave Field Expanding-Hemispheric Lens system consists of a hemifield prism of 12.00 prism diopters. It is positioned similar to other prism systems with the base of the prism toward the field defect. (Courtesy of Inwave Optics, Inc., Janesville, WI.)**

4. Alternate methods of testing visual fields include
   (a) finger wiggle confrontation
   (b) penlight field test
   (c) functional field test
   (d) all of the above

5. Observation of behavioral changes may frequently be the best indicator that diplopia is present or that neutralization of the diplopia has been attained.
   True or False

6. Unilateral inattention is always accompanied by a visual field loss.
   True or False

7. The most accurate test for unilateral inattention is
   (a) confrontation testing
   (b) observation of functional activity performance
   (c) drawing tests
   (d) penlight field test
   (e) a combination of all of the above

8. The recommended treatment for unilateral inattention is
   (a) increase awareness by incorporating prism
   (b) increase awareness by incorporating borders
   (c) increase awareness by incorporating verbal cues
   (d) practice scanning patterns
   (e) a combination of all of the above

REFERENCES

1. Falk NS, Aksionoff EB. The primary care optometric evaluation of the traumatic brain injury patient. J Am Optom Assoc 1992; 63:547–553.
2. Bouska MJ, Gallaway M. Primary visual deficits in adults with brain damage: management in occupational therapy. Occup Ther Pract J 1991;3:1–11.
3. Butter CM, Kirsch N. Combined and separate effects of eye patching and visual stimulation on unilateral neglect following stroke. Arch Phys Med Rehabil 1992;73:1133–1139.
4. Cohen AH, Soden R. An optometric approach to the rehabilitation of the stroke patient. J Am Optom Assoc 1981;52: 795–800.

5. Waiss B, Soden R. Head trauma and low vision: clinical modifications for diagnosis and prescription. J Am Optom Assoc 1992; 63:559–563.
6. Abreu B. Perceptual Motor Skills: Assessment and Intervention Strategies. American Occupational Therapy Association Self-Study Series: Cognitive Rehabilitation. Rockville, MD: The American Occupational Therapy Association, 1994.
7. Greene HA. Objective Methods for the Evaluation of Visual Field Enhancement. Presented at the Neuro-Optometric Rehabilitation Association Conference, Washington, DC, April 1993.
8. Bouska MJ, Kauffman NA, Marcus SE. Disorders of the Visual Perceptual System. In DA Umphred (ed), Neurological Rehabilitation. Philadelphia: Mosby, 1990;705–749.
9. Roberts SP. Visual disorders of higher cortical function. J Am Optom Assoc 1992;63:723–732.
10. Grovier WM, Cottam G, Webster JS, et al. Behavioral interventions with stroke patients for improving wheelchair navigation. Int J Clin Neuropsychol 1984;6:186–190.
11. Halligan PW, Cockburn J, Wilson BA. The behavioral assessment of visual neglect. Neuropsychol Rehabil 1991;1:5–32.
12. Robertson IH, North N. Spatio-motor cueing in unilateral left neglect: the role of hemispace, hand and motor activation. Neuropsychologia 1992;30:553–563.
13. Rossi PW, Kheyfets S, Reding MJ. Fresnel prisms improve visual perception in stroke patients with homonymous hemianopsia or unilateral neglect. Neurology 1990;40:1597–1599.
14. Webster JS, Jones S, Blanton P, Gross R. Visual scanning training with stroke patients. Behav Ther 1984;15:129–143.
15. Greene HA. Objective Methods for the Evaluation of Near Point Functional Effects of Visual Field Loss and the Benefit of Treatment Techniques. Presented at the Pennsylvania College of Optometry Low Vision Symposium: Brain Injury and Stroke Management and Rehabilitation. Philadelphia, October 1993.
16. Stone SP, Halligan PW, Greenwood RJ. The incidence of neglect phenomena and related disorders in patients with an acute right or left hemisphere stroke. Age Ageing 1993;22:46–52.
17. Hugonnier R, Hugonnier S, Troutman S. Strabismus Heterophoria and Ocular Motor Paralysis. St. Louis: Mosby, 1969.
18. Birnbaum MH. Noncomitant strabismus: evaluation and management. J Am Optom Assoc 1984;11:758–764.
19. Brilliant RL. Special Low Vision Devices for Special Tasks. Presented at the Scheie Eye Institute Symposium on Low Vision. Philadelphia, October 1986.
20. Moradiellos DP, Parrish DE. A clinical technique for correcting diplopia with prism. J Am Optom Assoc 1986;57:740–743.
21. Gottlieb D, Freeman P, Williams M. Clinical research and statistical analysis of a visual field awareness system. J Am Optom Assoc 1992;63:581–588.
22. Gottlieb D. Enhancing Awareness, Increasing Safety and Returning to Driving for Patients with Visual Field Loss and Neglect. Presented at the Neuro-Optometric Rehabilitation Association Conference, Washington, DC, April 1993.
23. Warren, M. Visuospatial Skills: Assessment and Intervention Strategies. American Occupational Therapy Association Self-Study Series: Cognitive Rehabilitation. Rockville, MD: The American Occupational Therapy Association, Inc. 1994.

Appendix A

MANUFACTURERS AND SUPPLIERS

Fresnel Prism & Lens Company
(Fresnel Prisms)
7975 North Hayden Rd., Suite A106
Scottsdale, AZ 85258-3242
(602) 596-3998
800-544-4760

Vision Training Products, Inc.
(Hart Chart and Broken Wheel Cards)
4016 N. Home St.
Mishawaka, IN 46545
(219) 259-2070
800-348-2225

Inwave Optics, Inc.
(The Inwave Field-Expanding Hemispheric Lens)
29 West Milwaukee Street
Post Office Box 5113
Janesville, WI 53547-5113
(608) 752-8181
800-957-8400

Jardon Eye Prosthetics, Inc.
(Mirror Systems)
17100 West 12 Mile Rd.
Southfield, MI 48076
(810) 424-8560

Western Psychological Services
(Rivermead Behavioral Inattention Test)
12031 Wilshire Blvd.
Los Angeles, CA 90025-1251
800-648-8857

REKINDLE
(Visual Field Awareness System)
Gottlieb Vision Group
Medical Center and Sports Medicine Complex
5462 Memorial Dr., Suite 101
Stone Mountain, GA 30083
(404) 296-6000
800-666-7484

CHAPTER EIGHTEEN

Practice Management

Kathleen Fraser Freeman,
Glenn S. Corbin, and
Charles Hollander

Once a practitioner has determined the need for low vision rehabilitation services in his or her community, a number of practice management issues must be addressed. The practitioner must set up a referral base, add the necessary equipment and devices, make adjustments in the schedule to accommodate the service, train staff, and establish a fee schedule. Interacting with agencies in the community is also helpful, but this often occurs later, after one has become proficient and comfortable with the low vision process. This chapter outlines some of the practice management issues to consider and address when starting a low vision practice or adding it to an existing practice.

EQUIPMENT AND DEVICES

Standard optometric equipment, including a trial lens set, appropriate lighting, and a comfortable chair, is needed for the basic vision and magnification assessment, but the magnification and low vision evaluation of optical devices requires equipment that would not be found in most practitioners' offices. To adequately evaluate visually impaired patients, certain specialized equipment is required, including low vision charts and a stock of diagnostic low vision lenses and devices of various types, equivalent powers, and levels of sophistication. Eighty percent of low vision cases can be managed with a self-made trial kit similar to that seen in Appendix A. It is neither necessary nor productive to have every lens or device that is available. In many cases, several different manufacturers will offer telescopes, spectacles, or magnifiers that are optically similar or identical (Appendix B). Often more sophisticated design systems, such as spectacle-mounted telescopes, can be rented from the manufacturer to evaluate appropriate patients and therefore need not be purchased outright unless there is a consistent demand. For the beginning practitioner, a basic supply of diagnostic and loaner devices is recommended to allow for minimal investment as well as the opportunity to gain experience with the type of population that will be served. In addition, sophisticated and expensive low vision devices should probably not be purchased until the practitioner is comfortable with his or her low vision skills and certain that he or she wants to provide these more sophisticated systems, which are more difficult to evaluate and fit. A list of various categories of lenses, devices, and equipment for the office are as follows:

1. *Trial frame and lenses.* A full-diameter trial lens set (as compared to the small-aperture, corrected curve type) is quite useful for evaluating high-powered spectacle corrections as well as high adds. The trial frame is also useful for quickly evaluating and comparing various tinted lenses and filters. Information on the performance of a trial frame refraction as well as the advantages and disadvantages of using this system is available in Chapter 3.

2. *Charts and lighting.* Distance and near charts specifically designed for low vision are recommended. A music stand used to support a distance acuity chart is an inexpensive and versatile way of taking acuities at various distances. Permanently installed ceiling or track lights with a rheostat could provide optimum illumination for testing. A gooseneck floor lamp will also allow for flexibility in chart illumination.

3. *Microscopes.* Microscopes are high plus reading lenses that are commonly prescribed devices. Half-eye spectacles with base-in prism incorporated in each lens may allow a patient to maintain binocularity up to approximately +12.00 D. Aspheric lenticular lenses are commonly prescribed as monocular systems from +12.00 D and above. Doublet microscopic lenses can be considered at any power but are generally most appreciated by patients in higher powers, +20.00 D and above.

4. *Loupes and visors.* Clip-on loupes and visor-type devices are frequently overlooked inexpensive and effective options that are often readily accepted by the patient for near needs (see Figure 10-10).

5. *Hand magnifiers.* There is a greater variety of handheld magnifiers than any other type of low vision device. By the time they are seen, most patients have found very low powered magnifiers in the +4.00 to +6.00 D range, and are in need of stronger powers. Patients invariably ask for stronger lenses in larger diameters, so it is advisable to have several good optical quality magnifiers with the largest possible lens diameter, as well as inexpensive pocket magnifiers in a variety of strengths and illuminated versions.

6. *Stand magnifiers.* Both nonilluminated and illuminated stand magnifiers of many equivalent powers are available. It must be noted that in most cases accommodation, bifocal addition, or a reading lens must be used in combination with stand magnifiers.

7. *Telescopes.* Handheld as well as spectacle-mounted telescopic devices can be used without going to very sophisticated designs. Most telescopic devices dispensed in busy low vision practices are of the handheld Keplerian type.

8. *Telemicroscopes.* Near-focus telescopes are available as stock devices from several manufacturers, or they can be custom designed. For telescopes requiring reading caps, the practitioner can temporarily attach a trial lens to the front of the telescope with tape, which prevents having to inventory numerous lens caps.

9. *Sun filters and tinted lenses.* Plastic, wraparound sun filters, such as the NoIR sun lens (NoIR Medical Technologies, South Lyon, MI) are useful for determination of the most appropriate color and transmission, whether they are prescribed to be worn over spectacles or as prescription sunglasses. Frames with side shields or top shields should be considered for patients who are very photophobic.

10. *Nonoptical devices.* Many nonoptical devices are available to make activities of daily living easier. A few of the more universally used devices are felt-tipped pens, bold-lined paper, typoscopes and signature guides, large-print telephone dials and buttons, large-print playing cards, large-print timers, large-print checks, and High Marks (Kentucky Industries for the Blind, Louisville, KY) (for marking stove dials and other appliances).

11. *Electronic devices.* Closed-circuit television reading machines (CCTV) are available from a number of sources, with a variety of technical options for the patient. As many patients are sophisticated consumers and aware of advances in technology, it might be prudent for the practitioner to have at least one demonstration unit that patients can work with. Most companies have programs whereby the practitioner can dispense CCTVs from the practice. If this is not something the practitioner wants to become involved in, sales representatives are often willing to visit the patient in his or her home to demonstrate the device. The practitioner should establish contact with the area sales representative to arrange these meetings. Some practitioners prefer to have the salesperson bring the CCTV to the office for evaluation and demonstration to appropriate patients, allowing various optical and nonoptical devices to be evaluated in conjunction with the CCTV. In addition, there may be CCTV systems in the community that are accessible to patients (such as at the public library, retirement centers, or in the school system) where patients can evaluate them at their convenience.

REFERRALS

If a low vision practice is being started from an existing practice, there are several sources within the office to generate a patient base. Patient histories may indicate family members having visual problems with conditions such as macular degeneration, diabetes, cataracts, or glaucoma. A description of low vision services and a pamphlet describing these services will generally be well received by the patient on behalf of his or her family member. Low vision pamphlets, large-print materials, business cards, and aesthetically pleasing signs placed throughout the office indicating the addition of low vision services are also very helpful.

Often, one must look beyond the present patient base and attempt to generate patients from outside sources. This can be accomplished through various means, such as professional referrals, agency referrals, speaking engagements, and publicity.

Speaking to local organizations, such as the Rotary and Lion's clubs, senior citizen centers, and support groups, is important. Such presentations emphasize the practitioner's presence in the community. Discussions about common pathologies and how low vision services may help an individual's functioning are always well received. Many of these organizations and centers may be aware of potential low vision patients and, in some cases, may even help with patient finances. In addition, these groups sometimes provide public service announcements in local newspapers, radio, and television as to their topics and speakers with the hope of informing the local community.

Special education departments in school districts as well as the education service centers in the practitioner's area are also in need of evaluation and recommendations for students with low vision. State agencies for the blind and disabled work with adults who have vocational or secondary education needs. Early on, it is imperative to establish a good working relationship with these referral sources, as future referrals will often depend on the outcome of the first few "test cases." For this reason, it might be prudent for the practitioner to refrain from agency networking until a level of expertise is developed that will allow the handling of more challenging cases.

Because of the nature of their problem, most low vision patients will be under the care of an ophthalmologist. It is, therefore, helpful to make contact with the ophthalmologists, in particular, the specialists (e.g., retina, glaucoma, neuro-ophthalmology, anterior segment, pediatric), as well as the local optometrists. The practitioner should make the community's primary eye care providers aware that he or she is offering low vision services, exactly what these services involve, and the type of patient who might benefit from low vision services. The referring doctors may want to be reassured that primary care will not be provided and that these patients will be returned to them at the completion of services. General practitioners (e.g., internists, family practitioners) as well as other types of medical specialists (e.g., endocrinologists, neurologists) are also a good source of referrals.

A system for facilitating referrals may be helpful. A form sent to the referring doctor's office to fill out, indicating the diagnosis; past, present, and planned medical or surgical intervention; and any specific concerns the doctor has for this patient is both quick and simple (Appendix C). This approach documents that the patient was indeed referred by another doctor and that appropriate medical intervention has already taken place. In turn, a letter goes back to the referring doctor regarding the outcome of the low vision evaluation, with copies to other doctors involved in the patient's systemic and ocular care. This copy will make a number of doctors aware of services that have been provided, and the role that the low vision practitioner has played in their patient's care. Referral letters must also go back to agencies and teachers (when the patient is referred by the school system). Letter writing is, therefore, an important part of the low vision process.

LETTER WRITING

Letter writing is an important aspect to stimulate and reinforce the referral process. It is also the most appropriate means to convey information to the doctor, counselor, or teacher. For doctor referrals, a letter to the referring doctor is required by Medicare and some insurance agencies if a consultation is billed. It should be kept in mind that the referring doctor may not have a lot of time to read every detail of the low vision examination and therefore these letters are best kept succinct. The letter (Appendix D) should contain the chief complaint, diagnosis, acuities, results of specialized testing, results of low vision evaluation and instruction, prognosis, and what has been planned for the patient. Also, with doctor referrals, a statement indicating that the patient has been advised to return to the referring doctor for continued care should be included.

For agencies, forms are often available and these are often required to be filled out before payment will be made for services rendered. Agencies will need a thorough history, diagnosis of the condition, low vision device evaluation for specific tasks and proficiency of use, and evaluation of the ability to do work-related activities. A statement as to the prognosis and whether the patient is legally blind may also be helpful. The emphasis of this letter is a bit different from the doctor's letter, as the goal of this evaluation may be more specific to vocational or educational needs.

For school personnel, a more functional approach is helpful. In the educational setting, questions arise regarding the capabilities of the student, as well as needs for glasses or low vision devices. How the glasses or low vision devices should be used, instructional tips in using the devices, and suggestions for preferential seating or modifications in the environment are some of the important statements that should be included. These reports tend to be more detailed (Appendix E), and should be written in lay terms, as they will be used by parents, teachers, therapists, and others who may not be knowledgeable about medical or ocular terminology. Broad statements, such as "this child needs large print," should be avoided. A statement regarding the size of print as well as the distance the material is held is much more helpful. Issues, such as efficiency, practicality, and student's acceptance of a low vision device, are all important pieces of information that may play a role in the student's educational setting.

As letter writing can be quite time-consuming, particularly in the busy practice, dictation becomes a necessity so that reports are processed in a timely and efficient manner. Although it takes a bit of time to become comfortable with dictating correspondence, it is strongly recommended by many doctors. The first 25–30 letters will need revision, but after that, the practitioner may wonder how he or she ever managed without it.

Statements of legal blindness are also often sought by patients for various purposes. A standard form on the practitioner's letterhead that allows for patient's name, date of birth, level of vision, and cause for visual impairment is acceptable (see Appendix 19C).

SCHEDULING THE PATIENT

When deciding how to schedule a low vision patient, one of the most important considerations is the amount of time required by that patient. For a variety of reasons, low vision patients require more time than the average patient. Typically, an initial consultation will require 1½–2 hours to assess visual and ocular functioning, evaluate low vision devices, and provide instruction. It is not necessary that the doctor do all of this, but the fact is, much of it is face-to-face doctor time. As it requires a different mind-set, patient flow, and use of staff time, it is suggested that a given day or portion of the day be set aside for low vision patient care. Some practitioners suggest breaking up the initial

workup into two 1-hour sessions scheduled on two separate visits. The first 1-hour session is devoted to history, acuities, ocular health, and special testing (e.g., visual fields, contrast sensitivity testing); the second 1-hour session is devoted to low vision device evaluation and instruction. This split session is inadvisable, in most cases, because the patient is hoping to obtain some help during the initial visit when enthusiasm and motivation are generally at the highest level. If a split session approach is chosen, it is helpful to introduce a low vision device on the first visit, thus allowing the patient to hopefully experience some initial visual improvement.

It is impossible to rush these patient visits. Many of the low vision patients will be elderly, and will need extra time simply to accomplish the required tests. Others will have several tasks with which they need assistance, and each must be addressed separately. It should be kept in mind that there is a lot of counseling involved in the patient management and there must be time allocated for discussion.

A major disadvantage of devoting a 2-hour time slot to one patient occurs when the patient does not show up for the appointment. A missed appointment might often be due to uncontrollable circumstances, such as the weather, transportation problems, and health problems, which might be more common with low vision patients. Therefore, it is important that the office have good lines of communication with the patient in terms of confirming an appointment. It should either be done in writing at the time of scheduling or a confirmation letter should be sent a few days before the scheduled appointment. This letter, preferably in large, bold print should state the following:

1. Date of the appointment
2. Time of the appointment
3. Length of appointment
4. Doctor's name and phone number

Phone confirmation by the receptionist 1 day before the appointment is also recommended.

A simple solution to a missed appointment is to schedule the low vision patient as the last patient of the day. If the patient cancels the appointment, the doctor now has some free time to make phone calls or complete the day's paper work. This scheduling not only allows extra time for the patient whose examination may require more than 2 hours but also prevents the appointment from interfering with the appointments of the primary care patients who are scheduled throughout the day.

Follow-up visits can be scheduled with the doctor or staff member after the initial visit. The follow-up visits are generally scheduled for 30 minutes to 1 hour, depending on the case complexity. If a low vision device is loaned, a follow-up visit should be scheduled for the patient to return within 1–2 weeks.

During the examination, family members and close friends should be encouraged to observe and ask questions as well. In many cases, the family members may be care providers and their observation will allow for a better understanding of the patient's visual problems and potential solutions. They may also help with reinforcing the doctor's explanations and instructions when the patient is at home. Many of the individuals who accompany the patient become excited and motivated by observing the success of the patient and they, in turn, may generate new referrals.

LOANER SYSTEM

Once a device has been tentatively recommended for the patient, it is advisable for the patient to evaluate it in the home or job environment if possible. For this reason, a device loaning system should be incorporated into the low vision practice.

The benefits of a loaner system are many:

1. Both doctor and patient feel more confident about the final prescription.
2. It is easier to have a loaned device returned than it is to explain to a displeased patient why his or her newly purchased device does not perform the same way it did during the examination.
3. It is very important that patients be familiar with the actual appearance of the devices as well as experience the advantages and disadvantages before making a decision. This experience will eliminate the potential dissatisfaction that may ensue if the patient thought he or she was getting a low vision device that resembled conventional eyewear.
4. The patient may have a collection of lenses and devices at home and the loaned device can then be compared under "true life" situations to determine which one is best. This comparison may be especially advisable for job-related tasks.
5. A patient may have fluctuating vision and the loaned device can then be evaluated on "good and bad" days.
6. It may take time for a patient to develop the skills required to efficiently use some low vision devices. It is expected that the proficiency in using a device will improve with each day of practice.

For the part-time low vision practice, there are some doctors who support the idea that the loaner system can be coordinated from the trial kit. Their recommendation is that the patient can borrow the device used during the examination. The patient is then scheduled for a follow-up visit on the subsequent day that low vision examinations are performed. For example, if low vision patients are scheduled on Monday and Thursday afternoons, the patient is loaned a device on Thursday. He or she is then scheduled for a visit on Monday afternoon, immediately preceding the full low vision examination. In this way, no additional equipment is needed and all devices are available for the next patient.

This system, however, does have some major drawbacks. If a patient misses a follow-up appointment for any reason, the loaned device would obviously not be available for the next incoming patient to evaluate. Also, if the patient returning a loaned device is scheduled as the second or third low vision patient of the day, the loaned device would not be available for the first patient seen that day.

For the busier low vision practice, it may be necessary to have a separate loaner stock. One set of devices is strictly for use during examinations (diagnostic set). The loaner stock can be continually replaced as the items are dispensed or the devices can stay in the loaner system with new devices ordered as needed for dispensing. In the case of the former, it is important to inform the patient beforehand that the device being loaned is new and could be dispensed if desired. The advantage to this method is that the patient does not have to wait while a device is on order. It also allows for a constant turnover of stock so that the loaner has less chance of being returned scratched or broken. In either case, low vision lenses generally should not be loaned for more than 2 weeks. This amount of time is generally enough for a patient to fully evaluate any system. Limiting the longer period to 2 weeks also ensures that any problems that arise are addressed quickly, thereby reducing the potential for further frustration.

With any loaner system, accurate documentation is required (Appendix F). A form listing devices loaned, responsibilities of the patient, and expected return date should be signed by both the patient and the doctor. This form should be in triplicate, with one page going to the patient, one page for the record, and the last page placed in a "tickler file" with the expected return date. In some practices, the doctor may feel more comfortable requiring a deposit from the patient.

RECALL SYSTEM

Recall of patients is necessary to monitor visual status and ocular health, as well as to monitor the effectiveness of previously prescribed devices. If the low vision patient does not have an eye care practitioner, then routine follow-up care can easily be scheduled on a yearly basis. If the low vision patient is being monitored by a referring eye care practitioner, it is good policy to involve the referring practitioner in the determination of recall options for his or her patient. In such situations, it should be emphasized to the referring doctor that the patient is being recalled for a low vision progress evaluation as opposed to routine vision care. The emphasis of this evaluation would be to determine if previously prescribed devices are performing at optimal levels as well as to explore any new lenses or devices that have recently become available.

Another mechanism for encouraging periodic return evaluations is an informative patient newsletter that discusses low vision issues, pathology, and new developments in optical and nonoptical devices. All printed materials sent to patients should be in large print with good contrast.

FEES

Fees for low vision services must take into account the doctor's chair time, instruction time, letter writing time, and, of course, overhead. Professional fees may include office visits or consultations, visual field testing or other specialized testing to help assess visual functioning, low vision refraction, magnification assessment, and training. Some services will not be covered by third-party payers. There are a number of sources of payment for services, including private payment:

1. *Medicare.* Medicare does not (at the time of this writing) cover refraction, low vision services, nor low vision lenses or devices. An office visit or consultation visit can be billed provided that a medical diagnosis is made or confirmed. Specialized testing that helps make or confirm the diagnosis is also appropriate to bill. The low vision refraction and magnification assessment, as well as the instructional session, are noncovered services and must be billed directly to the patient. It is imperative that this be understood before the appointment and reiterated at the time of the visit. A standard form acknowledging noncovered services should be signed by the patient. In addition, glasses and low vision devices are noncovered (with the exception of the first pair of aphakic spectacles).

2. *Insurance.* Secondary insurance companies will generally follow Medicare guidelines on noncovered services but will often pick up the deductible. For patients who are not Medicare eligible, an insurance company may cover the refraction and instruction, but this varies with individual carriers. Although Medicare does not cover low vision devices, sometimes insurance companies will cover these in part, if it is explained (in a letter) that the devices are not regular glasses but are prosthetic devices specifically designed to improve the functioning of a malformed or damaged eye or visual system.

3. *Medicaid.* Medicaid will cover refraction and glasses for eligible patients but, in most cases, will not cover low vision services or devices. Again, office visits and consultation as well as appropriate specialized testing should be covered with a medical diagnosis.

4. *School districts and education service centers.* In some cases, school districts or the local education service center will have funds allocated for low vision evaluations for special education students. Reimbursement levels will depend on contractual agreements determined before the provision of services, with each individual entity. It is not unusual to work out a contract agreeing on a set fee for each student evaluated, specifying a certain number of students annually at the beginning of each school year.

5. *Rehabilitation agencies.* Every state in the United States has a state rehabilitation agency that has funds for low vision evaluations as well as funds for low vision devices. Each agency may operate slightly differently from state to state; however, in all cases, prior authorization (from agency to the doctor) for services and devices is required. These agencies operate on fiscal calendars and, invariably, funds will run out at certain times of the year, which may affect recommendations for patients.

Once fees have been established, a policy should also be developed to cover lenses and devices that are returned after a short period. There are various reasons for this occurring, including the following:

1. The patient had experienced a dramatic and permanent decrease in his or her vision.
2. The patient could not adapt to the device.
3. The device did not perform up to expectations.
4. The patient was not happy with the final appearance of the device.
5. Due to fluctuating vision, the "lenses are not as clear" as they once were.

Many practitioners fail to establish a policy for refunds and so, after a lot of time and hard work, a case that initially appeared to be successful can turn into a nightmare.

COMMUNITY SERVICES

Community services are an important resource that patients may want to take advantage of. These include local library services as well as state libraries for the blind and physically handicapped that have materials in large print, on recorded disc, and on tape. These are free services for which patients may qualify. Aside from the state rehabilitation agencies, there may also be nonprofit agencies that teach independent living services. In larger communities, there are often consumer groups, such as local councils for the blind, support groups, and parent groups, that are important sources of information and advocacy for visually impaired children and adults. Many national groups send out newsletters and have written information concerning the visually impaired (see Appendix 19B). Newsletters, booklets, and information regarding these national groups can be displayed in the waiting room, making them available to all patients. It is important that the practitioner be aware of the variety of community resources in the area, and, conversely, to be recognized by those services as a resource as well (see Chapter 19).

SELF-ASSESSMENT QUESTIONS

1. When establishing low vision rehabilitation as a specialty service in your practice, it is best to initially purchase all of the low vision devices that are available so that patients can be evaluated with the appropriate devices during the initial visit.
   True or False

2. When scheduling a patient with low vision, when is it best to schedule him or her?
   (a) As the first patient of the day, before "normal sighted" patients, because you have more energy in the morning for patients who may be more difficult to please.
   (b) As the last patient of the day because he or she will not interfere with the schedule if the appointment takes longer than expected.
   (c) On a separate day when only patients with low vision are seen.
   (d) All of the above.
   (e) b and c

3. When providing low vision services, letter writing
   - (a) is not necessary for all patients
   - (b) is an important aspect to stimulate and reinforce the referral process
   - (c) is an appropriate means to convey information to a doctor, counselor, or teacher about a patient.
   - (d) all of the above
   - (e) b and c

4. In a well-established low vision practice, it is recommended that loaners *not* be available to patients because it becomes too costly to the practitioner.
   True or False

5. Which of the following *may* pay the practitioner for low vision services?
   - (a) a private insurance company
   - (b) Medicare
   - (c) a state rehabilitation agency
   - (d) all of the above
   - (e) a and c

Appendix A

BASIC LOW VISION KIT

The following is a list of diagnostic low vision devices that will allow the practitioner to manage a majority of low vision cases.

   I. Distance low vision chart
   II. Near visual acuity card (metric system recommended) and near continuous text reading card
   III. Telescopes
      A. 2.8× (Galilean) binocular sport glasses
      B. 2.8× (Keplerian) handheld telescope
      C. 4.0× (Keplerian) handheld telescope
      D. 6.0× (Keplerian) handheld telescope
      E. 4× or 7× (Keplerian) binocular Beecher Mirage (Beecher Research Co., Schaumburg, IL)
   IV. Microscopes
      A. +6/8 base-in (BI) prism half eye
      B. +8/10 BI prism half eye
      C. +10/12 BI prism half eye
      D. +12/14 BI prism half eye
      E. +12.00 D full-diameter microscope OU
      F. +16.00 D full-diameter microscope OU
      G. +20.00 D full-diameter microscope OU
      H. +24.00 D full-diameter microscope OU
   V. Magnifiers
      A. 2×, 3×, and 5× handheld magnifiers (nonilluminated)
      B. 4×, 5×, and 7× handheld magnifiers (illuminated)
      C. 4× and 7× stand magnifiers (nonilluminated)
      D. 4×, 6×, and 10× stand magnifiers (illuminated)
   VI. Sun filters or absorptive lenses (a few different colors and transmission levels)
   VII. Nonoptical
      A. Typoscope
      B. Bold-line paper
      C. Felt-tip pen
      D. Large-print checks
      E. Large-print playing cards
      F. Large-print reading material (e.g., *Reader's Digest*, Bible, crossword puzzles)
      G. Acetate filters
   VIII. Gooseneck lamp

Appendix B

MANUFACTURERS AND SUPPLIERS OF OPTICAL AND NONOPTICAL SYSTEMS

Note. The information in this appendix does not denote a complete list of manufacturers and suppliers in the United States.

American Printing House for the Blind
1839 Frankfort Ave.
P.O. Box 6085
Louisville, KY 40206
(502) 895-2405
800-223-1839

Beecher Research Co.
906 Morse Ave.
Schaumburg, IL 60193
(708) 893-0187
800-934-8765

Bernell Corp.
750 Lincolnway E.
South Bend, IN 46618
(219) 234-3200
800-348-2225

Choice Magazine Listening
85 Channel Dr.
Port Washington, NY 11050
(516) 883-8280

Christian Association for Rehabilitation
Education Ministries (CARE)
P.O. Box 1830
Starkville, MS 39760
(601) 323-4999

Corning Medical Optics
Caller Service 1511
Elmira, NY 14902
800-742-5273

Designs for Vision
760 Koehler Ave.
Ronkonkoma, NY 11779
(516) 585-3300
800-345-4009

Donegan Optical Co., Inc.
P.O. Box 14308
Lenexa, KS 66215
(913) 492-2500

Doubleday Large Print Home Library
Membership Service Center
6550 E. 30th St.
Box 6325
Indianapolis, IN 46206
(317) 541-8920

Edmund Scientific Co.
101 E. Gloucester Pike
Barrington, NJ 08007-1380
(609) 573-6260

Edwards Optical
P.O. Box 3299
Virginia Beach, VA 23454
(804) 481-6285

Electronic Visual Aid Specialists
16 David Ave.
P.O. Box 371
Westerly, RI 02891
(401) 596-3155
800-872-3827

Eschenbach Direct
904 Ethan Allen Highway
Ridgefield, CT 06877
(203) 438-7471
800-487-5389

Franel Optical Supply Co.
P.O. Box 940096
Maitland, FL 32794-0096
800-327-2070

General Scientific Corp.
77 Enterprise Dr.
Ann Arbor, MI 48103
(313) 996-9200
800-959-0153

Mark F. Goodkin & Associates
4918 Shamrock Ct. SW
Mableton, GA 30059
(404) 944-8226
800-759-6275

Gulden Ophthalmics
225 Cadwalader Ave.
P.O. Box 7154
Elkins Park, PA 19027-2097
(215) 884-7950
800-659-2250

Heine USA Ltd.
3500 Regency Park Way
Cary, NC 27511
(919) 380-8090

Independent Living Aids
27 East Mall
Plainview, NY 11803
800-537-2188

Keeler Optical Co.
456 Park Way
Broomall, PA 19008
(610) 353-4350
800-523-5620

Large Print Books-By-Mail (Macmillan Publishing)
Front and Brown Streets
Riverside, NJ 08075
800-257-5755

The Lighthouse, Inc.
Low Vision Products
36-02 Northern Blvd.
Long Island City, NY 11101
(718) 937-6959
800-453-4923

L.S.&S. Group Inc.
P.O. Box 673
Northbrook, IL 60065
(708) 498-9777
800-468-4789

Luxo Lamp Corp.
36 Midland Ave.
Port Chester, NY 10573
800-222-5896

Luzerne Optical
Low Vision Aids
180 North Wilkes-Barre Blvd.
P.O. Box 998
Wilkes-Barre, PA 18703
800-233-9637

Matilda Ziegler Magazine for the Blind
80 8th Ave., Room 1304
New York, NY 10011
(212) 242-0263

Mattingly International
5590 Hamill Ave.
San Diego, CA 92120
(619) 741-0767
800-826-4200

Maxi Aids
42 Executive Blvd.
P.O. Box 3209
Farmingdale, NY 11735
(516) 752-0521
800-522-6294

M-Tech Optics Corp.
44514 N. Woodard Ave.
Royal Oak, MI 48073
(313) 266-2181

Meditec
3322 S. Oneida Way
Denver, CO 80224
(303) 758-6978

New York Times Mail Subscriptions
Large Type Weekly
P.O. Box 5792
New York, NY 10087
800-631-2580

NoIR Medical Technologies
6155 Pontiac Trail
P.O. Box 159
South Lyon, MI 48178
(313) 769-5565
800-521-9746

Ocutech, Inc.
P.O. Box 625
Chapel Hill, NC 27515
(919) 967-6460
800-326-6460

Optical Designs, Inc.
14441 Memorial Dr.
Suite 13
Houston, TX 77079
(281) 497-2988

Optical Technology
Franel Optical Supply Co.
P.O. Box 96
Maitland, FL 32751
(407) 831-4000
800-327-2070

Orascoptic Research, Inc.
7 N. Pinckney St.
Suite 305
Madison, WI 53703
800-369-3698

Random House
400 Hahn Rd.
Westminster, MD 21157
800-726-0600

Reader's Digest Association
Large Type Publications
Box 241
Mount Morris, IL 61054
800-877-5293

Science Products
Box 888
Southeastern, PA 19399
800-888-7400

Selsi Co. Inc.
194 Greenwood Ave.
Midland Park, NJ 07432
(201) 612-9200
800-275-7357

Tech-Optics International Corp.
59 Hanse Ave.
Freeport, NY 11520
(516) 546-7480
800-678-4277

Unilens Corp. USA
10431 72nd Street N.
Largo, FL 34647
(813) 544-2531
800-446-2020

Walters, Inc.
30423 Canwood St.
Suite 126
Agoura Hills, CA 91301
(818) 706-2202
800-992-5837

Yorktowne Optical
Industrial Park
P.O. Box 276
Emigsville, PA 17318
(717) 767-6406
800-233-1990

Appendix C

PATIENT CONSULTATION AND REFERRAL FORM

Patient name: _____   Date seen: _____

Address: _____   Telephone (h): _____ (o): _____

[ ] Please call patient for appointment

[ ] Patient will call for an appointment

Diagnosis   OD: _____

OS: _____

Distance acuity (best visual acuity): [ ] with Rx [ ] without Rx

OD: _____ OS: _____

Near acuity (best visual acuity): [ ] with Rx [ ] without Rx

OD: _____ OS: _____

Patient's visual concerns   1. _____

2. _____

3. _____

4. _____

Doctor's comments: _____

_____

Doctor's name: _____   UPIN # _____

Address: _____   Phone # _____

Consultant's Report

Diagnosis and treatment plan: _____

_____

_____

_____

_____

Dr. _____   Date: _____

Appendix D

SAMPLE LETTER TO REFERRING DOCTOR

Dear Dr. Smith:

Thank you for your kind referral of Mrs. Jones, whom I had the pleasure of seeing on August 1, 1992. The history of visual impairment secondary to age-related macular degeneration in this 76 year old is well known to you. Mrs. Jones identified the primary concerns for this visit as improvement in near vision for reading, writing, and activities of daily living. In addition, she would like to be able to see television more easily.

Entering acuities with her present glasses were:

OD +2.00 − 0.50 × 90/+2.50 = 10/120−

OS +2.00 − 0.25 × 90/+2.50 = 10/60

At near she was able to see 0.40/4 M OD (20/200 at 40-cm equivalent) and 0.40/3.2 M OS (20/150 at 40-cm equivalent). There was no improvement of distance acuity on refraction, and this was again explained to the patient. Visual field testing with the tangent screen and a 6/1,000 mm white target showed a 5-degree scotoma located superior to fixation in the better seeing left eye. Tangent testing of the right eye was deferred. On the Amsler's grid, the disturbance was noted as a dim area superior to fixation in the left eye; with the right eye the entire right half of the grid was obscured.

For reading, we are working with a +10.00 D half-eye reading lens that enabled her to read 0.8 M (20/40 equivalent) print at 12 cm. During the instructional session Mrs. Jones was able to read samples of regular typewritten print as well as newspaper print and television guide listings provided illumination was adequate (80 foot-candles). Because she initially had some difficulty with the close working distance required, equivalent-powered handheld and stand magnifiers were also evaluated. Mrs. Jones preferred, however, to use spectacles as she can perform writing and other hands-free tasks more easily. The half eyes have been loaned, along with a pair of 2.5× sport glasses to evaluate for television viewing. The sport glasses provided 10/25 acuity OU.

I am looking forward to seeing Mrs. Jones for a follow-up visit in several weeks. If the loaner devices meet her needs, they will be dispensed and she will be asked to return to your office for further care. Otherwise, we will investigate other options. In the meantime, please feel free to contact the office should you have additional concerns that I can assist with. I do appreciate the opportunity to participate in her care.

Sincerely,

Kathleen Fraser Freeman, O.D., F.A.A.O.

Appendix E

SAMPLE LETTER TO TEACHER

Dear Teacher:

I had the pleasure of seeing Johnny Student for a low vision evaluation on March 19, 1993. As you know, this 7-year-old boy has a history of congenital visual impairment secondary to bilateral optic atrophy and is followed by John Q. Pediatrician, M.D. Johnny's mother reports that he is mainstreamed and in the second grade; however, he reads at the fourth-grade level and is doing well in school. He reads standard print without difficulty, but purple dittos and some dictionary-size print cause some difficulty. In addition, he is having problems seeing the blackboard even when seated in the front of the room. The primary concerns for this evaluation were to assess the present level of vision and to determine if glasses or low vision devices will improve his visual functioning, especially with school related activities.

Entering (unaided) acuities were as follows:
OD (right eye): 10/100 (head to right and squinting) (20/200 equivalent)
OS (left eye): 10/600 (20/1200 equivalent)

At near, he was able to see 0.5 M (20/25 equivalent) print at 6 cm with both eyes. At 20 cm, he was able to see 1.6 M (20/80 equivalent or large-print sized).

Refraction indicated a significant amount of myopia (nearsightedness); however, there was only a slight improvement in his distance vision (10/100+ in the right eye). There was no improvement of acuity in the left eye. It is reported that Johnny has had a nearsighted correction in the past but he did not wear it, and this is consistent with the facts that (1) the spectacle correction will not improve distance acuity and (2) he will see better at near without the correction, as he has a "built-in reading lens" (myopia). I have recommended that he be encouraged to wear his spectacles as much as possible for distance, to give him the advantage of not having to squint as well as for protection of his eyes. It is hoped that Johnny will accept this compromise.

Motility examination revealed a variable nystagmus (oscillating eye movements) and a left esotropia (left eye turned inward). Johnny asked about the "quivering" of his eyes and how this affects his vision. Apparently, he has had some questions from his peers regarding this and has become preoccupied with it. I explained the nystagmus and assured him that the eye movements alone were not causing him to see poorly and that this was associated with his optic nerve condition. Johnny is not binocular and uses the right eye for all tasks. Color vision testing with the Farnsworth D-15 showed normal sequencing. Visual field testing was done with an arc perimeter and showed moderate constrictions in the inferior, nasal, and temporal quadrants of the right eye, with marked constriction (to within 10 degrees fixation) in the superior quadrant. Johnny is very aware that his "side vision" and "bottom vision" are good, but states that his "top vision" is not very good. With this type of visual field impairment, I would not expect him to have any difficulty with independent travel, and indeed, no significant orientation and mobility problems have been noted.

For distance vision improvement, a 6× handheld telescope is recommended. With this device, he was able to see 10/20, and during the training session he could read 1-cm letters written on a blackboard from 14 ft. He demonstrated good spotting, scanning, and focusing skills with the device, and thought it would be useful not only in the classroom but also for recreational activities. It should be noted that the handheld telescope will focus for Johnny's nearsightedness; therefore, it will not look clear to the average observer (looking through) when Johnny has the telescope focused properly for his eye (without his spectacles). It is important to be aware of this when checking his focusing skills.

At near, Johnny's functioning was initially evaluated without glasses or low vision devices. He was able to read samples of regular typewritten print, newspaper print, and a fifth-grade reader from 9 cm to 10 cm. Average reading speed with these materials was 101 words per minute, with overhead room illumination of 40 foot-candles (average room illumination). Extra illumination on the page was helpful but not necessary. Yellow acetate filters placed on top of pages with purple ditto print improved contrast and allowed Johnny to read with comfort. He was not interested in working with handheld or stand magnifiers.

The following recommendations have been made to maximize Johnny's efficiency:

1. Spectacles should be encouraged for distance use but will not be adequate for seeing print on the blackboard. Instead, he should use the 6× handheld telescope that will allow him to read the print with more comfort and efficiency.
2. No lenses or low vision devices are recommended for reading or writing. Johnny should be permitted and encouraged to get as close to his work as he thinks necessary (within 10 cm) and to hold his head and eye in whatever position he finds comfortable.
3. Poor-quality purple dittos as well as other low-contrast printed materials should be avoided. If these materials cannot be improved, perhaps by photocopying, then a yellow acetate filter used with good lighting is recommended.

4. Contrast and lighting go hand in hand; if Johnny is able to sit near a window (with the window to his left or behind him), he will benefit from optimum lighting on his work. He should not face a window, however, because this would create bothersome glare and worsen his vision problems.
5. Consideration should be given to allowing Johnny to use his typing skills for some of his written work. It is possible that this would help with his efficiency.

I appreciate the opportunity to see Johnny and hope you will feel free to contact me should you have additional questions or concerns. Johnny should continue to see Dr. Pediatrician on an annual basis, and I will be happy to see him again should his needs or vision change. Thanks again for this kind referral.

Sincerely,

Kathleen Fraser Freeman, O.D., F.A.A.O.

cc: John Q. Pediatrician, M.D.
    Mother and Father Student

_____ Appendix F _____

LOANER FORM

Patient name: _____

Address: _____

Home telephone #: _____Work telephone #: _____

Date	Device Loaned	Date Returned
_____	_____	_____
_____	_____	_____
_____	_____	_____
_____	_____	_____
_____	_____	_____
_____	_____	_____
_____	_____	_____

To be signed by patient:

I acknowledge receipt of a low vision device(s) from Dr. _____. I understand that this device is being loaned to me for a 2-week period after which I will return for a follow-up visit. By accepting this loaned device, I am accepting full responsibility for the return of this device to Dr. _____. Should I experience difficulty using this device, I will contact Dr. _____'s office by telephone or report the problems at my follow-up appointment.

Should any of the loaned devices be lost or broken, I understand that I will be responsible for the cost of replacement.

Patient signature: _____ Date: _____

Staff signature: _____ Date: _____

CHAPTER NINETEEN

The Vision-Related Rehabilitation Network

Laura A. Edwards,
Maureen A. Duffy,
and John S. Ray

Individuals with vision impairment often require a broad range of comprehensive, holistic, and interdisciplinary vision-related rehabilitation services that may vary (1) across the individual's life span, (2) within individual rehabilitation programs, and (3) within individual plans of instruction. Although the low vision evaluation can be a valuable resource to ensure the efficient and effective use of residual vision, there are a number of other vision-related rehabilitation services within the rehabilitation network that play equally significant roles in the holistic rehabilitation of individuals with vision impairment. These services include counseling (e.g., adjustment to vision loss, psychotherapy, vocational, and genetic), communication skills training (e.g., the use of large print, braille, or assistive computer technology), orientation and mobility therapy (e.g., cane travel, dog guides, or electronic travel devices, as well as instruction in sighted guide and pre-cane skills), rehabilitation teaching (e.g., home management, personal management, communication skills, activities of daily living, leisure activities, and indoor orientation skills), and vocational rehabilitation (e.g., vocational evaluation and training, job-seeking skills training, work adjustment training, job modification and restructuring, job development, and job placement). To ensure that all components of the vision-related rehabilitation network provide coordinated, comprehensive, and effective services to individuals who are blind or have low vision, it is critical to maintain ongoing communication between the individual and all related service providers. This chapter describes the range of services available within the vision-related rehabilitation network and emphasizes the interdisciplinary role of the low vision service provider.

THE REHABILITATION SERVICES NETWORK: HISTORY AND OVERVIEW

Vision-related rehabilitation services to individuals with low vision may be provided through a variety of federal, state, and private rehabilitation programs. Most services in the vision-related rehabilitation network originate within the federal/state vocational rehabilitation system. This system provides organized and federally-mandated linkages between federal, state, and public-private rehabilitation services and programs.

The acceleration of vocational education and rehabilitation programs was viewed as a critical need when the first wave of blind and disabled veterans emerged from World War I. Between 1918 and 1920, eight states passed laws that established civilian vocational rehabilitation programs. The first significant federal legislation for vocational rehabilitation programs began in 1920 when Congress passed the Smith-Fess Act (PL 66-236), also known as the *Civilian Vocational Rehabilitation Act*, which authorized a joint federal/state vocational rehabilitation program for disabled civilians. Throughout the years, the presence of the federal government in state rehabilitation programs has ensured a common sequence of services to individuals with disabilities and a common national reporting system. Statistics demonstrate that rehabilitation services lead to gainful employment, increase the number of taxpayers, and reduce the number of individuals who otherwise would be dependent on families, Social Security disability insurance, workman's compensation insurance, or the public welfare system.

From 1920 to 1973 in the federal/state rehabilitation system, the goal of all services provided by federal and state rehabilitation agencies was to help adults with disabilities to obtain and maintain gainful employment. Even when state societies for the blind or state commissions for the blind were initially allowed to participate in the federal/state rehabilitation system in 1943, they were required to develop rehabilitation units with specific service goals of achieving "gainful employment" for adults who were blind or visually impaired. When Congress passed the Rehabilitation Act of 1973 and Rehabilitation Act Amendments in 1978, however, state rehabilitation programs were required to give priority service to individuals with severe disabilities, and independent living became a necessary additional goal for individuals with disabilities.

State Rehabilitation Programs and Services

States can provide vision-related rehabilitation services through either of the following structures: (1) a generic rehabilitation agency with a separate unit serving individuals who are blind or visually impaired or (2) a separate agency devoted to providing vision-related rehabilitation services. These agencies may stand alone or may operate within the Department of Public Welfare, Department of Education, Department of Labor, or Department of Human Resources. The federal office overseeing all federal/state programs is known as the Rehabilitation Services Administration, operating within the U.S. Department of Education, Office of Special Education and Rehabilitation Services.

Although all states are mandated to provide rehabilitation services, there is considerable variation in the administration and organization of these services and programs from state to state. The actual provision of service may be accomplished through the use of one or all of the following service delivery models: (1) a specific office within the state rehabilitation agency, (2) a state-sponsored comprehensive rehabilitation center, or (3) a rehabilitation unit within the state commission for the blind and visually impaired.

The state rehabilitation agency authorizes services from a range of community resources, including eye care providers. Some state-sponsored comprehensive rehabilitation centers may specialize in services to adults who are blind or visually impaired and provide residential accommodation during the rehabilitation training program; others may serve persons with multiple disabilities and devote a small portion of their services to persons who are blind or visually impaired. The rehabilitation unit within the state commission for the blind and visually impaired is the component that concentrates on services for working-age persons. Other units within the state commission, typically within the social services component of the agency, may provide services for children, adults who do not have specific vocational goals, and older adults.

Determination of Eligibility and Development of the Service Plan

To be eligible for services from the state rehabilitation agency, an applicant must have a disability defined in the Rehabilitation Act as a *physical or mental impairment impeding employment or limiting one or more major life activities.* The rehabilitation counselor can use existing documentation, such as school records of disability status or Social Security Disability Insurance records, to determine eligibility. Even if eligibility has been determined from such documentation, the rehabilitation counselor may require additional medical, optometric, psychological, social, and vocational data to develop an individualized plan for vision-related rehabilitation services that will address the applicant's specific needs. The state agency generally has a medical consultant on call to respond to questions counselors may have in interpreting medical data.

Program assessment, typically conducted through the joint efforts of the client and the rehabilitation counselor, is the next step in the eligibility and planning process. This process determines which major vision-related rehabilitation services the individual will receive, and results in the Individualized Written Rehabilitation Plan (IWRP). The IWRP identifies specific vocational or independent living goals and the specific vision-related rehabilitation services that are required for the individual to attain these goals. In addition, the IWRP must include projected timelines for goal achievement, professional disciplines involved in goal attainment, specialized or adapted equipment and materials required, and specific outcome measures (i.e., criteria for success). Once the plan is agreed to and signed by both parties, the rehabilitation counselor may authorize any or all of the following vision-related rehabilitation services: eye surgery, medications, optical devices for near or distance, electrodiagnostic testing, technology assessment for nonoptical devices or equipment, follow-up visits for eye care practitioners or a low vision rehabilitation center, counseling, communication skills training, orientation and mobility therapy, rehabilitation teaching or training in activities of daily living, and vocational rehabilitation assessment and training.

Provision of Vision-Related Rehabilitation Services

The range of appropriate service providers is extensive. Although licensure or certification, or both, are available in most of these disciplines, some vision-related rehabilitation service providers do not require either as a condition of employment and may allow prospective employees to substitute on-the-job or inservice training. This practice of on-the-job training or inservice training is not recommended, because it may impact on the quality and scope of vision-related rehabilitation services that are provided to the client.

REHABILITATION COUNSELORS. Rehabilitation counselors coordinate all services related to vocational goals, including authorizing services from vendors such as eye care providers and private rehabilitation facilities. Vocational goals may include competitive employment (full- or part-time), supported employment, homemaker (to permit a spouse to return to work rather than staying at home with a dependent spouse), family unpaid worker, or other vocational outcome. A typical annual caseload for a rehabilitation counselor may include 150 or more individuals who may be participating in some or all of the following phases of the rehabilitation process: evaluation, medical or psychological services, counseling and guidance, mobility training, life skills training, vocational training, rehabilitation technology training, work adjustment training, job-seeking skill development, and job placement. Certified rehabilitation counselors possess a master of science degree in rehabilitation counseling and a documented level of experience in helping individuals with impairments enter, return to, or remain in gainful employment. Rehabilitation counselors work in state agencies, state rehabilitation facilities, and private rehabilitation programs, including those linked to workmen's compensation insurance programs.

EYE CARE PROVIDERS. Optometrists and ophthalmologists provide diagnostic, therapeutic, and rehabilitative services to individuals who are blind or visually impaired. Generally, there is a wide range of experience and professional training that these eye care providers bring to the vision-related rehabilitation setting. Some practitioners hold diplomate status in low vision rehabilitation and some have master of science degrees in low vision rehabilitation. Others may have experience in a 1-year residency program and still others may have received one semester of clinical training in a low vision service. The American Academy of Optometry offers a diplomate in low vision, which requires extensive clinical experience in low vision rehabilitation, submission of case reports, and successful completion of written, oral, and practical examinations. Eye care providers may identify themselves as low vision specialists and may be listed in the *Blue Book of Optometrists*[1] or the *Red Book of Ophthalmologists*.[2] In addition, the American Foundation for the Blind (AFB) publishes the *AFB Directory of Services for Blind and Visually Impaired Persons in the United States and Canada*,[3] which identifies low vision, rehabilitation, education, and other services by state and lists the addresses and telephone numbers for key national professional and consumer organizations and resources.

REHABILITATION TEACHERS. Rehabilitation teachers are university-trained professionals who address the broad range of skills needed by individuals who are blind or visually impaired to live independently at home, to obtain employment, and to participate in community life. Rehabilitation teachers provide instruction in the following areas to facilitate independence in all aspects of daily life: home management, personal management, communication and education, activities of daily living, leisure activities, and indoor orientation skills.[4] Certification is offered through Division 11 of the Association for Education and Rehabilitation of the Blind and Visually Impaired (AER), an international professional membership organization. Rehabilitation teachers may provide instruction in rehabilitation centers, outpatient facilities, and individual clients' homes.

ORIENTATION AND MOBILITY THERAPISTS. Orientation and mobility therapists are university-trained professionals who specialize in teaching travel skills to individuals who are blind or visually impaired. Orientation and mobility techniques are a set of specific skills and strategies that help individuals move about safely and efficiently while traveling in a variety of environments, including school, work, home, and recreational settings. Instruction can include the use of canes, guide dogs, or electronic travel devices, as well as instruction in sighted guide and pre-cane skills and techniques.[5] Orientation and mobility therapists may provide these services in rehabilitation centers, outpatient facilities, and individual clients' homes. Certification is offered through Division 9 of the AER.

LOW VISION THERAPISTS. Low vision therapists instruct individuals in the use of residual vision with optical devices, nonoptical devices, and assistive technology, and help in determining the need for appropriate environmental modifications in the home, workplace, or school. Professionals who provide this service do so in conjunction with eye care practitioners and may be rehabilitation teachers, orientation and mobility therapists, occupational therapists, educational specialists, and other vision-related rehabilitation professionals who possess a master of science degree or certificate in low vision rehabilitation. Low vision therapists may provide services in schools, low vision centers, rehabilitation centers, outpatient facilities, hospitals, and individual client's homes. Certification is offered through Division 7 of the AER.

OCCUPATIONAL AND PHYSICAL THERAPISTS. Occupational and physical therapists work with physical disorders that may have sensory implications. In cases of multiple impairments, such as those caused by traumatic brain injury and stroke, the services of occupational and physical therapists—in conjunction with physiatrists (physicians who specialize in rehabilitation medicine)—may be required to increase fine and gross motor skills, build strength and muscle tone, integrate the use of all senses, learn usage of adaptive equipment, and develop overall physical functioning as it relates to independent living goals. Occupational therapists in particular have a special interest in vision-related rehabilitation because of their emphasis on sensory integration activities. Both types of professionals may provide services in hospitals, rehabilitation centers, outpatient facilities, and individual client's homes, and must possess certification and licensure to practice.

SOCIAL WORKERS AND CASE WORKERS. Social workers and case workers, especially in commissions for the blind or low vision centers, provide individual and group counseling and facilitate consumer access to appropriate community-based support services, including public assistance programs, rehabilitation programs, senior centers, hospitals, and clinics. They use self-help techniques to assist blind and visually impaired children and adults who may be economically, physically, mentally or socially in need of vision-related rehabilitation services. Social work certification is offered through the National Association of Social Workers and the Academy of Certified Social Workers. In some instances, state licensure or certification, or both, may be required to practice in certain settings.

VOCATIONAL EVALUATORS, PLACEMENT SPECIALISTS, AND JOB COACHES. Vocational evaluators, placement specialists, and job coaches assist counselors and clients in determining and achieving employment goals. Vocational evaluators administer tests and work samples to evaluate vocational interests and aptitudes. Placement specialists develop, analyze, and modify jobs for the placement of rehabilitation agency clients. Their objective is to enhance the employer's understanding of the individual's specific visual requirements. Job coaches work side-by-side in industries and businesses with individuals with disabilities. These individuals may be developmentally or physically disabled and may require intensive one-on-one training, coaching, and direct job supervision.

Private Rehabilitation Programs

In some states, the state rehabilitation agency provides vision-related rehabilitation services through contractual agreements with private, nonprofit, volunteer programs or Industries for the Blind. The private program may be a part of a national or statewide network or association, such as the Pennsylvania Association for the Blind (PAB). Participating PAB member agencies offer similar services in their respective geographic areas, which may include social services, transportation, vocational evaluation, work adjustment training, rehabilitation teaching and activities of daily living, orientation and mobility therapy, counseling services, and recreational activities. One additional feature of such programs is the provision of work activities that have been contracted with local manufacturers or businesses. This arrangement enables vocational evaluators to assess skills of visually impaired individuals on real work samples, and in some instances becomes a source of employment when the individual is unable to compete in the job market, with or without supported employment services.

Rehabilitation counselors may also work in the private sector as facilitators of workmen's compensation cases. Unlike the federal/state rehabilitation system, counselors in the private sector are able to provide services with fewer time delays and less paperwork. Eligibility determination is eliminated and only essential services are provided to return a previously employed worker—who is either temporarily or permanently disabled—back to the same job or to a comparable one.

Federal/State Programs for Veterans

The Veterans Administration serves veterans who are blind or visually impaired in one of three ways: visual impairment services (VIS), vision impairment centers to optimize remaining sight (VICTORS), and regional blind rehabilitation centers. The VIS program provides help in adjusting to loss of sight and its functional implications for the veteran and his or her family. The VIS coordinator also provides information on services, resources, and benefits available to veterans with visual impairment. The VICTORS program addresses the needs of veterans with partial sight (best-corrected visual acuity from 20/50 to 20/200 or visual fields >20 degrees) who are not eligible for other services. The VICTORS program provides holistic interdisciplinary services from the fields of ophthalmology, optometry, low vision rehabilitation, social work, and audiology in addition to other services authorized by the VICTORS coordinator. Regional blind rehabilitation centers are found in Veterans Affairs medical centers in Alabama, Arizona, Connecticut, Georgia, Illinois, Puerto Rico, Texas, and Washington. Veterans are generally in residence at the center for a 6-week period to receive a range of vision-related rehabilitation services, including low vision, orientation and mobility therapy, rehabilitation teaching and activities of daily living, alternative communications training (including assistive technology), and referrals to appropriate community resources, such as state rehabilitation services and the Blinded Veterans Association.

Federal/State Programs for Older Adults

The 1965 Older Americans Act (OAA) provided the structural framework for today's array of programs for older persons. Program objectives are geared to health, housing, employment opportunities, community services, research, and independence. The Administration on Aging under the U.S. Department of Health and Human Services oversees funding and implementation by state and local governments and advocates for the interests and concerns of older Americans. Eye care providers can assist older Americans through appropriate, timely referrals to the array of programs authorized by the OAA. Area agencies on aging (AAAs) may offer protective services, housing repair or modifications, friendly visitors (i.e., senior companions), home delivered meals, adult day care, eye care, therapies, medical equipment and supplies, nursing and home health care, personal emergency response service, transportation, career counseling, job search seminars, family caregiver support, and information and referral services. To confirm services available in the client's area, the state or local AAA should be contacted.

The 1978 amendments to the Rehabilitation Act of 1973 added Title VII, Part C, which authorized grants to state vocational rehabilitation agencies to provide independent living services to older blind and visually impaired persons. In the current Rehabilitation Act Amendments of 1992, the program for older Americans is now Title VII, Chapter 2. Specific guidelines for funds include the definition that an older blind individual includes any person age 55 years or older whose severe visual impairment makes gainful employment extremely difficult to obtain, but for whom independent living goals are feasible. It is also stipulated that the designated state agency be the only program within that state that would be eligible for program funds. Through this program, states have provided such services as training in orientation and mobility therapy, rehabilitation teaching, communication, daily living skills, use of low vision devices, peer and family counseling, and outreach to rural older people and minority groups who have had limited access to vision-related rehabilitation services.[6]

Federal/State Educational Services for Students with Visual Impairments

The educational network for the blind and visually impaired school-age population includes regular and special educational instruction, early intervention programs and services, and teachers who are certified in vision. Students may receive services in special classrooms, resource rooms, itinerant programs in public, private, parochial, or tribal schools, or residential schools for blind and visually impaired children.

The Individuals with Disabilities Education Act (IDEA) (formerly the Education for all Handicapped Children Act of 1975) entitles children with disabilities that adversely affect their educational performance, including visual impairment, to a free and appropriate public education in the least restrictive environment. In addition, the law requires states to provide essential related educational services, including transportation; physical, occupational, and speech therapy; and audiologic and psychological services. IDEA also mandates coverage of all or part of low vision clinical evaluations, training in the use of low vision devices, and other related services, such as orientation and mobility training for visually impaired children.[7]

Transition planning begins at age 14 years to ensure that students with disabilities receive appropriate educational support to prepare for college, employment, or community living, or all. Rehabilitation counselors from the federal/state rehabilitation system participate in transition planning and services designated in the plan, especially after graduation. Children with disabilities not covered under IDEA may be covered under the Rehabilitation Act Section 504 or the Americans with Disabilities Act of 1990.

For states to receive federal funding, the Department of Education requires that local educational institutions develop and maintain an Individualized Education Plan (IEP) for each child. The IEP contains the following information: specific educational goals, projected timelines for goal achievement, related educational services required, professional disciplines involved, and specialized or adapted equipment and materials. When planning services for students with vision impairments, a multidisciplinary team will meet with the parent or child, or both, to develop an appropriate IEP. Input from a low vision specialist who has observed and evaluated the child is essential to ensure that the child is capable of achieving the goals developed in the IEP. School systems are expected to provide necessary services, devices, and environmental modifications that will facilitate access and learning for the student who is blind or visually impaired. Parents have the right to participate in an appeals process and to arrange for an independent educational evaluation if they disagree with the IEP goals, methods, or content.

Services for students who are blind or visually impaired include braille training and equipment, large-print resources, listening skills, orientation and mobility training, life skills training, vocational counseling, evaluation and training, and assisitive technology as needed to enhance learning and IEP goals. Itinerant vision teachers travel to schools on a regular basis and meet with students to review their educational goals, provide adaptive resources and instruction, and monitor progress toward achievement of those goals. Some students in the public school system may participate in specialized classrooms or work with a special educator in a resource room for part of the school day. A state vision consultant or a special education unit in a state department or division of education generally oversees activities related to working with visually impaired children. The American Printing House for the Blind (APH) receives an annual appropriation from Congress to provide textbooks and educational resources for students who are blind or visually impaired. APH produces books and other learning materials in braille, large print, and audiotape. State commissions for the blind may supplement the services of APH as necessary. When students who are blind or visually impaired graduate or reach working age, they may be referred for vocational rehabilitation assistance from the state rehabilitation agency or unit.

Other Related Programs and Services

The Client Assistance Program is designed specifically for advocacy between clients and state rehabilitation units and agencies. This program, found in most states, is an objective third party that helps clarify the rehabilitation process, reaffirms the rights of clients of rehabilitation services, and facilitates the resolution of conflicts between rehabilitation counselors and clients. The rights of clients include: (1) the right to a fair and complete evaluation, (2) the right to know the reasons for a determination that an individual is not eligible for services, (3) the right to an appeals process, (4) the right to confidentiality of records, (5) the right to be a partner in planning goals and services, and (6) the right to continuous involvement of the counselor throughout the vocational rehabilitation process. If any of the rights have been violated, the client assistance program can advocate on the client's behalf.

The National Library Service for the Blind and Physically Handicapped, a division of the Library of Congress,

administers a free library program of braille and recorded materials circulated to eligible borrowers through a network of cooperating libraries. Any individual who is unable to read or use standard printed materials as a result of temporary or permanent visual or physical limitations is eligible to receive this service. Reading material and playback equipment are available for loan free of charge and are exchanged through the mail as "Free Matter for the Blind or Handicapped." Information about this service is available through state and local blindness agencies, the Library of Congress, local public libraries, or the telephone directory.

The National Association of Radio Reading Services (NARRS) is an organization that provides audio access to individuals who are unable to read or use standard printed materials as a result of temporary or permanent visual or physical limitations. Radio reading services are typically broadcast on a subcarrier of an FM radio station. When individuals register with this service, they obtain a closed-circuit radio receiver that transmits a variety of programs, including news, features, sports, business, advertisements, and public affairs programming. Receivers are loaned to listeners for an indefinite period, and a deposit may be required. Information about this service is available through NARRS, state and local rehabilitation agencies, area agencies on aging, senior centers, or the telephone directory.

Communities providing public transportation services in a given geographic area to residents must make them accessible to people with disabilities or provide an alternative form of transportation. These services can transport individuals with disabilities to and from a variety of services, including employment, health care, social services, rehabilitation, and places of worship. Costs and eligibility criteria may vary, and certification of impairment is required. Applications are available from most local public transportation systems. In addition, reduced transit fares may be available on public transportation systems for individuals with disabilities, and are generally offered during off-peak hours of operation. Some public and private rehabilitation agencies have volunteers who provide limited transportation services for clients. Large clinical facilities may also provide transportation to and from appointments at their sites. Information is available through local public transportation systems, state and local rehabilitation agencies, local clinical facilities, AAAs, and senior centers.

Federal housing subsidies are available to assist persons with disabilities—including blindness or visual impairment—in accessing affordable, appropriate housing facilities. The rent for an individual unit is determined by the cost of the unit, a fixed percentage of the individual's income, and a federal subsidy. Eligibility criteria for such facilities may vary, and certification of visual status may be required. Information about this type of housing is available through state and local rehabilitation agencies, local clinical facilities, AAAs, and senior centers.

Directory assistance privileges and operator-assisted dialing are available in most communities free of charge to individuals who are certified as legally blind. Applications may be obtained from the local telephone company.

THE LOW VISION PRACTITIONER'S ROLE IN THE VISION-RELATED REHABILITATION SERVICES NETWORK

Once authorized to conduct an ocular and visual examination, the eye care practitioner is expected to provide reports that will verify the potential client's ocular and visual status. The information requested typically includes visual acuity, visual fields, ocular health, and prognosis. It is important to clearly summarize the functional implications of the visual impairment in terms of the individual's rehabilitation goals. Does the individual have a progressive disease that will result in total blindness? Does the individual have sufficient vision to continue driving? Does the individual have sufficient vision to be able to read under appropriate lighting with or without an optical device? Should the individual be monitored closely or referred for further evaluation? Will the individual benefit from a low vision evaluation? Prompt reporting in lay—as well as in technical—terms will facilitate the client's timely progress through his or her rehabilitation program.

In addition, the low vision eye care practitioner evaluates visual functioning, determines visual goals, prescribes appropriate optical devices and suggests appropriate nonoptical devices as part of the client's IWRP. For example, if an individual needs to read regular-size print for his or her chosen vocation, the practitioner may prescribe a spectacle microscope to attain that goal. The practitioner should be aware that if the goal of the funding agency is to enable the client to obtain or retain employment, recommendations for services or devices should include a discussion of how the service or device will enable the individual to achieve those goals. Once the recommendation is made and the client's performance with the device is well-documented in terminology that is objective and understandable, the doctor requests an authorization from the rehabilitation counselor. If the request is approved, the state agency will assist the client in purchasing the device and related services, such as instruction in the use of optical devices that are necessary for its continued use. A sample letter for the request of a microscope is illustrated in Appendix A.

Although rehabilitation counselors have the major responsibility for the job placement phase of the rehabilitation plan, they may also require assistance from the eye care practitioner in interpreting the visual demands of a specific job. For example, job modification or environmental modifications may involve adjusting the position and wattage of lighting, as well as changing print size, color, and contrast.

Building a Referral Network

In some states, rehabilitation agencies refer clients to the low vision eye care practitioner with whom they have established reliable working relationships. By introducing him- or herself to the staff of the rehabilitation agency in his or her area, a low vision practitioner will gain valuable information that will facilitate the implementation of an ongoing referral relationship with the state agency. In other states, rehabilitation agencies may formalize the relationship with practitioners by developing a written contract or cooperative agreement regarding responsibilities and fees. Some states may use a credentialing process that may include a required number of low vision patient care experiences, completion of a residency in low vision rehabilitation, or documented evidence of continuing education courses. Qualifications to become a vendor are not automatic and may have certain limitations of service scope and location. Information on becoming a vendor and specific vendor responsibilities may be obtained from the state or local rehabilitation or blindness agency.

Vendor-Agency Relationship

When an eye care practitioner accepts an authorization for services, payment is provided directly from the state agency rather than from the client or the client's insurance company. As a vendor, the doctor agrees to provide visual diagnostic written reports to document the eye condition, provide services and, when authorized, dispense devices to agency clients. Some states may contract with a low vision service for its clients in a given locale while allowing one-time vendors to serve clients who are in rural settings or would have difficulty accessing a contracted vendor. Alternatively, clients may request that they receive services and devices from their regular eye care practitioner, but this arrangement requires prior approval before services and devices can be rendered.

Ensuring Accessibility to Services

A practitioner who is interested in becoming a low vision service provider for a rehabilitation agency should reassess the clinical environment for its accessibility to persons with disabilities. Signs should contain high-contrast letters of sufficient size to be read by individuals with reduced visual acuity and should be adequately illuminated. Numbers on elevators should be in large print and braille. The practitioner should ensure that the facility is accessible to people using assistive mobility devices such as canes, wheelchairs, and walkers. Examination rooms and restrooms should be accessible to wheelchairs. The parking lot should have an appropriate number of parking spaces for persons with disabilities. Water fountains and pay phones should also be accessible to people in wheelchairs. The practitioner should be prepared to provide interpretation services when requested to do so by patients with hearing impairments. Since the inception of the Rehabilitation Act of 1973 and its subsequent amendments and the Americans with Disabilities Act of 1990, failure to comply with these adaptations could lead to significant financial penalties.

FINANCIAL RESOURCES

A number of entitlements are available to individuals with visual impairments. Entitlements are public funds available for all persons who meet eligibility requirements. These entitlements provide funding for health care and provide income to eligible individuals. They include Social Security disability income (SSDI), supplemental security income (SSI), Medicare, and Medical Assistance/Medicaid.

SSDI is a federal program that benefits nonworking disabled individuals and their dependents. Eligibility is not only based on disability but also on having paid into the Social Security System for a specified number of years. Each state has medical staff working in its disability service to help determine medical disability for participation in SSDI. Application for this entitlement is made through the Social Security Administration.

SSI is a federal income maintenance program for legally blind, disabled, or older adults. Individuals must be unable to work and must meet income eligibility criteria. Application is made through the Social Security Administration and certification of disability is necessary.

Medicare provides medical insurance coverage to persons 65 years old and older, or to individuals already receiving SSDI. Generally, after the deductible is met, services are reimbursed at 80% of Medicare allowable fees if there is a medical diagnosis related to the service. Refractive services are not included. For those patients with vision impairment in need of ocular health services, Medicare may be used.

Medical Assistance/Medicaid is a state-administered program often associated with public assistance and SSI. This program provides financial coverage for services received from contracted providers. To participate in this program, the practitioner contracts with the state program and agrees to accept the level of reimbursement provided. There are generally limits to the number of visits allowed through this program. Medicaid is available for financially eligible persons and is administered by the department of public assistance in each state. If low vision services are not in the standard list of covered services, the practitioner may be able to obtain authorization for services or devices by submitting information to the state's department of public assistance indicating that these services or devices are medically necessary in the management of the individual's care.

Individuals who are certified as legally blind by an optometrist or ophthalmologist are eligible to claim one additional exemption when filing their federal income tax return. A form of certification is required documentation (see Appendix B).

Public service organizations that may provide funding (on an individual basis) for services and low vision devices include the Lions, Kiwanis, Rotary, Elks, and Variety clubs; Masons organizations; and religious and civic groups. Traditionally, Lions clubs have dedicated the majority of their fundraising efforts to assist individuals with vision problems. It is advised that the patient or eye care practitioner contact an officer or designated person of the organization for assistance. It is also beneficial for the doctor to present a lecture to these organizations and provide them with information on how their funds would benefit a par-

ticular patient. These service organizations can serve as valuable resources for funding and increase referral sources by enhancing public awareness of the need for low vision rehabilitation services.

CONSUMER ORGANIZATIONS

Consumers have developed a number of national organizations to address specific issues. Two generic organizations of consumers who are blind or visually impaired are the American Council of the Blind (ACB) and the National Federation of the Blind (NFB). NFB seeks to improve the social and economic conditions of blind individuals. They publish *The Braille Monitor* and *Future Reflections*. The ACB promotes effective participation of blind people, including those with low vision, in all aspects of society. Its major publication is *The Braille Forum*. ACB has as one of its divisions the Council of Citizens with Low Vision International. This group promotes education and research in low vision issues and facilitates networking to address problems of people with low vision.

Some consumer organizations are sports-oriented, such as the American Blind Bowling Association, the American Blind Skiing Foundation, and the United Association for Blind Athletes. Other consumer organizations are vocationally oriented, such as the American Blind Lawyers Association, Blinded Veterans Association, Blind Enterprise Program, and National Association of Vision Professions. Organizations for parents include the National Association of Parents of the Visually Impaired and the American Council of Blind Parents. Organizations specific to diseases and disorders include, but are not limited to, National Organization for Albinism and Hypopigmentation and the Foundation Fighting Blindness. See Appendix C for selected organizations, their addresses, telephone numbers, and where available, World Wide Web addresses.

The American Foundation for the Blind (AFB), while not a consumer organization, has been a leader in increasing the visibility and positive image of people who are blind or visually impaired and in supporting the growth and development of vision-related rehabilitation professionals. AFB sponsors seminars for leadership and professional development and publishes recent research results and legislative updates in its *Journal of Visual Impairment and Blindness*. AFB provides advocacy, leadership in legislative issues, information and referral, consultations, and books and publications.

SELF-ASSESSMENT QUESTIONS

1. The backbone of the federal/state rehabilitation program is (are)
   (a) financial assistance
   (b) gainful employment
   (c) counseling services
   (d) all of the above
   (e) a and b

The Vision-Related Rehabilitation Network 375

2. The Individuals with Disabilities Education Act entitles children with disabilities to receive a free and
appropriate public education in the least restrictive
environment.
True or False

3. Specialized transportation services will typically provide transportation for persons with disabilities to and
from
   (a) work
   (b) medical and rehabilitation appointments
   (c) places of worship
   (d) grocery shopping
   (e) all of the above

4. A client requiring instruction in the use of a low vision
device may receive assistance from which of the following specialists?
   (a) rehabilitation teacher
   (b) low vision therapist
   (c) orientation and mobility therapist
   (d) occupational therapist
   (e) all of the above

5. Entitlements are public funds that are available for
health care and providing income to eligible individuals.
True or False

REFERENCES

1. Blue Book of Optometrists. Who's Who in Optometry (46th ed).
VT: Jobson Publishing, 1998.
2. Red Book of Ophthalmologists. Who's Who in Ophthalmology
(42nd ed). VT: Jobson Publishing, 1997.
3. American Foundation for the Blind. AFB Directory of Services
for Blind and Visually Impaired Persons in the United States and
Canada (24th ed). New York: AFB Press, 1997.
4. Crews JE, Luxton L. Rehabilitation Teaching for Older Adults. In
AL Orr (ed), Vision and Aging: Crossroads for Service Delivery.
New York: American Foundation for the Blind, 1992;233–253.
5. Blasch BB, Weiner WR, Welsh RL (eds). Foundations of Orientation and Mobility (2nd ed). New York: AFB Press, 1997.
6. American Foundation for the Blind. Fact Sheet: Independent Living
Services for Older Individuals Who Are Blind Program (Title VII,
Chapter 2 of the Rehabilitation Act). New York: AFB Press, 1997.
7. Orr AL. An overview of the blindness system. In AL Orr (ed),
Vision and Aging: Crossroads for Service Delivery. New York:
American Foundation for the Blind, 1992;159–183.

_____Appendix A_____

SAMPLE LETTER FOR THE REQUEST OF A LOW VISION SYSTEM FROM A STATE AGENCY

Ms. Iris Coloboma
Commission for the Blind
2041 Main Street
Metropolis, Anystate 77777

Re: Mr. Seymour Sharp
DOB: 7/14/21

Dear Ms. Coloboma:

Your client, Mr. Seymour Sharp, presented for a low vision evaluation on June 24, 1998. As you know, Mr. Sharp has an ocular diagnosis of bilateral age-related macular degeneration that first presented in the right eye 4 years ago and 2 years ago in the left eye. The remaining ocular history is unremarkable. He further reports his general health to be excellent. The history is also negative for systemic or ocular surgery and any medications. Mr. Sharp reports that his primary goal is to improve his visual acuity for reading, most specifically, reading his bills and writing checks.

Visual acuities were found to be best with his present spectacle correction and were recorded as 10/120 (20/240 equivalent) in the right eye and 10/100 (20/200 equivalent) in the left. At near, through his +2.50 D bifocal, Mr. Sharp was able to see 0.40/4 M (20/200 equivalent at 40 cm) in each eye. A low vision refraction showed no improvement in his distance spectacle correction. Visual fields indicated the presence of bilateral central scotomas secondary to the macular degeneration.

A number of spectacle-mounted reading lenses and handheld magnifiers were evaluated. Mr. Sharp preferred a 2.5× reading spectacle, which incorporates base-in prism to allow him to read comfortably with both eyes. With this lens system, he was able to read 0.10/1 M (20/50 equivalent at 10 cm) continuous text print (magazine size print). His skills in using this device were excellent. Appropriate lighting was demonstrated, and Mr. Sharp worked best with direct illumination. Large-print checks were also shown, and Mr. Sharp was thrilled with the comfort and ease in using this type of check along with the ease in using the large-print balance sheet. He was able to use his present bifocal and flair-tip pen when writing a check.

An ocular health evaluation confirmed bilateral atrophic age-related macular degeneration along with slight nuclear cataracts in each eye. Mr. Sharp was told of his ocular condition and it was also explained to him that his reduced vision is due to the macular degeneration and that the cataracts are of no consequence at this time.

In conclusion, Mr. Sharp's ocular condition appears stable. It was recommended to him that he see a retinal specialist on a yearly basis. Mr. Sharp was pleased with the 2.5× reading lens. He thought that this lens system would allow him to maintain his independence. Prognosis for successful adaptation to this device is excellent. I therefore request authorization for this reading lens ($_____) on behalf of Mr. Sharp.

Thank you for your referral and for allowing me to participate in your client's vision rehabilitation. Please contact me if you have any questions concerning my findings and recommendations.

Sincerely,

Richard L. Brilliant, O.D., F.A.A.O.
Low Vision Specialist

Appendix B

STATEMENT OF LEGAL BLINDNESS

Note. On doctor's letterhead.

Re: <u>James S. Smith</u>
DOB: <u>1/18/37</u>
SS #:   <u>422 47 3632</u>

To whom it may concern:

<u>Mr. James S. Smith</u> was seen in this office on <u>January 4, 1998</u>. At that time, his/her best corrected visual acuities were:
OD <u>20/200</u>
OS <u>20/300</u>
and/or he/she had a visual field of _____ OD, _____ OS at its widest meridian.

This reduced vision is due to _____. This condition is permanent and irreversible. The level of vision loss qualifies the above named person as **legally blind**, and as such, he/she is entitled to all services and benefits available to the legally blind.

Please feel free to contact this office should additional information be required.

Sincerely,

Claire Ize, O.D., F.A.A.O.
Low Vision Rehabilitation Specialist

Appendix C

RESOURCE LIST FOR LOW VISION CONSUMERS AND PROVIDERS*

Note. This information does not denote a complete list of low vision resources in the United States.

American Blind Lawyers Association
See American Council of the Blind for current information

American Bioptic Certified Drivers (ABCD)
23872 Innisbrook
Laguna Niguel, CA 92677
(714) 495-3334

American Council of the Blind
1155 15th St. NW, Suite 720
Washington, DC 20005
(202) 467-5081
800-424-8666
Fax: (202) 467-5085

American Council of Families with Visual Impairment
See American Council of the Blind for current information

American Foundation for the Blind
11 Penn Plaza, Suite 300
New York, NY 10001
(212) 502-7600

American Printing House for the Blind
P.O. Box 6085
1839 Frankfort Ave.
Louisville, KY 40206-0085
(502) 895-2405
800-223-1839
Fax: (502) 899-2274

American Society of Human Genetics
9650 Rockville Pike
Bethesda, MD 20814
(301) 571-1825

Architectural and Transportation Barriers
Compliance Board
1331 F St. NW, Suite 1000
Washington, DC 20004-1111
(202) 272-5434

Association for Education and Rehabilitation
of the Blind and Visually Impaired
4600 Duke St., Suite 430
P.O. Box 22397
Alexandria, VA 22304
(703) 823-9690
www.aerbvi.org

Association for Macular Diseases
210 E. 64th St.
New York, NY 10021
(212) 605-3719

Association for Persons with Severe Handicaps
29 W. Susquehanna Ave., Suite 210
Baltimore, MD 21204
(410) 828-8274
(410) 828-1306 TTY
www.tash.org

Association of Radio Reading Services
c/o Pittsburgh Radio Information Service
2100 Wharton St., #140
Pittsburgh, PA 15203
[address changes with current president]
800-280-5325 (number stays the same)

Bible Alliance, Inc.
P.O. Box 1549
Bradenton, FL 34206
(941) 748-3031

Blind and Visually Impaired Division
Rehabilitation Services Administration
330 C St. SW, Room 3227
Washington, DC 20202
(202) 205-9902

Blinded Veterans Association
477 H St. NW
Washington, DC 20001-2694
(202) 371-8880

Clovernook Printing House for the Blind
7000 Hamilton Ave.
Cincinnati, OH 45231
(513) 522-3860
888-234-7156

Corneal Dystrophy Foundation
1926 Hidden Creek Dr.
Kingwood, TX 77339
(713) 358-4227

Council of Citizens with Low Vision International
See American Council of the Blind for current information

Descriptive Video Service
WGBH Educational Foundation
125 Western Ave.
Boston, MA 02134
(617) 492-2777, ext. 3490
800-333-1203
Fax: (617) 787-0714

Equal Employment Opportunity Commission
Headquarters and Office of Legal Counsel
1801 L St. NW
Washington, DC 20507
(202) 663-4900
www.eeoc.gov
[For nearest field office, dial 800-669-4000 or
800-669-6820 TDD]
[For publications, dial 800-669-3362 or 800-669-3302 TDD]

Fight for Sight National Council to Combat Blindness
160 E. 56th St., 8th Floor
New York, NY 10022
(212) 751-1118

Foundation Fighting Blindness
11350 McCormick St.
Hunt Valley, MD 21031
(410) 785-1414
800-683-5555

Glaucoma Research Foundation
490 Post St., Suite 830
San Francisco, CA 94102
800-826-6693

Helen Keller National Center for Blind Youths and Adults
111 Middle Neck Rd.
Sands Point, NY 11050
(516) 944-8900

Institute for Families of Blind Children
P.O. Box 54700 (mail stop #111)
Los Angeles, CA 90054
(213) 669-4649

International Society on Metabolic Eye Disease
1200 5th Ave.
New York, NY 10029
(212) 427-1246

Jewish Braille Institute of America
110 E. 30th St.
New York, NY 10016
800-433-1531
(212) 889-2525
[cassettes and large-type materials also]

Lighthouse Center for Education
111 E. 59th St.
New York, NY 10022
800-829-0500

Lutheran Library for the Blind
1333 S. Kirkwood Rd.
Saint Louis, MO 63122
(314) 965-9000

National Information Center for Children and Youth
with Disabilities
P.O. Box 1492
Washington, DC 20036
800-695-0285

National Alliance of Blind Students
See American Council of the Blind for current information

Schepens Eye Research Institute of the Retina Foundation
20 Stanford St.
Boston, MA 02114
(617) 742-3140

National Association of Area Agencies on Aging
1112 16th St. NW, Suite 100
Washington, DC 20036
(202) 296-8130

National Association of Blind Teachers
See American Council of the Blind for current information

National Association for Parents of the Visually Impaired
P.O. Box 317
Watertown, MA 02272-0317
(617) 972-4441
800-562-6265

National Association for the Visually Handicapped
22 W. 21st St., 6th Floor
New York, NY 10010
(212) 889-3141
Fax: (212) 727-2931

National Council on Disability
1331 F St. NW, 10th Floor
Washington, DC 20004-1107
(202) 272-2004
Fax: (202) 267-3232 and TTY

National Council of Private Agencies for the Blind
c/o Hadley School for the Blind
700 Elm St.
Winnetka, IL 60093
(847) 446-6175
(847) 446-8111

National Eye Institute
National Institutes of Health
Building 31, Room 6A03
Bethesda, MD 20892
(301) 496-2234

National Federation of the Blind
1800 Johnson St.
Baltimore, MD 21230
(410) 659-9314
Fax: (410) 685-5653
www.nfb.org

National Institute on Disability and Rehabilitation Research
Office of Special Education and Rehabilitation Services
U.S. Department of Education
330 C St. SW
Washington, DC 20202
(202) 205-8134

National Library Service for the Blind and Physically Handicapped
The Library of Congress
1291 Taylor St. NW
Washington, DC 20542
(847) 491-8305

National Multiple Sclerosis Society
733 3rd Ave., 6th Floor
New York, NY 10017
(212) 986-3240
800-344-4867

National Organization for Albinism and Hypopigmentation
1530 Locust St., No. 29
Philadelphia, PA 19102-4415
800-473-2310
www.albinism.org

National Rehabilitation Information Center
8455 Colesville Rd., Suite 935
Silver Spring, MD 20910-3319
800-346-2742
www.naric.org

National Health Information Center
Office of Disease Prevention and Health Promotion
U.S. Health and Human Services
P.O. Box 1133
Washington, DC 20013
800-336-4797
Fax: (301) 984-4256
www.nhic-nt.health.org

Prevent Blindness America
500 E. Remmington Rd.
Schaumburg, IL 60173
(847) 843-2020

Recording for the Blind and Dyslexic
20 Roszel Rd.
Princeton, NJ 08540
(609) 452-0606
www.rfbd.org

Rehabilitation Services Administration
Office of Special Education and Rehabilitative Services
U.S. Department of Education
330 C St. SW
Washington, DC 20202
(202) 205-5482

Research to Prevent Blindness, Inc.
645 Madison Ave.
New York, NY 10022
(212) 752-4333
800-621-0026

Resources for Rehabilitation
33 Bedford St., Suite 19A
Lexington, MA 02420
(781) 862-6455

Taping for the Blind
3935 Essex Ln.
Houston, TX 77027
(713) 622-2767

U.S. Association of Blind Athletes
33 N. Institute St., West Hall
Colorado Springs, CO 80903
(719) 630-0422
Fax: (719) 630-0616
www.saba.org

Vision Foundation, Inc.
818 Mt. Auburn St.
Watertown, MA 02172
(617) 926-4232

Xavier Society for the Blind (publishing company)
154 E. 23rd St.
New York, NY 10010
(212) 473-7800

CHAPTER TWENTY

Case Studies

Richard L. Brilliant

There is a maxim that is very relevant to life in general and, in many cases, may be very pertinent to the field of low vision rehabilitation:

Tell me and I will forget
Show me and I will remember
Involve me and I will understand

Chapters 1–19 have provided both the student and the practitioner with the basic information on low vision rehabilitation or the "tell me" section of this aphorism. What follows in this chapter are three case studies that will demonstrate to the student and practitioner how the basic information is used to help the patient with low vision. In essence, it is the "show me" section of the triad. The final portion of this adage is only achieved through direct patient care and a love for and commitment to low vision rehabilitation. It is here that the practitioner will achieve a true understanding of this critical field of eye care. Only through "involvement" does all of this information come together in a meaningful way.

CASE I

Case History

AW, a 15-year-old high school student, presented for a low vision evaluation. She was referred by a local optometrist who had been providing care for her for the previous 10 years. AW was last seen by her optometrist 6 weeks before this visit. He had explained to her that he had provided her with the best care that he was capable of giving and that a low vision evaluation would now be required to meet her new needs. AW was very satisfied with her previous eye care and was now looking forward to the low vision examination. She was a very mature, motivated young woman.

AW was accompanied to the examination by her mother. During the initial history, AW reported that her general health was excellent. She had no history of systemic or ocular surgery. She took no medication other than acetaminophen for occasional headaches and "aches and pains." Both AW and her mother appeared to be quite vocal and concerned about AW's future. AW, an only child, lived at home with her mother, who was divorced. AW was in the tenth grade and had a previous history of doing very well throughout her school career. She was now, however, reporting difficulty with distance-related tasks, especially seeing the blackboard (even though she was already sitting in the front of the class). AW was receiving itinerant vision services 1 day each week from the county's intermediate unit. AW said that the emphasis was on reading large print, and both she and her mother were not satisfied. AW's mother was working with the county to try to improve these services for her daughter.

AW reported that she was very familiar with her ocular condition of albinism and nystagmus. AW had been wearing glasses for the past 10 years and she thought that there was a slight improvement with them on. She was instructed by her optometrist to wear them full time. AW had been evaluated and dispensed a pair of rigid corneal lenses by her optometrist approximately 2 years earlier. After a few months of wearing them, she decided they were not for her. She thought that they did not provide any increase in her vision over her own spectacles. She also thought that they were slightly uncomfortable and required more time and effort to maintain than her spectacles. One other problem noted by AW was that the contact lenses increased her sensitivity to light even though they had a dark blue tint. Aperture control lenses (pinhole lenses) were discussed and demonstrated to AW, but she was not interested in pursuing them. She was advised to contact her optometrist if she would like to evaluate new contact lenses (gas-permeable or toric soft) in the future. AW informed me that her family, teachers, and friends were all aware of her visual impairment and that she perceived herself as being a "fully sighted" individual.

In further discussing her vision, AW reported that she had fluctuations in vision and that her vision was better under dim, nonglare situations. She also reported that headaches were common when she was in bright lighting for a period (approximately 15 minutes or longer). She used "photosun" lenses, prescribed by her optometrist, when outdoors, and these had been extremely helpful for comfort as well as reducing the number of headaches.

AW was able to read standard-size print in school at what she described as a "comfortable distance" (approximately 8 in.). She thought that her reading skills were good and she saw no reason to read any other way (as mentioned before, her itinerant teacher had her reading large print). When reading very small print (newspaper print) for long periods, AW found a handheld magnifier useful. This device was recommended by her optometrist along with a clip-on telescope for watching television. AW preferred, however, to watch television without the telescope. Her mother purchased a 27-in. color television, and by sitting approximately 5 ft away, AW thought that she was able to see very well.

When AW was not in school, she enjoyed movies, theater, and watching school marching bands. Her future goals were to finish high school and to enter college with the goal of becoming a lawyer. She wanted to one day provide legal representation for handicapped individuals.

In conclusion, AW reported no mobility problems day or night, and she thought that her general health was good. Her chief concerns were listed as the following, in priority order:

1. Seeing the blackboard
2. Help with seeing theater events (recognizing facial detail at a play) and marching bands (recognizing faces and costumes at a distance)
3. Reading small print for long periods without a handheld magnifier
4. Driving a car in the future

Diagnostic Findings

The distance chart used throughout the examination was a Designs for Vision number chart (Designs for Vision, Inc., Ronkonkoma, NY). It was illuminated by two reflector lamps housing 75-W incandescent bulbs angled overhead. This arrangement created direct illumination, providing even lighting with no glare. A rheostat was used to vary the illumination on the chart. At near, the Lighthouse Near Visual Acuity Chart (Lighthouse, Inc., New York, NY) (reduced version of the Ferris-Bailey Early Treatment Diabetic Retinopathy Study [ETDRS] chart) was used. A Luxo floor lamp housing a 60-W incandescent bulb (a 100-W bulb was found to be too bright) provided the illumination. AW was allowed to angle the lamp for the appropriate illumination without creating glare.

Unaided Visual Acuity

	Distance	Near
OD	10/60 − 2	0.20/0.8 M (metric system)
OS	10/80	0.20/0.8 M − 1
OU	10/60 − 2	0.20/0.8 M

Aided Visual Acuity (with habitual prescription)

	Distance	Near
OD	10/60 + 1	0.20/0.8 M
OS	10/60 + 1	0.20/0.8 M
OU	10/60 + 1	0.20/0.8 M

Habitual Prescription

OD	OS
+1.75 − 3.00 × 180	+2.00 − 3.50 × 180

Visual Acuity through Previously Owned Devices

2.8× clip-on telescope over habitual prescription: OD 10/20

+5.00 D handheld magnifier with habitual prescription: OU 0.5 M − 2

AW was very quick and precise in her responses. She favored her right eye when acuities were recorded. There was no head turn or eccentric viewing noted. Her nystagmus was consistent in all meridians of gaze at both distance and near.

Keratometry
Keratometry was performed without either eye being occluded (because of the nystagmus).

OD	OS
−3.50 × 180 axis meridian (AM) 42.75	−3.75 × 180 AM 43.00

Retinoscopy

OS		OS	
+1.25 − 3.00 × 180	10/60	+2.00 − 3.50 × 180	10/60

Subjective
A bracketing technique with just noticeable difference was used when doing the subjective. A ±1.25 cross cylinder was also used.

OD	OS
+1.75 − 3.00 × 180	+2.00 − 3.50 × 180
10/60 + 1	10/60+1

Visual Fields
Amsler's grid testing was performed to provide some quantitative and qualitative analysis of the macular area. Even though a scotoma was not an expected finding, the test was important because one of AW's concerns was reading small print for long periods. The grid was held before each eye at a 33-cm test distance with the patient's spectacles in place. AW was able to see the central fixation dot on the grid, and she reported that all four corners of the grid were present and all the vertical and horizontal lines appeared straight. Her responses were rated as good.

Because Amsler's grid screening demonstrated no scotomas and visual field losses are not associated with albinism, it was deemed unnecessary to perform a tangent screen evaluation. Because of AW's wish to drive in the future, some record of her peripheral fields would be beneficial. An arc perimeter was used because of its relative simplicity and speed in obtaining information on any possible peripheral defects. Testing was performed with AW's spectacle correction in place using a 6/330-W isopter. Peripheral fields proved to be full and normal in all meridians of each eye.

Color Vision
The Farnsworth dichotomous (D-15) test was used to evaluate AW's color vision. A Macbeth lamp was used for illumination, and AW used her spectacle correction to see the colored chips at a distance of 20 cm. Evaluating each eye separately, AW demonstrated normal color vision.

Evaluation of Low Vision Devices

Due to the length of time taken for the initial visit, the decision was made to concentrate on a device (or devices) for AW's distance needs during the visit, as most of her concerns were distance related. When questioned about her previously owned 2.8× clip-on telescope, AW said that when she used it in school for the blackboard, it did allow her to read most of the print. Her performance with the device, however, depended on the print size and color of the chalk used (yellow chalk providing best acuity; blue being the worst—the board was dark green). She also complained that the clip-on was awkward and had a tendency to slide to one side of her glasses. AW was not concerned about using a telescope in the classroom because she thought that all the students knew of her visual situation and she was determined to "do well in school."

Due to the patient's visual acuities and visual demands, a 4.2× Keplerian handheld focusable telescope was evaluated. AW was able to obtain 20/25 acuity in each eye through the telescope and her spectacle correction. She did not notice any difference in field of view or clarity when asked to look through the telescope without her spectacle correction. AW, in fact, preferred to wear her spectacle correction. AW demonstrated excellent skills in localization and scanning with the handheld telescope. She was loaned this device for a 2-week period and told to evaluate it at home and in school.

Ocular Health Evaluation

An ocular health evaluation was performed at the end of the first visit to confirm the diagnosis and stability of the disorder.

Externals
AW demonstrated a horizontal pendular nystagmus with no null point in each eye. Iris transillumination was present in each eye. There was no sign of paresis or paralysis of the extraocular muscles in all positions of gaze. The lids, lashes, conjunctiva, cornea, and lens were normal in appearance OU. The anterior chamber was open and quiet in each eye.

Intraocular Pressure
Due to the nystagmus, a Tono-Pen was used. Pressures were found to be 19 mm Hg in the right eye and 20 mm Hg in the left. Applanation tonometry was performed at 11:30 A.M.

Ophthalmoscopy
Dilated fundus evaluation revealed clear media in each eye. Retinal hypopigmentation was noted with accompanying prominence of the choroidal vascular network. The optic nerve heads were slightly pale and there was no foveal reflex in either eye. All other structures were normal.

Due to AW's physical appearance and the ocular findings (pendular nystagmus, iris transillumination, and absence of pigment in the retina and choroid), a diagnosis of oculocutaneous albinism was confirmed.

At the completion of the first visit, a summary of the results was discussed with AW and her mother. She was reassured that her condition was stable.

Follow-Up Visits

On her follow-up visit, AW indicated that her goals were the same as that of her first visit and that she had used the loaned 4.2× telescope extensively both at home and at school. She was very pleased with the results because she was able to see everything on the blackboard. She was also very successful when using it in the auditorium during a school presentation. AW thought that this magnification provided her with enough facial detail to recognize peo-

ple at a distance, which became evident when she was able to see her friends in the school marching band. Because the power of the telescope was appropriate for all her needs, the various treatment options were discussed and demonstrated to AW. Three different types of 4× spectacle-mounted telescopes were demonstrated and all provided an acuity of 20/25 in each eye. AW preferred a 4× binocular bioptic because she was using both eyes and it could be worn full time. Binocularity was determined to be present through the telescopes by use of a Worth four-dot test. A +4.00 D cap was placed on the telescopic objective of the right eye (her preferred eye) and AW was able to see 0.25/0.5 M. She was also able to read a newspaper with this telemicroscope in normal lighting (60-W bulb in a Luxo floor lamp).

A spectacle microscope was also demonstrated for reading. Because AW was already able to see 0.20/0.8 M and because of her young age and ability to see binocularly (Worth four-dot testing at near), +4.00 D and +6.00 D half-eyes with base-in prism were compared. Through the +4.00 D half-eye, AW was able to see 0.20/0.8 M + 2 OU and through the +6.00 D half-eye, she was able to see 0.20/0.5 M − 1 OU. When her cylindrical correction was held behind the +4.00 D and +6.00 D half-eyes, AW did not notice any difference in clarity or ease in reading. A magazine and newspaper were provided so that AW could compare the two lenses for contrast, print size, and composition. During this component of the low vision evaluation, AW was also introduced to nonoptical systems. Various filters of colored acetate, to be used over her reading material, were evaluated as well as the use of a typoscope and clipboard to hold her reading material. Proper lighting was also discussed and demonstrated. AW thought that the +6.00 D half-eye glasses with 8 prism diopters base in and good lighting were all that were necessary for comfortable reading.

Based on the preceding results with all the low vision devices and that all of AW's goals or concerns were addressed, it was mutually agreed that a conclusion could be reached on the final prescriptions. AW liked the binocular bioptic telescope because it provided the appropriate acuity, allowed her to use both eyes, and could be worn full time. She was also hopeful that the bioptic telescope could be used in the future for driving (assuming she lived in a state that allowed bioptic driving). For reading standard-size print for long periods, AW preferred the +6.00 D half-eye prism spectacles. She did not like the restricted field of the telemicroscope, and therefore the reading cap for the telescope was ruled out. AW was also evaluated with a number of absorptive lenses. Various tints, NoIR lenses (NoIR Medical Technologies, South Lyon, MI) and Corning Protective Filter (CPF) (Corning Medical Optics, Elmira, NY) lenses were demonstrated, but she preferred her own photosun prescription lenses.

On the dispensing visit, AW was able to attain 20/25+ acuity in each eye through the telescope. Each telescope had her distance prescription incorporated into the eyepiece to obtain maximum clarity. The +6.00 D half-eyes provided 0.19/0.5 M acuity OU. Both systems were adjusted to provide maximum comfort, and AW was very pleased with the results. She was instructed in the proper care and maintenance of these devices. AW was told to return to her local optometrist for her continued ocular health evaluations. She was also told that a letter would be sent to her and her optometrist summarizing her visits.

Discussion and Conclusion

AW was very sure of her goals and concerns and appeared to be very motivated and mature for her young age. She had also been very well prepared for the low vision evaluation by her optometrist. AW was aware of her visual and physical condition and appeared to be able to cope with no difficulty.

As expected, the areas of concern for an albinotic patient would be that of providing magnification to increase acuity (caused by an underdeveloped macular area) and a sun lens evaluation to reduce photophobia (caused by lack of pigment). AW did very well in responding to magnification and exhibited excellent visual skills in adapting to the telescope and half-eye reading glasses. Her decision of initially preferring the versatility of a mounted telescope again demonstrated her maturity and awareness of her goals for the present and future.

There were a number of reasons for deciding on the 4× telescope:

1. Because AW's best visual acuity (with conventional lenses) was 20/120, a 3× telescope would be predicted to improve her vision to 20/40 (20/40 or 20/50 is the normal target acuity unless otherwise specified). AW already owned a 2.8× telescope; however, this magnification was not sufficient to see the print on the blackboard in all circumstances. When contrast was poor (blue chalk on a green blackboard), AW was unable to see the print on the blackboard. Through increased magnification, AW attained better visual acuity (20/25), thus making it easier for her to read the print on the blackboard in all situations, even when seated farther from the board.

2. AW's other concerns were seeing facial detail of an actor at a play and recognizing faces and costumes in a marching band. These concerns required greater distances than 20 ft and, therefore, better acuity than 20/40 or 20/50 would be required.

3. Because AW's condition was stable and she planned to attend college, where lecture halls would perhaps be larger than her classroom, it would be advantageous for her to have better acuity than 20/40 or 20/50. This would allow AW to sit in a lecture hall and see the lecturer as well as the details of any film or slide presentation.

AW was provided with all the information necessary to apply for a driver's permit and license. AW resides in the state of New Jersey, which allows the use of a bioptic telescope to obtain a driver's license. New Jersey requires 20/50 acuity or better through either eye using the telescope, with no standards established for fields. Color vision requirements in the state consist of the applicant's ability to distinguish between red, amber, and green.

For reading, because of AW's age and expected high amplitude of accommodation, low-powered reading glasses were prescribed. Because of AW's refractive error (+1.75 D OD and +2.00 D OS), the +6.00 D half-eye spectacle was, in reality, providing approximately 4.00 D of accommodative relief. Because AW was holding her reading material at 20 cm, she was providing approximately 1.00 D of accommodation (through the +4.00 D lens), certainly a very reasonable amount for long-term reading. The astigmatic correction was not incorporated into the half-eye spectacle because AW did not demonstrate any subjective or objective improvement in reading when she was trial framed with the cylinder correction in place.

As for the expected photophobia, AW's needs were met for outdoor use by previously prescribed sun lenses. She did not experience any glare problems when indoors, and therefore no absorptive lenses were recommended for indoor use.

In conclusion, AW was a young, very mature patient with low vision. Her diagnosed condition was that of oculocutaneous albinism. She had been provided with excellent optometric services that had allowed her to remain active and competitive at home and in school. At age 15 years, her visual demands began to increase, and her optometrist thought it was necessary for a low vision referral. AW adapted very well to low vision devices and her visual prognosis is excellent.

CASE II

Case History

WS, a 43-year-old woman, presented for an initial low vision evaluation. She was referred by the local state rehabilitation agency. WS's history indicated that she was recently separated from her husband and that she has two daughters ages 8 and 6 years. WS thought that her separation was partly due to her ocular condition and the stress it created on her family life. Both she and her husband were receiving family counseling through their local church. WS had a high school degree and 1 year of college. She was working as a district court clerk; however, she was forced to quit work due to her failing vision. She wanted to resume working, perhaps in the field of computers (word processing).

WS reported that she was very familiar with her ocular condition. She identified her disorder as retinitis pigmentosa. This condition was initially diagnosed by her ophthalmologist when she was 18 years old. Her visual complaints at that time were poor night vision as well as light and dark adaptation problems that were most notable when she attended movies with her friends. WS thought that her condition had gradually worsened over the years to the point that she had to give up driving 1 year ago. This change left her feeling totally dependent on her husband and parents, who lived nearby. In further discussing her visual problems, WS indicated that she was bumping into objects more often and that her mobility had definitely deteriorated in unfamiliar surroundings, most noticeably in the last year. She also reported having fluctuations in vision, with her vision being the best under "normal home lighting" (incandescent bulbs in her lamps) where there was nonglare situations. WS was also bothered by the bright sunlight (more so in the summer months), especially when she first walked outside. The only protective sun lenses that she wore outdoors were a pair of "store-bought" Polaroid lenses that her ophthalmologist had recommended. WS reported that they were somewhat helpful outdoors but did not totally eliminate her photophobia and glare complaints.

WS reported that her distance vision was fair and improved slightly when she wore her spectacle prescription. She also stated that she was still able to read standard-size print at a distance of approximately 8 in. When reading, WS preferred to read with her spectacles and she also found it easier to read magazine print than newspaper print. She said most of her reading was done at a desk where she was able to use a tensor lamp.

The remainder of her history indicated that her general health was excellent. There was no family history of retinitis pigmentosa or any other ocular condition. She had two older sisters and two older brothers, and all appeared to have "normal vision." WS had no history of ocular surgery or medications. She last saw her ophthalmologist 2 years before this examination and had no plans to see him in the near future. WS had never had a low vision examination and was hopeful that some of her visual concerns could be addressed. Her chief concerns were listed in priority order as follows:

1. To see print on a computer screen with greater ease and comfort
2. To address glare and photophobia complaints both indoors and outdoors
3. To read newspaper print more comfortably
4. To improve mobility in unfamiliar surroundings
5. To spot her young children while they played in the playground (she had difficulty identifying them in the playground when they were a distance away and when there were many children in the playground)

Diagnostic Findings

The distance chart used throughout the examination was a Designs for Vision number chart. It was illuminated by a reflector lamp housing two 75-W incandescent bulbs angled 45 degrees to the chart. This arrangement created direct illumination on the chart and provided even lighting without glare. The amount of illumination was controlled by a rheostat that is incorporated into the light switch. At near, the Lighthouse Near Visual Acuity Chart (reduced version of the Ferris-Bailey ETDRS chart calibrated for 40 cm) was used. A Luxo floor lamp housing a 75-W incandescent bulb provided the illumination. WS was allowed to angle the lamp for the appropriate illumination without creating glare. A fluorescent lamp was also evaluated at near; however, as expected, it produced a glare that could not be eliminated at any angle the in which lamp was positioned.

Unaided Visual Acuity

	Distance	Near
OD	10/40	0.20/1.2 M
OS	10/50 – 1	0.20/1.6 M
OU	10/40	0.20/1.2 M

Habitual Prescription

OD	OS
Plano (pl.) −1.00 × 45	Pl. −1.50 × 135

Acuities through Habitual Prescription

	Distance	Near
OD	10/25	0.20/1.0 M
OS	10/30 + 2	0.20/1.0 M
OU	10/25	0.20/1.0 M

WS was quick and precise in her responses. She thought that her right eye was slightly better as was demonstrated by her acuities. There was no head turn or eccentric viewing noted.

Keratometry

Keratometry was performed to confirm the amount of corneal astigmatism that was present and to see if there was a possibility of more astigmatism. The quality of the mires was good. From the findings, it appeared that all of her astigmatism lay within the cornea and was corrected by her habitual spectacle prescription.

OD	OS
−1.50 × 45 AM 42.50	−1.75 × 135 AM 42.50

Retinoscopy

OD	OS
+0.25 − 1.25 × 45	+0.25 − 1.50 × 135
10/25	10/30 + 2

Subjective

A bracketing technique with just noticeable difference was used when doing the subjective.

OD	OS
+0.50 − 1.00 × 45	+0.50 − 1.50 × 135
10/25 + 1	10/30 + 2

Visual Fields

Amsler's grid testing was performed to provide some analysis of WS's macular area, as two of WS's ocular complaints concerned reading small print (goals 1 and 3). The grid was held before each eye at a 33-cm test distance with the patient's spectacles in place. WS was able to see the central fixation dot on the grid and she reported all four corners of the grid to be present and all the vertical and horizontal lines to appear straight. She reported no areas of the grid missing. Her responses were rated as excellent.

Because improved mobility was another one of her concerns (and because of her diagnosis of retinitis pigmentosa), it was imperative that the extent of her central and peripheral fields be fully investigated. Tangent screen testing was performed using a 5/1,000-W isopter. Results indicated a peripheral constriction in each eye with the remaining field extending from point of fixation out to approximately 20 degrees in all meridians of each eye. For peripheral fields, an arc perimeter was used because of its relative simplicity and speed in identifying any possible peripheral defects. Testing was performed with WS's spectacle correction in place using a 5/330-W isopter. The results confirmed the loss of peripheral fields with no islands of vision in either eye. WS was able to see the wand at approximately 25 degrees from fixation in each eye, which was consistent with the tangent screen testing.

Because WS's initial concern involved seeing print on the computer screen and eliminating glare from the screen, the EZ computer magnifier (Less Gauss, Inc., Rhineback, NY) was thought to be an ideal device to evaluate. The EZ computer magnifier provides approximately 2× magnification and is easily attached to a computer screen (see Figure 14-1). By holding the EZ computer magnifier at the focal distance from the computer screen, WS was able to sit 16 in. from the lens and easily read the print. By placing a continuous-text reading card against the computer screen (behind the EZ computer magnifier) and providing appropriate illumination with a floor lamp, WS's near acuity was measured at 0.5 M with each eye through her (distance) spectacle prescription. WS was very pleased with the results because she was able to sit at a comfortable distance from the computer screen and obtain the necessary acuity with the elimination of glare. The possibility of using large-print software was also discussed, but WS was so pleased with the EZ computer magnifier that she was not interested in using the software at that time.

In regard to WS's problem with photophobia and glare, she was evaluated both indoors and outdoors with Corning CPF lenses and a variety of NoIR lenses. Indoors (in the examination room) lighting was adjusted to simulate the illumination in WS's home. When WS thought that there was comparable illumination (approximately 40 foot-candles of incandescent lighting) the various lenses were evaluated. She chose CPF 527 trial lenses that were attached to her prescription lenses by the use of Halberg clips. WS thought that these lenses provided the most comfort from glare and was pleasantly surprised by the improvement in the overall contrast of objects in the room. A similar evaluation was performed outdoors. It was a bright and sunny winter's day, and WS thought that 32% gray NoIR lenses were best under these circumstances. She was told to come back one day in the summer when the sun would be brighter to reevaluate the sun lenses. (WS did return during the summer to reevaluate the absorptive lenses and she preferred 4% plum NoIR lenses for the bright, sunny, summer days.)

For WS's reading concerns, trial lenses with a prescription of $+2.50 - 1.00 \times 45$ OD and a $+2.50 - 1.50 \times 135$ OS were shown in a trial frame. She was able to see $0.18/0.8$ M + 3 with each eye. With the aid of a yellow acetate filter, typoscope, and proper illumination (75-W incandescent bulb in a Luxo lamp), WS was able to read magazines and newspapers with no problem. Low-powered handheld and stand magnifiers were discussed and demonstrated; however, WS preferred the reading spectacle lens. She thought this lens was the easiest to use as well as the most normal in appearance. The use of a bifocal was also discussed, but it was thought that it might interfere with her mobility. To evaluate this, a +2.00 D Fresnel lens (which was cut similar to a flat-top 28 bifocal) was attached to her spectacle prescription and she walked around in the hallway, outside of the examination room. She agreed that it created a problem by interfering with her inferior field, thereby interfering with her mobility, which reinforced the decision to use a separate pair of reading glasses.

In regard to WS's concern in being able to spot her children on a playground, a 2.8× Keplerian handheld telescope was initially evaluated. This telescope was used over her distance prescription glasses, and with the right eye she was able to see 20/20. WS's skills with the telescope (focusing and localization) were excellent.

Ocular Health Evaluation

The ocular health evaluation was deemed necessary during this visit because WS had not seen her ophthalmologist in 2 years, and a confirmation of the initial diagnosis had to be made. This part of the evaluation was performed at the end of the examination to minimize the bleaching out of her photoreceptor cells, thereby minimizing visual difficulty during the initial visual evaluation.

Externals
There was no sign of paresis or paralysis of WS's extraocular muscles in all positions of gaze. Her pupils were equal and reacted to light, both direct and consensual. Her lids, lashes, conjunctiva, and cornea were normal. The lens showed early changes of a posterior subcapsular cataract (greater in the left than the right). The anterior chamber was open and quiet in each eye.

Intraocular Pressure
Pressures were found to be 17 mm Hg in each eye, measured by Goldmann applanation tonometry at 3:15 P.M.

Ophthalmoscopy
A dilated fundus evaluation revealed pigment clumping throughout the retina with some bone spicule pigmentation along the retinal vessels. There was some attenuation of the retinal arteries and the optic nerve appeared to have a slight waxy pale appearance in each eye. There was no foveal reflex in either eye. All other structures were normal.

At the completion of ophthalmoscopy, a summary of the results was discussed with WS. She was told that her diagnosis of retinitis pigmentosa was correct and that she had the beginnings of a cataract in each eye. She was also told that it was not possible to predict the rate at which her fields might further constrict but that she should be reevaluated on a regular basis, especially for the progression of her cataracts.

At this point, the initial visit was completed. The various optical and nonoptical devices that were evaluated during this visit were reviewed and it was explained to her that the lenses with which she appeared to have had the most success would be reevaluated at her next visit. She was also told that her mobility concerns would be addressed at the next visit. She was loaned a 2.8× handheld telescope to evaluate at home for 2 weeks and was instructed to call if she had any problems before her next follow-up visit.

Follow-Up Visits

WS returned for a follow-up visit and reported no changes in her visual concerns. Her unaided visual acuity was measured as 10/40 OD and 10/50 OS (similar to her first visit). She reported that the 2.8× telescope was extremely useful in helping her locate her children in the playground. She also thought it was very helpful for other tasks that she had not previously thought of, such as seeing the menu behind the counter of fast food restaurants and reading the signs in the aisles of a grocery store. By wearing the telescope on a neck string, WS found it very accessible, and she thought that she "could not live without it." Spectacle-mounted telescopes were demonstrated, which provided the same 20/20 acuity in each eye. WS, however, preferred the ease of the handheld telescope but appreciated knowing that other devices were available. The CPF and NoIR lenses were reevaluated with the same results, as was the reading lens with a typoscope and yellow acetate filter. During the remainder of this visit, WS's field and mobility problems were addressed. A Wide-Angle Mobility Light (Farallon Industries, Belmont, CA) was initially demonstrated. WS was impressed by the bright and wide path of light it afforded but she thought it was too heavy, even with the shoulder strap. She also commented that she does not go anywhere at night without being accompanied. Use of a flashlight at night if the need should ever arise was also discussed. Mounted 1.7× and 2.2× reverse Galilean bioptics were demonstrated and WS noticed the increased functional field but was extremely disappointed by the reduction in acuity (10/50 OD and 10/60 OS). Amorphic telescopes were also demonstrated, and functionally, WS preferred the −1.6×. When walking around with these lenses (in bioptic form), however, WS did not think that they dramatically improved her mobility. She also commented that she was slightly nauseated from wearing them. The use of Fresnel prisms was discussed next, and when she was presented with 30 prism diopter Fresnel prisms placed on the temporal aspect of her distance prescription lenses, she was able to observe the displacement of objects. During the instructional procedure, it became necessary to reduce the size of the prism to the point at which there was just a sliver of the lens left on each eye. It was mutually agreed that the prism was not providing any benefit over WS's normal scanning and, therefore, the use of prism was discontinued. Use of a long cane, mobility lessons, and sighted guide techniques as well as activities of daily living

were discussed. She appeared interested, and she was informed that these services would be requested for her through the state agency. In addition to these services, the following were requested:

1. A 2.8× Keplerian handheld variable focus telescope
2. Distance prescription with CPF 527 lenses
3. 32% gray NoIR sun lenses (and later, in July, requested 4% plum NoIR lenses)
4. Reading prescription: OD +2.50 − 1.00 × 45; OS +2.50 − 1.50 × 135 (she was provided with a typoscope and yellow acetate filter)
5. Luxo lamp
6. EZ computer magnifier

Six weeks later, the authorization was received for all of the requested devices as well as the rehabilitation services (mobility and activities of daily living). WS returned for a dispensing visit. Through the 2.8× handheld telescope, she was able to see 20/20 using the right eye. The reading glasses provided 0.19/0.6 M acuity in each eye, and with the yellow acetate, typoscope, and Luxo lamp, WS was able to read all types of print extremely well. The EZ computer magnifier provided the comfort and ease to see print on the computer monitor. She also found that the CPF prescription lenses and 32% gray NoIR lenses (worn over her habitual clear distance prescription) provided comfort indoors and outdoors, respectively. All the spectacle devices were adjusted to provide maximum comfort, and WS was very pleased with the results. She was instructed in the proper care and maintenance of these devices. She was told that a mobility instructor as well as a rehabilitation teacher would be contacting her regarding the mobility instruction and activities of daily living services. It was again reinforced that if she had any problems with the low vision devices she was to call immediately, and she was also told to return to her ophthalmologist for routine ocular health evaluations.

Discussion and Conclusion

This case represents a straightforward evaluation and management of a low vision patient, yet also demonstrates the complexity involved in prescribing for a patient with retinitis pigmentosa. WS had very definite ocular concerns that required the need for multiple prescriptions and services. The patient required solutions to her glare and contrast problems as well as some magnification needs and, most characteristically, solutions to compensate for peripheral field constrictions. Common presenting concerns of retinitis pigmentosa patients include photophobia, glare, and contrast problems. These were evident in WS's case as all five of her concerns dealt to some extent with these problems. By eliminating glare and improving contrast, the EZ computer magnifier was helpful for seeing print comfortably on the computer monitor, and the typoscope, yellow acetate filter, and Luxo lamp were also extremely helpful in providing comfort when reading. For indoor and outdoor comfort from glare and photophobia, three different lenses were prescribed: 32% gray NoIRs, 4% plum NoIRs, and CPF 527 lenses. These lenses were expected to be of some help as well in WS's orientation and mobility, as she adapted to different environmental levels of illumination.

In this particular case, WS's ocular disorder was beginning to create real problems and concerns. Her peripheral fields were constricted to the point at which they impacted her mobility, especially in unfamiliar environments. When evaluated by tangent screen and arc perimeter, however, the fields were not reduced to the point that field expansion devices (reverse and Amorphic telescopes) or peripheral awareness systems (Fresnel prisms) would be of any benefit. From experience, a patient generally has to have less than a 20-degree field remaining before these systems are of any benefit. In this and similar situations, however, it is important for a patient to experience these systems. It gives him or her some reassurance that options are available as the condition worsens but, most important, each patient may respond differently to his or her disorder and to low vision devices. There have been patients that I have worked with in the past (and I am sure I will see in the future) that responded favorably to treatment options that were not initially expected to help them. Therefore, as long as the patient is willing, all possible treatment options should be discussed and demonstrated to them. In this case, as well as in similar cases, it is important to work in conjunction with other professionals to meet the patient's needs. WS's mobility would be greatly improved with the services of an orientation and mobility instructor. I also believed that WS was not fully aware of some problems that might have existed in her home environment (activities of daily living); therefore, a rehabilitation teacher would provide additional benefit to her.

In regard to the optical devices recommended, WS had very good visual acuity remaining at distance and near and, therefore, did not require much magnification. Because WS was able to read 1 M and held her reading material at 20 cm, there was 5.00 D of accommodation required. With the +2.00 D in her reading spectacle, she was left with 3.00 D of accommodation. This was certainly a very reasonable amount that would allow WS a greater range in which to hold her reading material. In addition to the relief on her accommodative system, the use of yellow acetate (to enhance contrast and eliminate glare) and a typoscope (to maintain her place and relieve glare), as well as good, direct lighting, were the most important factors in her reading success.

At distance, the 2.8× handheld telescope provided the necessary acuity to solve WS's concerns. The more she used the device, the more she was aware of its many benefits, which again goes back to the philosophy of discussing and demonstrating different treatment options (devices and or services) that might not have been initially requested so that the patient is better educated and more informed. (This was also reflected in the decision to demonstrate spectacle-mounted telescopes.)

In conclusion, WS presented with many ocular concerns that were all approachable from a rehabilitation

point of view. Her condition had progressed to a predictable point at which she required optical and nonoptical devices as well as other professional services (mobility instructor and rehabilitation teacher) to all work in tandem. She was provided with experiences and information that would help her in the future as well. She was also encouraged to maintain routine ophthalmologic care. Her prognosis in the use of her low vision devices and services was excellent at the time of dispensing.

CASE III

Case History

JS was 16 years old when she first presented for a low vision evaluation. She was referred by the local state rehabilitation agency. JS was confined to a wheelchair and was accompanied by her mother. Her mother was very helpful in providing additional information as to JS's history. JS, who lived with her parents, was an only child and attended the local high school. She had just completed tenth grade. JS reported that she did well in school and that her grades were excellent; however, she was forced to miss a lot of school due to chronic illness. JS had a tutor throughout the years who visited her at home and in the hospital so that she was able to keep up with her school work. JS reported having poor vision all of her life and most of her learning was done through talking books and large-print reading material that the school provided. She used a stand magnifier (which she did not like) in conjunction with the large-print material. JS also received itinerant vision services 1 day per week from the county's intermediate unit. (Her itinerant teacher was the one who recommended the large-print material and provided her with the stand magnifier).

JS had a medical history of spina bifida and hydrocephalus. She underwent surgery at 3 months of age at which time a shunt was inserted. The hydrocephalus, however, had an effect on JS's vision, resulting in secondary optic atrophy. Her mother reported that JS's vision deteriorated slowly over the years until approximately age 8 years, when it appeared to have stabilized. In further discussing her ocular history, JS reported no fluctuating vision but an extreme sensitivity to sunlight outdoors. She had been prescribed a pair of gray photochromatic lenses by her ophthalmologist, but they were only somewhat helpful outdoors on bright sunny days. She had never worn glasses (other than the photochromatic lenses), and she had no history of ocular surgery or ocular medications. JS spent most of her day doing school work, even in the summer months, and she enjoyed watching television. She preferred to watch television (25-in. color television set) from a distance of 3 ft and was able to see some facial detail of the characters but was unable to read any written words on the screen. JS enjoyed going to the movies but had a difficult time seeing the detail on the screen when she was forced to sit toward the back of the movie theater because of her wheelchair. She also enjoyed sightseeing when going for weekend car rides with her parents.

JS's general health was considered to be fair. She was not taking any medications at the time of her initial visit.

When JS was asked to prioritize her visual goals and concerns she presented them in the following order:

1. To see the blackboard and teacher in the front of the classroom (she sat in the front row approximately 12 ft from the blackboard)
2. To see the words on a television screen and to see detail on a movie screen
3. To see small print (textbooks and math problems) at a "normal distance" (JS defined a normal distance at approximately 10 in.)
4. To address glare and photophobic complaints when outdoors
5. To see the scenery when she went on car rides with her parents

Diagnostic Findings

The distance chart used throughout the examination was a Designs for Vision number chart. It was illuminated by a reflector lamp housing two 75-W incandescent bulbs angled 45 degrees to the chart. This arrangement created direct illumination on the chart and provided even lighting without glare. The amount of illumination was controlled by a rheostat that was incorporated into the light switch. At near, the Lighthouse Near Visual Acuity Chart (designed with Sloan letters calibrated for 40 cm [LNHV-1]) and a continuous-text reading card were used. A Luxo floor lamp housing a 75-W incandescent bulb, provided the illumination. JS was encouraged to position the lamp at the appropriate distance and angle so that comfortable illumination was present without glare.

Unaided Visual Acuity

	Distance	Near
OD	10/80	0.40/4 M+
OS	10/350	0.40/13 M
OU	10/80	0.40/4 M+

JS was slow and deliberate in her responses. She was very concerned about giving the correct answers. There was no head turn or eccentric viewing noted. She was encouraged to move her eyes and head around to find the optimum viewing point. JS thought there was no improvement noted in either eye with eccentric viewing.

JS did not have habitual spectacles. She had never had a prescription for glasses; she had been told by ophthalmologists that there was no need for one. Through her own Jupiter stand magnifier (The Lighthouse, Inc., Long Island City, NY), equivalent power of 9.00 D, JS was able to read 2 M continuous text print.

Keratometry
Keratometry was performed to determine the integrity of JS's corneas. The mires were rated as good. Most impor-

tant, however, because she had never worn spectacles, the test was performed to rule out the possibility of JS having a large amount of corneal astigmatism that may have been undetected. Obviously, from the findings, this was not the case.

OD	OS
−0.75 × 180 AM 43.75	−0.50 × 180 AM 44.00

Retinoscopy

OD	OS
+0.50 − 0.25 × 90	+0.50 spherical (sph.)
10/80	10/350

Subjective
A bracketing technique incorporating just noticeable difference was used when doing the subjective. A ±1.25 cross cylinder was used to determine a subjective response for astigmatism.

OD	OS
Pl. sph. 10/80	Pl. sph. 10/350

Contrast Sensitivity Testing
With the use of a Vistech (Consultants, Inc., Dayton, OH) contrast sensitivity chart for distance, JS demonstrated a loss at the mid and high spatial frequency ranges OD and was unable to respond with her left eye. The test was performed at 10 ft with uniform lighting of the chart.

Visual Fields
Amsler's grid testing was initially performed to provide some analysis of her macular area because some of JS's visual concerns centered around reading. In addition, because fields are unpredictable in optic atrophy cases, it was important to thoroughly evaluate her central and peripheral fields. The Amsler's grid was held before each eye at a 33-cm test distance with a +3.00 D sphere (using a trial frame) in place. JS was unable to see the central fixation dot on the grid. A grid with an X drawn on the fixation target was used. JS was instructed to look at the area where she thought the lines cross in the X. With the right eye, JS reported that all four corners of the grid were present and that all the vertical and horizontal lines appeared straight. She also exhibited a large central scotoma (greater loss on the right side of fixation) in that same eye. With her left eye, JS was able to see the four corners but exhibited a large central and paracentral scotoma. Her responses were rated as good.

Tangent screen testing was performed using a 8/1,000-W isopter on the right eye. The tangent field on the left eye was not evaluated because it was quite evident that concentration would be solely on the right eye for the low vision devices (both the acuity and field of the left eye were greatly reduced over that of the right eye). Results of the right eye confirmed a central scotoma (6 degrees to the right of fixation and 4 degrees to the left). The remainder of the field appeared to be intact.

Peripheral field testing was performed on each eye to gather information that might be related to any mobility problems. An arc perimeter was used with a 6/330-W isopter. The results confirmed a 10-degree central scotoma in the right eye and a 20-degree central scotoma in the left eye. The peripheral fields appeared normal in each eye. The responses were considered reliable in both the tangent screen and arc perimeter testing.

Evaluation of Low Vision Systems

Because most of JS's concerns centered around distance vision improvement, telescopes were evaluated first. It was determined that in JS's school setting, the blackboard varied from 12 ft away in one classroom to 21 ft away in another. In my experience, a patient would require 20/40 to 20/25 acuity to read most print on a blackboard. She was also looking for detail acuity when sitting at the back of a movie theater (confined to the back of the theater because of her wheelchair) and when going on car rides and seeing scenery at distances of greater than 20 ft away. A 6× Keplerian handheld telescope was initially introduced using the right eye. She was able to see 20/30+, but JS did not like the idea of holding a telescope for all of her distance needs. A 6× Keplerian bioptic telescope was then evaluated, and JS was able to attain 20/30+ through the right eye. JS performed well with the telescope in regard to localization and focusing. Her initial reaction to the appearance (bioptic form) and the use of a telescope was very favorable. An 8× Keplerian bioptic telescope was also evaluated, and JS was able to see 20/25+. JS believed that the 8× telescope was slightly more difficult to use, and she did not think that this telescope provided her with much better vision than the previous (6×) telescope. She did, however, agree to compare both these bioptic telescopes for watching television and reading words on a blackboard. A classroom setting was simulated in the waiting room by placing a blackboard 20 ft from JS, and various colors of chalk were used for the printed words on the board. She decided that the 6× telescope met her visual needs and still provided her with enough field to function efficiently. She was also very happy with the ability to focus the telescope for different distances. JS's instruction with the telescope was all related to her visual concerns. All the activities started out with simple, large, high-contrast targets and progressed to more detailed, very discriminating visual tasks. For example, a large letter was initially written on the blackboard. JS was able to successfully locate the object and focus the telescope appropriately. As she progressed, smaller letters were identified until eventually words and sentences were successfully read. When JS completed this aspect of the instruction, she was then shown moving targets. She was instructed to spot the target without the telescope, align the telescope with her eye's line of sight (she did not have to eccentrically view), and to focus the telescope on the moving target. JS was also instructed on how to accurately track moving targets (move her head and body slowly and smoothly without moving her eyes) and finally how to scan her environment (to search her environment for objects that she could not see without the telescope). She had no problem in adapting to the con-

cept of wearing the bioptic full time so that the telescope would be at her disposal at any time for as long as she needed it.

Ocular Health Evaluation

An ocular health evaluation was performed at the end of the examination to minimize the amount of bright light entering the eye, thereby reducing visual fatigue.

Externals
There was no sign of paresis or paralysis of JS's extraocular muscles in all positions of gaze, nor was there any sign of nystagmus. Her pupils were equal and reacted to light, both direct and consensual; however, her left pupil appeared to react more slowly than the right. There was no sign of an afferent pupillary defect. Her lids, lashes, conjunctiva, lens, and cornea appeared normal in each eye. The anterior chamber was open and quiet in both eyes.

Intraocular Pressure
Pressures were found to be 19 mm Hg and 17 mm Hg in the right eye and left eye, respectively, measured by Goldmann applanation tonometry at 10:30 A.M.

Ophthalmoscopy
A dilated fundus evaluation revealed pale white optic nerve heads in each eye, with both appearing equal in paleness. The blood vessels in each eye were very tortuous with an artery to vein ratio equal to one-third. There were no foveal reflexes noted in either eye. All other structures of the fundus were normal.

At the completion of ophthalmoscopy, a summary of the results were discussed with JS and her mother. JS was told that her diagnosis of optic atrophy was correct and that her condition appeared stable. She was also told that she would be evaluated with additional low vision devices on her next visit, and she was encouraged to bring in some of her textbooks for evaluation with the low vision devices.

Follow-Up Visits

On her return visit, it was determined that the print size of JS's textbooks was 1 M (by using the rule of 1,000; see section on predicting near magnification in Chapter 10). JS was therefore evaluated with a +10.00 D microscope and her visual acuity with the right eye was 0.10/1.2 M +2 (single letters). The +10.00 D microscope was predicted as the initial lens based on JS's near acuity at 40 cm. Because she was able to read 4 M (single letters) at 40 cm, she would be expected to read 1 M at 10 cm with the appropriate accommodation or reading lens. The +10.00 D lens was therefore used because she had no refractive error to account for. This lens also eliminated the need for her to accommodate (at 10 cm). With a +12.00 D lens, JS was able to see 0.08/1 M − 1, but she was only able to read 1.5 M slowly with a continuous-text reading card. A +16.00 D microscope provided 0.06/0.8 M + 2 visual acuity and permitted JS to read 1.0 M continuous text. She experienced difficulty in reading her own textbooks, however. A +20.00 D microscope was also evaluated, and it allowed JS to attain 0.05/0.6 M acuity. This microscope provided the necessary clarity to read her textbooks. Throughout the whole near-point evaluation, JS was allowed to position the Luxo lamp to provide maximum illumination without glare. A fluorescent lamp was also evaluated; however, JS preferred the incandescent lamp because she thought it produced less glare. Because JS did not want to read at such a close distance (5 cm), and she did not like the idea of using a handheld or stand magnifier, two other options were discussed and evaluated. A +4.00 D reading cap was placed on the 6× bioptic telescope (equivalent power is 24.00 D), which enabled JS to see 0.6 M + 3 acuity at 25 cm and also allowed her to read her textbooks at this distance. She was thrilled by the results of reading her textbook at a "normal distance." JS's skills with this telemicroscope were surprisingly good given that the telemicroscope reduces the brightness and field of view when compared to an equivalent-powered microscope. She did, however, experience some difficulty in maintaining the correct reading distance when holding her textbook for a few minutes. A reading stand remedied this problem. The final device demonstrated at near was a closed-circuit television (CCTV). With 6× magnification on the screen and a working distance of 14 in. (equivalent power is +17.14 D), she was able to read her textbooks and write with comfort and ease. JS preferred reverse polarity (white print on a black background) at all times.

As many devices were evaluated and JS was feeling fatigued, it was mutually decided to defer an outdoor sun lens evaluation until the next visit. JS was scheduled for a follow-up visit in 3 weeks because some time was needed to design and make a reading stand that could be attached to her wheelchair. JS returned for her third visit and reported no changes in her vision or visual concerns. Her unaided visual acuity was measured at 10/80+ OD and 10/350 OS (similar to her first visit). The 6× bioptic was reevaluated for distance and she attained 20/25 acuity, a slight improvement in acuity over her last visit. With a +4.00 D cap on the telescope and a reading stand attached to her wheelchair, JS was able to read her textbooks, and she was also able to write notes at a distance of 10 in. with little difficulty. (The reading stand consisted of a reading platform with three "goose neck" cables attached to it, which then attached to a clamp that fastened to the arm of the wheelchair. Two goose neck cables were initially evaluated but it did not provide the rigidity required for supporting heavy textbooks and for writing.) JS was able to achieve these results with normal room, glare-free illumination (measured with a light meter at 50 foot-candles). The CCTV was also reevaluated and JS performed equally as well as she did on her initial evaluation with this device. She again preferred reverse polarity and she believed that this device would be ideal for her long-term reading and writing, especially for math homework.

In regard to JS's problem with photophobia and glare, she was evaluated outdoors with Corning CPF and NoIR lenses. It was a bright, sunny, summer day (the type of day on which JS had the most problems) and JS preferred 19% green NoIRs. Once the selection of sun lenses was completed, all of JS's visual concerns had been addressed and successfully resolved. A letter was written to the state agency for blindness and visual services requesting the following devices:

1. A 6× monocular Keplerian bioptic with a +4.00 D reading cap
2. A CCTV
3. 19% green NoIR sun lenses
4. Custom-designed reading stand that attached to the wheelchair

Approximately 5 weeks later, the authorization was received for all of the above devices, and JS returned for a dispensing visit. The dispensing was routine, and JS was provided with information on the care and maintenance of the devices. She was also told to continue seeing her eye care practitioner for all of her ocular health evaluations.

Discussion and Conclusion

JS was a patient with specific visual concerns and a strong determination to succeed. These are two important factors required in the success of using low vision devices. Most of JS's visual concerns centered around improvement of her distance vision—more specifically, improvement of distance vision for extended periods (e.g., watching television, classroom and blackboard use, seeing scenery). For those reasons, a spectacle-mounted telescope was the most appropriate device. The telescope also had the advantage of being converted into a telemicroscope by use of a +4.00 D cap. This system enabled JS to work at a comfortable distance while reading and writing. The reading stand attached to her wheelchair provided a stable platform at the correct distance. The 6× telescope with +4.00 D reading cap provided JS with the equivalent of +24.00 D. Initially, this appeared to be more magnification than was necessary (her visual acuity at near was 0.40/4.00 M OD), but as was seen by her microscopic evaluation, she required more magnification than was initially predicted. This might be explained by the following:

1. Visual acuity or single-letter acuity is generally easier to see, with better results obtained, than reading acuity for most low vision patients. With reading acuity, there is less space between each individual letter (crowding phenomenon) and many times patients generally complain of words running together. Therefore, these patients require more magnification to read continuous text than they would need to read individual letters. JS appears to be a perfect example of a low vision patient requiring more magnification to read continuous text than was necessary to see individual letters that were equivalent in size.

2. A second factor might have been her large central scotoma that extended on the right side of fixation. Because JS did not appreciate the need to eccentrically view, increased magnification was required to cope with the irregularly shaped, large scotoma.

3. It is generally expected that patients with an optic nerve disorder commonly show an overall loss of contrast sensitivity. Because JS's contrast sensitivity testing showed poor results in the mid and high frequency range, glare control, greater magnification, and greater brightness and contrast were expected to be needed. This loss of contrast sensitivity was substantiated by the fact that JS performed so well with the CCTV with which she was able to control polarity, brightness, and contrast. With the CCTV, it was determined that she required approximately +17.00 D of equivalent power to read her textbooks.

In conclusion, JS benefited tremendously from a number of low vision devices. Her skills and determination were truly commendable and enabled her to attain her goals. Her prognosis was excellent with the use of low vision devices.

Answers to Questions

Chapter 1

1. c
2. b
3. a
4. c
5. d

Chapter 2

1. False
2. denial or shock, anger, depression, bargaining, acknowledgment/coexistence
3. type of vision loss, life stage, family reaction, personality, self-concept, recent significant life events
4. e
5. True

Chapter 3

1. False
2. True
3. False
4. True
5. True
6. True
7. False
8. False
9. True
10. True

Chapter 4

1. e
2. d
3. False
4. True
5. c
6. True
7. False
8. False
9. True
10. False
11. True
12. False
13. True
14. False
15. False
16. True

Chapter 5

1. False
2. d
3. b
4. False
5. True
6. False

Chapter 6

1. b
2. a
3. c
4. b
5. c
6. d
7. a
8. c
9. c
10. d

Chapter 7

1. e
2. c
3. c
4. b
5. d
6. c
7. d
8. c

Chapter 8

1. d
2. b
3. d
4. True
5. False
6. e
7. b
8. a
9. e
10. c

Chapter 9

1. a
2. b
3. e
4. c
5. b
6. e
7. b
8. e
9. c
10. c

Chapter 10

1. c
2. b
3. False
4. d
5. False
6. a
7. True
8. b
9. e
10. e

Chapter 11

1. e
2. True
3. False
4. e
5. c
6. b
7. False

Chapter 12

1. b
2. e
3. d
4. b
5. c

6. e
7. d

Chapter 13

1. c
2. b
3. e
4. a
5. d
6. a
7. b
8. b
9. c
10. c
11. c
12. b

Chapter 14

1. d
2. a
3. True
4. True
5. e
6. True

7. b
8. False
9. False
10. a

Chapter 15

1. False
2. True
3. c
4. d
5. True
6. e
7. True

Chapter 16

1. False
2. b
3. e
4. False
5. d
6. c
7. e

Chapter 17

1. d
2. d
3. e
4. d
5. True
6. False
7. e
8. e

Chapter 18

1. False
2. e
3. d
4. False
5. e

Chapter 19

1. b
2. True
3. e
4. e
5. True

Index